Are You Eating Right?

Analyze Your Diet
Using the
Nutrient Content of More Than 5,000 Foods

Judi Sakimoto Morrill Sheri Cimino Bakun Suzanne Pierce Murphy

Printed on Recycled Paper.

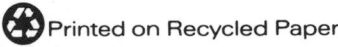

Cover Design: Lorenzo Ramos

Orange Grove Publishing
1239 Bellair Way
Menlo Park, CA 94025-6612

ISBN 0-9657951-9-5

Printed by Litho Communications, Inc.

Table of Contents

The Impatient User's Guide

Step 1: Record everything you eat and drink for 24 hours.

Step 2: Fill in Table 2 (pp. 18-19) using food labels and the Food Composition Table.

For the **Recommended Amounts** row:

- **Protein** (grams): Divide your weight in pounds by 3. *If you're under age 19, or overweight, or a strict vegetarian, or pregnant or nursing,* *see page 17.*

- **% of Daily Value**: Use the values from Table 3 on page 20.

Step 3: Compare your intake with the recommended amounts, using the information in Table 2. Also, fill in the boxes below:

- 30% or less of your calories should come from fat. Calculate your %, using your *total grams of fat* and *total calories* from Table 2:

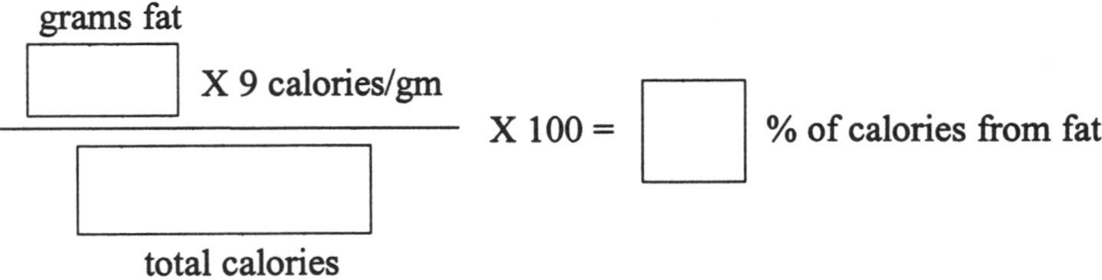

- Less than 10% of your calories should come from saturated fat. Calculate your %, using your *total grams saturated fat* and *total calories* from Table 2:

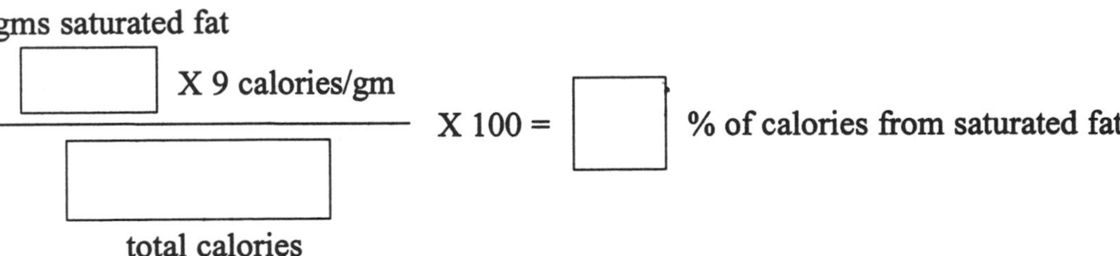

That's it! If you want to know more, you can't be so impatient!

Introduction

Chances are, magazine articles and food labels—or your mother—have made you insecure about your diet. For starters, you may wonder if your diet is deficient in nutrients or excessive in fat.

A detailed analysis of your diet may not be necessary. But by doing such an analysis, you can assure yourself that you are, in fact, "eating right." Or if you find that your diet can be improved, you'll know how to make the appropriate changes.

This book is divided into sections:

- **Dietary Recommendations**: The guidelines put forth by expert committees
- **Your Diet Analysis**: Step-by-step directions
- **Additional Information**: Calculating nutrient content from recipes, etc.
- **Food Composition Table**: Nutrient content of more than 5,000 foods
- **Food Index**: Quickly find a particular food

We hope that after assessing your diet, you'll eat with less worry and more pleasure.

Dietary Recommendations

One goal of a healthy diet is to eat enough; another is to avoid eating too much.

The first question—does my diet have all the nutrients I need?—is the easier question. Scientists know in much detail what nutrients we need, their functions, and how much we need. There are, of course, many unanswered questions, but not as many as advertisements for dietary supplements would have you believe.

The other question—does my diet have too much of some nutrients?—is harder to answer. This question has to do with "chronic disease," such as heart disease, cancer, and diabetes—diseases which are far more complex than those caused by the lack of a nutrient.

A high-fat diet, for example, is linked with a higher risk of heart disease and some cancers. Though it isn't always certain that this is a cause-and-effect link, most of us have much to gain from following the advice to eat a low-fat diet. Such advice is the basis of the "prudent diet"—there are good reasons to believe that following the advice is healthful, and there are few, if any, reasons to believe it's harmful.

Meeting Nutrient Needs

The Recommended Dietary Allowances (RDAs)

The RDAs are the amounts of nutrients that our experts have decided are adequate and safe—amounts that should meet the needs of the general U.S. population, yet not be so much as to risk toxicity.

- **The RDAs are for daily averages,** since diets vary from day to day. You aren't expected to get the recommended amounts every single day. Practically speaking, your average nutrient intake, over several days, should meet the RDA.

- **The RDAs are generous**. They allow for such things as individual variations in need, amounts lost in food preparation, and how efficiently the nutrients are absorbed into the body. The RDAs also provide for reserves in the body.

- **The RDAs are for healthy people**. If you have a long-term illness, they may not apply to you.

- **There are 18 sets of the RDAs,** differing by age, sex, and whether a woman is pregnant or nursing.

- **The RDAs are revised periodically** to incorporate new information. The 10th and latest edition was published in 1989.

As the RDA Committee states, the RDAs are *"designed for the maintenance of good nutrition of practically all healthy people in the United States.... The allowances, expressed as average daily intakes over time, are intended to provide for individual variations among most normal persons as they live in the United States under usual environmental stresses."*

The Daily Values

In 1973, the Food and Drug Administration created standards for nutrient labeling of foods. **These standards are called Daily Values on food labels.**

Why Daily Values are needed:

- Nutrients are measured in metric units (grams, milligrams, micrograms), which are unfamiliar to most U.S. consumers.
- If told how much of the nutrient is in a food, e.g., 1 milligram of zinc, we can't tell if it's a trivial amount or a lot, unless we know the recommended amount.
- It isn't practical to put the many sets of RDAs on a label.

The Daily Values as a solution:

- **One Daily Value set was made from several sets of RDAs** by taking the highest RDA from the 1968 edition (the most current at the time) for each nutrient for people 4 years old or older, excluding pregnant or nursing women. This is the set used for most labels.

  There are three other sets of Daily Values: for infants up to 12 months old, children under 4 years, and pregnant women. These are for products intended specifically for these groups, e.g., the set for infants is used for labeling baby food.

- **Nutrient content is given as a percentage of the Daily Value**, e.g., the Daily Value for niacin is 20 mg, so a food having 10 mg of niacin is said to have 50% of the Daily Value. This makes the nutrient content easier to understand.

A Guide to Daily Food Choices

- **Grain Group: 6 or more portions for adolescents and adults**; 6 or more smaller portions for children; 7 or more portions for pregnant or nursing women. Emphasize whole grains.

  1 portion = 1 small pancake, slice of bread, tortilla; half a hamburger or hot dog bun; half a bagel or English muffin; 5 saltine crackers; 4 graham crackers; 1 oz dry cereal (= 1 C* cornflakes, ⅔ C shredded wheat; ¼ C Grape Nuts); ½ C cooked rice, pasta, cereal, grits.

- **Vegetable Group: 3 or more portions for adolescents and adults**; 3 or more smaller portions for children; 4 or more portions for pregnant or nursing women (see below for portion sizes).

- **Fruit Group: 2 or more portions for adolescents and adults**: 2 or more smaller portions for children; 3 or more portions for pregnant or nursing women.

  1 portion = 1 medium fruit or vegetable (e.g., apple, carrot, banana, potato); 1 C raw, leafy green vegetable (e.g., lettuce); ½ C fruit or other vegetable (e.g., broccoli, canned peaches, cooked spinach); ¾ C (6 fl oz)* fruit or vegetable juice. (½ C beans or peas counts as 1 portion in the vegetable group or ½ portion in the meat group.)

  Include 1 portion of a fruit or vegetable rich in vitamin C (e.g., orange, grapefruit, strawberries, green pepper, broccoli) and 1 portion of a carotene-rich (dark green or orange-colored) fruit or vegetable (e.g., carrot, spinach, pumpkin, broccoli, apricot, cantaloupe; the orange in orange juice isn't carotene).

- **Milk Group: 2 portions for adults age 25 and older** and children ages 1 to 10; **3 portions for ages 11-24** and women who are pregnant or nursing.

  1 portion = 1 C milk, yogurt, pudding, custard; 1½ C ice cream, ice milk, frozen yogurt; 2 C cottage cheese; ¼ C parmesan cheese; 1½ oz (1 oz = 1″ cube) regular cheese (e.g., cheddar, swiss, mozzarella); 2 oz processed cheese (e.g., Velveeta). Cream cheese doesn't count here; it's more like butter.

- **Meat or Meat-substitute Group: 2 portions for adolescents and adults**; 2 smaller portions for children; 3 portions for pregnant or nursing women.

  1 portion = 2 to 3 oz† cooked poultry, fish, meat; 2 frankfurters; 2 eggs; 1 C peas, beans, lentils, soybean curd (tofu); ½ C nuts, sunflower seeds; ¼ C (4 Tbs)* peanut butter.

---

* 1 C (cup) = 16 Tbs (tablespoons); fl oz = fluid ounce; a 12 fl oz can of soda, beer = 1½ C.

† 3 oz lean, cooked poultry, fish, meat is about the size of a deck of cards; a "regular slice" of pre-sliced luncheon meats like bologna = 0.8 oz.

Most of us don't want to—and shouldn't have to—add up % Daily Values to be assured of getting enough of each nutrient. **A Guide to Daily Food Choices** (see opposite page) was set up by the U.S. Department of Agriculture to help us select a good diet.

- **We're advised to eat a certain number of servings per day from 5 food groups**, shown graphically as the **Food Guide Pyramid** (see below), with the most servings coming from the Grain Group, and the least from foods high in fat and/or sugar, shown as the small "6th group" at the tip of the pyramid.

- **Each food group is particularly rich in certain nutrients,** e.g., foods in the Milk Group are generally good sources of calcium, riboflavin, and high-quality protein.

- The idea is that if you include the advised number of servings from each food group and eat a variety of foods, you can be quite sure that you're meeting your nutrient needs.

- **The serving sizes are made to be equivalent in terms of certain nutrients,** e.g., 1 serving in the Milk Group is an amount that has about 300 mg of calcium: 1 cup of milk or 1½ oz of cheddar cheese or 2 cups of cottage cheese.

A serving is called a [nutrient] portion in the Guide on the opposite page, because the amounts aren't always realistic servings, e.g., most of us don't think of 2 cups of cottage cheese as one serving.

- **Try to average—over several days—the advised portions per day.**

- **The key is to eat a lot of plant foods, and get your nutrients from a variety of foods.**

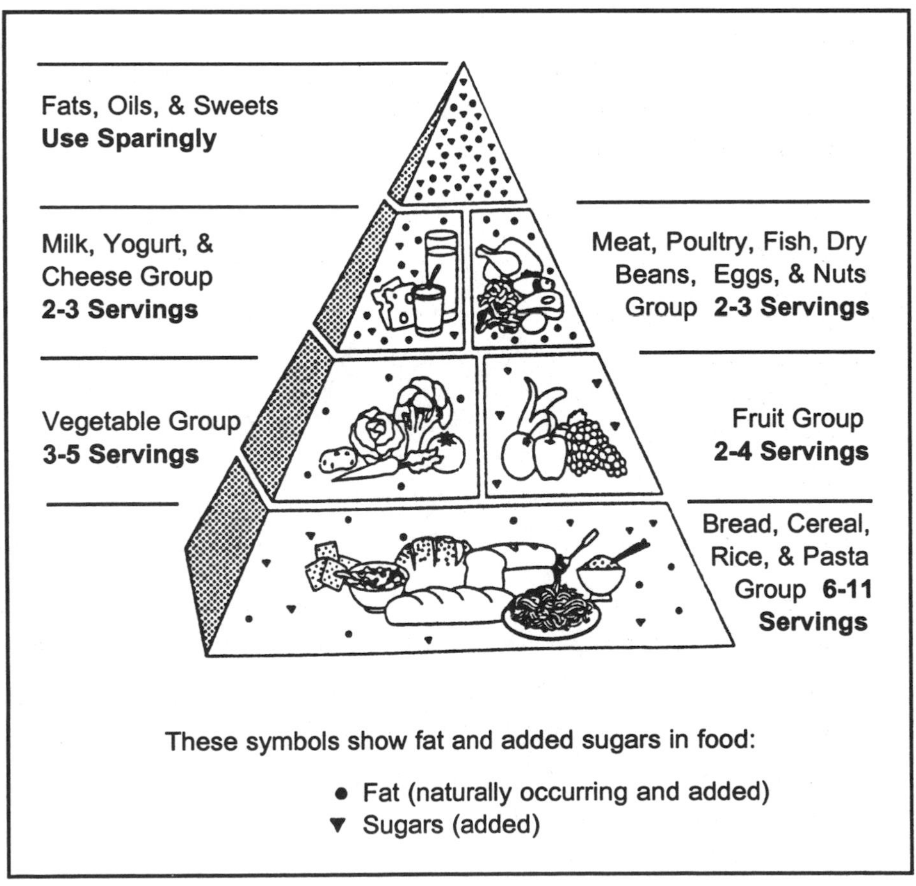

Maintaining Good Health

There's already a lot of scientific evidence that one's diet can affect the risk of such diseases as heart disease, chronic liver disease, and cancer of the stomach, colon, breast, lung, and esophagus. The American Heart Association, American Cancer Society, and various government committees evaluating the scientific evidence all give similar dietary advice.

We're bombarded with advice from many sources, such as advertisements, diet and health books, and sports and fitness magazines, not all of which are based on scientific evidence. Often, the advice is tied in with products to sell. This—together with a steady stream of news reports of studies that sometimes seem in conflict—can leave us bewildered. What dietary advice can science give us so far?

The Dietary Guidelines Advisory Committee (composed of our most knowledgeable experts), established jointly by the U.S. Department of Agriculture and U.S. Department of Health and Human Services, recommends a set of *Dietary Guidelines for Americans* for healthy Americans ages 2 years and over. First published in 1980, they were revised in 1985, 1990, and 1995 to reflect new scientific knowledge. On the opposite page, the guidelines are in bold print, followed by a brief explanation.

Dietary Guidelines for Americans

- **Eat a variety of foods.** Get your nutrients and other healthful substances from a wide variety of foods rather than from only a few foods, highly fortified foods, or dietary supplements.
- **Balance the food you eat with physical activity; maintain or improve your weight.** You're more likely to develop health problems if you're too thin or too fat —especially if you've got a "big belly." Putting on excess weight is usually from not being active enough. Even losing a few of the excess pounds is healthful; if you aren't losing, try to keep from gaining more. "Healthy weights" are given on the next page.
- **Choose a diet with plenty of grain products, vegetables, and fruits.** These are rich in vitamins, minerals, fiber, and a variety of substances that lower the risk of heart disease and some cancers. They also tend to be low in fat. Foods rich in fiber can lower the risk of chronic constipation, diverticulosis, and hemorrhoids.
- **Choose a diet low in fat, saturated fat, and cholesterol.** Excessive amounts may raise the risk of heart disease, certain cancers, and obesity. This guideline, in particular, isn't for children under 2 years old, since a low-fat diet may not meet their nutrient needs.
- **Choose a diet moderate in sugars.** Sugars provide a concentrated source of calories without otherwise contributing to nutrient intake. Sugars also contribute to tooth decay.
- **Choose a diet moderate in salt and sodium.** Most Americans eat more salt (sodium chloride) than needed; excessive amounts may lead to high blood pressure in some people.
- **If you drink alcoholic beverages, do so in moderation.** Alcohol in excessive amounts raises the risk of several diseases such as cirrhosis of the liver and cancer of the esophagus. Women who are pregnant or trying to conceive shouldn't drink any alcohol; alcohol can damage the unborn child.

  Moderate drinking = no more than 1 drink/day for women; no more than 2 for men.
  One drink = about ½ oz pure alcohol, e.g., a 12-oz bottle of beer or wine cooler, 5 oz wine, 1 jigger (1½ oz) vodka, rum, whisky, or gin.

A Healthy Weight

Height	Weight
4'10"	91-119
4'11"	94-124
5'0"	97-128
5'1"	101-132
5'2"	104-137
5'3"	107-141
5'4"	111-146
5'5"	114-150
5'6"	118-155
5'7"	121-160
5'8"	125-164
5'9"	129-169
5'10"	132-174
5'11"	136-179
6'0"	140-184
6'1"	144-189
6'2"	148-195
6'3"	152-200
6'4"	156-205
6'5"	160-211
6'6"	164-216

- **See if your weight** (without clothes) **is within the range suggested for your height** (without shoes).

  The range in weight for a given height allows for different amounts of muscle and bone. Since men have more muscle and bone, the upper end of the range generally applies to men, and the lower end to women.

  Weighing just under the range may be healthy for some people. But unintentional weight loss can be an early sign of a health problem.

- **See if your waist is smaller or no bigger than your hips.** Excess abdominal fat—a "big belly"—is a bigger health risk than excess fat on the hips and thighs, and is linked to high blood pressure, diabetes, early heart disease, and some cancers. Smoking and excessive alcohol tend to put on abdominal fat; vigorous exercise tends to reduce it.

  Measure your waist near your naval while standing relaxed, not pulling in your stomach. Measure your hips where they are biggest, over your buttocks. Divide your waist measurement by your hip measurement to get your waist-to-hip ratio. **A ratio above 0.8 for women and 0.95 for men suggests an excess of abdominal fat.**

  $$\frac{\text{your waist in inches}}{\text{your hips in inches}} = \frac{\square}{\square} = \square$$

  Ratio

- If your weight is within the suggested range, your waist-to-hip ratio isn't high, you've gained less than 10 pounds since reaching your adult height, and you don't have a health problem for which your doctor advises weight loss or gain there's no apparent health advantage to changing your weight.

Other Dietary Advice

Several organizations and government agencies give dietary advice, e.g., the American Heart Association has a set of recommendations, as does the American Cancer Society. In 1988, there was the Surgeon General's Report on Nutrition and Health. In 1989, the Committee on Diet and Health (19 experts from the U.S. and Canada) came out with advice for lowering risk of chronic disease. It's reassuring that the experts from these various groups have come up with remarkably similar advice.

Most of the dietary recommendations are covered by the Food Guide Pyramid and the Dietary Guidelines for Americans. Here are a couple more made by the Committee on Diet and Health:

- **Maintain protein intake at moderate levels** (not more than twice the RDA). A high-protein diet has been linked to a higher risk of heart disease, certain cancers, and osteoporosis.
- **Maintain an optimal intake of fluoride,** particularly during the years when baby and adult teeth are forming, to lower risk of tooth decay. Fluoride in the drinking water at 1 ppm (1 part fluoride per million parts of water) is advised. Dentists and pediatricians can prescribe fluoride drops or tablets for children drinking unfluoridated water.

Eating for Health and Pleasure

- **Use the Dietary Guidelines for Americans when choosing foods in the Food Guide Pyramid.** For example, if you drink low-fat or nonfat milk instead of whole milk, you are following the guideline to choose a diet lower in fat, saturated fat, and cholesterol. Also, since nonfat and low-fat milk have fewer calories, this choice can help you improve your weight (another guideline) if you're overweight.

- **Make changes gradually**. For example, it's hard to switch abruptly from whole milk to non-fat milk. Switch gradually by combining whole milk and low-fat milk, gradually increasing the proportion of low-fat milk. Then combine low-fat milk and nonfat milk. Once the switch to nonfat milk is made, even low-fat milk may taste like cream. Low-fat milk can then substitute for cream in coffee, etc.

- **Keep in mind that it's the overall diet, not individual foods, that are "good" or "bad."** Think in terms of being free to eat anything you want—just make a habit of eating foods like candy, hot dogs, and potato chips in smaller amounts or not as often.

- **Eating for health and eating for pleasure can be the same!** Eating is one of life's pleasures, but people often think of healthy food as bland and "boring." Many cuisines show us otherwise. What could be less boring, yet so in keeping with dietary guidelines, than a burrito topped with a hearty portion of a zesty salsa made of red tomatoes, purple onions, bright green cilantro, chili peppers, lime juice, and a dash of olive oil and salt?

Assessing Your Diet

The Plan

- **Record everything you eat and drink for 24 hours** on a typical day. A 3-day record is more accurate, but this can be too tedious for a "first-timer." If needed, make changes afterwards to reflect a more typical day.

- **Categorize the foods you eat by food group, and evaluate your diet using the Guide to Daily Food Choices**. Generally speaking, if you meet the recommendations of this guide, your diet is adequate in nutrients.

- **Do a more detailed analysis of your diet** by tabulating the amounts of the various nutrients in your diet, first using food labels and then the Food Composition Table.

- **Compare your nutrient intake with the recommended amounts.**

- **See how your diet compares to the Dietary Guidelines.** If needed, see what specific changes you can make to improve your diet.

Quick Diet Analysis Using the Food Guide Pyramid

- **On Table 1, record everything you eat and drink for 24 hours,** selecting a day in which your diet is typical. If you eat at a fast-food chain (e.g., McDonald's), ask for their booklet that shows the nutrient content of their foods (for use in Table 2).

  Include everything—coffee, tea, added sugar and cream, diet drinks, the oil you cook something in, the mayonnaise on the sandwich bread, etc.

  Be as accurate as you can in recording amounts in ounces, cups, etc.; we tend to underestimate. For perspective, a can of soda is 12 fluid ounces, which is 1½ cups. See page 33 for conversions and abbreviations, e.g., 1 cup = 16 Tbs; 1 oz = 28 grams.

- **Tabulate the number of portions you had in each food group** (see the Guide on page 6 for portion sizes). Note that a portion isn't necessarily a typical serving size, e.g., 2 cups of cottage cheese = 1 portion (½ cup of cottage cheese = ¼ of a portion in the milk group).

  If the item (e.g., candy) isn't in a food group, put a checkmark in the *not in a group* column.

- **For each food group, fill in your recommended number of portions** (see page 6).

- **Answer the questions at the bottom of Table 1.** If you answered yes to these questions, it's likely that you met your nutrient needs.

Table 1: Diet Analysis Using the Food Guide Pyramid

Food or Drink Consumed		Number of Portions					√ if not in a group
Amount	Food	Grain	Veg	Fruit	Milk	Meat	
12 fl oz	orange juice			2			
1 cup	Cheerios	1					
½ cup	non-fat milk				½		
16 fl oz	coffee						√
1	McDonald's Big Mac	2			½	1½	
21 fl oz	diet Coke						√
1	banana			1			
2	bean-cheese burritos	2			1	1	
1	carrot		1				
1 cup	iceburg lettuce		1				
2 Tbs	Italian dressing						√
1 cup	non-fat milk				1		
4	Oreo cookies						√
Total number of portions for the day		5	2	3	3	2½	
Your recommended portions		6+	3+	2+	2	2	

Did you eat the recommended number of portions from each of the 5 food groups? yes (no)

Did you eat a vitamin C-rich fruit or vegetable? (yes) no

Did you eat a carotene-rich (dark green of orange colored) fruit or vegetable? (yes) no

Did you eat a variety of foods? (yes) no

Table 1: Diet Analysis Using the Food Guide Pyramid

Food or Drink Consumed		Number of Portions					√ if not in a group
Amount	Food	Grain	Veg	Fruit	Milk	Meat	
Total number of portions for the day							
Your recommended portions							

Did you eat the recommended number of portions from each of the 5 food groups? Yes No

Did you eat a vitamin C-rich fruit or vegetable? Yes No

Did you eat a carotene-rich (dark green or orange-colored) fruit or vegetable? Yes No

Did you eat a variety of foods? Yes No

Detailed Diet Analysis

- **Copy your foods and amounts from Table 1** (page 15) **onto Table 2** (pages 18-19).
- **Fill in the nutrient content of your foods. First use values from labels** (and pamphlets if you ate at fast-food chains). Write these in a color or use a highlighter. You can calculate % calories from fat: (calories from fat X 100)/total calories = % cal fat.

  For unlabeled food (e.g., apples), use the food composition table, first reading pages 45-46. If the food isn't listed, use a similar food. Note portion sizes, e.g., is your apple much larger or smaller than what's listed?

  If the amount you ate isn't the same as that given in the food composition table or for one serving on the label, adjust the values accordingly—except for the % of calories from fat (% cal fat), e.g., eggs have 60% cal fat, no matter how many you eat. If, for example, the listed bagel is 2 oz, and yours is 3 oz, multiply the values (except % cal fat) for the listed bagel by 1.5 (=3 oz/2 oz).

  For nutrients not listed on the label or pamphlet, find a similar food in the food composition table to get approximate values and give its food #. **Don't leave any blanks, and don't put in zeroes unless you know them to be zeroes.** Be sure all the units are the same in each column (e.g., fat is in grams, iron is as % Daily Value).
- **List any supplements separately** where indicated on Table 2. Nutrient content is on the label. If you take prenatal supplements, adjust the % Daily Value on the label (see how on page 35); they're based on values specified for pregnant women.
- **Fill in your recommended amounts** as given on page 17 for protein, and page 20 for others.

Table 2: Detailed Diet Analysis

Food No.	Food Amount & Description	wt gm	wt oz	cal	% cal fat	prot gm	carbo gm	fiber gm
116	12 fl oz Minute Maid orange juice, from concentrate	374	13.2	165	1%	0	40	0
3548	1 cup Cheerios	30	1.0	110	14%	3	22	3
559	½ cup Lucerne non-fat milk	122	4.3	45	5%	4	6	0
295	16 fl oz cup coffee, black	480	17	11	0%	0	3	0.0
7922	1 McDonald's Big Mac	215	7.9	530	47%	25	47	3.0
209	21 fl. oz (medium) diet Coke	621	22	0	0%	0	0	0
2030	1 banana	114	4.0	105	5%	1	27	2.7
8100	2 Tina's frozen bean-cheese burritos	142	10	680	26%	24	104	16
2439	1 carrot	50	1.8	21	4%	1	5	1.5
2538	1 cup iceburg lettuce	55	1.9	7	14%	1	1	0.8
5527	2 Tbs Wishbone Italian dressing	29.0	1.0	80	88%	0	3	0
559	1 cup Lucerne non-fat milk	245	8.6	90	5%	9	13	0
1227	4 Oreo reduced-fat cookies	43	1.6	173	23%	3	33	1
	Total from food:			2017		71	304	28
	Total from supplements: Safeway "One Tablet Daily"			0		0	0	0
	Total from food and supplements:			2017		71	304	28
	Recommended amount (Sue: 120 lb, age 25):					43		20-35

- **Calculate** (below) **and fill in** (on Table 2) **your recommended protein intake.**

  Recommendations are based on age, sex, and normal body weight.

  If you're overweight, pregnant, or nursing, use an adjusted body weight:

  If overweight, use a weight within the range given for your height on page 10.

  If pregnant or nursing, use your pre-pregnancy weight.

  Grams protein recommended = body weight X gm/lb (see table just below):

	☐	actual or adjusted body weight
X	☐	gm/lb
=	☐	**grams protein recommended***

Age	**Female**	**Male**
years	*gm/lb*	*gm/lb*
19 and up	0.36	0.36
15-18	0.36	0.41
7-14	0.45	0.45
4-6	0.50	0.50

***Pregnant:** Add 10 grams to your recommended amount.

***Nursing:** Add 15 grams to your recommended amount during the first 6 months of nursing; add 12 grams thereafter.

						% of Daily Value													
Food No.	fat gm	sat fat gm	choles mg	sodium mg	potas mg	vit A	vit E	vit C	thia	ribo	niac	vit B-6	fola	vit B-12	calc	phos	mag	iron	zinc
116	0	0	0	0	720	12	1	300	15	4	4	9	22	0	3	6	9	0	2
3548	2	0	0	280	95	25	1	25	25	25	25	25	25	0	4	10	8	45	25
559	0	0	2	65	203	5	0	2	3	10	0	2	2	8	15	12	4	0	4
295	0	0	0	11	259	0	0	0	0	0	5	0	0	0	0	0	5	3	0
7922	28	10	80	880	460	6	9	4	27	30	38	18	10	45	20	35	11	25	37
209	0	0	0	40	0	0	0	0	2	9	0	0	0	0	2	5	2	2	4
2030	1	0	0	1	451	1	1	17	3	7	3	33	5	0	1	2	8	2	1
8100	18	6	8	1200	757	0	11	0	43	34	17	14	49	9	8	63	26	20	26
2439	0	0	0	17	161	140	1	8	3	2	2	4	2	0	1	2	2	1	1
2538	0	0	0	5	87	2	1	4	2	1	1	1	8	0	1	1	1	2	1
5527	8	1	0	490	4	0	14	0	0	0	0	0	0	0	0	0	0	0	0
559	0	0	4	130	406	10	0	4	6	20	1	5	3	15	30	25	7	0	7
1227	5	1	0	280	86	0	2	0	8	6	6	0	2	0	0	8	4	8	2
	62	18	94	3399	3689	201	41	364	137	148	102	111	128	77	85	173	87	108	110
	0	0	0	0	0	100	100	100	100	100	100	100	100	100	0	0	0	0	0
	62	18	94	3399	3689	301	141	464	237	248	202	211	228	177	85	173	87	108	110
			Less than 300	500-2400	3500 or more	80	36	100	73	76	75	80	45	33	80	80	70	83	80

Table 2: Detailed Diet Analysis

Food No.	**Food Amount & Description**	wt gm	wt oz	calories	% cal fat	prot gm	carbo gm	fiber gm
	Total from food:							
	Total from supplements:							
	Total from food and supplements:							
	Recommended amounts:							

						% of Daily Value													
Food No.	fat gm	sat fat gm	choles mg	sodium mg	potas mg	vit A	vit E	vit C	thia	ribo	niac	vit B-6	fola	vit B-12	calc	phos	mag	iron	zinc
			Less than 300																

Your Recommended Amounts of Nutrients

As in the food composition table, fiber, sodium, and potassium are given by weight, and the other nutrients that follow are given as % Daily Values. These percentages reflect the RDAs for your particular age-and-sex group, as specified by a committee of the National Academy of Sciences. For adults who aren't pregnant or nursing, the committee recommends the range shown for sodium, and an intake of potassium that meets or exceeds the given amount (the amounts for children and pregnant or nursing women are extrapolated values). The ranges for fiber are from recommendations of the American Academy of Pediatrics and the National Cancer Institute.

Example: Sue, age 25, wants to know how the % Daily Value for calcium applies to her. The table below shows, for females age 25-50, the number **80** in the calcium (calc) column. The Daily Value for calcium is 1000 mg. The RDA is 800 mg calcium for women ages 25-50. This makes **80** the recommended % Daily Value for calcium for women ages 25-50 (800 mg is 80% of 1000 mg). If Sue's diet has 80% of the Daily Value for calcium, she meets her RDA for calcium.

				% of Daily Value													
Age	fiber gm	sodium mg	potassium mg	vit A	vit E	vit C*	thia	ribo	niac	vit B-6	fola	vit B-12	calc	phos	mag	iron	zinc
Children																	
4-6	9-16	300-1400	2400+	50	32	75	60	65	60	55	19	17	80	80	30	56	67
7-10	12-20	400-1900	2800+	70	32	75	67	71	65	70	25	23	80	80	43	56	67
Males																	
11-14	16-24	500-2400	3500+	100	45	83	87	88	85	85	38	33	120	120	68	67	100
15-18	20-28	500-2400	3500+	100	45	100	100	106	100	100	50	33	120	120	100	67	100
19-24	20-35	500-2400	3500+	100	45	100	100	100	95	100	50	33	120	120	88	56	100
25-50	20-35	500-2400	3500+	100	45	100	100	100	95	100	50	33	80	80	88	56	100
51+	20-35	500-2400	3500+	100	45	100	80	82	75	100	50	33	80	80	88	56	100
Females																	
11-14	16-24	500-2400	3500+	80	36	83	73	76	75	70	38	33	120	120	70	83	80
15-18	20-28	500-2400	3500+	80	36	100	73	76	75	75	45	33	120	120	75	83	80
19-24	20-35	500-2400	3500+	80	36	100	73	76	75	80	45	33	120	120	70	83	80
25-50	20-35	500-2400	3500+	80	36	100	73	76	75	80	45	33	80	80	70	83	80
51+	20-35	500-2400	3500+	80	36	100	67	71	65	80	45	33	80	80	70	56	80
Pregnant	20-35	600-2400	3500+	80	45	117	100	94	85	110	100	37	120	120	80	167	100
Nursing																	
1st 6 months	20-35	700-2400	3500+	130	55	158	107	106	100	105	70	43	120	120	89	83	127
2nd 6 months	20-35	700-2400	3500+	120	50	150	107	100	100	105	65	43	120	120	85	83	107

*** For adult smokers, the recommended vitamin C is 165%, rather than 100%, of the Daily Value.**

Comparing Your Diet to the Recommendations

- **CALORIES:** Your body weight indicates whether the calories you use are in balance with what you eat. Your food intake as recorded on Table 2 is probably less than usual. We tend to underestimate how much we eat and overestimate how active we are. Also, when we record what we eat, we tend to eat less. Calculate your baseline calories on p. 38.

✎ Are your calories on Table 2 at least 1.3 times your baseline need? ☐
If not, you probably ate less than your daily average. Add more food to Table 2 for a more realistic assessment of your diet.

✎ Are your weight and waist-to-hip ratio healthy, according to the Table on p. 10? ☐

✎ If not, what changes in your diet and/or physical activity could you make? Be realistic!

If you need to lose weight, be more active and/or eat less. You're especially encouraged to be more active. As you lose weight, you tend to lose muscle as well as fat. Being more active not only increases the calories used each day, but helps prevent the loss of muscle as you lose weight.

Being more active doesn't necessarily mean taking up a sport; e.g., you can use stairs instead of elevators at work or school, use your own power to mow the lawn (vs. a power mower), etc. Modest changes are more likely to be long-lasting. Most of the health benefits of physical activity occurs in going from "sedentary" to "moderately active."

Unless under medical supervision, avoid weight-loss diets with calorie counts lower than your baseline requirement (see pp. 38-39). The recommended rate of loss is ½ to 1 pound per week. Weight loss is slow (the same way you gained it), but there's a much better chance of maintaining the loss.

- **ALCOHOL:** If you drink alcoholic beverages, do so in moderation. Women who are pregnant or trying to conceive shouldn't drink any alcohol, since alcohol can damage the unborn child.

  Moderate drinking = no more than 1 drink/day for women; no more than 2 for men.
  One drink = about ½ oz pure alcohol, e.g., a 12-oz can or bottle of beer or wine cooler, 5 oz table wine, 1 jigger (1½ oz) vodka, rum, whisky, or gin.

✎ You drink: ☐ not at all ☐ moderately ☐ heavily

If you had alcohol on this day, adjust your total calories on Table 2 to exclude calories from alcohol (as shown below). Use this adjusted total calories to calculate the % of calories in your diet that come from carbohydrates, fat, and saturated fat.

Alcohol content is given in the food composition table as part of the description of the beverage, and is given in grams. There are 7 calories in a gram of alcohol.

✎ Add up the number of grams of alcohol you drank, and multiply the total grams by 7 to get the number of calories that came from alcohol:

Your Calories From Alcohol =

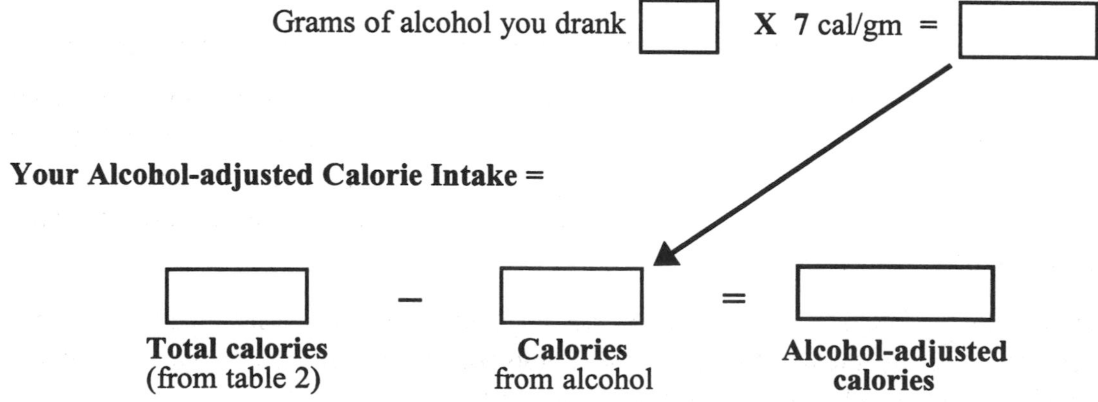

Grams of alcohol you drank
X 7 cal/gm =
Your Alcohol-adjusted Calorie Intake =
–
=
Total calories
(from table 2)
Calories
from alcohol
Alcohol-adjusted
calories

• **PROTEIN** in your diet should be adequate (meets the recommendation) but not excessive (doesn't exceed twice the recommendation).

✎ Do you eat at least the recommended amount?

✎ Do you eat more than twice the recommended amount?

✎ If needed, how can you adjust your diet to bring your protein intake to an "adequate but not excessive" amount, while keeping the calories the same?

Chronically excessive protein intake has been shown to cause kidney damage in some animal studies. Whether this is a cause for concern in humans is uncertain. What's somewhat worrisome is that some athletes and others take large, self-prescribed doses of amino acid and/or protein supplements over many years. The popularity of this practice is relatively recent, so long-term effects, if any, aren't known.

Dietary protein is absorbed from the intestine as amino acids. Excesses aren't stored in the body as amino acids: the amino part of the amino acid comes off and forms urea, which is excreted in the urine. The calorie-containing part can be stored as fat or can be broken down to provide energy. Excretion of urea uses water (we urinate more). It follows that we need more water when we eat protein excessively.

- **CARBOHYDRATE:** The Dietary Guidelines say to choose a diet with plenty of grains, vegetables, and fruits, and a diet moderate in sugars. We're advised to get 55% or more of our calories from carbohydrate—mostly from grains, vegetables, and fruits.

Calculate your % of calories from carbohydrate, using your *total grams of carbohydrate* and *total calories* from Table 2 (or *alcohol-adjusted calories* from page 22):

$$\frac{\boxed{}_{\text{gms carbohydrate}} \textbf{ X 4 calories/gm}}{\boxed{}_{\text{total calories}}} \textbf{ X 100 } = \boxed{}$$ **% of calories from carbohydrate**

Does 55% or more of your calories come from carbohydrate? ☐

Does most of it come from vegetables, fruit, and grain, rather than from candy, desserts, soft drinks, etc.? ☐

What changes, if any, might you make to improve the amount and sources of carbohydrate in your diet?

- **FIBER:** There are many kinds of dietary fiber, and they're only found in plants. The typical American diet is low in fiber, and we're advised to choose a diet with plenty of grains, vegetables, and fruits. This not only gives us more fiber, but more carbohydrates, vitamins, and minerals.

✎ Was the amount of fiber in your diet within the suggested range? ☐

✎ Did the fiber come mainly come from a variety of vegetables, fruits, and grain products (rather than from fiber-fortified breakfast cereal, for example)? ☐

✎ What changes, if any, are needed to bring your fiber intake within the suggested range and to vary your sources of fiber? Look down the column for fiber in the food composition table to find foods higher (or lower) in fiber.

A low-fiber diet raises the risk of constipation and diverticulosis (outpouchings in the colon wall). Also, people who eat low-fiber diets tend to have higher rates of colon cancer. But don't go to extremes in eating fiber. Fiber can hamper absorption of minerals. As usual, moderation makes good sense.

- **FAT:** A high-fat diet is linked to a higher risk of obesity and some cancers. It's advised that not more than 30% of our calories come from fat.

Where does most of the fat in your diet come from (see the fat/gm column in Table 2)?

Calculate your % of calories from fat, using your ***total grams of fat*** and ***total calories*** from Table 2 (or ***alcohol-adjusted calories*** from page 22):

$$\frac{\boxed{}_{\text{gms fat}} \times 9 \text{ calories/gm}}{\boxed{}_{\text{total calories}}} \times 100 = \boxed{} \text{ \% of calories from fat}$$

Does 30% or less of your calories come from fat?

If not, what are practical changes that you can make?

Saturated fat is solid at room temperature; unsaturated fat is liquid. Fat is a mix of saturated, monounsaturated, and polyunsaturated fats. Whether a fat is solid or liquid depends on which predominates: beef fat (solid) is mostly saturated, corn oil (liquid) mostly polyunsaturated, olive oil (liquid, but thicker than corn oil) mostly monounsaturated.

- **SATURATED FAT** can raise blood-cholesterol. Because a high blood-cholesterol raises the risk of heart disease, we're advised to keep our calories from saturated fat to less than 10% of our total calories.

✎ Where does most of the saturated fat in your diet come from?

✎ Calculate your % of calories from saturated fat, using your *total grams of saturated fat* and *total calories* from Table 2 (or *alcohol-adjusted calories* from page 22):

$$\frac{\text{gms saturated fat} \; \square \; \mathbf{X\ 9}\ \text{calories/gm}}{\square \; \text{total calories}} \; \mathbf{X\ 100} = \square \; \textbf{\% of calories from saturated fat}$$

✎ Does less than 10% of your calories come from saturated fat?

✎ If not, what are some changes you can make?

- **CHOLESTEROL** is found only in animal foods. It's not found in plants. A lot of cholesterol in the diet can raise cholesterol levels in the blood. It's advised that, on average, you limit your intake of cholesterol to less than 300 mg per day.

✎ Is your cholesterol intake less than 300 mg for this day? ☐

✎ Where does most of the cholesterol in your diet come from?

✎ Would you say that your cholesterol intake averages less than 300 mg per day? ☐

✎ If not, what dietary changes might you make?

Cholesterol in the diet doesn't raise blood-cholesterol as much as saturated fat does. This is why it's misleading to label a product "cholesterol-free" when it's high in saturated fat.

The amounts of fat, saturated fat, and cholesterol in food aren't proportional, e.g., salad oil is 100% fat—very high in fat—but low in saturated fat, and has no cholesterol; shrimp is low in fat but rich in cholesterol. Look through the food composition table to confirm this.

Since most of the cholesterol in a typical American diet comes from egg yolks, we're advised to limit egg yolks to 3 or 4 per week (there's no fat or cholesterol in egg whites).

- **SODIUM** is a required nutrient, but is excessive in the typical American diet. Most of it comes from salt (sodium chloride) in "fast food" and processed foods such as potato chips, olives, cold cuts, bacon, frankfurters, crackers, and frozen dinners.

  Excessive amounts of salt can raise the risk of high blood pressure in people who are genetically "salt-sensitive." But most people eating a high-salt diet don't develop high blood pressure as a result, presumably because of their genetics. Since there's no known advantage to a high-salt diet and it's not known beforehand who's salt-sensitive, we're advised to keep sodium intake to an adequate but not excessive amount.

✎ Which foods in Table 2 are the highest in sodium?

✎ Is your sodium intake within the recommended range?

✎ If not, what changes do you suggest?

- **POTASSIUM** is often low in the typical American diet. Fruits and vegetables are good sources. Those who *"choose a diet with plenty of grain products, vegetables, and fruits"* are eating a diet rich in potassium, a diet linked to a lower risk of high blood pressure and stroke. Your intake should meet or exceed the recommended amount.

✎ Does your potassium intake meet or exceed your recommended amount?

✎ If not, what changes do you suggest?

- **VITAMINS and MINERALS from FOOD** (vitamins and minerals from supplements will be considered separately)

✎ Check off those that meet or exceed the recommended amounts:

❑ Vitamin A	❑ Niacin	❑ Phosphorus
❑ Vitamin E	❑ Vitamin B-6	❑ Magnesium
❑ Vitamin C	❑ Folate	❑ Iron
❑ Thiamin	❑ Vitamin B-12	❑ Zinc
❑ Riboflavin	❑ Calcium	

If your **Vitamin A from food** looks extremely high, don't be concerned if most of it came from fruits and vegetables. Vitamin A can be very toxic in big doses, but the vitamin A values given for fruits and vegetables actually represent their carotene content. Vitamin A itself is not found in plants.

Carotene is the most common of about 20 yellow-to-deep-red plant pigments that can be converted to vitamin A in the body. But unlike vitamin A, large amounts aren't toxic. People who drink a lot of carrot juice, for example, get a lot of carotene. The excess isn't converted to vitamin A, but is stored in body fat, e.g., in the fat layer under the skin. As a result, the skin of those who drink a lot of carrot juice can have a distinct carrot-colored tone.

In the Guide to Daily Food Choices, we're advised to eat a lot of plant foods and to include one portion of a dark green or orange-colored fruit or vegetable each day. (In dark green vegetables, the color of carotene is masked by the dark green color of chlorophyll.) This provides us with carotene as well as other carotene-like substances.

Carotene is also found in some animal foods. Cows and chickens, for example, eat carotene-containing plants, which give a yellow-orange color to butter, egg yolks, and chicken skin. Carotene is added to margarine to give it the color of butter (margarine would otherwise be white.

If your **niacin** intake is low, you needn't be concerned if you meet your RDA for protein. This is because the body can make niacin from tryptophan, an amino acid in protein.

Vitamin B-12 isn't found in plant foods. Strict vegetarians can get vitamin B-12 as a supplement or in such foods as fortified cereals.

There are other required nutrients not covered here, mainly because the amounts in many foods haven't been measured. But if your diet is adequate in the nutrients given in Table 2, and the nutrients come from a variety of food rather than from supplements or from a few heavily fortified foods, you can be quite certain that your diet is nutritionally adequate.

✏ If you didn't meet all the vitamin/mineral recommendations, what foods might **you** eat to raise your intake to the advised level of each nutrient you're low in (e.g., if you're low in zinc, look down the zinc column in the food composition table for possibilities)?

- **DIETARY SUPPLEMENTS and/or heavily fortified food***

✏ Were the supplements appropriate in providing the nutrients which were low?

✏ Did you eat a heavily fortified food*?

✏ If yes, was it appropriate in providing nutrients that were low?

*Even if you don't take supplements, per se, you may be taking them in cereal, fruit drinks, etc., e.g., fiber and 100% of the Daily Value of vitamins and minerals are added to many breakfast cereals. Try to eat a diet that has the recommended amounts without having to rely on such heavily fortified foods. On the other hand, if you need a supplement, you could get it in the form of a fortified food, e.g., many cereals have a lot of added iron.

The Dietary Guidelines Committee says, "Supplements that are at or below the RDA are considered safe, but not usually needed by people who follow the Food Guide Pyramid." Getting your nutrients from food is best. There are many substances, many yet unidentified, in food which may be healthful, e.g., cabbage has indoles which may protect against cancer.

✏ **SUMMARY**: Give an overview and summary of your diet analysis, including discussion of this day's diet as compared to your usual diet.

In an overview, we see that improving our diet in one nutrient also improves our diet in other ways. For instance, you may have suggested eating more vegetables, fruit, and grain in several of the "answer boxes" that ask for ways to improve your intake of a specific nutrient By eating more of these plant foods, you get more fiber, vitamins, and minerals, including potassium. Also, these foods tend to be bulky and relatively low in fat and calories—you don't have as much "room" for "extras," making it easier to keep from becoming overweight.

Even by doing this diet analysis just once, you may have learned enough so you don't need to do it again. For a while, you may want to assess your "weak spots" (e.g., your fat and fiber intake). After that, your "nutrition consciousness" may be enough to keep you on track.

Once you assure yourself that you're "eating right," you're less vulnerable to the steady bombardment of diet-related advertisements, news reports, etc., that may have caused you anxiety. Also, knowing that your basic diet is good, there's no conflict in eating the likes of an occasional hot fudge sundae. You can eat with less worry and more pleasure.

Additional Information

Conversion Factors and Abbreviations

Weight

1 pound (lb) = 454 grams (gm)

1 pound (lb) = 16 ounces (oz)

1 ounce (oz) = 28 grams (gm)

100 grams (gm) = 3.5 ounces (oz)

1 kilogram (kg) = 2.2 pounds (lb)

1 kilogram (kg) = 1,000 grams (gm)

1 gm = 1,000 milligrams (mg)

1 mg = 1,000 micrograms (µ or mcg)

Volume

1 gallon (gal) = 4 quarts (qt)

1 quart (qt) = 2 pints = 4 cups (C)

1 cup (C) = 8 fluid ounces (fl oz)

1 cup (C) = 16 tablespoons (Tbs)

1 tablespoon (Tbs) = 3 teaspoons (tsp)

1 quart = 0.9464 liters (l)

1 liter (l) = 1.0567 quarts (qt)

1 liter (l) = 1,000 milliliters (ml)

Calories

Fat = 9 calories per gram (cal/gm)

Alcohol = 7 cal/gm

Carbohydrate = 4 cal/gm

Protein = 4 cal/gm

Length

Diameter = dia

Inch(es) = ″

Adult Recommended Dietary Allowances (RDAs) and Daily Value (DV)

	Adult RDA						
	Women (age)			**Men** (age)			Daily Value*
	19-24	25-50	51+	19-24	25-50	51+	
Fat-soluble vitamins:							
vitamin A (mcg)†	800	800	800	1000	1000	1000	1000
vitamin E (mg)†	8	8	8	10	10	10	22
Water-soluble vitamins:							
vitamin C (mg)**	60	60	60	60	60	60	60
thiamin (mg)	1.1	1.1	1.0	1.5	1.5	1.2	1.5
riboflavin (mg)	1.3	1.3	1.2	1.7	1.7	1.4	1.7
niacin (mg)	15	15	13	19	19	15	20
vitamin B-6 (mg)	1.6	1.6	1.6	2.0	2.0	2.0	2.0
folate (mcg)	180	180	180	200	200	200	400
vitamin B-12 (mcg)	2	2	2	2	2	2	6
Minerals:							
calcium (mg)	1200	800	800	1200	800	800	1000
phosphorus (mg)	1200	800	800	1200	800	800	1000
magnesium (mg)	280	280	280	350	350	350	400
iron (mg)	15	15	10	10	10	10	18
zinc (mg)	12	12	12	15	15	15	15

* Daily Values (see page 5) are for those age 4 or older (excluding pregnant or nursing women); are based on the 1968 RDA (the current one is the 1989 RDA); and are used for food labels, e.g., if a serving has 9 mg iron, the label says a serving has 50% of Daily Value (9 mg is 50% of the Daily Value of 18 mg iron).

† Vitamins A and E are sometimes given in international units (IU) on diet-supplement labels, in which case 5000 IU vitamin A = 1000 mcg vitamin A, and 30 IU vitamin E = 22 mg vitamin E.

** The RDA for those who smoke is 100 mg (rather than 60 mg) vitamin C.

Adjustment of % of Prenatal Daily Values for Use in Table 2

Some of the *% of [prenatal] Daily Values* on the labels of prenatal supplements must be adjusted for use in Table 2. (The values for vitamins E and C, niacin, iron, and zinc don't need to be changed.) For the nutrients listed below, the percentages given on the prenatal supplement labels should be adjusted as follows:

Vitamin A	☐	% prenatal Daily Value X 1.6 =	☐	Adjusted % Daily Value
Thiamin	☐	% prenatal Daily Value X 1.1 =	☐	Adjusted % Daily Value
Riboflavin	☐	% prenatal Daily Value X 1.2 =	☐	Adjusted % Daily Value
Vitamin B-6	☐	% prenatal Daily Value X 1.2 =	☐	Adjusted % Daily Value
Folate	☐	% prenatal Daily Value X 2.0 =	☐	Adjusted % Daily Value
Vitamin B-12	☐	% prenatal Daily Value X 1.3 =	☐	Adjusted % Daily Value
Calcium	☐	% prenatal Daily Value X 1.3 =	☐	Adjusted % Daily Value
Phosphorus	☐	% prenatal Daily Value X 1.3 =	☐	Adjusted % Daily Value
Magnesium	☐	% prenatal Daily Value X 1.1 =	☐	Adjusted % Daily Value

For example, 800 mcg of folate would be listed on prenatal supplements as 100% of the Daily Value because 800 mcg is the Daily Value for pregnant women. The regular Daily Value (for those 4 years or older who aren't pregnant or nursing) is 400 mcg of folate. Thus, the 100% of prenatal Daily Value for folate is 200% of the regular Daily Value (100% X 2.0 = 200%). This 200% is the adjusted value for folate to use in the row for supplements on Table 2.

Vitamins and Minerals Assessed

There are other vitamins and required minerals besides those in the food composition table, but you can be quite certain that your diet is nutritionally adequate if it's adequate in the nutrients assessed in Table 2, and if the nutrients come from a variety of foods rather than from dietary supplements or a few heavily fortified foods.

The table on the opposite page gives for each of the vitamins and minerals assessed:

- **The Name of the Nutrient**, with alternate names in parenthesis.
- **Some Functions.** A common function of vitamins and minerals is to take part in a cell's chemical reactions, which are collectively called *metabolism*. For example, vitamin B-6 takes part in amino acid metabolism—chemical reactions involving amino acids.
- **Some Sources**. Foods or groups of foods that are examples of good sources of each nutrient. (Better yet, look for yourself in the food composition table.)
- **Deficiency symptoms**. Some diseases are caused by severe deficiencies of specific nutrients. *Xerophthalmia*, for example, is an inflammation of eye tissue caused by a severe deficiency of vitamin A. In some developing countries, it's a common cause of blindness in children.

  Nutrient deficiencies often cause vague symptoms, an ideal situation for selling supplements. Bleeding gums, for example, can be from a vitamin C deficiency, but a much more common cause is periodontal disease. Similarly, a vitamin deficiency can cause fatigue, but so can depression, lack of sleep, etc. In other words, if you have a symptom of a deficiency, don't automatically conclude you have the deficiency. Besides, you would know from your diet analysis whether you're likely to be deficient.

- **Possible Toxicity from Excessive Amounts**. In general, such excessive amounts come from taking supplements, e.g., birth defects are more common in infants born to women taking high doses of vitamin A. There are exceptions, such as the iron-toxicity disease hemochromatosis, which stems from a genetic defect in which iron is absorbed more efficiently than normal. The result can be severe—even fatal—damage from iron accumulating in various tissues. In genetically susceptible people, the disease occurs more commonly in men, since women regularly "get rid of" iron via menstruation (blood is rich in iron).

Nutrient	Functions	Sources	Deficiency	Large Excess
Sodium	Water balance	Salty foods, softened water	Weakness, cramps	High blood pressure
Potassium	Nerve function	Citrus fruits, bananas, apricots	Weakness, irregular heartbeat	Irregular heartbeat
Vitamin A	Night vision, maintain various tissues	Liver, yellow-orange and dark-green fruits and vegetables	Night blindness, xerophthalmia	Fatigue, nausea, headache, hair loss
Vitamin E	Antioxidant	Plant oils, whole grains, almonds	Hemolytic anemia	Cramps, diarrhea, dizziness
Vitamin C (ascorbic acid, ascorbate)	Antioxidant, synthesis of connective tissue	Citrus fruits, berries, potatoes, red and green peppers	Scurvy, loose teeth, bleeding gums	Diarrhea, kidney stones
Thiamin (vitamin B-1)	Helps in carbohydrate metabolism	Pork, legumes, whole and enriched grains, liver, nuts	Beriberi, impaired nervous system	Headache, weakness, irritability
Riboflavin (vitamin B-2)	Helps in energy and protein metabolism	Liver, meat, dairy products, enriched grains, eggs	Sore, red tongue, inflamed skin, eye disorders	None reported
Niacin (nicotinic acid, niacinamide)	Helps in energy metabolism	Liver, meat, fish, whole and enriched grains, legumes	Pellagra (diarrhea, inflamed skin, dementia)	Flushing of face and hands, liver damage
Vitamin B-6 (pyridoxine)	Helps in amino acid metabolism	Liver, meat, legumes, potatoes, organ meats	Inflamed skin, convulsions in infants	Weak and numb muscles, nerve damage
Folate (folic acid, folacin)	Helps in cell division	Liver, legumes, oranges, green leafy veggies, whole grains	Anemia. risk of neural tube defects in fetus	High folate can delay diagnosing B-12 deficiency
Vitamin B-12	Helps in cell division	Animal products (meats, eggs, milk)	Anemia, nerve damage	Diarrhea
Calcium	Bone/teeth structure, muscle and nerve function	Milk/milk products, soft fish bones, leafy green vegetables	Stunted growth, malformed bones	Less absorption of Iron and Zinc
Phosphorus	Bone/teeth formation, energy production	Meat, fish, poultry, milk, eggs, legumes, cereals, nuts	Irritability, weakness, muscle ache	Poor bone mineralization if low calcium intake
Magnesium	Helps in metabolism	Whole grains, nuts, legumes, green leafy vegetables	Weakness, muscle pain, cramps, spasms	Loss of reflexes, respiratory failure
Iron	Carries oxygen in blood	Liver, meats, whole grains, legumes	Anemia, fatigue	Hemochromatosis
Zinc	Helps in metabolism, development	Oysters, beef, lamb, legumes, whole grains	Retarded growth	Nausea, cramps, diarrhea, fever

Calorie Requirements

First, estimate the calories you need just to breathe, maintain body temperature, blood circulation, muscle tone, etc. (your baseline requirement) by multiplying your **body surface area** (see opposite page) by a **basic calorie factor** based on your age and sex (see table below).

Your **body surface area** is an indication of your size and the amount of surface from which your body can lose heat. The bigger you are and the greater your surface area, the more baseline calories you need.

Your **basic calorie factor** is affected by whether you're growing and how lean you are. Lean tissue uses more calories than fat tissue. Men are generally leaner than women. Also, as we age, we become less lean. Your basic calorie factor (cal/day/m2) is the estimated calories used each day for basic functions for each square meter of body surface.

[ ] m2 X [ ] cal/day/m2 = [ ] calories/day

your body surface area **your basic calorie factor** **Your Baseline Requirement**

What you use, on average, for daily activities varies from about 30% more for the very lightly active to about 100% more for the heavily active (e.g., strenuous activity several hours daily). To estimate what you use, multiply your baseline requirement by an activity factor ranging from 1.3 (very lightly active) to 2.0 (heavily active).

[ ] cal/day X [ ] = [ ] calories/day

your baseline requirement **your activity factor (1.3 to 2.0)** **Your Daily Use**

Basic Calorie Factors (cal/day/m2) by Age and Sex

Age	Male	Female	Age	Male	Female	Age	Male	Female
6	1270	1215	**15**	1100	960	**28-29**	955	855
7	1260	1180	**16**	1095	930	**30-34**	945	850
8	1245	1130	**17**	1075	910	**35-39**	930	845
9	1215	1100	**18**	1040	880	**40-44**	910	845
10	1165	1090	**19**	1015	875	**45-49**	895	840
11	1130	1085	**20-21**	995	870	**50-54**	880	815
12	1120	1065	**22-23**	980	865	**55-59**	865	795
13	1110	1030	**24-25**	965	860	**60-64**	850	785
14	1105	995	**26-27**	960	855	**65 +**	835	775

Your Body Surface Area

Draw a straight line between your height and weight. Read the intersect for your body surface area in square meters (m2), reading to the 2nd decimal point (each segment between numbers is 0.02). The dotted line: a 135-lb, 5′5″ person = 1.67 m2 estimated body surface.

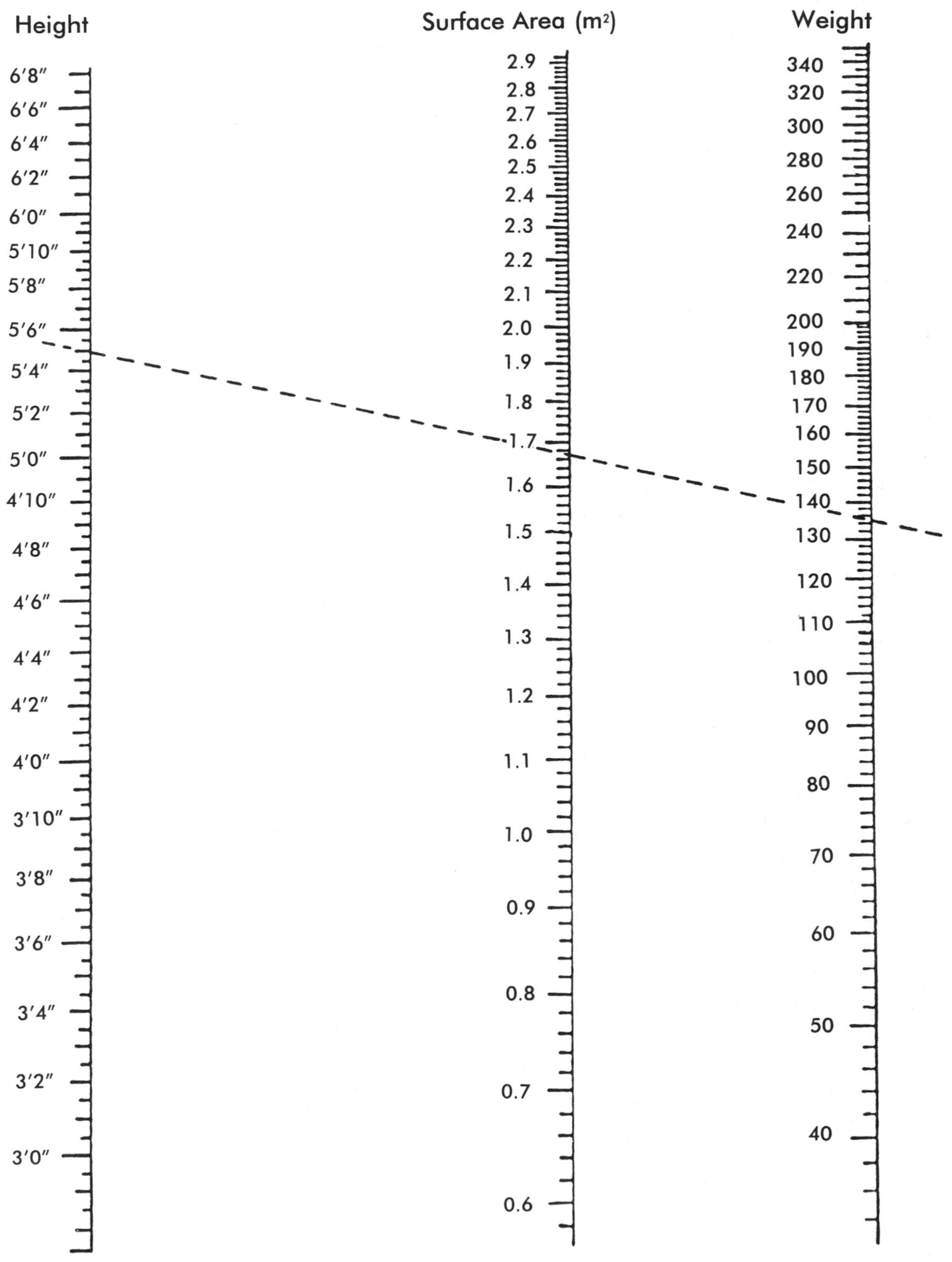

Nutrition Facts on Food Labels

Required*	**Optional****
Calories per Serving	
Calories from Fat	Calories from Saturated Fat
Total Fat	
Saturated Fat	Polyunsaturated Fat
	Monounsaturated Fat
Cholesterol	
Sodium	Potassium
Total Carbohydrate	
Dietary Fiber	Soluble Fiber
	Insoluble Fiber
Sugars	Sugar Alcohol (e.g., sorbitol)
Protein	
Vitamin A	
Vitamin C	
Calcium	
Iron	Other Vitamins and Minerals

*Except for certain foods, e.g., a soft drink label needn't give values for fat.

**Required if they've been added or if the label makes claims about them, e.g., the % Daily Value for vitamin D is required if it's been added to the food.

Nutrition Facts

Serving Size: ½ cup (114 g)
Servings Per Container: 4
Calories per serving: 90
Calories per serving from Fat: 30

Amount Per Serving		% Daily Value*
Total Fat	3 g	5%
Saturated Fat	2 g	10%
Cholesterol	0 mg	0%
Sodium	300 mg	13%
Total Carbohydrate	13 g	4%
Dietary Fiber	2 g	8%
Sugars	4 g	
Protein	3 g	
Vitamin A		80%
Vitamin C		50%
Calcium		4%
Iron		4%

* Percent Daily Values are based on a 2,000 calorie diet. Your Daily Values may be higher or lower depending on your calorie needs:

Nutrient		2,000 *Calories*	2,500 *Calories*
Total Fat	Less than	65 g	80 g
Sat Fat	Less Than	20 g	25 g
Cholesterol	Less Than	300 mg	300 mg
Sodium	Less Than	2,400 mg	2,400 mg
Total Carbohydrate		300 g	375 g
Fiber		25 g	30 g

1 gram of Fat = 9 calories
1 gram of Carbohydrates = 4 calories
1 gram of Protein = 4 calories

% Daily Value (DV) shows how a food fits in your overall diet. Some DVs are maximums, e.g., fat (65 g *or less*), some are minimums, e.g., carbohydrate (300 g *or more*); some are recommended amounts, e.g., vitamin C (60 mg).

A 50% DV of vit. C means that 1 serving gives you 50% (30 mg) of what you need to get the recommended amount (60 mg).

For most of us, the goal is to choose foods that add up to about 100% of the DV for total carbohydrate, dietary fiber, vitamins, and minerals.

Many women, teenage girls, and less active men use about 2,000 calories/day.

Many men, teenage boys, and very active women use about 2,500 calories/day.

Calculating Nutrient Content from Recipes

As shown for this example of Pumpkin Pie Squares, calculating the nutrient content from recipes involves adding up what's in the recipe and dividing it by the number of servings. Be sure to use the information from the labels first. There are extra lines at the end of the sections in the food composition table for you to add what you've calculated for your recipes (e.g., you can add the nutrient content of this recipe to the end of the desserts/sweets section).

You can, of course, adjust this recipe to your liking and convenience. If you don't have whole wheat flour and non-fat milk, white flour and low-fat or whole milk work fine. You can adjust the amount of spices, and add ginger according to your taste (the nutrient content of such small amounts of these spices is trivial, and isn't included in the analysis). You can substitute margarine for butter, brown sugar for white, 2 egg whites for an egg, etc.

In doing nutrient analyses of your recipes (and your diet), you can learn a lot by being observant. Looking at the nutrient content of the ingredients in this recipe, for example, you see that only plant foods have fiber; only animal foods have cholesterol and B-12; and sugar and fat have lots of calories relative to their nutrient content. Note also that you get more than 100% of the Daily Value for vitamin A from one pumpkin square. Pumpkin is a rich source of carotene, which shows as vitamin A in the analysis. Carotene can be converted to vitamin A in the body; plants don't have vitamin A, per se.

Food No.	Food Description & Amount	wt gm	wt oz	cal	% cal fat	prot gm	carbo gm	fiber gm
3132	1 cup whole wheat flour	132	4	480	4	20	88	16
3427	½ cup oats	39	1.4	140	18	5	26	4
1832	½ cup dark brown sugar	96	3.4	360	0	0	96	0
5403	½ cup butter (1 cube)	112	4	800	100	0	0	0
2723	29 oz canned pumpkin	822	29	270	12	13	61	34
1839	1 cup sugar	192	7	720	0	0	192	0
index	½ teaspoon salt	3	0	0	0	0	0	0
969	3 eggs	150	5.4	210	57	18	3	0
559	1½ cups non-fat milk	368	13	135	5	14	20	0
	Total			3125	32*	70	486	54
	Total/15 = 1 piece (3" x 2½")			208	32	5	32	4

*Calculated value: (112 gm fat X 9 cal/gm)/3115 cal = 0.32 = 32% of calories from fat

Pumpkin Pie Squares

1 cup whole wheat flour
½ cup oats (dry oatmeal)
½ cup brown sugar
½ cup softened butter (1 cube)

Mix dry ingredients, and then mix in butter until crumbly (butter at room temperature is about the right softness). Press into 13 X 9" pan. Bake at 350° until lightly browned (about 15 minutes).

1 large (29 oz) can pumpkin
1 cup sugar
½ teaspoon salt
1½ teaspoon cinnamon
¼ teaspoon nutmeg
¼ teaspoon ground cloves
3 eggs
1½ cups non-fat milk

Mix pumpkin, sugar, salt, and spices (you can use same bowl that you made crust in). Mix in eggs, and then milk. Pour over crust. Bake at 350° until knife inserted about 1" from side of pan comes out clean (about 45-55 minutes). Cut into 15 pieces (3 X 2½").

For a fancier version, add a layer of whipped cream before cutting, with lightly toasted chopped walnuts or pecans sprinkled on top. For other changes to recipe, see page 42.

						% of Daily Value													
Food No.	fat gm	sat fat gm	choles mg	sodium mg	potas mg	vit A	vit E	vit C	thia	ribo	niac	vit B-6	fola	vit B-12	calc	pho s	mag	iron	zinc
3132	4	0	0	0	486	0	7	0	40	8	32	20	13	0	0	42	41	32	23
3427	3	0	0	0	142	0	2	0	15	2	2	3	4	0	2	15	10	10	8
1832	0	0	0	0	326	0	0	0	0	0	0	0	0	0	7	3	7	10	0
5403	88	64	240	680	32	64	8	0	0	0	0	0	0	0	0	0	0	0	0
2723	3	0	0	34	1688	2358	40	54	13	27	13	23	23	0	27	30	47	67	10
1839	0	0	0	0	0	0	0	0	0	0	0	0	0	0	0	0	0	0	0
index	0	0	0	1180	0	0	0	0	0	0	0	0	0	0	0	0	0	0	0
969	14	4	645	195	183	18	6	0	6	45	0	9	18	24	6	27	3	12	12
559	0	0	6	195	609	15	0	6	9	30	2	8	4	22	45	38	10	0	10
	112	68	891	2284	3528	2455	63	60	83	112	49	63	62	46	87	155	118	131	63
	7	5	59	152	235	164	4	4	6	7	3	4	4	3	6	10	8	9	4

References

American Cancer Society. *Guidelines for Diet, Nutrition, and Cancer Prevention*, 1996 (see http://www.cancer.org).

National Research Council, National Academy of Sciences. *Diet and Health: Implications for Reducing Chronic Disease Risk.* Washington DC: National Academy Press, 1989.

National Research Council, National Academy of Sciences. *Recommended Dietary Allowances*, 10th Edition. Washington DC: National Academy Press, 1989.

U.S. Department of Agriculture. *Preparing Foods and Planning Menus Using the Dietary Guidelines*. Home and Garden Bulletin No. 232-8. Washington DC: U.S. Government Printing Office.

U.S. Dept. of Agriculture and U.S. Dept. of Health and Human Services. *The Food Guide Pyramid.* Home and Garden Bulletin No. 252. Washington DC: U.S. Government Printing Office, 1992.

U.S. Dept. of Agriculture and U.S. Dept. of Health and Human Services. *Nutrition and Your Health: Dietary Guidelines for Americans*, 4th Edition. Home and Garden Bulletin No. 232. Washington DC: U.S. Government Printing Office, 1995.

U.S. Dept. of Agriculture, Agricultural Research Service, Dietary Guidelines Advisory Committee. *Report of the Dietary Guidelines Advisory Committee on the Dietary Guidelines for Americans, 1995, to the Secretary of Health and Human Services and the Secretary of Agriculture* (the revised, current guidelines were issued in January, 1996; see http://www.os.dhhs.gov).

U.S. Dept. of Health and Human Services. *Eating to Lower Your High Blood Cholesterol*, 1992.

About the Food Composition Table

The Database

The table is adapted from food composition data provided by the Agricultural Research Service, United States Department of Agriculture (USDA) in January 1997. The USDA compiled the data for evaluating the nutritional adequacy of diets in the United States.

They used many food samples for each determination of nutrient content, and the values are averages. There are no missing values in the database; when a chemical analysis of a nutrient in a food was unavailable, they estimated a likely level. The nutrient values are reasonable estimates, not hard-and-fast numbers.

The Nutrient Values

The following nutrient values are given for each food: calories, the percent of calories from fat, the grams or milligrams of protein, carbohydrate, fiber, fat, saturated fat, cholesterol, sodium, potassium, and the percent of the Daily Value for 14 nutrients—vitamins A, E, and C, the B-vitamins (thiamin, riboflavin, niacin, B-6, folate, B-12), and calcium, phosphorus, magnesium, iron, and zinc.

The values have been rounded, and this can appear to result in discrepancies. For example, if the amount of fat is less than ½ gm, it is rounded to zero, but the trace amount is still used to calculate the % of calories from fat. This can make the % of calories from fat appear abnormally high if thc food is cxtrcmcly low in calories.

Portion Size

A description of the portion size for each food is given in parentheses after the name of the food. The weight of the portion, given in grams and ounces, applies only to the edible portion of the food (e.g., an orange without the peel, or a rib steak without the bone).

Unless you weigh your food on a scale, it's probably easier to use the description of the portion size, rather than trying to estimate its weight. An ounce is 1/16 of a pound, and, for most foods, isn't the same as a fluid ounce, which is what we measure in a measuring cup (see page 33 for abbreviations and conversions). There are 8 fluid ounces in a cup, but a cup of most foods doesn't weigh exactly 8 ounces (e.g., a cup of milk weighs more than 8 ounces, while a cup of potato chips weighs much less). **Pay close attention to portion sizes**, e.g., does your candy bar weigh the same as what's listed in the food composition table; is that ¾ cup or 1 cup of rice on your plate?

Variation in Foods

Prepared foods can vary a lot. Even batches of spaghetti sauce made by the same person using the same recipe vary. New products are introduced constantly, changes are often made in existing products, and food composition tables can hardly keep up. This is why **you should first use nutrient values from labels**, and then look up a similar food in the food composition table to approximate missing nutrient values. For your deli sandwich, it's of course more accurate to list the parts separately, rather than using the values for a generic version.

Foods vary even in their natural state, not only between varieties but within one variety, e.g., the nutrient content of an apple on one side of a tree isn't identical to one on the other. And of course the sizes of apples, carrots, etc., also vary. Canned tuna of the same brand and description can vary so much that different labels are used, depending on when and where the tuna was caught. Other variations (e.g., storage and cooking times) also come into play. As mentioned earlier, nutrient values are reasonable estimates, not hard-and-fast numbers.

There are sections in the food composition table for you to add foods. You may want to add brand-name foods that you eat often, but aren't specifically listed in the table. As noted earlier, if there are missing nutrient values on the food labels, booklets from a fast-food eatery, etc., you should estimate the values by looking up similar foods in the food composition table. Some food companies have a toll-free number and address listed on the label, which you can use to inquire about nutrient content.

You may also want to add foods made from your favorite recipes (see pages 42-43). Some newspapers, magazines, and cookbooks provide nutrient information, including % of Daily Values, for their recipes.

The Food Index helps you find a particular food.

Beverages, Dairy, Eggs

Beverages, Dairy, Eggs

Food No.	Food Description & Amount	wt gm	wt oz	cal	% cal fat	prot gm	carbo gm	fiber gm
	Juices							
1	Acerola juice [1 cup]	249	8.8	52	13%	1	12	0.7
2	Aloe vera juice [1 cup]	251	8.9	100	5%	2	23	0.5
3	Ambrosia juice (Include Knudsen's) [1 cup]	245	8.6	153	14%	1	32	0.6
4	Apple cider (Include sparkling cider) [1 cup]	248	8.7	117	2%	0	29	0.2
5	Apple cider-flavored drink, made from powdered mix, low calorie, with vitamin C added [1 cup]	240	8.5	2	0%	0	1	0.0
6	Apple cider-flavored drink, made from powdered mix, with sugar and vitamin C added [1 cup]	250	8.8	66	0%	0	17	0.0
7	Apple drink with vitamin C added [1 cup]	250	8.8	117	0%	0	30	0.0
8	Apple drink [1 cup]	250	8.8	118	0%	0	30	0.0
9	Apple juice drink [1 cup]	250	8.8	126	0%	0	32	0.1
10	Apple juice [1 cup]	248	8.7	117	2%	0	29	0.2
11	Apple juice, with added vitamin C [1 cup]	248	8.7	117	2%	0	29	0.2
12	Apple juice with added vitamin C and calcium [1 cup]	248	8.7	116	2%	0	29	0.2
13	Apple-cherry drink (Include apple-grape, apple-raspberry, apple-pineapple)	250	8.8	117	0%	0	30	0.1
14	Apple-cherry juice [1 cup]	250	8.8	117	2%	1	29	1.4
15	Apple-cranberry-grape juice drink [1 cup (8 fl oz)]	251	8.9	109	2%	0	28	0.1
16	Apple-grape juice [1 cup]	244	8.6	128	2%	1	32	0.2
17	Apple-grape-raspberry juice [1 cup]	250	8.8	130	3%	1	32	0.3
18	Apple-orange-pineapple juice drink [1 cup (8 fl oz)]	251	8.9	131	1%	0	34	0.2
19	Apple-raspberry juice [1 cup]	239	8.4	108	4%	0	26	0.2
20	Apple-pear juice [1 cup]	248	8.7	119	2%	0	30	0.2
21	Apple-white grape juice drink, low calorie, with vitamin C added (Include cocktail) [1 cup]	240	8.5	54	2%	0	13	0.1
22	Apricot nectar [1 cup]	251	8.9	141	1%	1	36	1.5
23	Apricot-orange juice [1 cup]	250	8.8	123	2%	1	30	1.0
24	Apricot-pineapple juice drink [1 cup]	250	8.8	128	1%	0	32	0.4
25	Banana nectar [1 cup]	250	8.8	177	2%	1	45	2.1
26	Banana-orange drink [1 cup]	250	8.8	126	0%	0	32	0.2
27	Black cherry drink [1 cup]	250	8.8	117	0%	0	30	0.4
28	Black cherry drink with vitamin C added [1 cup]	250	8.8	117	0%	0	30	0.4
29	Blackberry juice [1 cup]	250	8.8	93	15%	1	20	0.3
30	Cantaloupe nectar [1 cup]	250	8.8	155	2%	1	39	0.8
31	Celery juice [1 cup]	236	8.3	42	8%	2	9	3.8
32	Cherry drink with vitamin C added [1 cup]	250	8.8	117	0%	0	30	0.4
33	Citrus drink with vitamin C added [1 cup]	250	8.8	127	0%	0	33	0.0
34	Citrus fruit juice drink (60% fruit juice) (Include 5 Alive Citrus) [1 cup]	247	8.7	114	1%	1	28	0.1
35	Citrus juice drink, calcium fortified (Include Citrus Hill Grapefruit Juice Beverage Plus Calcium) [1 cup]	240	8.5	112	2%	1	28	0.1
36	Citrus juice drink, low calorie (Include TreeSweet Lite grapefruit, orange, citrus combo) [1 cup]	240	8.5	72	0%	1	18	0.2
37	Coconut beverage, Puerto Rican [1 cup]	240	8.5	173	41%	2	25	4.3
38	Cranberry juice drink with vitamin C added (Include cocktail) [1 cup]	253	8.9	144	2%	0	36	0.3
39	Cranberry juice drink, low calorie, with vitamin C added (Include low-calorie cranberry juice cocktail) [1 cup]	240	8.5	46	0%	0	11	0.0
40	Cranapple-citrus juice drink, low calorie [1 cup]	240	8.5	59	0%	0	15	0.2
41	Cranberry juice, unsweetened [1 cup]	253	8.9	124	4%	1	32	0.3
42	Cranberry-apple juice drink with vitamin C added (Include cocktail; Crantastic; blueberry-cranberry, raspberry-cranberry, cranberry-apricot, and cranberry-grape juice drink) [1 cup]	253	8.9	170	0%	0	43	0.3
43	Cranberry-apple juice drink, low calorie, with vitamin C added (Include cocktail, low calorie raspberry-cranberry, cranberry- blueberry, and cranberry-apricot juice drinks) [1 cup]	240	8.5	46	0%	0	11	0.2

Food no.	fat gm	sat fat gm	choles mg	sodium mg	potas mg	% of Daily Value													
						vit A	vit E	vit C	thia	ribo	niac	vit B-6	fola	vit B-12	calc	phos	mag	iron	zinc
1	1	0	0	7	242	13	0	6640	3	9	5	0	9	0	2	2	7	7	2
2	1	0	0	73	733	1	0	36	15	9	5	28	3	0	6	11	9	6	3
3	2	2	0	11	342	1	1	42	7	4	3	9	8	0	3	3	7	4	2
4	0	0	0	7	295	0	0	4	3	2	1	4	0	0	2	2	2	5	0
5	0	0	0	7	0	0	0	105	0	0	0	0	0	0	3	3	1	0	0
6	0	0	0	8	1	0	0	110	0	0	0	0	0	0	3	3	1	1	1
7	0	0	0	12	47	0	0	46	2	4	0	0	1	0	2	1	1	4	2
8	0	0	0	13	48	0	0	0	2	4	0	0	1	0	2	1	1	4	2
9	0	0	0	7	75	0	0	138	1	1	0	1	0	0	1	0	1	1	1
10	0	0	0	7	295	0	0	4	3	2	1	4	0	0	2	2	2	5	0
11	0	0	0	7	295	0	0	177	3	2	1	4	0	0	2	2	2	5	0
12	0	0	0	17	312	0	0	143	0	2	0	4	0	0	28	2	3	4	1
13	0	0	0	7	31	0	0	1	0	1	0	0	0	0	1	0	1	1	1
14	0	0	0	6	307	1	1	6	4	4	3	4	1	0	2	2	3	5	1
15	0	0	0	6	121	0	0	15	2	2	1	3	1	0	1	1	2	2	1
16	0	0	0	7	303	0	0	2	4	4	2	5	1	0	2	2	4	4	1
17	1	0	0	5	335	1	2	18	5	7	5	6	6	0	3	3	6	5	3
18	0	0	0	7	167	0	0	20	3	2	1	3	3	0	1	1	2	3	1
19	0	0	0	6	309	1	0	11	3	3	2	4	1	0	2	2	4	6	1
20	0	0	0	12	347	0	0	5	2	3	3	2	2	0	2	2	4	5	1
21	0	0	0	12	145	0	0	1	0	1	0	2	0	0	1	1	2	2	1
22	0	0	0	8	286	33	1	3	2	2	3	3	1	0	2	2	3	5	2
23	0	0	0	6	361	19	1	73	6	3	4	7	6	0	2	3	5	6	1
24	0	0	0	5	161	5	0	16	4	2	2	5	5	0	2	1	4	2	1
25	0	0	0	5	347	1	1	13	3	5	2	25	4	0	1	2	7	2	1
26	0	0	0	6	61	0	0	13	1	1	0	2	2	0	1	0	1	0	1
27	0	0	0	7	34	0	0	1	0	1	1	0	0	0	1	1	1	1	1
28	0	0	0	7	34	0	0	136	0	1	1	0	0	0	1	1	1	1	1
29	2	0	0	3	425	4	2	42	3	4	4	5	7	0	3	3	13	13	3
30	0	0	0	13	277	24	1	49	2	1	3	5	2	0	1	2	3	1	1
31	0	0	0	215	670	3	4	24	7	7	4	10	13	0	10	6	7	6	2
32	0	0	0	7	34	0	0	136	0	1	1	0	0	0	1	1	1	1	1
33	0	0	0	7	48	0	0	132	0	1	0	1	0	0	1	0	1	3	1
34	0	0	0	7	275	1	0	111	2	2	2	3	1	0	2	3	4	15	1
35	0	0	0	4	196	0	0	133	4	2	2	3	1	0	32	2	4	1	1
36	0	0	0	7	266	1	0	108	2	3	2	2	1	0	2	2	4	15	1
37	8	7	0	218	589	0	1	9	5	7	1	4	3	0	5	7	15	6	3
38	0	0	0	5	46	0	0	149	2	1	0	2	0	0	1	1	1	2	1
39	0	0	0	7	53	0	0	129	1	1	0	2	0	0	2	0	1	1	0
40	0	0	0	6	166	0	0	118	1	3	1	2	1	0	2	2	2	8	1
41	1	0	0	3	162	1	1	29	3	3	1	8	1	0	2	2	3	3	2
42	0	0	0	5	68	0	0	135	1	3	1	3	0	0	2	1	1	1	1
43	0	0	0	5	65	0	0	128	0	3	1	2	0	0	2	1	1	1	1

Beverages, Dairy, Eggs

Food No.	Food Description & Amount	wt gm	wt oz	cal	% cal fat	prot gm	carbo gm	fiber gm
44	Cranberry-white grape juice mixture, unsweetened (Include Knudsen Cranberry Nectar) [1 cup]	253	8.9	142	2%	1	36	0.3
45	Fluid replacement, electrolyte solution (Include Pedialyte) [1 cup]	240	8.5	24	0%	0	7	0.0
46	Fluid replacement, 5% glucose in water [1 cup]	242	8.5	44	0%	0	12	0.0
47	Frozen daiquiri mix, from frozen concentrate, reconstituted [1 fl oz]	29	1.0	19	1%	0	5	0.1
48	Frozen daiquiri mix, frozen concentrate, not reconstituted [1 fl oz]	36	1.3	101	1%	0	26	0.5
49	Fruit drink (Include fruit punches and fruit ades, Hawaiian Punch made from canned or frozen) [1 cup]	248	8.7	117	0%	0	30	0.2
50	Fruit drink, low calorie [1 cup]	240	8.5	43	0%	0	11	0.0
51	Fruit juice blend, 100% juice, all flavors (Include Juicy Juice, Hi-C 100) [1 cup]	250	8.8	132	2%	1	33	0.3
52	Fruit punch, fruit drinks, or fruitades, with vitamin C added (Include Hi-C) [1 cup]	247	8.7	116	0%	0	29	0.2
53	Fruit punch, made with fruit juice and soda [1 cup]	245	8.6	110	1%	0	28	0.2
54	Fruit punch, made with soda, fruit juice, and sherbet or ice cream [1 cup]	256	9.0	164	6%	1	39	0.5
55	Fruit-flavored beverage, dry concentrate, low calorie, not reconstituted (Include Crystal Light) [1 Tbs]	12	0.4	26	0%	1	9	0.0
56	Fruit-flavored beverage, dry concentrate, low sugar, not reconstituted (Include Gatorade) [1 Tbs]	13	0.4	46	0%	0	12	0.0
57	Fruit-flavored beverage, low sugar (Include Gatorade, Quick Kick) [1 cup]	240	8.5	60	0%	0	15	0.0
58	Fruit-flavored concentrate, dry, with vitamin C added (Include Kool-Aid, Hawaiian Punch) [1 Tbs]	13	0.4	48	0%	0	12	0.0
59	Fruit-flavored drink, low calorie, calcium fortified (Include Supri drink mix) [1 cup]	240	8.5	3	0%	0	1	0.0
60	Fruit-flavored drink, made from powdered mix with high vitamin C added, low calorie (Include Sugar Free Tang) [1 cup]	240	8.5	7	1%	0	2	0.0
61	Fruit-flavored drink, made from powdered mix with vitamin C added, no sugar or low calorie sweetener (Include Kool-Aid, Wyler's) [1 cup]	240	8.5	90	0%	0	23	0.0
62	Fruit-flavored drink, made from powdered mix, with sugar and vitamin C added (Include Kool-Aid, Wylers) [1 cup]	250	8.8	88	0%	0	22	0.0
63	Fruit-flavored drink, non-carbonated, made from low calorie powdered mix (Include Sugar Free Crystal light) [1 cup]	240	8.5	3	0%	0	1	0.0
64	Fruit-flavored drink, non-carbonated, made from powdered mix, with sugar (Include Fla-vor-Aid) [1 can (12 fl oz)]	356	12.6	125	0%	0	32	0.0
65	Fruit-flavored drinks, made from powdered mix, mainly sugar, with high vitamin C added (Incl. Borden's Instant Breakfast Drink, Keen, Tang Instant Breakfast Juice Drink) [1 cup]	240	8.5	119	0%	0	30	0.0
66	Fruit-flavored drinks, punches, ades, low calorie, with vitamin C added (Include low calorie Hi C, Kool-Aid, Wylers) [1 cup]	240	8.5	43	0%	0	11	0.0
67	Fruit-flavored thirst quencher beverage, low calorie [1 cup]	240	8.5	26	0%	0	7	0.0
68	Fruit-flavored drink, vitamin and mineral fortified [1 cup]	240	8.5	50	0%	0	14	0.0
69	Gelatin drink, powder, flavored, with low-calorie sweetener, reconstituted (Include Nutri System Orange Drink) [1 packet dry mix with 1 cup water]	255	9.0	51	0%	13	0	0.0
70	Grape juice drink [1 cup]	250	8.8	125	0%	0	32	0.3
71	Grape drink with vitamin C added [1 cup]	250	8.8	113	0%	0	29	0.0
72	Grape juice, unsweetened or low-cal sweetener [1 cup]	250	8.8	153	1%	1	37	0.3
73	Grape juice, unsweetened, with added vitamin C [1 cup]	250	8.8	152	1%	1	37	0.3
74	Grape juice, with sugar, with added vitamin C [1 cup]	250	8.8	128	2%	0	32	0.3
75	Grape-tangerine-lemon juice [1 cup]	245	8.6	128	2%	1	32	0.4
76	Grapeade and grape drink [1 cup]	250	8.8	107	0%	0	28	0.0
77	Grapefruit juice drink [1 cup]	250	8.8	128	1%	0	32	0.1
78	Grapefruit juice drink with vitamin C added [1 cup]	250	8.8	128	1%	0	32	0.1
79	Grapefruit juice drink, low calorie, with vitamin C added [1 cup]	231	8.1	32	2%	0	7	0.1
80	Grapefruit juice, canned or bottled, unsweetened or sweetened with low-cal sweetener (Include Ocean Spray) [1 cup]	247	8.7	94	2%	1	22	0.2

Food no.	fat gm	sat fat gm	choles mg	sodium mg	potas mg	% of Daily Value													
						vit A	vit E	vit C	thia	ribo	niac	vit B-6	fola	vit B-12	calc	phos	mag	iron	zinc
44	0	0	0	6	265	0	0	12	4	4	2	8	1	0	2	3	5	3	1
45	0	0	0	250	187	0	0	0	0	0	0	0	0	0	2	2	1	0	0
46	0	0	0	7	0	0	0	0	0	0	0	0	0	0	0	0	1	0	0
47	0	0	0	23	6	0	0	1	0	0	0	0	0	0	0	0	0	0	0
48	0	0	0	123	34	0	0	5	1	1	0	0	0	0	0	1	0	1	1
49	0	0	0	55	62	0	0	23	3	3	0	0	1	0	2	0	1	3	2
50	0	0	0	50	50	0	0	129	2	3	0	0	1	0	2	0	1	4	2
51	0	0	0	7	328	1	0	100	5	4	3	7	3	0	2	2	5	4	1
52	0	0	0	54	62	0	0	122	4	3	0	0	1	0	2	0	1	3	2
53	0	0	0	10	165	0	0	22	5	2	2	6	7	0	2	1	4	3	1
54	1	1	3	30	272	1	1	60	7	4	2	6	12	1	5	4	5	2	3
55	0	0	0	1	447	0	0	99	0	0	0	0	0	0	33	15	0	0	0
56	0	0	0	84	19	0	0	0	0	0	0	0	0	0	0	2	0	0	0
57	0	0	0	96	26	0	0	0	1	0	0	0	0	0	0	2	1	1	0
58	0	0	0	15	1	0	0	25	0	0	0	0	0	0	2	3	0	0	0
59	0	0	0	11	4	0	0	0	0	0	0	0	0	0	32	1	1	0	0
60	0	0	0	10	71	17	0	112	0	11	11	11	22	0	1	1	2	0	0
61	0	0	0	13	0	0	0	50	0	0	0	0	0	0	1	1	1	0	0
62	0	0	0	34	1	0	0	47	0	0	0	0	0	0	4	5	1	1	1
63	0	0	0	7	45	0	0	10	0	0	0	0	0	0	4	2	1	0	0
64	0	0	0	49	2	0	0	67	0	0	0	0	0	0	5	7	1	1	1
65	0	0	0	12	51	57	0	210	0	2	0	0	37	0	6	4	1	1	1
66	0	0	0	50	50	0	0	129	2	3	0	0	1	0	2	0	1	4	2
67	0	0	0	84	24	0	0	25	0	0	0	0	0	0	0	2	1	1	0
68	0	0	0	26	50	1	33	51	0	0	30	16	31	30	0	0	2	0	0
69	0	0	0	37	2	0	0	0	0	2	0	0	1	0	1	1	1	1	1
70	0	0	0	3	88	0	0	67	2	1	1	3	1	0	1	1	3	1	1
71	0	0	0	15	13	0	0	142	1	1	0	1	0	0	1	0	1	2	2
72	0	0	0	8	330	0	0	0	4	5	3	8	2	0	2	3	6	3	1
73	0	0	0	7	330	0	0	100	4	5	3	8	2	0	2	3	6	3	1
74	0	0	0	5	53	0	1	100	3	4	2	5	1	0	1	1	3	1	1
75	0	0	0	14	331	2	0	34	6	4	3	7	3	0	3	3	6	3	1
76	0	0	0	7	33	0	0	0	1	1	0	1	0	0	1	0	1	1	1
77	0	0	0	5	115	0	0	37	2	1	1	1	2	0	1	1	2	1	1
78	0	0	0	5	115	0	0	132	2	1	1	1	2	0	1	1	2	1	1
79	0	0	0	5	127	0	0	137	2	1	1	1	2	0	1	1	2	1	1
80	0	0	0	2	378	0	1	120	7	3	3	2	6	0	2	3	6	3	1

Beverages, Dairy, Eggs

Food No.	Food Description & Amount	wt gm	wt oz	cal	% cal fat	prot gm	carbo gm	fiber gm
81	Grapefruit juice, canned, with sugar [1 cup]	250	8.8	115	2%	1	28	0.3
82	Grapefruit juice, fresh [1 cup]	247	8.7	96	2%	1	23	0.2
83	Grapefruit juice, frozen, unsweetened (reconstituted with water) [1 cup]	247	8.7	101	3%	1	24	0.3
84	Grapefruit juice, frozen, with sugar (reconstituted with water) [1 cup]	248	8.7	118	3%	1	28	0.3
85	Grapefruit-orange juice, canned, unsweetened [1 cup]	247	8.7	106	2%	1	25	0.2
86	Grapefruit-orange juice, canned, with sugar [1 cup]	249	8.8	127	2%	1	31	0.2
87	Grapefruit-orange juice, fresh [1 cup]	247	8.7	104	3%	1	24	0.4
88	Grapefruit-orange juice, frozen, unsweetened (reconstituted with water) [1 cup]	247	8.7	106	2%	2	25	0.4
89	Guava drink [1 cup]	250	8.8	131	1%	0	33	2.0
90	Guava nectar [1 cup]	250	8.8	149	1%	0	38	2.0
91	Lemon juice, canned or bottled [1 Tbs]	15	0.5	3	12%	0	1	0.1
92	Lemon juice, fresh [1 Tbs]	15	0.5	4	0%	0	1	0.1
93	Lemon juice, frozen [1 Tbs]	15	0.5	3	13%	0	1	0.1
94	Lemon-limeade [1 cup]	248	8.7	133	1%	0	35	0.3
95	Lemonade with vitamin C added [1 cup]	248	8.7	131	1%	0	34	0.3
96	Lemonade, low calorie [1 cup]	240	8.5	43	0%	0	11	0.2
97	Lemonade-flavored drink, made from low-cal powdered mix, with vitamin C added (Include Sugar Free Country Time) [1 cup]	240	8.5	5	1%	0	1	0.0
98	Lemonade-flavored drink, made from sugar and powdered mix, with vitamin C added (Include Country Time) [1 cup]	250	8.8	90	0%	0	24	0.0
99	Lemonade [1 cup]	248	8.7	99	1%	0	26	0.2
100	Lemonade, frozen concentrate, not reconstituted [1 can (6 fl oz)]	219	7.7	396	1%	1	103	0.9
101	Lime juice, fresh or frozen [1 Tbs]	15	0.5	4	3%	0	1	0.1
102	Lime juice, canned or bottled [1 Tbs]	15	0.5	3	10%	0	1	0.1
103	Limeade [1 cup]	248	8.7	135	0%	0	36	0.3
104	Mango nectar [1 cup]	250	8.8	146	2%	1	38	1.8
105	Orange breakfast drink [1 cup]	250	8.8	110	0%	0	27	0.0
106	Orange breakfast drink, calcium fortified [1 cup]	252	8.9	136	0%	0	33	0.3
107	Orange breakfast drink, low calorie [1 cup]	250	8.8	15	0%	0	4	0.5
108	Orange breakfast drink, made from frozen concentrate (Include Orange Plus, Awake) [1 cup]	250	8.8	117	1%	0	29	0.1
109	Orange drink (Include orange ade, Yabba Dabba Dew, Sunny Delight) [1 cup]	249	8.8	115	0%	0	31	0.0
110	Orange drink and orangeade with vitamin C added [1 cup]	249	8.8	127	0%	0	32	0.2
111	Orange juice drink, vitamin-fortified [1 cup]	249	8.8	132	0%	0	33	0.0
112	**Orange juice, fresh** [1 cup]	248	8.7	112	4%	2	26	0.5
113	Orange juice, canned, unsweetened [1 cup]	249	8.8	105	3%	1	25	0.5
114	Orange juice, canned, with sugar [1 cup]	250	8.8	131	2%	1	31	0.5
115	Orange juice, canned, with calcium added, bottled or in a carton, unsweetened [1 cup]	248	8.7	111	1%	2	27	0.5
116	**Orange juice, frozen, unsweetened (reconstituted with water)** (Include reduced acid) [1 cup]	249	8.8	113	1%	2	27	0.6
117	Orange juice, frozen, unsweetened, with calcium added (reconstituted with water) [1 cup]	249	8.8	113	1%	2	27	0.6
118	Orange juice, frozen, unsweetened, not reconstituted [1 Tbs]	18	0.6	28	1%	0	7	0.1
119	Orange juice, frozen, with sugar (reconstituted with water) [1 cup]	250	8.8	126	1%	2	31	0.6
120	Orange juice, frozen, with sugar, not reconstituted [1 Tbs]	18	0.6	32	1%	0	8	0.1
121	Orange-apricot juice drink [1 cup]	249	8.8	127	2%	1	32	0.2
122	Orange-banana juice [1 cup]	250	8.8	142	3%	2	35	1.9
123	Orange-white grape-peach juice [1 cup]	248	8.7	117	2%	1	28	0.5
124	Orange-cranberry juice drink [1 cup]	249	8.8	118	1%	0	31	0.1
125	Orange-cranberry juice drink, low calorie, with vitamin C added [1 cup]	240	8.5	29	3%	0	7	0.4
126	Orange-lemon drink [1 cup]	249	8.8	125	0%	0	32	0.1
127	Orange-grape-banana juice drink [1 cup]	234	8.3	100	2%	1	25	0.5
128	Orange-mango juice drink [1 cup]	238	8.4	103	1%	0	27	0.1

Food no.	fat gm	sat fat gm	choles mg	sodium mg	potas mg	% of Daily Value													
						vit A	vit E	vit C	thia	ribo	niac	vit B-6	fola	vit B-12	calc	phos	mag	iron	zinc
81	0	0	0	5	405	0	1	112	7	3	4	3	7	0	2	3	6	5	1
82	0	0	0	2	400	0	1	156	7	3	2	5	6	0	2	4	7	3	1
83	0	0	0	7	334	0	1	138	7	3	3	5	2	0	2	3	7	2	1
84	0	0	0	7	329	0	1	136	7	3	3	5	2	0	2	3	7	2	1
85	0	0	0	7	390	3	1	120	9	4	4	3	9	0	2	3	6	6	1
86	0	0	0	7	384	3	1	118	9	4	4	3	9	0	2	3	6	6	1
87	0	0	0	2	447	3	1	181	11	4	4	5	13	0	2	4	7	3	1
88	0	0	0	7	405	1	1	150	10	3	3	5	15	0	2	4	7	2	1
89	0	0	0	7	104	3	2	111	1	1	2	3	1	0	1	1	1	1	1
90	0	0	0	7	93	2	2	78	1	1	2	2	1	0	1	1	1	1	1
91	0	0	0	3	16	0	0	6	0	0	0	0	0	0	0	0	0	0	0
92	0	0	0	0	19	0	0	12	0	0	0	0	0	0	0	0	0	0	0
93	0	0	0	0	14	0	0	8	1	0	0	0	0	0	0	0	0	0	0
94	0	0	0	7	45	0	0	18	1	2	0	0	1	0	1	1	1	2	1
95	0	0	0	8	48	1	0	21	1	4	0	1	2	0	1	1	1	3	1
96	0	0	0	7	38	0	0	27	2	1	0	0	2	0	1	0	1	2	0
97	0	0	0	7	0	0	0	10	0	0	0	0	0	0	5	2	1	1	0
98	0	0	0	13	23	0	0	19	0	0	0	0	1	0	5	2	1	1	1
99	0	0	0	8	37	1	0	16	1	3	0	1	1	0	1	0	1	2	1
100	0	0	0	9	147	2	0	65	4	12	1	3	5	0	2	2	3	9	1
101	0	0	0	0	17	0	0	8	0	0	0	0	0	0	0	0	0	0	0
102	0	0	0	2	12	0	0	2	0	0	0	0	0	0	0	0	0	0	0
103	0	0	0	5	43	0	0	14	0	0	0	0	1	0	1	0	1	0	1
104	0	0	0	6	141	29	5	32	3	3	3	6	2	0	1	1	3	1	1
105	0	0	0	160	103	10	0	54	20	1	1	1	5	0	1	1	2	1	1
106	0	0	0	136	209	10	0	101	20	1	1	3	12	0	25	2	3	1	1
107	0	0	0	138	45	11	0	53	21	0	0	0	1	0	1	0	1	0	1
108	0	0	0	23	323	0	0	258	19	80	2	5	17	0	19	7	4	1	1
109	0	0	0	7	44	0	0	14	1	1	0	1	1	0	1	0	1	1	1
110	0	0	0	40	45	0	0	142	1	0	0	1	1	0	1	0	1	4	1
111	0	0	0	5	105	1	0	62	63	63	62	62	2	62	0	1	2	2	0
112	0	0	0	2	496	5	1	207	15	4	5	5	19	0	3	4	7	3	1
113	0	0	0	5	436	4	1	143	10	4	4	11	11	0	2	3	7	6	1
114	0	0	0	5	425	4	1	139	10	4	4	11	11	0	2	3	7	6	1
115	0	0	0	2	471	2	2	161	13	3	3	5	27	0	30	4	6	1	1
116	0	0	0	7	479	2	1	163	13	3	3	6	28	0	3	4	6	1	1
117	0	0	0	7	478	2	1	163	13	3	3	5	28	0	30	4	6	1	1
118	0	0	0	1	120	0	0	41	3	1	1	1	7	0	1	1	2	0	0
119	0	0	0	7	474	2	1	162	13	3	3	6	27	0	3	4	6	1	1
120	0	0	0	1	109	0	0	37	3	1	1	1	6	0	1	1	1	0	0
121	0	0	0	5	199	14	0	83	3	1	2	3	4	0	1	2	2	1	1
122	0	0	0	3	604	2	2	131	12	6	4	22	24	0	2	4	9	2	1
123	0	0	0	30	409	7	1	14	8	6	3	6	4	0	3	3	6	6	1
124	0	0	0	6	95	1	0	30	2	1	1	3	2	0	1	1	2	1	1
125	0	0	0	35	110	1	0	115	3	1	1	3	3	0	1	1	2	2	1
126	0	0	0	8	41	0	0	13	1	1	0	1	1	0	1	0	1	1	1
127	0	0	0	6	226	1	0	41	4	3	2	8	4	0	1	2	4	3	1
128	0	0	0	7	74	4	1	19	2	1	1	2	2	0	1	1	2	1	1

Beverages, Dairy, Eggs

Food No.	Food Description & Amount	wt gm	wt oz	cal	% cal fat	prot gm	carbo gm	fiber gm
129	Orange-peach juice drink [1 cup]	240	8.5	122	2%	1	30	0.2
130	Orange-raspberry juice drink [1 cup]	249	8.8	107	1%	0	28	0.1
131	Papaya juice/drink [1 cup]	248	8.7	141	2%	0	36	1.5
132	Papaya juice/nectar [1 cup]	249	8.8	134	0%	1	35	1.5
133	Papaya nectar [1 cup]	250	8.8	143	2%	0	36	1.5
134	Passion fruit juice (Include yellow, Lilikoi) [1 cup]	247	8.7	137	2%	1	35	0.5
135	Passion fruit nectar [1 cup]	250	8.8	167	0%	0	44	0.2
136	Pear nectar [1 cup]	250	8.8	150	0%	0	39	1.5
137	Pear-white grape-passion fruit juice, with added vitamin C [1 cup]	246	8.7	149	1%	1	38	0.8
138	Pina Colada mix, nonalcoholic [1 fl oz]	30	1.1	32	16%	0	7	0.1
139	Pineapple juice, unsweetened [1 cup]	250	8.8	140	1%	1	34	0.5
140	Pineapple juice, unsweetened, with added Vitamin C [1 cup]	250	8.8	140	1%	1	34	0.5
141	Pineapple juice, with sugar [1 cup]	252	8.9	158	1%	1	39	0.5
142	Pineapple-apple-guava juice, with added vitamin C [1 cup]	244	8.6	120	1%	1	30	0.7
143	Pineapple-grapefruit juice drink with vitamin C added [1 cup]	250	8.8	118	2%	1	29	0.3
144	Pineapple-grapefruit juice, canned, unsweetened [1 cup]	250	8.8	118	2%	1	28	0.4
145	Pineapple-grapefruit juice, canned, with sugar [1 cup]	250	8.8	134	1%	1	33	0.4
146	Pineapple-grapefruit juice, frozen (reconstituted with water) [1 cup]	250	8.8	116	2%	1	28	0.4
147	Pineapple-orange juice drink with vitamin C added [1 cup]	250	8.8	125	0%	3	30	0.3
148	Pineapple-orange juice, canned, unsweetened [1 cup]	250	8.8	123	2%	1	30	0.5
149	Pineapple-orange juice, canned, with sugar [1 cup]	250	8.8	139	2%	1	34	0.5
150	Pineapple-orange juice, frozen (reconstituted with water) [1 cup]	250	8.8	121	1%	1	30	0.5
151	Pineapple-orange-banana juice [1 cup]	250	8.8	127	1%	1	31	0.8
152	Pineapple juice-non-citrus juice blend, unsweetened, with added vitamin C [1 cup]	249	8.8	132	1%	1	33	0.9
153	Pineapple-orange-grapefruit juice drink with vitamin C added [1 cup]	251	8.9	122	1%	2	29	0.3
154	Prune juice, unsweetened [1 cup]	256	9.0	182	0%	2	45	2.6
155	Prune juice, with sugar [1 cup]	258	9.1	199	0%	2	49	2.5
156	Raspberry-flavored drink [1 fl oz]	28	1.0	14	0%	0	4	0.0
157	Soursop (Guanabana) nectar [1 cup]	250	8.8	160	1%	0	41	1.2
158	Strawberry juice [1 cup]	237	8.4	71	12%	1	17	0.2
159	Strawberry-banana-orange juice [1 cup]	234	8.3	126	5%	1	29	2.6
160	Strawberry-flavored drink [1 cup]	250	8.8	126	0%	0	32	0.0
161	Strawberry-flavored drink with vitamin C added [1 cup]	250	8.8	88	0%	0	22	0.0
162	Tamarind drink, Puerto Rican (Refresco de tamarindo) [1 cup]	250	8.8	267	1%	2	69	2.9
163	Tang, dry concentrate [1 Tbs]	14	0.5	52	0%	0	13	0.0
164	Tangerine juice, canned, unsweetened [1 cup]	247	8.7	106	4%	1	25	0.5
165	Tangerine juice, canned, with sugar [1 cup]	249	8.8	125	4%	1	30	0.5
166	Tangerine juice, frozen, unsweetened (reconstituted with water) [1 cup]	248	8.7	107	4%	1	25	0.5
167	Tomato juice [1 cup]	243	8.6	41	3%	2	10	1.0
168	Tomato juice, low sodium [1 cup]	243	8.6	41	3%	2	10	1.9
169	Tomato juice cocktail [1 cup]	243	8.6	46	4%	2	11	1.9
170	Tomato and vegetable juice, mostly tomato (Include V-8) [1 cup]	242	8.5	46	4%	2	11	1.9
171	Tomato and vegetable juice, mostly tomato, low sodium [1 cup]	242	8.5	46	5%	1	11	1.9
172	Tomato juice with clam or beef juice [1 cup]	242	8.5	35	6%	2	8	0.7
173	Vegetable juice, mixed (vegetables other than tomato) [1 cup]	246	8.7	70	8%	4	15	4.4
174	Watermelon juice [1 cup]	238	8.4	76	12%	1	17	1.2
	Soft Drinks and Miscellaneous Drinks							
200	Ale-type soft drink (Include Ale-8) [1 can (12 fl oz)]	360	12.7	216	2%	1	48	0.0
201	Atole (corn meal beverage) [1 cup]	249	8.8	210	17%	4	41	0.8
202	Carbonated citrus juice drink (75% juice) [1 can (12 fl oz)]	372	13.1	110	3%	2	26	0.4
203	Carbonated noncitrus juice drink (70% juice) [1 can (12 fl oz)]	372	13.1	141	2%	1	35	0.3
204	Carbonated water, sweetened (Include tonic, quinine water) [1 can (12 fl oz)]	366	12.9	124	0%	0	32	0.0

Food no.	fat gm	sat fat gm	choles mg	sodium mg	potas mg	vit A	vit E	vit C	thia	ribo	niac	vit B-6	fola	vit B-12	calc	phos	mag	iron	zinc
						% of Daily Value													
129	0	0	0	5	192	14	0	80	3	1	2	3	3	0	1	2	2	1	1
130	0	0	0	6	78	1	0	39	2	2	1	3	2	0	1	1	2	1	1
131	0	0	0	12	77	3	0	12	1	1	2	1	1	0	2	0	2	5	2
132	0	0	0	17	100	6	0	22	0	2	4	1	1	0	1	1	2	3	1
133	0	0	0	13	78	3	0	13	1	1	2	1	1	0	3	0	2	5	3
134	0	0	0	15	687	39	1	99	0	17	23	7	5	0	1	5	10	4	1
135	0	0	0	10	279	7	0	50	0	8	7	3	2	0	1	1	5	2	1
136	0	0	0	10	33	0	1	5	0	2	2	2	1	0	1	1	2	4	1
137	0	0	0	9	201	3	1	133	2	4	4	5	1	0	2	2	4	3	1
138	1	0	0	2	21	0	0	2	1	0	0	1	1	0	0	0	1	0	0
139	0	0	0	3	335	0	0	45	9	3	3	12	14	0	4	2	8	4	2
140	0	0	0	3	335	0	0	100	9	3	3	12	14	0	4	2	8	4	2
141	0	0	0	3	331	0	0	44	9	3	3	12	14	0	4	2	8	4	2
142	0	0	0	5	337	3	0	134	7	3	3	7	4	0	2	2	4	4	1
143	0	0	0	35	153	1	0	192	5	2	3	5	7	0	2	2	4	4	1
144	0	0	0	3	359	0	0	83	8	3	3	7	10	0	3	2	7	3	2
145	0	0	0	3	352	0	0	81	8	3	3	7	10	0	3	2	7	3	2
146	0	0	0	8	339	0	0	95	9	3	3	7	4	0	3	3	7	3	2
147	0	0	0	8	115	13	0	94	5	3	3	6	7	0	1	1	4	4	1
148	0	0	0	4	386	2	1	94	10	4	4	12	13	0	3	3	8	5	2
149	0	0	0	4	379	2	1	92	9	4	4	11	13	0	3	3	7	5	1
150	0	0	0	8	410	1	1	107	12	3	3	7	17	0	3	3	7	3	2
151	0	0	0	3	433	1	1	100	12	3	3	11	16	0	2	3	7	3	1
152	0	0	0	3	361	3	0	147	11	3	3	11	7	0	3	2	6	4	2
153	0	0	0	21	134	7	0	143	5	3	3	6	7	0	2	1	4	4	1
154	0	0	0	10	707	0	0	17	3	11	10	28	0	0	3	6	9	17	4
155	0	0	0	10	698	0	0	17	3	10	10	28	0	0	3	6	9	17	4
156	0	0	0	1	0	0	0	0	0	0	0	0	0	0	0	0	0	0	0
157	0	0	0	11	95	0	1	9	1	1	2	1	1	0	1	1	2	1	1
158	1	0	0	2	393	0	2	112	3	8	2	6	5	0	3	5	6	5	2
159	1	0	0	33	517	0	1	34	19	10	4	20	9	0	3	4	9	7	2
160	0	0	0	7	1	0	0	0	0	0	0	0	0	0	0	0	1	0	1
161	0	0	0	34	1	0	0	47	0	0	0	0	0	0	4	5	1	1	1
162	0	0	0	21	360	0	2	3	16	5	6	2	2	0	5	7	14	9	1
163	0	0	0	2	23	25	0	93	0	1	0	0	16	0	3	2	0	0	0
164	0	0	0	2	440	10	1	121	9	3	1	5	3	0	4	3	5	3	0
165	0	0	0	2	443	10	1	91	10	3	1	4	3	0	4	3	5	3	0
166	0	0	0	2	441	10	1	122	9	3	1	5	2	0	4	3	5	3	0
167	0	0	0	877	535	14	10	74	8	4	8	13	12	0	2	5	7	8	2
168	0	0	0	24	535	14	10	74	8	4	8	13	12	0	2	5	7	8	2
169	0	0	0	656	469	28	4	112	7	4	9	17	13	0	3	4	7	6	3
170	0	0	0	653	467	28	4	112	7	4	9	17	13	0	3	4	7	6	3
171	0	0	0	169	467	28	4	112	6	4	9	17	13	0	3	4	7	6	3
172	0	0	0	852	432	10	8	55	6	4	8	10	9	1	2	4	5	6	2
173	1	0	0	132	794	199	6	108	11	10	6	15	32	0	14	10	14	20	6
174	1	0	0	5	276	9	2	38	13	3	2	17	1	0	2	2	7	2	1
200	0	0	0	47	29	0	0	3	4	10	20	5	13	1	2	8	6	1	0
201	4	2	15	56	188	3	1	2	9	14	4	3	2	6	14	12	6	4	4
202	0	0	0	24	453	3	1	146	9	4	4	7	10	0	3	3	7	5	2
203	0	0	0	31	329	0	0	2	4	4	2	6	1	0	3	2	5	4	1
204	0	0	0	15	0	0	0	0	0	0	0	0	0	0	0	0	0	0	2

Beverages, Dairy, Eggs

Food No.	Food Description & Amount	wt gm	wt oz	cal	% cal fat	prot gm	carbo gm	fiber gm
205	Carbonated water, unsweetened (Include flavored; club soda, Perrier, seltzer water) [1 can (12 fl oz)]	355	12.5	0	0%	0	0	0.0
206	Chocolate-flavored soda [1 can (12 fl oz)]	369	13.0	155	0%	0	39	0.0
207	Chocolate-flavored soda, sugar-free or sweetened with low-cal sweetener (Include Canfield's Diet Chocolate Fudge Soda) [1 can (12 fl oz)]	355	12.5	4	0%	0	0	0.0
208	**Cola-type soft drink**, plain or flavored, with or without caffeine [1 can (12 fl oz)]	369	13.0	151	0%	0	38	0.0
209	**Cola-type soft drink, sugar-free**, with or without caffeine [1 can (12 fl oz)]	355	12.5	4	0%	0	0	0.0
210	Corn beverage with chocolate and milk (Champurrado, Atole de Chocolate) [1 cup (8 fl oz)]	254	9.0	283	26%	5	51	1.9
211	Cream soda (Include Almond Smash) [1 can (12 fl oz)]	371	13.1	189	0%	0	49	0.0
212	Cream soda, sugar-free [1 can (12 fl oz)]	355	12.5	0	0%	0	0	0.0
213	**Fruit-flavored soft drink** (Include orange, lemon, lime, cherry, grape, strawberry, Tom Collins mixer, 7-Up, Sprite, Mellow Yellow, Mountain Dew, Big Red, 7-Up Gold) [1 can (12 fl oz)]	372	13.1	149	0%	0	39	0.0
214	**Fruit-flavored soft drink, sugar-free** (Include Diet Mountain Dew, Diet 7-Up Gold) [1 can (12 fl oz)]	355	12.5	0	0%	0	0	0.0
215	Ginger ale [1 can (12 fl oz)]	366	12.9	124	0%	0	32	0.0
216	Ginger ale, sugar-free [1 can (12 fl oz)]	355	12.5	0	0%	0	0	0.0
217	Guava juice drink with vitamin C added (Include Ocean Spray Mauna Lai, Guava Passion Fruit Drink) [1 cup]	253	8.9	132	1%	0	34	2.0
218	Horchata, Puerto Rican (made with almonds, sesame seeds, sugar, water) [1 cup]	240	8.5	246	46%	5	32	2.1
219	Mavi drink [1 can (12 fl oz)]	369	13.0	140	0%	0	38	0.0
220	Oatmeal beverage, Puerto Rican [1 cup]	240	8.5	104	2%	1	25	0.5
221	Oatmeal beverage with milk (Atole de avena) [1 cup]	255	9.0	209	18%	5	40	0.7
222	Rice beverage, Mexican (Horchata) [1 cup]	240	8.5	98	0%	0	25	0.3
223	**Root beer** [1 can (12 fl oz)]	369	13.0	151	0%	0	39	0.0
224	Root beer, noncarbonated, made from powdered mix, with sugar [1 cup]	240	8.5	84	0%	0	22	0.0
225	Root beer, sugar-free [1 can (12 fl oz)]	355	12.5	0	0%	0	0	0.0
226	Sugar cane beverage, Puerto Rican [1 cup]	247	8.7	169	0%	0	44	0.0
227	Tonic water, sugar-free [1 can (12 fl oz)]	355	12.5	0	0%	0	0	0.0
228	Whiskey sour mix, nonalcoholic (Include Lemix) [1 fl oz]	31	1.1	26	1%	0	7	0.0
	Coffee and Tea							
280	Bean beverage [1 cup]	230	8.1	81	0%	6	14	0.0
281	Cappuccino [¾ cup]	196	6.9	64	47%	3	5	0.2
282	Cappuccino, decaffeinated [¾ cup]	180	6.3	59	47%	3	5	0.2
283	Cereal beverage (Include Pero, Break Away, Kafix) [¾ cup]	180	6.3	9	8%	0	2	0.2
284	Cereal beverage with beet roots, powdered instant, dry (Include Kafix) [1 tsp, dry]	1	0.0	4	8%	0	1	0.1
285	Chicory [¾ cup]	180	6.3	4	2%	0	1	0.0
286	Coffee and chicory, dry powder [1 tsp, dry]	1	0.0	2	2%	0	0	0.0
287	Coffee and chicory, made from ground [¾ cup]	180	6.3	4	0%	0	1	0.0
288	Coffee and chicory, made from powdered instant (Include Luzianne) [¾ cup]	180	6.3	4	2%	0	1	0.0
289	Coffee and cocoa (mocha) mix, dry powder with whitener and low-cal sweetener (Include Sugar Free Irish Mocha Mint and Suisse Mocha) [1 tsp, dry]	6	0.2	28	60%	1	3	0.1
290	Coffee and cocoa (mocha) mix, dry powder, with whitener and low-cal sweetener, decaffeinated [1 tsp, dry]	2	0.1	8	60%	0	1	0.0
291	Coffee and cocoa (mocha) mix, dry powder with whitener, presweetened (Include Irish Mocha Mint, Suisse Mocha) [1 tsp, dry]	6	0.2	26	33%	0	4	0.1
292	Coffee and cocoa (mocha), made from powdered mix, with whitener and low-cal sweetener (Include Sugar Free Irish Mocha Mint, Suisse Mocha) [¾ cup]	180	6.3	27	60%	1	3	0.1
293	Coffee and cocoa (mocha), made from powdered mix, with whitener, presweetened (Irish Mocha Mint, Suisse Mocha) [¾ cup]	180	6.3	48	33%	0	8	0.1
294	Coffee and cocoa (mocha), made from powdered mix, with whitener and low-cal sweetener, decaffeinated [¾ cup]	179	6.3	27	60%	1	3	0.1
295	**Coffee, made from ground**, regular (Include flavored) [¾ cup]	180	6.3	4	0%	0	1	0.0

Food no.	fat gm	sat fat gm	choles mg	sodium mg	potas mg	% of Daily Value													
						vit A	vit E	vit C	thia	ribo	niac	vit B-6	fola	vit B-12	calc	phos	mag	iron	zinc
205	0	0	0	75	7	0	0	0	0	0	0	0	0	0	2	0	1	0	2
206	0	0	0	325	185	0	0	0	0	0	0	0	0	0	1	0	1	2	4
207	0	0	0	21	0	0	0	0	1	5	0	0	0	0	1	3	1	1	2
208	0	0	0	15	4	0	0	0	0	0	0	0	0	0	1	4	1	1	0
209	0	0	0	21	0	0	0	0	1	5	0	0	0	0	1	3	1	1	2
210	8	4	15	61	256	4	2	2	10	16	5	4	2	5	16	16	12	7	6
211	0	0	0	45	4	0	0	0	0	0	0	0	0	0	2	0	1	1	2
212	0	0	0	57	7	0	0	0	0	0	0	0	0	0	1	4	1	1	1
213	0	0	0	41	4	0	0	0	0	0	0	0	0	0	1	0	1	1	1
214	0	0	0	57	7	0	0	0	0	0	0	0	0	0	1	4	1	1	1
215	0	0	0	26	4	0	0	0	0	0	0	0	0	0	1	0	1	4	1
216	0	0	0	57	7	0	0	0	0	0	0	0	0	0	1	4	1	1	1
217	0	0	0	7	105	3	2	142	1	1	2	3	1	0	1	1	1	1	1
218	13	1	0	8	158	0	15	0	7	8	5	5	4	0	13	14	20	11	9
219	0	0	0	10	0	0	0	0	0	0	0	0	0	0	1	0	1	0	1
220	0	0	0	7	16	0	0	0	2	1	0	0	0	0	1	2	2	1	1
221	4	2	15	58	189	3	1	2	5	11	1	3	2	6	14	13	6	2	4
222	0	0	0	7	6	0	0	0	1	0	1	0	0	0	1	0	1	2	1
223	0	0	0	48	4	0	0	0	0	0	0	0	0	0	2	0	1	1	2
224	0	0	0	33	1	0	0	45	0	0	0	0	0	0	4	5	1	1	1
225	0	0	0	57	7	0	0	0	0	0	0	0	0	0	1	4	1	1	1
226	0	0	0	43	40	0	0	0	6	2	0	0	0	0	1	1	2	13	1
227	0	0	0	57	7	0	0	0	0	0	0	0	0	0	1	4	1	1	1
228	0	0	0	32	9	0	0	1	0	0	0	0	0	0	0	0	0	0	0
280	0	0	0	5	775	0	0	0	23	14	7	12	35	0	4	21	28	16	6
281	3	2	14	51	204	3	0	1	2	9	2	2	1	5	12	9	5	1	3
282	3	2	12	47	187	3	0	1	2	9	1	2	1	4	11	9	4	1	2
283	0	0	0	7	42	0	0	0	1	0	2	1	0	0	0	1	2	1	0
284	0	0	0	1	18	0	0	0	0	0	1	0	0	0	0	1	1	0	0
285	0	0	0	6	61	0	0	0	0	0	2	0	0	0	1	1	2	1	0
286	0	0	0	0	35	0	0	0	0	0	1	0	0	0	0	0	1	0	0
287	0	0	0	4	97	0	0	0	0	0	2	0	0	0	0	0	2	1	0
288	0	0	0	6	58	0	0	0	0	0	2	0	0	0	1	0	2	1	0
289	2	2	0	19	111	0	0	0	0	4	1	0	0	0	1	3	2	1	1
290	1	0	0	5	32	0	0	0	0	1	0	0	0	0	0	1	1	0	0
291	1	1	0	16	62	0	0	0	0	0	1	0	0	0	0	2	1	1	0
292	2	1	0	23	106	0	0	0	0	3	1	0	0	0	1	3	2	1	1
293	2	2	0	34	113	0	0	0	0	0	1	0	0	0	1	3	2	1	1
294	2	1	0	23	105	0	0	0	0	3	1	0	0	0	1	3	2	1	1
295	0	0	0	4	97	0	0	0	0	0	2	0	0	0	0	0	2	1	0

Beverages, Dairy, Eggs

Food No.	Food Description & Amount	wt gm	wt oz	cal	% cal fat	prot gm	carbo gm	fiber gm
296	Coffee, made from liquid concentrate [1/8 cup]	30	1.1	0	2%	0	0	0.0
297	Coffee, made from powdered mix, with whitener and low calorie sweetener, instant (Include Sugar Free Cafe au Lait, French Style Coffee, Orange Cappuccino, Cafe Amaretto, and Viennese Coffee mixes) [¾ cup]	180	6.3	57	60%	1	6	0.3
298	Coffee, made from powdered mix, with whitener and sugar, instant (Include Cafe au Lait, French Style Coffee, Orange Cappuccino, Cafe Amaretto, and Viennese coffee mixes) [¾ cup]	180	6.3	57	43%	0	8	0.0
299	Coffee, made from powdered (Include decaffeinated, acid neutralized) [¾ cup]	180	6.3	4	2%	0	1	0.0
300	Coffee, Cuban (Include sweetened expresso) [1/8 cup]	30	1.1	9	0%	0	2	0.0
301	Coffee, dry powder, regular or decaffeinated (Include Kava) [1 tsp, dry]	1	0.0	2	2%	0	0	0.0
302	Coffee, dry powder, with whitener and low-cal sweetener (Include Sugar Free Cafe au Lait, French Style Coffee, Orange Cappuccino, Cafe Amaretto, and Viennese Coffee Mixes) [1 tsp, dry]	5	0.2	22	60%	0	2	0.0
303	Coffee, dry powder, with whitener and sugar (Include Cafe au Lait, French Style Coffee, Orange Cappuccino, Cafe Amaretto, and Viennese Coffee Mixes) [1 tsp, dry]	5	0.2	23	43%	0	3	0.0
304	Coffee, expresso (Include demi-tasse) [¼ cup]	60	2.1	1	0%	0	0	0.0
305	Coffee, latte [¾ cup]	181	6.4	73	48%	4	6	0.0
306	Coffee, liquid concentrate [1 tsp]	5	0.2	2	2%	0	0	0.0
307	Coffee, Mexican, unsweetened (no milk; not cafe con leche) [¾ cup]	177	6.2	4	0%	0	1	0.0
308	Coffee, Mexican, sweetened (no milk; not cafe con leche) [¾ cup]	182	6.4	52	0%	0	13	0.0
309	Coffee, pre-lightened, no sugar (Include from vending machine) [¾ cup]	180	6.3	27	50%	0	3	0.0
310	Coffee, presweetened with sugar (Include from vending machine) [¾ cup]	180	6.3	29	0%	0	7	0.0
311	Coffee, presweetened with sugar, pre-lightened (Include coffee, light, with sugar, from vending machine) [¾ cup]	180	6.3	51	26%	0	9	0.0
312	Coffee, turkish (Include Mexican coffee) [½ cup]	120	4.2	47	0%	0	12	0.0
313	Coffee, with cereal, regular or decaffeinated (Include with barley) [¾ cup]	180	6.3	4	2%	0	1	0.0
314	Corn beverage [1/8 cup]	30	1.1	9	0%	0	3	0.0
315	Mate, sweetened beverage made from dried green leaves (Include Paraguay tea) [1 fl oz]	31	1.1	6	0%	0	2	0.0
316	Postum [¾ cup]	180	6.3	9	0%	0	2	0.0
317	Postum, dry powder [1 tsp, dry]	1	0.0	4	8%	0	1	0.1
318	Rice beverage (Include rice tea) [1/8 cup]	31	1.1	18	13%	0	4	0.3
319	Tea, camomile [¾ cup]	180	6.3	2	0%	0	0	0.0
320	Tea, herb [¾ cup]	180	6.3	2	0%	0	0	0.0
321	Tea, leaf, presweetened with low-cal sweetener (Include flavored) [¾ cup]	184	6.5	5	0%	0	1	0.0
322	Tea, leaf, presweetened with sugar (Include flavored) [¾ cup]	184	6.5	37	0%	0	10	0.0
323	Tea, leaf, regular or decaffeinated (Include tea bags, green tea, black tea, spiced and flavored teas) [¾ cup]	180	6.3	2	0%	0	1	0.0
324	Tea, made from caraway seeds [¾ cup]	180	6.3	2	0%	0	0	0.0
325	Tea, made from frozen concentrate (Include flavored) [¾ cup]	180	6.3	2	0%	0	1	0.0
326	Tea, made from frozen concentrate, presweetened with low calorie sweetener (Include flavored) [¾ cup]	184	6.5	5	0%	0	1	0.0
327	Tea, made from powdered instant (Include flavored) [¾ cup]	180	6.3	3	1%	0	1	0.0
328	Tea, made from powdered instant, presweetened with low-cal sweetener (Include flavored; Lipton Fruit Tea; Crystal Light Fruit Tea) [¾ cup]	184	6.5	4	0%	0	1	0.0
329	Tea, made from powdered instant, presweetened with sugar (Include flavored) [¾ cup]	184	6.5	18	0%	0	5	0.0
330	Tea, powdered instant, sweetened, dry [1 tsp, dry]	1	0.0	4	0%	0	1	0.0
331	Tea, powdered instant, unsweetened, dry (Include lemon- or other fruit-flavored) [1 tsp, dry]	1	0.0	3	1%	0	1	0.0
332	Tea, Russian (made with sugar, orange drink mix, powdered tea, cloves, cinnamon) [¾ cup]	184	6.5	107	0%	0	27	0.1

Food no.	fat gm	sat fat gm	choles mg	sodium mg	potas mg	% of Daily Value													
						vit A	vit E	vit C	thia	ribo	niac	vit B-6	fola	vit B-12	calc	phos	mag	iron	zinc
296	0	0	0	1	6	0	0	0	0	0	0	0	0	0	0	0	0	0	0
297	4	3	0	43	224	0	0	0	0	8	3	0	0	0	1	5	4	2	2
298	3	2	0	60	122	0	0	0	0	0	2	0	0	0	1	3	2	1	0
299	0	0	0	6	58	0	0	0	0	0	2	0	0	0	1	0	2	1	0
300	0	0	0	1	22	0	0	0	0	0	0	0	0	0	0	0	1	0	0
301	0	0	0	0	35	0	0	0	0	0	1	0	0	0	0	0	1	0	0
302	1	1	0	41	50	0	0	0	0	0	1	0	0	0	0	1	1	0	0
303	1	1	0	23	50	0	0	0	0	0	1	0	0	0	0	1	1	0	0
304	0	0	0	1	32	0	0	0	0	0	1	0	0	0	0	0	1	0	0
305	4	2	16	58	211	4	1	2	3	11	1	2	1	6	14	11	5	1	3
306	0	0	0	0	35	0	0	0	0	0	1	0	0	0	0	0	1	0	0
307	0	0	0	4	96	0	0	0	0	0	2	0	0	0	0	0	2	0	0
308	0	0	0	8	136	0	0	0	0	0	2	0	0	0	1	0	3	2	0
309	1	1	0	13	91	0	0	0	0	0	2	0	0	0	1	2	2	1	1
310	0	0	0	6	56	0	0	0	0	0	2	0	0	0	1	0	2	1	0
311	1	1	0	13	88	0	0	0	0	1	2	0	0	0	1	2	2	1	1
312	0	0	0	2	59	0	0	0	0	0	1	0	0	0	0	0	1	0	0
313	0	0	0	6	58	0	0	0	0	0	2	0	0	0	1	0	2	1	0
314	0	0	0	42	25	0	0	2	0	1	1	0	2	0	0	1	1	0	1
315	0	0	0	1	11	0	0	0	0	0	0	0	0	0	0	0	0	0	0
316	0	0	0	7	43	0	0	0	1	0	2	1	0	0	1	1	2	1	0
317	0	0	0	1	18	0	0	0	0	0	1	0	0	0	0	1	1	0	0
318	0	0	0	11	6	0	1	0	1	0	1	1	0	0	0	1	2	0	1
319	0	0	0	2	16	0	1	0	1	0	0	0	0	0	0	0	0	1	0
320	0	0	0	2	16	0	0	0	1	0	0	0	0	0	0	0	0	1	0
321	0	0	0	6	68	0	0	0	0	2	0	0	2	0	0	0	1	0	0
322	0	0	0	5	65	0	0	0	0	2	0	0	2	0	0	0	1	0	0
323	0	0	0	5	67	0	0	0	0	1	0	0	2	0	0	0	1	0	0
324	0	0	0	2	16	0	0	0	1	0	0	0	0	0	0	0	0	1	0
325	0	0	0	5	67	0	0	0	0	1	0	0	2	0	0	0	1	0	0
326	0	0	0	6	68	0	0	0	0	2	0	0	2	0	0	0	1	0	0
327	0	0	0	11	37	0	0	0	0	1	0	0	0	0	0	0	1	0	0
328	0	0	0	18	31	0	0	0	0	1	0	0	1	0	0	0	1	1	0
329	0	0	0	6	47	0	0	0	0	0	0	0	0	0	0	0	1	0	1
330	0	0	0	0	10	0	0	0	0	0	0	0	0	0	0	0	0	0	0
331	0	0	0	1	66	0	0	0	0	0	1	0	0	0	0	0	1	0	0
332	0	0	0	7	50	20	0	72	0	1	0	0	13	0	3	2	1	1	0

Beverages, Dairy, Eggs

Food No.	Food Description & Amount	wt gm	wt oz	cal	% cal fat	prot gm	carbo gm	fiber gm
	Alcoholic Beverages							
380	Alexander [1 cocktail] (18 gm alcohol)	74	2.6	176	9%	0	8	0.0
381	Bacardi cocktail [1 cocktail] (14 gm alcohol)	63	2.2	117	0%	0	6	0.1
382	Beer (Include ale) [1 can or bottle (12 fl oz)] (13 gm alcohol)	360	12.7	148	0%	1	13	0.7
383	Beer, lite [1 can or bottle (12 fl oz)] (12 gm alcohol)	360	12.7	101	0%	1	5	0.0
384	Black Russian [1 cocktail] (26 gm alcohol)	90	3.2	244	0%	0	16	0.0
385	Bloody Mary [1 cocktail] (15 gm alcohol)	148	5.2	123	1%	1	5	0.4
386	Bourbon and soda (Include scotch and soda, rum and soda) [1 cocktail] (15 gm alcohol)	116	4.1	105	0%	0	0	0.0
387	Brandy (Include applejack, cognac, tequila) [1 fl oz] (9 gm alcohol)	28	1.0	65	0%	0	0	0.0
388	Champagne punch [4 fl oz] (10 gm alcohol)	116	4.1	100	0%	0	7	0.0
389	Coquito, Puerto Rican (coconut, rum) [4 fl oz] (13 gm alcohol)	125	4.4	301	27%	5	20	0.3
390	Cordial or liqueur (Incl. amaretto, anisette, benedictine, chartreuse, cointreau, creme de menthe, curacao, drambuie, grenadine, kahlua, kirsh, kummel, sloe gin, tia maria, triple sec) [1 fl oz] (8 gm alcohol)	30	1.1	106	1%	0	13	0.0
391	Daiquiri [1 cocktail] (14 gm alcohol)	61	2.2	113	0%	0	4	0.1
392	Frozen daiquiri [1 drink] (21 gm alcohol)	231	8.1	430	0%	0	16	0.0
393	Fuzzy Navel (peach schnapps and orange juice) [1 cocktail] (14 gm alcohol)	213	7.5	254	1%	1	38	0.3
394	Gibson [1 cocktail] (23 gm alcohol)	71	2.5	158	0%	0	0	0.0
395	Gimlet [1 cocktail] (19 gm alcohol)	71	2.5	132	0%	0	1	0.1
396	Gin and Tonic [1 cocktail] (16 gm alcohol)	225	7.9	171	0%	0	16	0.1
397	Gin fizz [1 cocktail] (17 gm alcohol)	225	7.9	139	0%	0	6	0.1
398	Gin Rickey [1 cocktail] (16 gm alcohol)	205	7.2	114	0%	0	1	0.1
399	Gin [1 jigger] (16 gm alcohol)	42	1.5	110	0%	0	0	0.0
400	Glug (Include glogg, gluhwein) [1 drink (4 fl oz)] (10 gm alcohol)	116	4.1	113	0%	0	11	0.0
401	Gold Cadillac [1 cocktail] (25 gm alcohol)	125	4.4	377	9%	1	44	0.0
402	Grain alcohol [1 fl oz (no ice)] (26 gm alcohol)	28	1.0	179	0%	0	0	0.0
403	Grasshopper [1 cocktail] (10 gm alcohol)	64	2.3	164	20%	1	15	0.0
404	High ball [1 cocktail] (15 gm alcohol)	160	5.6	105	0%	0	0	0.0
405	Irish Coffee (Include Coffee Royale) [1 fl oz] (2 gm alcohol)	26	0.9	26	45%	0	1	0.0
406	Long Island iced tea [1 drink (5 fl oz)] (15 gm alcohol)	150	5.3	142	0%	0	11	0.1
407	Mai Tai [1 cocktail] (27 gm alcohol)	126	4.4	305	0%	0	29	0.1
408	Manhattan [1 cocktail] (17 gm alcohol)	57	2.0	128	0%	0	2	0.0
409	Margarita [1 cocktail] (18 gm alcohol)	77	2.7	170	0%	0	11	0.1
410	Martini [1 cocktail] (23 gm alcohol)	71	2.5	158	0%	0	0	0.0
411	Mexican eggnog, alcoholic (Rompope) [1 fl oz]	30	1.1	51	29%	1	5	0.0
412	Mint julep [1 cocktail] (20 gm alcohol)	65	2.3	156	0%	0	4	0.0
413	Nonalcoholic malt beverage [1 can or bottle (12 fl oz)] (1 gm alcohol)	360	12.7	216	2%	1	48	0.0
414	Old fashioned [1 cocktail] (20 gm alcohol)	60	2.1	156	0%	0	4	0.0
415	Pina Colada [1 cocktail] (13 gm alcohol)	133	4.7	231	10%	1	30	0.4
416	Rum and cola [1 cocktail] (14 gm alcohol)	211	7.4	159	0%	0	16	0.1
417	Rum [1 jigger] (14 gm alcohol)	42	1.5	97	0%	0	0	0.0
418	Rum, hot buttered [1 drink] (28 gm alcohol)	251	8.9	315	34%	0	4	0.2
419	Rum cooler [1 bottle (12.6 fl oz)] (13 gm alcohol)	390	13.8	217	2%	1	33	0.3
420	Sangria [1 drink] (11 gm alcohol)	228	8.0	156	0%	0	21	0.1
421	Sangria, Puerto Rican style [1 drink] (10 gm alcohol)	180	6.3	120	0%	0	16	0.1
422	Screwdriver (Include Harvey Wallbanger, Slo-Screw) [1 cocktail] (15 gm alcohol)	213	7.5	182	1%	1	18	0.3
423	Singapore Sling [1 cocktail] (26 gm alcohol)	225	7.9	229	0%	0	12	0.1
424	Sloe gin fizz [1 cocktail] (16 gm alcohol)	222	7.8	122	0%	0	3	0.1
425	Stinger [1 cocktail] (29 gm alcohol)	92	3.2	283	0%	0	21	0.0
426	Tequila Sunrise [1 cocktail] (19 gm alcohol)	172	6.1	189	1%	1	15	0.2
427	Tom Collins (Include Vodka Collins) [1 cocktail] (16 gm alcohol)	222	7.8	122	0%	0	3	0.1
428	Vodka [1 jigger] (14 gm alcohol)	42	1.5	97	0%	0	0	0.0

										% of Daily Value									
Food no.	fat gm	sat fat gm	choles mg	sodium mg	potas mg	vit A	vit E	vit C	thia	ribo	niac	vit B-6	fola	vit B-12	calc	phos	mag	iron	zinc
380	2	1	6	8	23	2	0	0	1	1	0	0	0	1	2	2	0	0	1
381	0	0	0	11	12	0	0	2	1	0	0	0	0	0	0	0	0	0	0
382	0	0	0	18	90	0	0	0	1	6	8	9	5	1	2	4	5	1	0
383	0	0	0	11	65	0	0	0	2	6	7	6	4	1	2	4	5	1	1
384	0	0	0	3	12	0	0	0	0	0	0	0	0	0	0	0	0	0	0
385	0	0	0	332	216	5	4	34	3	2	3	5	5	0	1	2	3	3	1
386	0	0	0	16	2	0	0	0	0	0	0	0	0	0	0	0	0	0	1
387	0	0	0	0	1	0	0	0	0	0	0	0	0	0	0	0	0	0	0
388	0	0	0	11	72	0	0	0	0	1	0	1	0	0	1	1	2	2	1
389	9	6	69	68	227	6	2	3	4	13	1	2	3	5	15	16	5	3	5
390	0	0	0	2	5	0	0	0	0	0	0	0	0	0	0	0	0	0	0
391	0	0	0	3	13	0	0	2	1	0	0	0	0	0	0	0	0	0	0
392	0	0	0	12	49	0	0	6	2	0	0	1	1	0	1	1	1	2	1
393	0	0	0	4	313	1	1	107	9	2	2	4	18	0	1	3	4	1	1
394	0	0	0	2	14	0	0	0	0	0	0	0	0	0	0	0	0	0	0
395	0	0	0	3	13	0	0	2	1	0	0	0	0	0	0	0	0	0	0
396	0	0	0	10	12	0	0	2	0	0	0	0	0	0	0	0	0	0	1
397	0	0	0	38	20	0	0	7	0	0	0	0	0	0	1	0	1	0	1
398	0	0	0	32	21	0	0	7	0	0	0	0	0	0	1	0	1	0	1
399	0	0	0	0	1	0	0	0	0	0	0	0	0	0	0	0	0	0	0
400	0	0	0	9	95	0	0	0	0	1	0	1	0	0	1	2	3	2	1
401	4	2	11	18	52	3	0	0	1	3	0	1	0	2	3	3	1	0	1
402	0	0	0	0	1	0	0	0	0	0	0	0	0	0	0	0	0	0	0
403	4	2	11	14	39	3	0	0	1	3	0	1	0	2	3	3	1	0	1
404	0	0	0	25	3	0	0	0	0	0	0	0	0	0	1	0	0	0	1
405	1	1	5	2	12	1	0	0	0	0	0	0	0	0	0	0	0	0	0
406	0	0	0	7	17	0	0	6	1	0	0	0	0	0	0	1	1	0	0
407	0	0	0	11	24	0	0	2	1	0	0	0	0	0	0	1	1	1	0
408	0	0	0	2	14	0	0	0	0	0	0	0	0	0	0	0	0	0	0
409	0	0	0	4	15	0	0	2	1	0	0	0	0	0	0	0	0	0	0
410	0	0	0	2	14	0	0	0	0	0	0	0	0	0	0	0	0	0	0
411	2	1	46	11	31	3	1	0	1	3	0	1	1	2	3	3	1	1	1
412	0	0	0	1	1	0	0	0	0	0	0	0	0	0	0	0	0	0	0
413	0	0	0	47	29	0	0	3	4	10	20	5	13	1	2	8	6	1	0
414	0	0	0	1	1	0	0	0	0	0	0	0	0	0	0	0	0	0	0
415	3	2	0	8	94	0	1	11	2	1	1	3	4	0	1	1	3	1	1
416	0	0	0	11	25	0	0	3	1	0	0	0	1	0	1	2	1	1	0
417	0	0	0	0	1	0	0	0	0	0	0	0	0	0	0	0	0	0	0
418	12	7	31	7	9	11	1	0	1	1	0	0	0	0	1	1	1	1	1
419	1	0	0	14	213	1	1	32	3	4	2	3	4	0	2	2	5	5	2
420	0	0	0	26	156	0	0	19	2	2	1	2	3	0	2	2	4	3	1
421	0	0	0	12	64	0	0	14	1	1	0	1	1	0	1	1	2	1	1
422	0	0	0	2	326	1	1	111	9	2	2	4	19	0	2	3	4	1	1
423	0	0	0	33	19	0	0	6	1	0	0	0	0	0	1	0	1	0	1
424	0	0	0	38	20	0	0	6	1	0	0	0	0	0	1	0	1	0	1
425	0	0	0	3	1	0	0	0	0	0	0	0	0	0	0	0	0	0	0
426	0	0	0	7	179	2	0	55	4	2	2	4	5	0	1	2	3	3	1
427	0	0	0	38	20	0	0	6	1	0	0	0	0	0	1	0	1	0	1
428	0	0	0	0	1	0	0	0	0	0	0	0	0	0	0	0	0	0	0

Beverages, Dairy, Eggs

Food No.	Food Description & Amount	wt gm	wt oz	cal	% cal fat	prot gm	carbo gm	fiber gm
429	Whiskey (Include bourbon, scotch, rye) [1 fl oz] (10 gm alcohol)	28	1.0	70	0%	0	0	0.0
430	Whiskey sour (Include scotch sour, vodka sour, soda sour, apricot sour, brandy sour) [1 cocktail] (15 gm alcohol)	90	3.2	123	1%	0	5	0.2
431	White Russian [1 cocktail] (26 gm alcohol)	100	3.5	257	4%	0	17	0.0
432	Wine cooler [1 drink (7 fl oz)] (8 gm alcohol)	210	7.4	105	0%	0	12	0.1
433	Wine spritzer [1 drink] (8 gm alcohol)	146	5.1	61	0%	0	1	0.0
434	Wine, Chinese [1 wine glass (3.5 fl oz)] (9 gm alcohol)	100	3.5	70	0%	0	1	0.0
435	Wine, cooking (after cooking) [1 fl oz] (0 gm alcohol)	29	1.0	8	0%	0	0	0.0
436	Wine, dessert, sweet (Include marsala, port, tokay, madeira, muscatel, angelica, sherry, sweet vermouth) [1 wine glass (3.5 fl oz)] (15 gm alcohol)	100	3.5	153	0%	0	12	0.0
437	Wine, light [1 wine glass (3.5 fl oz)] (7 gm alcohol)	102	3.6	51	0%	1	1	0.0
438	Wine, light, nonalcoholic [1 fl oz] (0 gm alcohol)	31	1.1	2	0%	0	0	0.0
439	Wine, nonalcoholic [1 fl oz] (0 gm alcohol)	29	1.0	2	0%	0	0	0.0
440	Wine, rice (Include sake) [1 fl oz] (5 gm alcohol)	30	1.1	40	0%	0	2	0.0
441	Wine, table, dry (Include burgundy, claret, chianti, sauterne, rhine, champagne, red wine, white wine, dry sherry) [1 wine glass (3.5 fl oz)] (9 gm alcohol)	100	3.5	70	0%	0	1	0.0
442	Zombie [1 cocktail] (46 gm alcohol)	193	6.8	372	0%	0	13	0.1
	Milk							
480	Buttermilk, dry [2 Tbs]	15	0.5	58	13%	5	7	0.0
481	Buttermilk, reconstituted from dry [1 cup]	245	8.6	93	13%	8	12	0.0
482	Buttermilk (Include Kefir milk) [1 cup]	245	8.6	99	20%	8	12	0.0
483	Buttermilk, 2% fat [1 cup]	245	8.6	137	32%	10	13	0.0
484	Chocolate milk (2%-fat milk with 2 Tbs chocolate syrup) [1 cup]	250	8.8	170	17%	8	30	0.6
485	Chocolate milk (non-fat milk with 2 Tbs chocolate syrup) [1 cup]	250	8.8	148	4%	8	30	0.6
486	Chocolate milk (whole milk with 2 Tbs chocolate syrup) [1 cup]	250	8.8	206	33%	8	30	0.6
487	Chocolate, instant, dry mix, fortified with vitamins and minerals, Puerto Rican style [1 Tbs]	8	0.3	29	9%	0	7	0.1
488	Chocolate drink, Spanish/Puerto Rican style (chocolate espanol) (Include chocolate milk beverage made with evaporated milk) [1 cup]	240	8.5	277	54%	10	25	1.1
489	Chocolate-flavored drink, whey- and milk-based (Include Yoo-hoo) [1 bottle (9 fl oz)]	274	9.7	145	7%	3	28	1.1
490	Cocoa, hot chocolate, not from dry mix (made with whole milk) [1 cup]	250	8.8	193	27%	10	29	2.0
491	Cocoa/chocolate powder with sugar (Include Hershey's Instant, Nestle's Quik) [1 Tbs]	8	0.3	29	8%	0	8	0.5
492	Cocoa/chocolate powder with low-cal sweetener [1 Tbs]	7	0.2	22	25%	1	4	1.6
493	Cocoa/chocolate powder with nonfat dry milk and sugar (Incl. Swiss Miss Hot Chocolate; Hershey's Hot Chocolate; Nestle's Hot Chocolate) [1 envelope]	28	1.0	101	10%	3	22	0.3
494	Cocoa/chocolate powder with nonfat dry milk and low-cal sweetener (Include Swiss Miss Sugar-Free Hot Cocoa Mix, Alba Sugar-Free Hot Cocoa Mix) [1 envelope]	17	0.6	54	8%	4	10	0.4
495	Cocoa beverage, Puerto Rican style (whole milk with 5 tsp sugar-cocoa mix fortified with vitamins and minerals) [1 cup]	250	8.8	212	35%	9	27	0.2
496	Cocoa beverage: 2%-fat milk with 2.5 tsp sugar-cocoa mix (Include Nestle's Quik, Hershey's Instant) [1 cup]	250	8.8	175	19%	8	30	1.2
497	Cocoa beverage: nonfat milk with 2.5 tsp sugar-cocoa mix (Include Nestle's Quik, Hershey's Instant) [1 cup]	250	8.8	152	6%	9	30	1.2
498	Cocoa beverage: whole milk with 2.5 tsp sugar-cocoa mix (Include Nestle's Quik, Hershey's Instant) [1 cup]	250	8.8	213	35%	8	29	1.2
499	Cocoa powder, unsweetened, (no dry milk) [1 Tbs]	5	0.2	12	54%	1	3	1.8
500	Cocoa beverage: water added to cocoa mix with nonfat dry milk and low cal sweetener (Include Sugar-Free Hot Cocoa Mix (Swiss Miss, Alba, Hills Bros. Old Fashioned), Nutri System Hot Chocolate) [1 packet plus 6 fl oz water]	197	6.9	49	8%	4	9	0.4

Food no.	fat gm	sat fat gm	choles mg	sodium mg	potas mg	% of Daily Value													
						vit A	vit E	vit C	thia	ribo	niac	vit B-6	fola	vit B-12	calc	phos	mag	iron	zinc
429	0	0	0	0	1	0	0	0	0	0	0	0	0	0	0	0	0	0	0
430	0	0	0	10	48	0	0	19	1	0	0	1	1	0	1	1	1	0	0
431	1	1	4	7	25	1	0	0	1	1	0	0	0	1	1	1	1	0	1
432	0	0	0	18	95	0	0	6	1	1	0	1	1	0	1	1	3	3	1
433	0	0	0	19	79	0	0	0	0	1	0	1	0	0	1	1	2	2	1
434	0	0	0	8	89	0	0	0	0	1	0	1	0	0	1	1	3	2	0
435	0	0	0	182	26	0	0	0	0	0	0	0	0	0	0	0	1	1	0
436	0	0	0	9	92	0	0	0	1	1	1	0	0	0	1	1	2	1	0
437	0	0	0	7	90	0	0	0	0	1	1	1	0	0	1	2	3	2	1
438	0	0	0	2	28	0	0	0	0	0	0	0	0	0	0	0	1	1	0
439	0	0	0	2	26	0	0	0	0	0	0	0	0	0	0	0	1	1	0
440	0	0	0	1	8	0	0	0	0	0	0	0	0	0	0	0	0	0	0
441	0	0	0	8	89	0	0	0	0	1	0	1	0	0	1	1	3	2	0
442	0	0	0	6	51	0	0	7	2	1	1	1	2	0	1	1	1	1	1
480	1	1	10	78	239	1	0	1	4	14	1	3	2	10	18	14	4	0	4
481	1	1	17	131	382	1	0	2	6	22	1	4	3	15	29	22	7	1	7
482	2	1	9	257	371	2	1	4	6	22	1	4	3	9	29	22	7	1	7
483	5	3	20	211	441	5	1	6	8	30	1	4	4	15	35	20	8	1	4
484	3	2	12	141	415	13	1	4	6	21	1	5	3	13	27	25	13	4	7
485	1	0	4	144	433	13	0	4	5	19	1	4	3	14	27	26	12	4	7
486	8	5	29	138	403	7	1	4	6	22	1	5	3	13	26	25	13	5	7
487	0	0	0	48	95	31	0	20	16	19	20	17	2	0	4	3	2	8	1
488	17	10	39	146	458	7	2	4	4	27	2	3	2	3	35	30	14	5	9
489	1	1	3	206	206	15	0	10	2	10	10	4	1	8	10	10	10	2	4
490	6	4	20	128	500	14	1	4	7	26	2	6	4	15	32	29	18	6	10
491	0	0	0	18	50	0	0	0	0	1	0	0	0	0	0	1	2	1	1
492	1	0	0	17	145	0	0	0	0	2	0	0	0	0	1	3	5	2	2
493	1	1	1	141	199	0	0	1	2	9	1	2	0	6	9	9	6	2	3
494	1	0	1	191	459	0	0	0	3	14	1	3	1	5	10	15	9	5	4
495	8	5	32	230	585	85	1	53	46	70	51	48	7	14	36	29	12	20	7
496	4	2	13	159	483	13	1	4	6	23	2	5	3	14	29	25	13	4	8
497	1	1	4	161	502	14	1	4	6	21	2	5	3	14	29	26	12	4	8
498	8	5	31	156	470	7	1	4	6	24	1	5	3	14	28	24	13	4	8
499	1	0	0	1	82	0	0	0	0	1	1	0	0	0	1	4	7	4	2
500	0	0	1	178	415	0	0	0	3	13	1	2	1	5	9	14	8	4	4

Beverages, Dairy, Eggs

Food No.	Food Description & Amount	wt gm	wt oz	cal	% cal fat	prot gm	carbo gm	fiber gm
501	Cocoa beverage: water added to high-calcium cocoa mix with nonfat dry milk and low-cal sweetener (Include Alba High Calcium Cocoa) [1 packet plus 6 fl oz water]	197	6.9	62	7%	5	10	0.5
502	Cocoa beverage: water added to cocoa mix with sugar, and dry milk (Incl. Swiss Miss Hot Chocolate; Hershey's Hot Chocolate; Nestle's Hot Chocolate; Carnation Hot Chocolate; mint-flavored) [1 oz packet plus 6 fl oz water]	206	7.3	102	10%	3	22	0.3
503	Cocoa-whey powder with low-cal sweetener, fortified, not reconstituted (Include Ovaltine Sugar-Free Hot Cocoa) [1 envelope]	12	0.4	37	8%	3	7	0.3
504	Cocoa-whey beverage: water added to dry mix with low-cal sweetener, fortified (Include Ovaltine Sugar-Free Hot Cocoa) [1 cup]	249	8.8	49	8%	4	9	0.4
505	Cocoa-whey beverage: 2%-fat milk added to dry mix with low-cal sweetener (Incl. Sugar-free Nestle's Quik, Swiss Miss Sugar-Free Chocolate Milk Maker) [1 cup]	250	8.8	124	30%	9	15	1.5
506	Cocoa-whey powder with low-cal sweetener (Incl. Sugar-Free Nestle's Quik, Swiss Miss Sugar-Free Chocolate Milk Maker) [1 envelope]	5	0.2	14	52%	1	3	1.3
507	Cream substitute, liquid or frozen (Include Coffee Whitner, Dairy Rich Moca Mix, mocha mix, Coffee Rich, Coffee Tone, Freezer Pak, Poly Perx, Poly Rich) [1 Tbs]	15	0.5	20	66%	0	2	0.0
508	Cream substitute, light, liquid [1 cup]	242	8.5	167	46%	2	22	0.0
509	Cream substitute, powdered (Include Coffee Mate, Coffee Tone, Cremora, instant coffee creamer, instant creamer, Please, Pream) [1 Tbs]	6	0.2	32	58%	0	3	0.0
510	Cream substitute, light, powdered [1 packet]	3	0.1	13	33%	0	2	0.0
511	Cream, half and half [2 Tbs]	30	1.1	39	79%	1	1	0.0
512	Cream, heavy (Include whipping cream) [2 Tbs]	30	1.0	103	97%	1	1	0.0
513	Cream, heavy, whipped, sweetened [1 cup]	119	4.2	413	90%	2	10	0.0
514	Cream, heavy, whipped, unsweetened [1 cup]	119	4.2	410	97%	2	3	0.0
515	Cream, light (Include coffee cream, table cream) [2 Tbs]	30	1.1	59	89%	1	1	0.0
516	Cream, light, whipped (unsweetened) (Include coffee cream, table cream) [1 cup]	120	4.2	351	95%	3	4	0.0
517	Cream, whipped, pressurized container (Include Reddiwip (red can), Fashion Whip, Quip) [1 cup]	60	2.1	154	78%	2	7	0.0
518	Eggnog, beads, reconstituted with whole milk [1 cup]	254	9.0	220	21%	8	37	0.8
519	Eggnog, made with 2%-fat milk [1 cup]	254	9.0	191	38%	12	17	0.0
520	Eggnog, made with whole milk [1 cup]	254	9.0	342	50%	10	34	0.0
521	Flavored milk drink, whey- and milk-based, flavors other than chocolate (Include Yoo-hoo) [1 bottle (9 fl oz)]	274	9.7	145	7%	3	28	1.1
522	High calorie milk beverage, powder (Include Nutrament) [2 Tbs]	15	0.5	57	4%	4	10	0.0
523	Imitation milk, fluid, non-soy, sweetened, chocolate flavor [1 cup]	250	8.8	153	24%	3	29	1.3
524	Instant breakfast, powder (Include Carnation Instant Breakfast, Lucerne) [1 envelope]	35	1.2	124	4%	7	23	0.1
525	Instant breakfast, powder, sugar-free (Include Sugar-free Carnation Instant Breakfast) [1 envelope]	20	0.7	72	13%	7	8	0.4
526	Meal replacement or nutritional supplement, Cambridge diet formula, powdered, nonfat milk solids base, dry [1 scoop (¼ cup)]	34	1.2	114	8%	11	15	0.1
527	Meal replacement, Nutrilite brand Positrim Drink Mix, powdered nonfat dry milk-based, dry, not reconstituted (Include all flavors) [1 packet (1.5 oz)]	43	1.5	162	23%	7	27	0.0
528	Meal replacement, protein type, milk-based, powdered (Include Slim-Fast, Joe Weider's Firmaloss Diet) [2 Tbs]	30	1.1	97	1%	5	19	0.6
529	Milk beverage beads, chocolate (Include PDQ) [2Tbs]	14	0.5	49	8%	0	13	0.8
530	Milk beverage beads, not chocolate [2 Tbs]	14	0.5	55	2%	0	14	0.4
531	Milk beverage with nonfat dry milk and low-cal sweetener, high calcium, water added, chocolate (Incl. Alba '77 High Calcium Shake) [1 packet dry mix]	12	0.4	4	8%	0	1	0.0
532	Milk beverage with nonfat dry milk and low-cal sweetener, water added, chocolate (Include Alba) [1 cup]	276	9.7	85	8%	7	14	0.5

Food no.	fat gm	sat fat gm	choles mg	sodium mg	potas mg	% of Daily Value													
						vit A	vit E	vit C	thia	ribo	niac	vit B-6	fola	vit B-12	calc	phos	mag	iron	zinc
501	0	0	4	165	425	8	0	1	4	17	1	1	0	4	33	24	11	0	5
502	1	1	1	148	202	0	0	1	2	9	1	2	0	6	10	9	6	2	3
503	0	0	1	76	313	4	0	0	2	10	1	2	0	4	17	19	6	3	3
504	0	0	1	107	413	5	0	0	3	13	1	2	1	5	22	25	9	4	4
505	4	2	14	161	502	14	1	4	7	25	2	6	4	15	30	27	14	4	8
506	1	0	0	7	123	0	0	0	1	2	1	0	0	0	1	4	6	4	2
507	1	0	0	12	29	0	1	0	0	0	0	0	0	0	0	1	0	0	0
508	8	2	0	145	428	0	0	0	0	0	0	0	0	0	0	18	0	8	1
509	2	2	0	11	48	0	0	0	0	1	0	0	0	0	0	2	0	0	0
510	0	0	0	7	27	0	0	0	0	0	0	0	0	0	0	0	0	0	0
511	3	2	11	12	39	3	0	0	1	3	0	1	0	2	3	3	1	0	1
512	11	7	41	11	22	13	1	0	0	2	0	0	0	1	2	2	1	0	0
513	41	26	153	42	85	47	3	1	2	7	0	1	1	3	7	7	2	0	2
514	44	27	163	45	90	50	3	1	2	8	0	2	1	4	8	7	2	0	2
515	6	4	20	12	37	5	0	0	1	3	0	0	0	1	3	2	1	0	1
516	37	23	133	41	116	35	3	1	2	9	0	2	1	4	8	7	2	0	2
517	13	8	46	78	88	12	2	0	1	2	0	1	0	3	6	5	2	0	1
518	5	3	26	154	354	11	1	4	6	22	1	5	3	14	28	22	8	2	6
519	8	4	194	155	369	20	3	3	7	32	1	7	8	19	27	27	8	4	8
520	19	11	149	138	420	20	3	6	6	28	1	6	1	19	33	28	12	3	8
521	1	1	3	206	206	15	0	10	2	10	10	4	1	8	10	10	10	2	4
522	0	0	1	34	183	10	0	9	8	3	9	8	9	5	13	11	8	9	8
523	4	3	0	245	78	5	0	0	0	1	1	0	1	0	4	5	4	1	3
524	0	0	4	135	331	52	23	45	20	4	25	20	25	10	10	15	20	25	20
525	1	0	9	143	341	54	23	46	20	4	26	20	25	10	10	10	21	3	21
526	1	0	19	507	680	51	31	34	34	34	34	34	34	34	34	34	34	34	34
527	4	1	3	106	395	45	21	30	30	10	35	30	35	20	25	20	25	35	30
528	0	0	3	110	254	40	34	32	32	11	37	32	21	21	16	16	26	37	32
529	0	0	0	29	83	0	0	0	0	1	0	0	0	0	1	2	3	2	1
530	0	0	3	22	1	0	0	0	0	0	0	0	0	0	0	0	0	1	0
531	0	0	0	10	28	0	0	0	0	1	0	0	0	0	2	1	1	1	0
532	1	1	2	229	637	10	0	1	2	32	2	2	3	11	26	24	16	12	7

Beverages, Dairy, Eggs

Food No.	Food Description & Amount	wt gm	wt oz	cal	% cal fat	prot gm	carbo gm	fiber gm
533	Milk beverage with nonfat dry milk and low-cal sweetener, water added, flavors other than chocolate (Include Alba) [1 cup]	276	9.7	104	7%	7	17	0.5
534	Milk beverage powder with sugar, dry milk, and egg white powder, dry mix (Include Banana Frost, Strawberry Frost) [2 Tbs]	26	0.9	99	0%	2	23	0.0
535	Milk beverage beads, chocolate, (Include PDQ), whole milk added [1 cup]	250	8.8	213	35%	8	29	1.2
536	Milk beverage, made with whole milk, flavors other than chocolate (Include strawberry Nestle's Quik) [1 cup]	250	8.8	221	31%	8	31	0.0
537	Milk beverage powder, dry mix, flavors other than chocolate (Include strawberry Nestle's Quik) [2 Tbs]	16	0.6	62	0%	0	16	0.0
538	Milk beverage powder with nonfat dry milk and low-cal sweetener, dry mix, chocolate (Include Alba) [2 Tbs]	16	0.6	48	8%	4	8	0.3
539	Milk beverage powder with nonfat dry milk and low-cal sweetener, dry mix, flavors other than chocolate (Incl. Alba) [2 Tbs]	14	0.5	46	7%	3	7	0.2
540	Milk fruit drink (Include licuado) made with whole milk, bananas, strawberries, sugar [1 cup]	209	7.4	150	18%	5	27	1.6
541	Milk fruit drink, Puerto Rican style (Champola de frutas) made with evap. whole milk, mashed papaya, sugar, lime juice [1 cup]	240	8.5	207	28%	6	32	0.4
542	Milk shake with malt (Include malted milk with ice cream) [10 fl oz]	283	10.0	404	32%	9	62	0.1
543	Milk shake, fountain type, chocolate [10 fl oz]	283	10.0	367	34%	9	57	1.8
544	Milk shake, fountain type, flavors other than chocolate [10 fl oz]	283	10.0	381	32%	8	60	0.5
545	Milk shake, thick, carry-out type, chocolate (Include thick shake mix, milk added; Wendy's Frosty) [12.5 fl oz]	313	11.0	398	26%	11	64	2.5
546	Milk shake, thick, carry-out type, flavors other than chocolate (Include thick shake mix, milk added) [12.5 fl oz]	313	11.0	347	24%	11	56	1.3
547	Milk shake, made with nonfat milk, chocolate [1 cup]	127	4.5	132	7%	5	28	1.9
548	Milk shake, made with nonfat milk, flavors other than chocolate [1 cup]	127	4.5	126	4%	5	27	1.2
549	Milk, chocolate, lowfat milk-based (Include chocolate milk drink) [1 cup]	250	8.8	175	23%	8	26	1.3
550	Milk, chocolate, nonfat milk-based [1 cup]	250	8.8	144	7%	9	27	1.5
551	Milk, chocolate, whole milk-based [1 cup]	250	8.8	208	37%	8	26	2.0
552	Milk, flavors other than chocolate, whole milk-based [1 cup]	250	8.8	221	31%	8	31	0.0
553	Milk, condensed, sweetened, undiluted [½ cup undiluted or 1 cup diluted]	306	10.8	982	24%	24	166	0.0
554	**Milk, cow's, 1% fat** (Include acidophilis milk, lactose-reduced milk, Lactaid) [1 cup]	245	8.6	103	23%	8	12	0.0
555	Milk, cow's, 1% fat, calcium-fortified (Include lactose-reduced milk, CalciMilk, CalciMilk with Lactaid) [1 cup]	247	8.7	103	23%	8	12	0.0
556	**Milk, cow's, 2% fat** (Include acidophilis milk, lactose-reduced milk, Hi-Protein milk, fortified milk) [1 cup]	245	8.6	122	35%	8	12	0.0
557	Milk, cow's, filled with vegetable oil, lowfat [1 cup]	245	8.6	113	29%	8	12	0.0
558	Milk, cow's, filled with vegetable oil, whole [1 cup]	244	8.6	153	49%	8	12	0.0
559	**Milk, cow's, nonfat** (Include lactose-reduced) [1 cup]	245	8.6	86	5%	8	12	0.0
560	**Milk, cow's, whole** (Include leche fresca) [1 cup]	244	8.6	150	49%	8	11	0.0
561	Milk, cow's, whole, calcium-fortified [1 cup]	247	8.7	151	49%	8	11	0.0
562	Milk, cow's, nonfat, calcium-fortified (Include lactose-reduced) [1 cup]	247	8.7	86	5%	8	12	0.0
563	Milk, cow's, whole, low-sodium [1 cup]	244	8.6	149	51%	8	11	0.0
564	Milk, dry, whole [2 Tbs]	16	0.6	79	48%	4	6	0.0
565	Milk, dry, lowfat [2 Tbs]	15	0.5	55	5%	5	8	0.0
566	Milk, dry, nonfat [2 Tbs]	8	0.3	30	2%	3	4	0.0
567	Milk, dry, reconstituted, whole [1 cup]	244	8.6	157	48%	8	12	0.0
568	Milk, dry, reconstituted, lowfat [1 cup]	245	8.6	84	4%	8	12	0.0
569	Milk, dry, reconstituted, nonfat [1 cup]	245	8.6	82	2%	8	12	0.0
570	Milk, evaporated, 2% fat [½ cup undiluted or 1 cup diluted]	244	8.6	117	19%	9	14	0.0
571	Milk, evaporated, filled with vegetable oil [½ cup undiluted or 1 cup diluted]	244	8.6	167	51%	9	13	0.0
572	Milk, evaporated, nonfat [½ cup undiluted or 1 cup diluted]	245	8.6	99	2%	10	14	0.0
573	Milk, evaporated, whole [½ cup undiluted or 1 cup diluted]	244	8.6	169	51%	9	13	0.0

Food no.	fat gm	sat fat gm	choles mg	sodium mg	potas mg	% of Daily Value													
						vit A	vit E	vit C	thia	ribo	niac	vit B-6	fola	vit B-12	calc	phos	mag	iron	zinc
533	1	1	4	256	701	9	0	1	2	6	2	2	3	13	29	5	17	14	8
534	0	0	1	38	81	3	0	0	1	6	0	1	1	3	5	4	1	0	1
535	8	5	31	156	470	7	1	4	6	24	1	5	3	14	28	24	13	4	8
536	8	5	31	120	348	7	1	4	6	23	1	5	3	14	27	21	8	1	6
537	0	0	0	6	0	0	0	0	0	1	0	0	0	0	0	0	0	0	0
538	0	0	1	125	358	6	0	0	1	18	1	1	2	6	14	14	8	7	4
539	0	0	2	109	308	4	0	0	1	3	1	1	1	6	12	2	7	6	3
540	3	2	11	67	400	7	1	36	5	16	2	14	5	8	17	14	8	2	4
541	7	4	25	94	388	5	2	49	5	17	2	3	8	2	23	18	7	1	5
542	14	9	55	216	499	14	1	4	12	34	6	8	5	16	32	28	12	2	8
543	14	9	47	182	538	14	2	4	6	25	2	6	5	13	28	29	19	10	9
544	13	8	54	147	422	14	1	26	6	26	2	6	3	14	29	23	8	4	9
545	12	7	41	304	626	7	1	2	12	45	3	8	3	18	35	32	13	5	9
546	9	6	34	257	545	10	1	4	9	34	3	8	3	19	38	32	9	2	8
547	1	1	5	97	302	1	0	2	4	13	1	3	2	9	17	15	7	3	5
548	0	0	4	96	237	1	0	2	4	12	1	2	2	9	17	13	4	1	4
549	5	3	15	151	423	14	1	4	6	24	2	5	3	14	28	25	8	3	7
550	1	1	4	121	486	14	1	4	6	20	1	5	3	15	29	27	11	4	8
551	8	5	31	149	417	7	1	4	6	24	2	5	3	14	28	25	8	3	7
552	8	5	31	120	348	7	1	4	6	23	1	5	3	14	27	21	8	1	6
553	27	17	104	389	1136	25	3	13	18	75	3	8	9	23	87	78	20	3	19
554	3	2	10	124	382	14	0	4	6	24	1	5	3	15	30	24	8	1	6
555	3	2	10	125	385	15	0	4	6	24	1	5	3	15	55	24	9	1	6
556	5	3	18	122	378	14	1	4	6	24	1	5	3	15	30	23	8	1	6
557	4	3	5	130	413	0	0	3	6	21	1	4	3	15	29	22	7	1	7
558	8	8	4	138	339	0	0	4	5	18	1	5	3	14	31	24	8	1	6
559	0	0	4	126	406	15	0	4	6	20	1	5	3	15	30	25	7	1	7
560	8	5	33	120	370	8	1	4	6	23	1	5	3	15	29	23	8	1	6
561	8	5	33	121	373	8	1	4	6	24	1	5	3	15	103	23	8	1	6
562	0	0	4	127	409	15	0	4	6	20	1	5	3	16	50	25	7	1	7
563	8	5	33	6	617	8	1	4	3	15	1	4	3	15	25	21	3	1	6
564	4	3	16	59	213	4	1	2	3	11	1	2	1	9	15	12	3	0	4
565	0	0	3	81	252	11	0	1	4	15	1	3	2	10	18	15	4	0	4
566	0	0	2	47	145	6	0	1	2	9	0	1	1	6	10	8	2	0	2
567	8	5	31	124	421	9	2	5	6	22	1	5	3	17	29	25	7	1	7
568	0	0	5	132	388	16	0	2	6	23	1	4	3	15	28	22	7	1	7
569	0	0	4	132	388	16	0	2	6	23	1	4	3	15	28	22	7	1	7
570	2	2	10	148	416	17	0	3	4	23	1	3	3	5	37	24	9	2	8
571	9	8	4	139	414	17	0	1	4	25	1	2	2	5	30	24	8	1	8
572	0	0	5	150	422	15	0	3	4	23	1	4	3	5	37	25	9	2	8
573	10	6	37	137	381	7	1	4	4	23	1	3	2	3	33	25	8	1	7

Beverages, Dairy, Eggs

Food No.	Food Description & Amount	wt gm	wt oz	cal	% cal fat	prot gm	carbo gm	fiber gm
574	Milk, goat's, whole [1 cup]	244	8.6	168	54%	9	11	0.0
575	Milk, human [1 cup]	246	8.7	171	57%	3	17	0.0
576	Milk, imitation, non-soy, corn-syrup based (Include Vitamite) [1 cup]	244	8.6	112	39%	4	13	0.0
577	Milk, imitation, soy based [1 cup]	244	8.6	150	50%	4	15	0.0
578	Milk, malted, dry mix, fortified, chocolate (Include Ovaltine) [2 Tbs]	16	0.6	57	9%	1	14	0.1
579	Milk, malted, dry mix, fortified, flavors other than chocolate (Include Ovaltine) [2 Tbs]	16	0.6	61	7%	1	13	0.1
580	Milk, malted, dry mix, unfortified, not reconstituted, chocolate [1 Tbs]	16	0.6	60	9%	1	14	0.1
581	Milk, malted, dry mix, unfortified, flavors other than chocolate [2 Tbs]	16	0.6	66	17%	2	12	0.1
582	Milk, malted, fortified, chocolate (Include Ovaltine) [1 cup]	235	8.3	177	26%	8	26	0.2
583	Milk, malted, fortified, natural flavor (Include Ovaltine) [1 cup]	235	8.3	182	25%	9	25	0.1
584	Milk, malted, unfortified, chocolate [1 cup]	235	8.3	180	26%	8	27	0.2
585	Milk, malted, unfortified, chocolate, made with nonfat milk [1 cup]	235	8.3	146	7%	8	27	0.2
586	Milk, malted, unfortified, natural flavor [1 cup]	235	8.3	188	29%	9	24	0.1
587	Milk, soy, canned or dry/reconstituted, not baby's (Include soyamel, soyagen) [1 cup]	245	8.6	81	52%	7	4	3.2
588	Milk, Tiger's, dry [2 Tbs]	15	0.5	53	5%	5	7	0.0
589	Milk-based fruit drink (Include orange julius, strawberry julius, pina colada julius) [1 cup]	262	9.2	214	2%	14	39	0.3
590	Diet beverage, liquid, canned (Include Metrecal, Sego Lite, Slender) [1 cup]	247	8.7	173	18%	9	27	0.0
591	Diet beverage, powder, reconstituted (Include Lookfit, Metrecal, Shape, Slender) [1 cup]	247	8.7	198	5%	13	34	0.0
592	High calorie beverage, canned or powdered, reconstituted (Include Nutrament, Sego) [1 cup]	250	8.8	235	25%	11	34	0.0
593	Instant breakfast, powder, whole milk added (Include Carnation Instant Breakfast; Lucerne) [1 cup]	247	8.7	224	20%	14	32	0.1
594	Meal supplement or replacement, canned, ready-to-drink (Include Ultra Slim Fast, all flavors) [1 cup]	248	8.7	174	18%	9	27	0.0
595	Meal supplement or replacement, milk-based, high protein, liquid (Include Sustacal Powder, reconstituted) [1 cup]	256	9.0	241	21%	15	33	0.0
596	Meal replacement formula, Cambridge diet, reconstituted, all flavors [1 cup]	272	9.6	107	8%	10	14	0.1
597	Nutrient supplement, milk-based, low calorie, powdered (Include Dietene) [2 Tbs]	20	0.7	72	2%	6	12	0.0
598	Nutrient supplement, milk-based, powdered (Include Sustagen) [2 Tbs]	16	0.6	62	8%	4	11	0.0
599	Protein supplement, milk-based, powdered (Include Meritene) [2 Tbs]	22	0.8	81	4%	6	13	0.0
600	Protein supplement, milk-based, powdered (Include Sustacal Powder) [1 packet]	57	2.0	206	1%	13	38	0.0
601	Protein supplement, milk-based, sodium controlled, powdered (Include Lonalac) [2 Tbs]	16	0.6	82	49%	4	6	0.0
602	Sour cream [2 Tbs]	29	1.0	62	88%	1	1	0.0
603	Sour cream, half and half [2 Tbs]	30	1.1	41	80%	1	1	0.0
604	Sour cream, reduced fat [2 Tbs]	32	1.1	58	70%	2	2	0.0
605	Sour cream, light [2 Tbs]	32	1.1	44	70%	1	2	0.0
606	Sour cream, fat free [2 Tbs]	32	1.1	24	0%	1	5	0.0
607	Sour cream, imitation (non-dairy) (Include Imo, Zero) [2 Tbs]	29	1.0	60	84%	1	2	0.0
608	Whey, sweet, dry [2 tbs]	18	0.6	64	3%	2	13	0.0
609	Whipped cream substitute, non-dairy, dietetic, made from powdered mix (Include Feather Weight Low Calorie Whipped Topping) [1 cup]	80	2.8	42	102%	1	8	0.0
610	Whipped cream substitute, non-dairy, made from powdered mix (Include Dream Whip, Lucky Whip, Smooth Whip) [1 cup]	80	2.8	151	59%	3	13	0.0
611	Whipped topping, nondairy, frozen (Include Cool Whip, Handiwhip Whipped Topping, Pet Whip) [1 cup]	75	2.6	239	72%	1	17	0.0
612	Whipped topping, non-dairy, frozen, lowfat [1 cup]	75	2.6	165	54%	2	18	0.0
613	Whipped topping, nondairy, pressurized can (Include Lucky Whip, Reddiwip (blue can)) [1 cup]	70	2.5	184	76%	1	11	0.0

Food no.	fat gm	sat fat gm	choles mg	sodium mg	potas mg	% of Daily Value													
						vit A	vit E	vit C	thia	ribo	niac	vit B-6	fola	vit B-12	calc	phos	mag	iron	zinc
574	10	7	28	122	499	14	1	5	8	20	3	6	0	3	33	27	9	1	5
575	11	5	34	42	126	16	10	21	2	5	2	1	3	2	8	3	2	0	3
576	5	1	0	134	366	15	0	0	0	0	1	0	0	0	20	24	1	1	2
577	8	2	0	191	279	0	12	0	2	13	0	0	0	0	8	18	4	5	19
578	1	0	1	95	191	63	0	40	33	39	41	35	4	1	7	6	4	15	1
579	0	0	3	65	155	51	0	34	32	34	39	29	2	2	6	6	3	15	1
580	1	0	1	40	99	0	0	0	2	2	2	1	1	1	1	3	3	2	1
581	1	1	3	79	121	1	0	1	5	9	4	3	2	2	5	6	4	1	1
582	5	3	20	218	558	83	1	50	43	65	48	45	7	14	34	28	12	19	7
583	5	3	22	183	516	70	1	44	42	60	46	38	5	16	33	28	10	18	6
584	5	3	20	155	451	11	1	4	8	23	3	6	4	14	27	24	10	3	7
585	1	1	5	158	474	14	1	4	7	20	3	6	4	14	28	25	9	3	7
586	6	4	22	200	477	12	1	4	12	30	6	8	5	16	32	27	12	1	7
587	5	1	0	29	345	1	0	0	26	10	2	5	1	0	1	12	12	8	4
588	0	0	0	50	263	0	0	0	49	45	23	28	2	30	33	24	5	16	4
589	0	0	7	198	936	1	1	102	18	35	3	10	21	24	47	38	14	2	11
590	3	1	5	420	450	30	18	20	20	20	20	20	20	20	20	20	20	20	20
591	1	1	7	227	662	53	27	30	30	23	30	28	32	31	32	33	28	30	33
592	7	1	0	163	360	34	21	23	23	24	23	23	23	23	23	23	23	23	23
593	5	3	22	232	641	59	22	45	24	24	24	23	26	22	35	34	26	24	24
594	3	1	5	422	451	30	18	20	20	20	20	20	20	20	20	20	20	20	20
595	6	1	0	220	494	29	20	22	24	24	22	23	22	22	24	22	22	22	22
596	1	0	18	483	638	48	29	32	32	32	32	32	32	32	32	32	32	32	32
597	0	0	4	78	233	26	23	21	21	14	25	21	18	7	14	14	18	25	21
598	1	0	2	42	113	5	0	18	9	9	9	9	4	9	11	8	4	4	5
599	0	0	3	109	259	19	15	15	14	11	16	14	17	7	19	18	11	17	13
600	0	0	9	201	591	41	0	35	28	12	36	29	35	18	31	26	28	35	28
601	4	4	0	0	0	5	0	0	4	16	1	0	0	0	14	13	3	1	0
602	6	4	13	15	41	6	1	0	1	3	0	0	1	1	3	2	1	0	1
603	4	2	12	12	39	3	0	0	1	3	0	0	1	2	3	3	1	0	1
604	5	3	11	22	68	4	1	0	1	5	0	0	1	2	5	3	1	0	1
605	3	2	11	23	68	3	0	0	1	2	0	0	1	2	5	2	1	0	1
606	0	0	3	45	41	3	0	0	1	3	0	0	1	2	4	3	1	0	1
607	6	5	0	29	46	0	0	0	0	0	0	0	0	0	0	1	0	1	2
608	0	0	1	196	377	0	0	0	6	24	1	5	1	7	14	17	8	1	2
609	5	3	0	85	21	0	0	0	0	0	0	0	0	0	0	2	0	0	0
610	10	9	8	53	121	4	1	1	1	6	0	1	1	3	7	7	2	0	1
611	19	16	0	19	14	6	1	0	0	0	0	0	0	0	0	1	0	1	0
612	10	8	2	54	76	3	0	0	1	4	0	1	1	3	5	6	1	0	1
613	16	13	0	43	13	3	1	0	0	0	0	0	0	0	0	1	0	0	0

Beverages, Dairy, Eggs

Food No.	Food Description & Amount	wt gm	wt oz	cal	% cal fat	prot gm	carbo gm	fiber gm
	Yogurt							
650	Yogurt, chocolate, whole milk [1-6 oz container]	170	6.0	172	28%	8	23	0.0
651	Yogurt, fruit and nuts [1-8 oz container]	227	8.0	268	23%	10	43	0.5
652	Yogurt, fruit variety, lowfat milk (Include custard style) [1-8 oz container]	227	8.0	231	10%	10	43	0.0
653	Yogurt, fruit variety, nonfat milk [1-8 oz container]	227	8.0	213	2%	10	43	0.0
654	Yogurt, fruit variety, nonfat milk, sweetened with low-calorie sweetener [1-6 oz container]	170	6.0	86	3%	7	14	0.9
655	Yogurt, fruit variety, whole milk (Include breakfast yogurt) [1-8 oz container]	227	8.0	270	25%	10	42	0.0
656	Yogurt, plain, lowfat milk [1-8 oz container]	227	8.0	144	22%	12	16	0.0
657	Yogurt, plain, nonfat milk [1-8 oz container]	227	8.0	127	3%	13	17	0.0
658	Yogurt, plain, whole milk [1-8 oz container]	227	8.0	139	48%	8	11	0.0
659	Yogurt, vanilla, lemon, maple, or coffee flavor, lowfat milk (Include liquid yogurt, LeShake, Tuscan) [1-8 oz container]	227	8.0	194	13%	11	31	0.0
660	Yogurt, vanilla, lemon, maple, or coffee flavor, nonfat milk [1-8 oz container]	227	8.0	207	2%	12	40	0.0
661	Yogurt, vanilla, lemon, maple, or coffee flavor, nonfat milk, sweetened with low calorie sweetener [1-8 oz container]	227	8.0	98	4%	9	17	0.0
662	Yogurt, vanilla, lemon, or coffee flavor, whole milk [1-8 oz container]	227	8.0	229	28%	11	31	0.0
	Ice Cream and Frozen Yogurt							
700	Ice cream bar or stick with fruit (Include Carnation Berry Swirl) [1 bar]	41	1.4	65	36%	1	10	0.8
701	Ice cream bar or stick, chocolate covered (Include ice cream nugget) [1 bar (3 fl oz)]	56	2.0	169	66%	2	14	0.2
702	Ice cream bar or stick, chocolate ice cream, chocolate covered (Include DoveBar) [1 bar]	101	3.6	339	61%	3	36	2.1
703	Ice cream bar or stick, chocolate or caramel covered, with nuts (Include Heavenly Sundae, Vanilla fudge nuts; Heavenly Sundae caramel; Heavenly Sundae) [1 bar]	54	1.9	177	63%	3	16	0.6
704	Ice cream bar or stick, not chocolate or cake covered [1 bar (3 fl oz)]	56	2.0	113	49%	2	13	0.0
705	Ice cream bar or stick, rich ice cream, thick chocolate covering (Include DoveBar) [1 bar]	81	2.9	261	57%	4	27	0.8
706	Ice cream bar or stick, rich ice cream, chocolate covered, with nuts [1 Haagen Dazs bar]	113	4.0	369	61%	6	34	1.9
707	Ice cream bar, cake covered [1 bar]	59	2.1	168	38%	3	25	0.7
708	Ice cream cone with nuts, chocolate ice cream [1 cone]	78	2.8	212	53%	5	23	1.8
709	Ice cream cone with nuts, flavors other than chocolate [1 cone]	78	2.8	205	57%	5	20	1.2
710	Ice cream cone, chocolate covered or dipped, chocolate ice cream [1 cone]	78	2.8	190	42%	3	27	1.1
711	Ice cream cone, chocolate covered or dipped, flavors other than chocolate [1 cone and single dip]	78	2.8	187	46%	3	24	0.6
712	Ice cream cone, chocolate covered, with nuts, chocolate ice cream [1 cone]	78	2.8	224	53%	5	25	2.0
713	Ice cream cone, chocolate covered, with nuts, flavors other than chocolate (Include Nutty Buddy) [1 cone and single dip]	78	2.8	217	57%	4	22	1.4
714	Ice cream cone, no topping, chocolate ice cream [1 cone and single dip (or 1 small cone)]	78	2.8	173	39%	3	25	0.7
715	Ice cream cone, no topping, flavors other than chocolate [1 cone and single dip (or 1 small cone)]	78	2.8	166	45%	3	21	0.1
716	Ice cream cookie sandwich (Include Chipwich) [1 sandwich]	59	2.1	144	35%	3	22	0.6
717	Ice cream pie (vanilla ice cream with whipped cream topping, no crust) [1/8 of 8" dia]	99	3.5	218	59%	3	21	0.0
718	Ice cream pie, with cookie crust, fudge topping, and whipped cream [1/8 of 8" dia]	230	8.1	695	45%	9	93	1.4
719	Ice cream sandwich (Include Oreo Ice Cream sandwich) [1 sandwich (5" x 1¾" x ¾")]	59	2.1	144	35%	3	22	0.6
720	Ice cream soda, chocolate [1 soda (10 fl oz)]	240	8.5	222	40%	3	35	1.0
721	Ice cream soda, flavors other than chocolate [1 soda (10 fl oz)]	240	8.5	203	30%	2	35	0.0
722	Ice cream sundae cone (Include Drumstick, all flavors) [1 cone]	107	3.8	284	51%	6	32	1.3

						% of Daily Value													
Food no.	fat gm	sat fat gm	choles mg	sodium mg	potas mg	vit A	vit E	vit C	thia	ribo	niac	vit B-6	fola	vit B-12	calc	phos	mag	iron	zinc
650	5	3	17	110	366	5	1	2	5	20	1	4	4	15	29	22	7	1	9
651	7	2	9	129	454	3	1	3	9	24	1	5	6	17	34	28	10	2	13
652	2	2	10	133	442	2	0	2	6	24	1	5	5	18	34	27	8	1	11
653	0	0	5	132	440	0	0	3	6	24	1	5	5	18	35	27	9	1	11
654	0	0	2	98	388	0	1	31	5	19	2	4	6	13	26	21	7	2	9
655	7	5	22	130	432	7	1	2	5	23	1	4	5	17	34	27	8	1	11
656	4	2	14	159	531	4	0	3	7	29	1	6	6	21	41	33	10	1	13
657	0	0	4	174	579	0	0	3	7	31	1	6	7	23	45	36	11	1	15
658	7	5	29	105	351	7	1	2	4	19	1	4	4	14	27	22	7	1	9
659	3	2	11	149	498	3	0	3	6	27	1	5	6	20	39	31	9	1	13
660	0	0	4	155	518	0	0	3	7	28	1	5	6	21	40	32	10	1	13
661	0	0	5	134	402	0	0	4	5	22	1	4	5	16	32	25	7	2	10
662	7	5	22	147	488	7	1	3	6	26	1	5	6	20	38	30	9	1	12
700	3	2	10	19	66	3	0	5	1	4	0	1	1	1	3	3	1	1	1
701	13	10	19	36	104	5	0	0	1	6	0	1	1	3	6	5	2	1	2
702	23	14	38	56	260	9	3	0	2	12	2	2	1	4	7	14	16	6	7
703	12	8	17	44	128	5	2	0	3	7	3	2	2	3	6	7	4	1	3
704	6	4	25	45	111	7	0	1	2	8	0	1	1	4	7	6	2	0	3
705	17	10	40	52	184	12	1	1	3	10	1	2	1	5	11	11	5	2	4
706	25	13	54	65	293	16	9	1	4	15	2	2	3	6	17	18	13	5	8
707	7	2	30	254	139	3	3	0	3	7	2	1	1	2	7	11	4	8	3
708	12	4	16	40	218	5	4	1	3	13	3	2	3	4	10	13	12	4	6
709	13	5	28	58	198	8	3	1	3	16	3	2	2	4	11	12	10	3	6
710	9	5	17	43	178	6	2	1	3	8	2	1	1	4	8	8	6	4	3
711	10	6	29	61	161	8	1	1	3	11	2	2	1	4	9	8	5	3	4
712	13	5	15	37	223	5	4	1	3	12	3	2	2	4	10	13	12	5	6
713	14	6	26	55	204	7	3	1	3	15	3	2	2	4	10	12	11	4	6
714	7	4	18	46	168	6	1	1	3	8	2	1	1	4	9	8	4	3	3
715	8	5	32	65	151	9	0	1	3	11	1	2	1	5	10	8	3	1	4
716	6	3	20	36	122	5	0	0	2	7	1	1	1	3	6	6	3	2	3
717	14	9	56	74	182	16	0	1	3	13	1	2	1	6	12	10	3	0	4
718	35	16	60	417	397	25	8	2	7	28	6	5	3	11	22	26	14	10	10
719	6	3	20	36	122	5	0	0	2	7	1	1	1	3	6	6	3	2	3
720	10	6	29	94	213	9	1	1	2	7	1	1	1	4	9	11	9	5	5
721	7	4	27	82	126	7	0	1	2	9	0	1	1	4	9	6	3	0	4
722	16	8	37	78	259	10	4	1	5	14	8	3	4	5	12	15	9	4	9

Beverages, Dairy, Eggs

Food No.	Food Description & Amount	wt gm	wt oz	cal	% cal fat	prot gm	carbo gm	fiber gm
723	Ice cream sundae, chocolate or fudge topping with whipped cream [1 sundae]	165	5.8	435	52%	6	52	0.6
724	Ice cream sundae, fruit topping with whipped cream [1 sundae]	165	5.8	386	42%	4	56	0.5
725	Ice cream sundae, fudge topping, with cake and whipped cream [1 sundae]	175	6.2	489	48%	7	62	0.7
726	Ice cream sundae, caramel or butterscotch topping with whipped cream [1 sundae]	165	5.8	402	51%	5	47	0.4
727	Ice cream sundae, prepackaged type, flavors other than chocolate [1 sundae (3.5 fl oz)]	65	2.3	120	29%	3	19	0.0
728	Ice cream with sherbet [1 cup]	163	5.7	267	31%	3	45	0.5
729	Ice cream, chocolate [1 cup]	133	4.7	273	42%	5	37	1.0
730	Ice cream, flavors other than chocolate [1 cup]	133	4.7	267	49%	5	31	0.0
731	Ice cream, rich, flavors other than chocolate [1 cup]	148	5.2	357	60%	5	33	0.0
732	Ice cream, fried [1 cup]	133	4.7	358	46%	5	46	0.8
733	Ice cream, imitation, chocolate (with vegetable fat) (Include Mellorine) [1 cup]	133	4.7	268	47%	5	33	1.0
734	Ice cream, imitation, flavors other than chocolate (with vegetable fat) (Include Mellorine) [1 cup]	133	4.7	265	46%	5	32	0.0
735	Ice cream, soft serve, chocolate [1 cup]	173	6.1	355	42%	6	48	1.3
736	Ice cream, soft serve, flavors other than chocolate [1 cup]	173	6.1	348	49%	6	41	0.0
737	Ice milk bar or stick, chocolate covered, with nuts (Include Buster bar) [1 bar]	149	5.3	441	65%	9	36	1.8
738	Ice milk bar or stick, with low-calorie sweetener, chocolate-coated (Include Sugar Free Eskimo Pie, Klondike Lite Sugar Free) [1 bar (2.5 fl oz)]	53	1.9	113	42%	3	14	1.1
739	Ice milk bar or stick, chocolate-coated [1 bar (3 fl oz)]	56	2.0	142	61%	2	14	0.2
740	Ice milk cone, chocolate [1 cone]	78	2.8	129	19%	4	23	0.5
741	Ice milk cone, flavors other than chocolate [1 cone]	78	2.8	116	18%	4	20	0.2
742	Ice milk creamsicle or dreamsicle [1 sicle (3 fl oz)]	66	2.3	91	20%	2	18	0.2
743	Ice milk sandwich (Include Dairy Queen) [1 sandwich]	60	2.1	118	20%	3	22	0.6
744	Ice milk sundae, chocolate or fudge topping with whipped cream (Include McDonald's sundaes) [1 sundae]	165	5.8	384	46%	6	51	0.6
745	Ice milk sundae, soft serve, chocolate or fudge topping, no whipped cream [1 cup]	142	5.0	257	26%	7	44	0.4
746	Ice milk sundae, fruit topping with whipped cream (Include McDonald's sundaes) [1 sundae]	165	5.8	335	33%	4	55	0.5
747	Ice milk sundae, soft serve, fruit topping, no whipped cream [1 cup]	142	5.0	173	15%	5	33	0.6
748	Ice milk sundae, caramel or butterscotch topping with whipped cream (Include McDonald's sundaes) [1 sundae]	165	5.8	366	28%	6	64	0.8
749	Ice milk sundae, soft serve, no fruit or chocolate topping, no whipped cream [1 cup]	142	5.0	269	19%	7	50	0.4
750	Ice milk, chocolate [1 cup]	131	4.6	189	20%	6	34	0.6
751	Ice milk, flavors other than chocolate [1 cup]	131	4.6	182	28%	5	30	0.0
752	Ice milk, fudgesicle [1 sicle (2.5 fl oz)]	73	2.6	104	29%	3	18	0.9
753	Ice milk, premium, chocolate (Include Breyers Light, Hood Light) [1 cup]	136	4.8	245	31%	6	38	0.6
754	Ice milk, premium, flavors other than chocolate (Include Breyers Light, Hood Light) [1 cup]	136	4.8	136	31%	4	21	0.0
755	Ice milk, soft serve, chocolate (Include frozen custard, Tastee Freeze, Dairy Queen, Dairy Queen Blizzard) [1 cup]	175	6.2	243	17%	8	45	0.8
756	Ice milk, soft serve cone, chocolate (Include Dairy Queen) [1 small fast food cone]	186	6.6	278	21%	11	51	3.7
757	Ice milk, soft serve, flavors other than chocolate (Include frozen custard, Tastee Freeze, Dairy Queen, Dairy Queen Blizzard) [1 cup]	175	6.2	221	19%	9	38	0.0
758	Ice milk, soft serve cone, flavors other than chocolate [1 small fast food cone (Include Dairy Queen)]	186	6.6	267	18%	9	47	0.3
759	Ice milk, with sherbet or ice cream [1 bar (2.5 fl oz)]	60	2.1	83	20%	1	16	0.2
760	Milk dessert bar, frozen, made from lowfat milk (Include Weight Watcher's Treat Bars) [1 bar (2.75 fl oz)]	81	2.9	88	10%	2	19	0.0
761	Milk dessert bar, frozen, made from lowfat milk and low-cal sweetener (Include sugar free Fudgsicle Fudge Pops) [1 bar (1.75 fl oz)]	41	1.4	24	13%	2	9	4.6

Food no.	fat gm	sat fat gm	choles mg	sodium mg	potas mg	% of Daily Value													
						vit A	vit E	vit C	thia	ribo	niac	vit B-6	fola	vit B-12	calc	phos	mag	iron	zinc
723	25	14	74	146	308	19	1	2	4	21	1	3	2	9	18	20	10	4	7
724	18	11	68	88	232	18	1	23	3	14	1	3	2	6	14	11	4	3	6
725	26	13	82	216	297	18	3	1	7	22	3	3	2	9	19	20	9	7	7
726	23	15	79	164	285	21	2	2	3	19	1	3	2	7	19	15	5	1	6
727	4	2	8	62	137	2	1	2	2	7	2	2	1	4	8	9	3	1	2
728	9	6	34	98	225	9	0	8	3	13	1	3	2	6	14	11	4	1	6
729	13	8	33	68	295	11	2	1	4	12	1	2	2	8	16	14	7	3	5
730	15	9	59	106	265	16	0	1	4	19	1	3	2	9	17	14	5	1	6
731	24	15	90	83	235	27	0	2	4	14	1	3	2	9	17	14	4	0	4
732	18	9	45	313	246	31	5	22	24	35	22	24	22	7	14	14	6	22	26
733	14	12	0	95	357	0	1	1	4	17	1	4	1	13	18	16	9	3	11
734	14	12	0	97	287	0	0	1	4	17	1	4	1	13	18	14	5	1	9
735	17	10	43	89	384	15	2	2	5	16	1	3	2	11	21	18	9	4	6
736	19	12	76	138	344	20	0	2	5	24	1	4	2	11	22	18	6	1	8
737	32	19	14	89	384	5	7	1	7	18	15	6	8	11	16	22	15	4	12
738	5	3	5	55	162	2	0	0	2	9	0	2	1	3	12	9	4	1	3
739	10	8	6	38	109	2	0	1	2	7	0	1	1	5	6	5	2	1	2
740	3	1	7	53	175	2	1	1	3	9	2	2	1	5	10	9	4	2	3
741	2	1	9	59	166	2	0	1	3	10	2	2	1	6	11	9	3	1	3
742	2	1	6	43	99	2	0	3	2	6	0	2	1	4	6	5	2	0	2
743	3	1	6	39	130	2	0	1	3	8	1	2	1	5	7	7	3	2	2
744	20	11	50	150	318	13	1	2	5	22	1	4	2	13	19	20	10	4	6
745	8	4	17	121	312	4	0	2	4	17	1	3	2	11	20	19	8	3	6
746	12	8	43	91	242	12	1	24	4	16	1	4	2	10	15	11	4	3	5
747	3	2	13	84	264	3	0	10	4	13	1	3	4	9	17	13	4	1	4
748	11	8	26	215	302	7	2	2	4	19	1	4	2	9	19	16	6	1	4
749	6	4	15	161	311	3	1	2	4	16	1	3	2	9	22	17	5	1	5
750	4	3	12	82	310	4	1	2	4	14	1	3	2	10	19	16	6	2	5
751	6	3	18	111	276	6	0	2	5	20	1	4	2	15	18	14	5	1	4
752	3	2	10	60	221	3	0	1	3	12	1	2	1	8	10	10	6	3	3
753	8	5	23	91	343	7	1	2	5	16	1	3	2	11	21	17	7	2	6
754	5	3	19	58	179	4	1	2	3	11	0	2	1	7	14	11	4	0	3
755	5	3	14	109	414	4	1	2	6	19	1	4	3	13	25	21	9	2	7
756	7	4	20	133	658	5	1	2	8	24	5	5	3	14	27	29	20	13	11
757	5	3	21	123	387	5	0	3	6	20	1	4	3	15	27	21	6	1	6
758	5	3	21	138	399	5	1	3	8	23	4	4	3	15	28	22	7	3	7
759	2	1	6	39	90	2	0	3	2	6	0	1	1	4	6	4	2	0	2
760	1	0	1	44	107	4	0	1	2	7	0	1	1	4	8	7	2	0	2
761	0	0	1	20	108	2	0	1	1	4	0	1	1	2	5	5	4	2	2

Beverages, Dairy, Eggs

Food No.	Food Description & Amount	wt gm	wt oz	cal	% cal fat	prot gm	carbo gm	fiber gm
762	Milk dessert bar or stick, frozen, with coconut (Include Frut Stix bar) [1 bar (4 fl oz)]	129	4.6	198	36%	7	27	2.2
763	Milk dessert sandwich bar, frozen, made from lowfat milk (Include Weight Watcher's Sandwich Bars) [1 sandwich bar (2.75 fl oz plus 2 wafers)]	77	2.7	135	9%	4	27	0.7
764	Milk dessert sandwich bar, frozen, with low-calorie sweetener, made from lowfat milk (Include 1 Eskimo Pie Sandwich) [1 Sandwich (3.2 fl oz)]	59	2.1	184	26%	3	31	1.2
765	Milk dessert, frozen, made with lowfat milk (Include Weight Watchers) [1 cup]	131	4.6	147	6%	6	29	0.0
766	Milk dessert, frozen, lowfat, made with low-calorie sweetener, flavors other than chocolate [1 cup]	137	4.8	156	10%	5	33	2.3
767	Milk dessert, frozen, nonfat, made with low-calorie sweetener, chocolate [1 cup]	144	5.1	153	16%	6	35	7.7
768	Milk dessert, frozen, nonfat, made with low-calorie sweetener, flavors other than chocolate [1 cup]	144	5.1	157	3%	4	36	1.2
769	Milk dessert, frozen, lowfat, flavors other than chocolate [1 cup]	144	5.1	174	3%	5	37	1.0
770	Milk dessert, frozen, milk-fat free, flavors other than chocolate [1 cup]	137	4.8	195	4%	5	43	4.1
771	Milk dessert, frozen, milk-fat free, chocolate [1 cup]	137	4.8	229	5%	6	52	2.7
772	Milk dessert, frozen, milk-fat free, made with Simplesse, flavors other than chocolate [1 cup]	179	6.3	240	0%	16	45	1.8
773	Milk dessert, frozen, milk-fat free, made with Simplesse, chocolate [1 cup]	179	6.3	279	3%	18	50	1.8
774	Milk dessert, frozen, made with low-calorie sweetener, flavors other than chocolate [1 cup]	129	4.6	183	40%	3	26	0.3
775	Milk dessert, frozen, made with low-calorie sweetener, chocolate [1 cup]	129	4.6	213	43%	6	34	5.6
776	Sherbet, all flavors [1 cup]	193	6.8	266	13%	2	59	1.0
777	Yogurt, frozen, carob-coated [1 bar]	41	1.4	100	42%	2	13	0.3
778	Yogurt, frozen, chocolate, whole milk [1 cup]	174	6.1	221	26%	5	38	4.0
779	Yogurt, frozen, chocolate, lowfat milk [1 cup]	193	6.8	219	15%	10	42	3.0
780	Yogurt, frozen, chocolate, nonfat milk [1 cup]	193	6.8	207	7%	11	43	3.0
781	Yogurt, frozen, chocolate, nonfat milk, with low-calorie sweetener [1 cup]	186	6.6	199	7%	8	37	3.7
782	Yogurt, frozen, chocolate-coated [1 bar]	41	1.4	109	56%	1	12	0.1
783	Yogurt, frozen, flavors other than chocolate, whole milk [1 cup]	174	6.1	221	26%	5	38	0.0
784	Yogurt, frozen, flavors other than chocolate, lowfat milk [1 cup]	193	6.8	203	12%	9	37	0.0
785	Yogurt, frozen, flavors other than chocolate, nonfat milk [1 cup]	193	6.8	191	1%	10	38	0.0
786	Yogurt, frozen, cone, chocolate [1 small cone]	78	2.8	168	39%	4	24	1.1
787	Yogurt, frozen, cone, chocolate, lowfat milk (Include McDonald's) [1 medium cone]	118	4.2	155	15%	6	29	1.9
788	Yogurt, frozen, cone, flavors other than chocolate [1 small cone]	78	2.8	147	26%	3	25	0.2
789	Yogurt, frozen, cone, flavors other than chocolate, lowfat milk (Include McDonald's) [1 medium cone]	118	4.2	99	20%	6	13	0.2
790	Yogurt, frozen, flavors other than chocolate, nonfat milk, with low-calorie sweetener [1 cup]	186	6.6	236	1%	9	52	1.8
791	Yogurt, frozen, sandwich [1 sandwich]	85	3.0	181	22%	4	32	0.4
	Cheese							
800	Cheese nuggets or pieces, breaded, baked, or fried (Include Banquet, Beatrice, Firesaver brands) [1 cup]	115	4.1	417	54%	30	17	0.5
801	Cheese spread, cheddar or American cheese base (Include Velveeta, Cheez Whiz (all flavors), Old English Smokey, Bacon, Yellow in a Jar) [2 Tbs]	31	1.1	89	66%	5	3	0.0
802	Cheese spread, cheddar or American cheese base, lowfat, low sodium (Include lowfat, low sodium Velveeta) [2 Tbs]	31	1.1	55	35%	8	1	0.0
803	Cheese spread, cream cheese or Neufchatel base [2 Tbs]	29	1.0	86	87%	2	1	0.0
804	Cheese spread, pressurized can [2 Tbs]	28	1.0	82	66%	5	2	0.0
805	Cheese spread, Swiss based (Include Swiss Almond cold pack cheese food) [1 oz]	28	1.0	81	66%	5	2	0.0
806	Cheese with nuts (Include cheese balls) [2 Tbs]	30	1.1	123	72%	8	1	0.1
807	Blue or Roquefort (Include Gorgonzola, Stilton) [2 Tbs, crumbled]	17	0.6	60	73%	4	0	0.0
808	Brick (Include Beer, Elbinger, Zweiteitige, Wilstermarsch, Bondost, Oka) [1 slice]	28	1.0	104	72%	7	1	0.0

Food no.	fat gm	sat fat gm	choles mg	sodium mg	potas mg	vit A	vit E	vit C	thia	ribo	niac	vit B-6	fola	vit B-12	calc	phos	mag	iron	zinc
						% of Daily Value													
762	8	7	9	165	425	2	1	2	5	16	1	6	3	12	24	19	7	2	7
763	1	1	3	55	183	0	0	1	3	7	1	2	1	7	10	10	4	2	3
764	5	1	2	233	130	0	3	0	6	8	5	1	1	3	5	8	6	8	3
765	1	1	7	122	312	1	0	1	3	15	1	3	0	15	22	18	5	1	4
766	2	1	8	78	310	2	0	29	4	14	1	4	3	9	18	14	5	1	4
767	3	1	2	137	570	6	1	2	4	11	4	3	3	7	16	17	13	6	7
768	0	0	2	68	212	7	0	2	3	10	1	2	1	7	14	11	3	0	3
769	1	0	4	98	344	12	0	0	4	18	1	1	1	4	19	16	5	6	6
770	1	1	0	121	255	9	0	0	4	15	1	2	1	7	18	14	5	1	4
771	1	1	0	133	456	3	0	2	5	21	1	3	2	13	21	17	15	0	4
772	0	0	30	131	401	3	0	1	4	31	1	3	3	10	19	14	7	1	6
773	1	1	20	150	465	3	0	3	6	34	3	4	3	12	22	18	9	4	6
774	8	5	30	52	157	11	1	2	2	9	0	2	1	6	12	10	3	0	3
775	10	6	29	42	559	10	1	1	3	12	2	3	2	4	11	20	23	16	9
776	4	2	10	89	185	3	1	14	3	8	1	3	2	4	10	8	4	2	6
777	5	4	1	38	125	2	1	1	1	5	1	2	1	3	7	5	2	1	3
778	6	4	23	110	407	5	1	19	5	18	1	3	5	2	17	15	11	4	3
779	4	2	10	113	621	3	0	2	5	23	2	4	5	15	30	30	19	9	14
780	2	1	3	123	655	0	0	2	6	25	2	5	6	16	33	32	19	10	15
781	1	1	7	151	631	0	0	2	5	20	2	4	6	15	30	24	19	0	6
782	7	5	1	28	74	2	0	0	1	4	0	1	1	2	5	4	1	1	1
783	6	4	23	110	271	5	1	2	5	18	1	3	2	2	17	15	4	4	3
784	3	2	10	118	393	3	0	2	5	21	1	4	5	16	31	24	7	1	10
785	0	0	3	129	429	0	0	2	5	23	1	4	5	17	33	26	8	1	11
786	7	4	1	84	197	4	1	1	5	11	3	3	1	3	10	12	8	5	4
787	3	1	6	75	365	1	1	1	4	15	3	3	3	9	17	18	11	7	8
788	4	2	1	90	158	4	1	1	5	11	3	3	1	3	10	10	3	3	2
789	2	1	7	88	267	2	1	1	4	15	2	3	3	10	20	17	5	2	7
790	0	0	3	129	424	0	0	2	6	23	1	4	5	17	32	25	8	1	10
791	4	2	1	57	151	4	1	1	3	9	2	3	2	3	10	10	3	2	2
800	25	13	93	684	150	20	8	0	9	27	6	4	4	10	75	55	9	9	22
801	6	4	17	410	74	6	1	0	1	8	0	2	1	2	17	22	2	1	5
802	2	1	11	2	55	2	1	0	1	7	0	1	1	4	21	25	2	1	7
803	8	5	26	195	32	10	1	0	0	3	1	1	1	2	2	3	0	2	1
804	6	4	16	378	68	5	1	0	1	7	0	2	0	2	16	20	2	1	5
805	6	4	15	377	68	5	1	0	1	7	0	2	0	2	16	20	2	1	5
806	10	5	26	175	43	7	1	0	1	6	0	2	1	5	23	16	3	1	6
807	5	3	13	235	43	4	0	0	0	4	1	1	2	3	9	7	1	0	3
808	8	5	26	157	38	8	1	0	0	6	0	1	1	6	19	13	2	1	5

Beverages, Dairy, Eggs

Food No.	Food Description & Amount	wt gm	wt oz	cal	% cal fat	prot gm	carbo gm	fiber gm
809	Brick with salami [1 slice]	28	1.0	100	72%	6	1	0.0
810	Brie [1 package]	128	4.5	427	75%	27	1	0.0
811	Camembert [1 wedge]	38	1.3	114	73%	8	0	0.0
812	Cheddar or American type (Include Coon, Longhorn, Wisconsin, New York, Pioneer, Hoop, Tillamook, sharp cheese, Chevres) [1 slice]	28	1.0	113	74%	7	0	0.0
813	Cheddar or American type, dry, grated [2 Tbs]	13	0.5	70	74%	4	0	0.0
814	Cheddar or Colby, low sodium [1 slice]	28	1.0	111	74%	7	1	0.0
815	Cheddar or Colby, low sodium, lowfat [1 slice]	28	1.0	48	36%	7	1	0.0
816	Cheddar or Colby, lowfat [1 slice]	28	1.0	48	36%	7	1	0.0
817	Colby [1 slice]	28	1.0	110	73%	7	1	0.0
818	Cottage cheese, creamed, large or small curd [1 cup]	210	7.4	217	39%	26	6	0.0
819	Cottage cheese, low sodium [1 cup]	225	7.9	232	39%	28	6	0.0
820	Cottage cheese, dry curd (Include baker's, pressed, dutch, skim, nonfat cottage cheese) [1 cup]	145	5.1	123	4%	25	3	0.0
821	Cottage cheese, farmer's [1 cup]	210	7.4	311	61%	25	5	0.0
822	Cottage cheese, lowfat (1-2% fat) (Include lowfat pot cheese) [1 cup]	226	8.0	164	13%	28	6	0.0
823	Cottage cheese, lowfat, lactose reduced [1 cup]	227	8.0	168	12%	28	7	1.4
824	Cottage cheese, lowfat, low sodium [1 cup]	225	7.9	162	13%	28	6	0.0
825	Cottage cheese, lowfat, with fruit or vegetables [1 cup]	226	8.0	174	15%	20	17	1.0
826	Cottage cheese, salted, dry curd [1 cup (not packed)]	145	5.1	121	4%	25	3	0.0
827	Cottage cheese, with gelatin dessert [1 cup]	240	8.5	199	26%	17	19	0.0
828	Cottage cheese, with gelatin dessert and fruit [1 cup]	240	8.5	214	19%	14	31	0.9
829	Cottage cheese, with gelatin dessert and vegetables [1 cup]	240	8.5	205	32%	21	14	0.5
830	Cottage cheese, with fruit (Include creamed or uncreamed; large or small curd) [1 cup]	226	8.0	279	25%	22	30	0.0
831	Cottage cheese, with vegetables [1 cup]	226	8.0	215	40%	25	7	0.0
832	Cream cheese [2 Tbs]	29	1.0	101	90%	2	1	0.0
833	Cream cheese, lowfat [2 Tbs]	29	1.0	68	69%	3	2	0.0
834	Cheese, Feta (Include goat cheese) [1 wedge]	38	1.3	100	73%	5	2	0.0
835	Fontina [1 slice]	28	1.0	109	72%	7	0	0.0
836	Goat cheese [2 Tbs, crumbled]	18	0.6	63	72%	4	0	0.0
837	Gouda or Edam (Include Caciocavallo, Delft, ball cheese) [1 slice]	28	1.0	100	70%	7	0	0.0
838	Gruyere [1 slice]	28	1.0	116	70%	8	0	0.0
839	Imitation cheese, American or cheddar type (Include Cheez-ola, Pretend, Country Meadow) [2 Tbs]	28	1.0	67	53%	5	3	0.0
840	Imitation cheese, American or cheddar type, low cholesterol [1 slice (2¾" x 1¼" x 3/16")]	11	0.4	44	74%	3	0	0.0
841	Imitation cheese spread (Include Count Down) [2 Tbs]	28	1.0	35	7%	5	3	0.0
842	Imitation cream cheese [2 Tbs]	29	1.0	67	83%	1	2	0.0
843	Imitation mozzarella cheese (Include Pizza Mate) [1 slice]	28	1.0	69	44%	3	7	0.0
844	Limburger [1 slice]	28	1.0	93	75%	6	0	0.0
845	Monterey [1 slice]	28	1.0	105	73%	7	0	0.0
846	Monterey, lowfat [1 slice]	28	1.0	89	62%	8	0	0.0
847	Mozzarella, (Include pizza cheese, string cheese, cheese sticks) [1 slice]	28	1.0	78	55%	8	1	0.0
848	Mozzarella, nonfat or fat free [1 cup, shredded]	113	4.0	168	0%	36	4	2.0
849	Mozzarella, low sodium [1 slice]	28	1.0	78	55%	8	1	0.0
850	Muenster [1 slice]	28	1.0	103	73%	7	0	0.0
851	Muenster, lowfat [1 slice]	28	1.0	77	58%	7	1	0.0
852	Muenster, low sodium [1 slice]	28	1.0	103	73%	7	0	0.0
853	Parmesan, dry grated (Include Romano) [2 Tbs]	13	0.4	57	59%	5	0	0.0
854	Parmesan, dry grated, low sodium [2 Tbs]	13	0.4	57	59%	5	0	0.0
855	Parmesan, hard (Include Romano) [1 cubic inch]	10	0.4	40	59%	4	0	0.0
856	Parmesan cheese topping, fat free [2 Tbs]	15	0.5	56	12%	6	6	0.0
857	Port du Salut [1 slice]	28	1.0	98	72%	7	0	0.0

Food no.	fat gm	sat fat gm	choles mg	sodium mg	potas mg	% of Daily Value: vit A	vit E	vit C	thia	ribo	niac	vit B-6	fola	vit B-12	calc	phos	mag	iron	zinc
809	8	5	26	171	40	8	1	0	1	6	1	1	1	7	17	12	2	1	5
810	35	22	128	806	195	23	4	0	6	39	2	15	21	35	24	24	6	4	20
811	9	6	27	320	71	10	1	0	1	11	1	4	6	8	15	13	2	1	6
812	9	6	29	174	28	8	0	0	1	6	0	1	1	4	20	14	2	1	6
813	6	4	18	108	17	5	0	0	0	4	0	1	1	2	13	9	1	1	4
814	9	6	28	6	31	8	0	0	0	6	0	1	1	4	20	14	2	1	6
815	2	1	6	6	31	2	0	0	0	0	0	1	1	4	20	14	2	1	6
816	2	1	6	171	18	2	0	0	0	4	0	1	1	2	12	14	1	1	3
817	9	6	27	169	35	8	0	0	0	6	0	1	1	4	19	13	2	1	6
818	9	6	31	850	177	10	1	0	3	20	1	7	6	22	13	28	3	2	5
819	10	6	34	29	189	11	1	0	3	21	1	8	7	23	14	30	3	2	6
820	1	0	10	19	47	1	1	0	2	12	1	6	5	20	5	15	1	2	5
821	21	13	61	801	167	21	3	0	3	19	1	7	6	21	12	26	3	2	5
822	2	1	10	918	193	2	1	0	3	22	1	8	7	24	14	30	3	2	6
823	2	1	9	499	195	2	1	0	3	21	1	8	7	24	12	30	3	2	6
824	2	1	9	29	194	2	1	0	3	21	1	8	7	24	14	30	3	2	6
825	3	2	12	594	218	6	4	3	3	17	3	6	5	17	10	23	3	3	5
826	1	0	10	580	47	1	1	0	2	12	1	6	5	20	5	15	1	2	5
827	6	4	19	570	110	6	1	0	2	13	1	4	4	13	8	19	2	1	3
828	4	3	15	437	160	6	2	3	2	10	2	6	4	10	7	16	3	2	3
829	7	5	24	673	190	23	1	14	3	16	2	7	6	16	10	23	3	2	4
830	8	5	25	915	151	8	1	0	3	17	1	6	5	19	11	24	2	1	4
831	9	6	32	911	194	17	1	15	2	17	1	6	6	18	13	29	2	1	4
832	10	6	32	86	35	13	1	0	0	3	0	1	1	2	2	3	0	2	1
833	5	3	16	87	49	6	1	0	0	5	0	1	1	3	3	4	1	3	1
834	8	6	34	424	23	5	0	0	4	19	2	8	3	11	19	13	2	1	7
835	9	5	32	224	18	8	0	0	0	3	0	1	0	8	15	10	1	0	7
836	5	3	13	72	14	7	0	0	1	8	1	1	0	1	8	8	1	2	1
837	8	5	27	258	47	6	1	0	1	6	0	1	1	7	20	15	2	1	7
838	9	5	31	94	23	8	0	0	1	5	0	1	1	7	28	17	3	0	7
839	4	2	10	378	68	4	0	0	1	7	0	2	0	2	16	20	2	1	5
840	4	1	2	76	6	2	0	0	0	2	0	0	1	2	8	6	1	0	2
841	0	0	1	394	82	0	0	0	1	8	0	2	1	2	15	22	2	1	5
842	6	1	0	245	127	0	14	0	0	0	0	0	0	0	0	10	0	1	2
843	3	1	0	192	127	12	3	0	0	7	0	1	1	4	17	16	3	1	4
844	8	5	26	227	36	9	1	0	2	8	0	1	4	5	14	11	1	0	4
845	8	5	25	150	23	7	0	0	0	6	0	1	1	4	21	12	2	1	6
846	6	4	18	160	23	9	1	0	0	6	0	1	1	4	20	13	2	1	6
847	5	3	15	148	27	5	1	0	0	6	0	1	1	4	20	15	2	0	6
848	0	0	20	797	120	23	1	0	2	20	1	5	3	17	100	74	9	2	30
849	5	3	15	4	27	5	1	0	0	6	0	1	1	4	20	15	2	0	6
850	8	5	27	176	38	9	1	0	0	5	0	1	1	7	20	13	2	1	5
851	5	3	18	168	38	5	0	0	0	6	0	1	1	7	15	13	2	1	5
852	8	5	27	5	38	9	1	0	0	5	0	1	1	7	20	13	2	1	5
853	4	2	10	233	13	2	0	0	0	3	0	1	0	3	17	10	2	1	3
854	4	2	10	8	13	2	0	0	0	3	0	1	0	3	17	10	2	1	3
855	3	2	7	165	9	2	0	0	0	2	0	0	0	2	12	7	1	0	2
856	1	0	3	173	90	7	0	0	1	0	0	1	1	3	12	11	2	4	3
857	8	5	34	150	38	10	1	0	0	4	0	1	1	7	18	10	2	1	5

Beverages, Dairy, Eggs

Food No.	Food Description & Amount	wt gm	wt oz	cal	% cal fat	prot gm	carbo gm	fiber gm
858	Processed cheese food [1 slice]	21	0.7	69	67%	4	2	0.0
859	Processed cheese, American and Swiss blends [1 slice]	21	0.7	79	75%	5	0	0.0
860	Processed cheese, American or cheddar type, lowfat, low sodium [1 slice]	21	0.7	38	35%	5	1	0.0
861	Processed cheese, American or cheddar type, lowfat [1 slice)]	21	0.7	38	35%	5	1	0.0
862	Processed cheese, American or cheddar type (Include American Cheese Slices; Cheezes; Cheez Kisses) [1 slice]	21	0.7	70	69%	4	1	0.0
863	Processed cheese, cheddar or American type, nonfat or fat free [1 slice]	21	0.7	31	5%	5	3	0.0
864	Processed cheese, American or cheddar type, low sodium [1 slice]	21	0.7	79	75%	5	0	0.0
865	Processed cream cheese product, nonfat or fat free [2 Tbs]	31	1.1	30	13%	5	2	0.0
866	Processed Mozzarella cheese, low sodium [1 slice]	21	0.7	59	55%	6	1	0.0
867	Processed Muenster cheese, lowfat, low sodium [1 slice]	21	0.7	35	38%	5	0	0.0
868	Processed Swiss cheese [1 slice]	21	0.7	70	67%	5	0	0.0
869	Processed Swiss cheese, low sodium [1 slice]	21	0.7	70	67%	5	0	0.0
870	Processed Swiss cheese, lowfat [1 slice]	21	0.7	36	27%	5	1	0.0
871	Processed cheese with vegetables (Include pepper cheese, pimiento) [1 oz]	28	1.0	105	75%	6	0	0.0
872	Processed cheese with wine [1 oz]	28	1.0	92	67%	5	2	0.0
873	Processed cheese product, American or cheddar type, reduced fat [1 slice]	34	1.2	82	53%	6	4	0.0
874	Processed cheese product, Swiss, reduced fat [1 slice]	21	0.7	44	45%	4	1	0.0
875	Provolone [1 slice]	28	1.0	98	68%	7	1	0.0
876	Provolone, reduced fat, reduced sodium [1 slice]	28	1.0	77	58%	7	1	0.0
877	Puerto Rican white cheese (queso del pais, blanco) [2 Tbs]	28	1.0	48	67%	3	1	0.0
878	Queso Anejo (aged Mexican cheese) [2 Tbs, crumbled]	17	0.6	62	72%	4	1	0.0
879	Queso Asadero (Include Oaxacan-style string cheese) [1 slice]	28	1.0	100	71%	6	1	0.0
880	Queso Chihuahua (Include Mennonite cheese) [1 slice]	28	1.0	105	71%	6	2	0.0
881	Queso Fresco (Include Hispanic-style farmer cheese) [1 oz]	28	1.0	41	52%	3	2	0.0
882	Ricotta [1 cup]	246	8.7	384	60%	28	10	0.0
883	Semi-soft cheese, low sodium [1 slice]	28	1.0	110	74%	7	0	0.0
884	Swiss (Include Emmentaler, Asiago, Jarlsburg, Samsoe, Danbo, Sweitzer) [1 slice]	28	1.0	105	66%	8	1	0.0
885	Swiss, low fat [1 slice]	28	1.0	50	26%	8	1	0.0
886	Swiss, low sodium [1 slice]	28	1.0	105	66%	8	1	0.0
887	Yogurt cheese [1 cup]	245	8.6	186	2%	19	25	0.0
	Eggs (Chicken eggs unless specified otherwise)							
925	Duck egg, cooked [1 egg]	70	2.5	130	67%	9	1	0.0
926	Egg casserole with bread, cheese, milk and meat [1 cup]	164	5.8	384	59%	20	18	0.9
927	Egg omelet or scrambled egg, with chicken [1 egg]	95	3.4	150	53%	15	2	0.0
928	Egg omelet or scrambled egg, plain [1 egg]	60	2.1	80	58%	6	1	0.0
929	Egg omelet or scrambled egg, with beef and onions [1 egg]	95	3.4	152	63%	11	3	0.1
930	Egg omelet or scrambled egg, with cheese and ham [1 egg]	78	2.8	156	65%	11	2	0.0
931	Egg omelet or scrambled egg, with cheese [1 egg]	67	2.4	127	66%	8	2	0.0
932	Egg omelet or scrambled egg, with chorizo [1 egg]	70	2.5	147	69%	9	2	0.0
933	Egg omelet or scrambled egg, with dark-green vegetables [1 egg]	84	3.0	110	63%	8	2	0.5
934	Egg omelet or scrambled egg, with fish [1 egg]	88	3.1	136	61%	11	2	0.0
935	Egg omelet or scrambled egg, with ham or bacon [1 egg]	70	2.5	130	64%	10	1	0.0
936	Egg omelet or scrambled egg, with mushrooms [1 egg]	69	2.4	88	63%	6	2	0.4
937	Egg omelet or scrambled egg, with onions, peppers, tomatoes, and mushrooms (Include Spanish omelet) [1 egg]	145	5.1	178	69%	8	6	1.1
938	Egg omelet or scrambled egg, with peppers, onion, and ham (Include Western omelet) [1 egg]	94	3.3	146	62%	11	3	0.2
939	Egg omelet or scrambled egg, with potatoes and/or onions (Tortilla Espanola, traditional style Spanish omelet) [1 egg]	156	5.5	199	50%	10	15	1.2
940	Egg omelet or scrambled egg, with sausage [1 egg]	87	3.1	204	71%	12	2	0.0
941	Egg omelet or scrambled egg, with sausage and cheese [1 egg]	85	3.0	189	70%	11	2	0.0
942	Egg omelet or scrambled egg, with sausage and mushrooms [1 egg]	95	3.4	167	67%	11	2	0.1

Food no.	fat gm	sat fat gm	choles mg	sodium mg	potas mg	% of Daily Value													
						vit A	vit E	vit C	thia	ribo	niac	vit B-6	fola	vit B-12	calc	phos	mag	iron	zinc
858	5	3	13	250	59	5	1	0	0	5	0	1	0	4	12	10	2	1	4
859	7	4	20	300	34	6	0	0	0	4	0	1	0	2	13	16	1	0	4
860	1	1	7	1	38	1	0	0	0	5	0	1	0	3	14	17	1	1	5
861	1	1	7	300	38	1	0	0	0	5	0	1	0	3	14	17	1	1	5
862	5	3	14	257	55	5	1	0	0	5	0	1	0	4	12	10	2	1	4
863	0	0	2	321	60	9	0	0	1	6	0	1	1	4	14	20	2	0	5
864	7	4	20	1	34	6	0	0	0	4	0	1	0	2	13	16	1	0	4
865	0	0	3	170	51	9	0	0	1	3	0	1	3	3	6	14	1	0	2
866	4	2	11	3	20	4	0	0	0	4	0	1	1	3	15	11	1	0	4
867	1	1	5	1	28	1	0	0	0	4	0	1	1	5	15	10	1	0	4
868	5	3	18	288	45	5	1	0	0	3	0	0	0	4	16	16	2	1	5
869	5	3	18	9	45	5	1	0	0	3	0	0	0	4	16	16	2	1	5
870	1	1	7	300	38	1	0	0	0	5	0	1	0	3	14	17	1	1	5
871	9	6	26	400	45	9	1	1	1	6	0	1	1	3	17	21	2	1	6
872	7	4	18	333	78	6	1	0	1	7	0	2	1	5	16	13	2	1	6
873	5	3	18	540	112	8	1	0	2	10	0	1	2	6	18	28	3	0	5
874	2	1	11	259	59	4	0	0	0	4	0	1	0	3	15	7	1	1	5
875	7	5	19	245	39	7	0	0	0	5	0	1	1	7	21	14	2	1	6
876	5	3	15	123	39	10	0	0	0	6	0	1	1	7	35	14	2	1	6
877	4	2	14	23	29	4	0	0	0	3	0	1	1	2	6	4	1	1	2
878	5	3	17	187	14	1	0	0	0	2	0	0	0	4	11	7	1	0	3
879	8	5	29	183	24	2	0	0	0	4	0	1	1	5	19	12	2	1	6
880	8	5	29	173	15	2	0	0	0	4	0	1	0	5	18	12	2	1	7
881	2	1	9	37	37	3	0	0	0	3	0	0	1	1	8	5	1	1	3
882	26	16	100	257	282	30	3	0	3	27	1	4	8	13	59	42	8	6	21
883	9	6	25	35	38	6	1	0	2	4	0	1	1	7	25	13	2	1	5
884	8	5	26	73	31	7	1	0	0	6	0	1	0	8	27	17	3	0	7
885	1	1	10	73	31	2	0	0	0	6	0	1	0	8	27	17	3	0	7
886	8	5	26	4	31	7	1	0	0	6	0	1	0	8	27	17	3	0	7
887	0	0	7	186	625	0	0	4	8	33	1	6	7	25	49	38	12	1	16
925	10	3	619	102	156	28	2	0	6	16	1	8	11	54	4	15	3	15	7
926	25	11	159	959	323	15	4	2	24	28	14	9	6	15	31	33	8	12	16
927	9	3	245	114	165	13	4	0	3	18	16	12	5	10	5	18	4	6	6
928	5	2	201	69	86	10	2	0	2	15	0	3	4	8	5	10	2	4	4
929	11	3	268	123	151	15	5	1	3	21	3	6	6	14	6	15	3	6	8
930	11	5	198	372	145	13	4	0	7	18	3	6	4	10	11	18	3	5	8
931	9	4	191	229	110	13	4	0	2	17	0	4	4	9	11	15	3	4	6
932	11	4	201	240	132	11	3	0	7	17	3	6	4	11	5	12	2	5	7
933	8	2	223	108	167	22	5	16	3	18	1	5	10	8	7	12	4	7	5
934	9	3	254	186	151	14	5	0	3	20	5	6	6	19	9	17	3	5	6
935	9	3	177	330	133	9	3	0	10	15	5	7	4	9	4	13	3	4	7
936	6	2	177	147	97	10	3	0	3	14	2	4	4	7	4	10	2	4	4
937	14	3	220	170	269	21	9	32	5	21	4	8	7	8	6	14	4	6	5
938	10	3	232	274	161	13	4	9	9	19	4	8	5	10	5	15	3	5	7
939	11	3	282	143	329	18	6	8	7	22	4	13	8	11	8	17	6	7	7
940	16	5	233	443	187	13	4	1	15	20	6	8	5	16	6	16	3	6	9
941	15	5	232	389	168	15	5	1	9	21	3	7	5	14	11	18	3	5	8
942	13	4	267	294	161	15	5	1	9	21	3	7	6	13	6	16	3	6	7

Beverages, Dairy, Eggs

Food No.	Food Description & Amount	wt gm	wt oz	cal	% cal fat	prot gm	carbo gm	fiber gm
943	Egg omelet or scrambled egg, with vegetables other than dark-green vegetables [1 egg]	64	2.3	84	62%	6	2	0.3
944	Egg omelet or scrambled, with chili, cheese, tomatoes, and beans [1 egg]	103	3.6	159	63%	10	4	0.6
945	Egg omelet with ripe plantain, Puerto Rican style (Tortilla de amarillo) [1 cup]	173	6.1	396	60%	11	32	2.2
946	Scrambled egg, made from cholesterol-free frozen mix (Include Egg Beaters) [1 cup, cooked]	153	5.4	252	65%	16	6	0.0
947	Scrambled egg, made from cholesterol-free frozen mix with cheese (Include Egg Beaters Cheese) [1 cup, cooked]	153	5.4	265	63%	17	7	0.0
948	Scrambled egg, made from cholesterol-free frozen mixture with vegetables [1 cup, cooked]	188	6.6	136	31%	17	5	0.3
949	Scrambled egg, made from dry eggs [1 cup]	214	7.5	461	80%	20	2	0.0
950	Scrambled egg, made from frozen mix (Include Egg Delight) [1 cup, cooked]	140	4.9	174	46%	15	9	0.0
951	Scrambled egg, made from packaged liquid mix (Include Second Nature) [1 cup, cooked]	210	7.4	214	47%	23	4	0.0
952	Scrambled egg, made from powdered mix (Include Eggstra) [1 cup, cooked]	188	6.6	361	66%	21	8	0.0
953	Scrambled eggs with jerked beef, Puerto Rican style (Revoltillo de tasajo) [1 cup]	140	4.9	375	64%	29	4	0.4
954	Shrimp-egg patty (Torta de Cameron seco) (Include dried shrimp patties) [1 patty (2" dia)]	18	0.6	77	67%	4	2	0.1
955	Egg salad [1 egg]	74	2.6	236	87%	7	1	0.0
956	Egg substitute (Include from powdered, frozen, or liquid) [1 cup, cooked]	210	7.4	256	51%	28	2	0.0
957	Eggs Benedict [1 egg]	155	5.5	288	55%	17	15	0.8
958	Egg, creamed [1 egg]	145	5.1	218	63%	11	8	0.2
959	Egg, deviled [½ egg]	31	1.1	63	73%	4	0	0.0
960	Egg, goose, cooked [1 egg]	144	5.1	267	65%	20	2	0.0
961	Egg, quail, canned [1 egg]	9	0.3	14	63%	1	0	0.0
962	Egg, white only, cooked, salted [1 white]	33	1.2	17	0%	3	0	0.0
963	Egg, white only, raw (Include cooked unsalted) [1 white]	33	1.2	17	0%	3	0	0.0
964	Egg, whole, baked, salted [1 egg]	45	1.6	75	61%	6	1	0.0
965	Egg, whole, boiled in salted water [1 egg]	50	1.8	78	62%	6	1	0.0
966	Egg, whole, fried (Include scrambled egg, no milk added) [1 egg]	46	1.6	91	68%	6	1	0.0
967	Egg, whole, pickled [1 egg]	47	1.7	73	62%	6	1	0.0
968	Egg, whole, poached in salted water (Include cooked and salted egg) [1 egg]	50	1.8	75	61%	6	1	0.0
969	Egg, whole, raw (Include cooked unsalted) [1 egg]	50	1.8	75	61%	6	1	0.0
970	Egg, yolk only, raw or cooked [1 yolk]	17	0.6	61	78%	3	0	0.0
971	Eggs a la Malaguena, Puerto Rican style (Huevos a la Malaguena) [1 egg]	123	4.3	126	43%	11	8	1.8
972	Huevos rancheros [1 egg]	118	4.2	139	51%	8	10	1.9
	Your Additions							

Food no.	fat gm	sat fat gm	choles mg	sodium mg	potas mg	% of Daily Value: vit A	vit E	vit C	thia	ribo	niac	vit B-6	fola	vit B-12	calc	phos	mag	iron	zinc
943	6	2	170	98	88	10	3	1	2	13	1	3	4	6	4	9	2	4	4
944	11	4	250	261	200	23	5	6	4	22	1	6	7	11	12	19	4	6	7
945	26	5	346	106	535	24	21	21	6	26	3	18	10	12	4	18	11	10	7
946	18	3	3	320	342	24	15	1	10	31	1	9	4	9	15	13	6	14	9
947	19	4	8	478	348	23	14	1	9	32	1	9	4	8	21	22	6	13	11
948	5	1	1	314	333	9	3	15	2	41	2	3	2	7	7	8	6	1	2
949	41	10	715	502	218	35	24	0	5	37	1	8	13	24	11	35	5	16	15
950	9	2	67	220	208	30	6	1	1	21	1	1	5	5	6	7	4	1	2
951	11	2	3	401	675	47	8	1	12	34	1	1	6	11	17	27	5	21	17
952	27	6	217	561	293	35	18	0	5	38	1	3	9	19	13	19	7	7	5
953	27	6	392	2247	409	16	20	2	7	32	17	17	10	38	5	27	8	23	28
954	6	1	86	145	42	4	5	0	2	5	2	2	2	5	2	4	2	4	2
955	23	4	235	188	73	11	14	0	2	16	0	9	6	11	3	10	1	4	4
956	15	3	2	489	763	57	10	0	14	39	1	0	6	10	12	28	5	27	20
957	17	6	226	1007	223	15	5	0	24	23	14	15	7	13	9	22	5	10	11
958	15	4	279	365	207	15	8	1	7	28	2	6	8	16	13	19	4	6	7
959	5	1	122	50	37	5	3	0	1	9	0	2	3	5	1	5	1	2	2
960	19	5	1227	199	302	55	5	0	12	31	1	16	20	104	9	30	6	29	13
961	1	0	75	47	12	1	0	0	1	4	0	1	1	2	1	2	0	2	1
962	0	0	0	54	47	0	0	0	0	8	0	0	0	1	0	0	1	0	0
963	0	0	0	54	47	0	0	0	0	9	0	0	0	1	0	0	1	0	0
964	5	2	212	63	60	10	2	0	2	14	0	3	4	7	2	9	1	4	4
965	5	2	212	62	63	8	2	0	2	15	0	3	6	9	3	9	1	3	4
966	7	2	212	85	61	11	4	0	2	14	0	3	4	7	3	9	1	4	4
967	5	2	199	58	59	8	2	0	2	14	0	3	5	9	2	8	1	3	3
968	5	2	213	63	61	10	2	0	2	13	0	3	4	7	2	9	1	4	4
969	5	2	213	63	61	10	2	0	2	15	0	3	6	8	2	9	1	4	4
970	5	2	218	7	16	10	2	0	2	6	0	3	6	9	2	8	0	3	4
971	6	2	231	513	303	17	6	14	9	19	6	9	9	8	4	15	5	8	7
972	8	2	217	249	199	14	6	21	4	16	3	8	7	7	8	15	5	8	6

Desserts and Sweets

Desserts & Sweets

Food No.	Food Description & Amount	wt gm	wt oz	cal	% cal fat	prot gm	carbo gm	fiber gm
	Cakes							
1000	Cake batter, raw, chocolate [2 Tbs]	28	1.0	88	38%	1	13	0.5
1001	Cake batter, raw, not chocolate [2 Tbs]	30	1.1	86	26%	1	15	0.2
1002	Cake, angel food, chocolate, no icing [1/12 of 10" dia]	57	2.0	141	2%	4	32	0.5
1003	Cake, angel food, with icing [1/12 of 10" dia]	77	2.7	207	1%	4	49	0.1
1004	Cake, angel food, no icing [1/12 of 10" dia]	57	2.0	143	1%	3	33	0.1
1005	Cake, applesauce with raisins, low calorie, no icing (Include Weight Watcher's Apple Raisin Spice Cake) [1 individual cake]	74	2.6	173	21%	4	32	1.6
1006	Cake, applesauce with raisins, with icing [1/12 of 10" dia]	108	3.8	399	30%	3	69	1.4
1007	Cake, applesauce with raisins, no icing (Include rhubarb, blueberry, apricot, blackberry, apple crunch cake) [1/12 of 10" dia]	87	3.1	313	33%	3	52	1.6
1008	Cake, banana, with icing [1/12 of 10" dia]	108	3.8	327	22%	4	61	1.4
1009	Cake, banana, no icing [1/12 of 10" dia]	87	3.1	262	27%	3	46	1.3
1010	Cake, Black Forest (chocolate-cherry) [1/12 of 2-layer, 8" dia]	71	2.5	187	43%	2	27	0.9
1011	Cake, Boston cream pie [1/12 of 8" dia]	69	2.4	174	30%	2	30	1.0
1012	Cake, butter, with icing [1/10 of 1-layer, 8" dia]	83	2.9	313	35%	3	50	0.7
1013	Cake, butter, no icing [1/10 of 8" dia]	53	1.9	193	41%	2	27	0.3
1014	Cake, carrot, low calorie (Include Weight Watcher's) [1 individual cake]	85	3.0	179	33%	4	28	1.2
1015	Cake, carrot, with icing (Include carrot cupcakes with icing) [1/10 of 1-layer, 8" dia]	80	2.8	328	46%	3	43	0.9
1016	Cake, carrot, no icing (Include carrot pudding) [1/10 of 8" dia]	58	2.0	242	50%	2	29	0.8
1017	Cake, chiffon, chocolate, with icing [1/12 of 10" dia]	92	3.2	328	41%	5	47	1.6
1018	Cake, chiffon, chocolate, no icing [1/12 of 10" dia]	66	2.3	227	41%	4	31	1.0
1019	Cake, chiffon, with icing [1/12 of 10" dia]	92	3.2	317	34%	4	49	0.3
1020	Cake, chiffon, no icing [1/12 of 10" dia]	66	2.3	219	36%	4	32	0.3
1021	Cake, chocolate, devil's food, or fudge, pudding-type mix, with icing (Include Pillsbury Plus, Duncan Hines, Betty Crocker Super Moist [1/12 of 2-layer, 8" dia]	109	3.8	401	38%	4	62	1.9
1022	Cake, chocolate, devil's food, or fudge, pudding-type mix, no icing (Include Pillsbury Plus, Duncan Hines, Betty Crocker Super Moist [1/10 of 8" dia]	42	1.5	147	48%	2	19	0.8
1023	Cake, chocolate, devil's food, or fudge, pudding-type mix, made by "Lite" recipe (eggs and water added to dry mix; no oil added), with icing [1/12 of 2-layer, 8" dia]	109	3.8	373	29%	4	66	2.1
1024	Cake, chocolate, devil's food, or fudge, pudding type mix, made by "no cholesterol" recipe (water, oil and egg whites added to dry mix), with "light" icing [1/10 of 1-layer, 8" dia]	66	2.3	220	29%	2	39	0.8
1025	Cake, chocolate, devil's food, or fudge, pudding type mix, made by "no cholesterol" recipe (water, oil and egg whites added to dry mix), no icing [1/10 of 8" dia]	42	1.5	136	40%	2	20	0.6
1026	Cake, chocolate, devil's food, or fudge, standard-type mix (eggs and water added to dry mix), with icing (Include Jiffy, Washington) [1/12 of 2-layer, 8" dia]	109	3.8	390	30%	4	69	1.7
1027	Cake, chocolate, devil's food, or fudge, standard-type mix (eggs and water added to dry mix), no icing [1/10 of 8" dia]	42	1.5	138	34%	2	22	0.7
1028	Cake, chocolate, devil's food, or fudge, with icing, made from home recipe or purchased ready-to-eat [1/12 of 2-layer, 8" dia]	109	3.8	410	35%	4	67	1.7
1029	Cake, chocolate, devil's food, or fudge, no icing or filling, made from home recipe or purchased ready-to-eat [1/10 of 8" dia]	42	1.5	152	42%	2	22	0.7
1030	Cake, chocolate, made with mayonnaise or salad dressing, with icing, coating, or filling [1/12 of 2-layer, 8" dia]	139	4.9	487	27%	4	89	2.3
1031	Cake, chocolate, made with mayonnaise or salad dressing, no icing or filling [1/10 of 8" dia]	53	1.9	161	28%	2	28	1.0
1032	Cake, chocolate, with icing, low calorie (Include Weight Watcher's Chocolate Cake) [1 individual cake]	71	2.5	217	25%	5	40	2.8
1033	Cake, coconut, with icing [1/12 of 2-layer, 8" dia]	109	3.8	388	26%	5	69	1.1

Food no.	fat gm	sat fat gm	choles mg	sodium mg	potas mg	% of Daily Value: vit A	vit E	vit C	thia	ribo	niac	vit B-6	fola	vit B-12	calc	phos	mag	iron	zinc
1000	4	1	12	95	49	1	2	0	3	3	2	1	1	1	3	4	2	4	1
1001	3	0	14	128	19	1	2	0	3	3	2	1	1	1	3	6	1	2	1
1002	0	0	0	275	91	0	0	0	3	7	1	0	1	0	5	13	3	2	1
1003	0	0	0	284	79	0	0	0	3	7	0	0	1	0	5	13	1	1	0
1004	0	0	0	283	75	0	0	0	3	7	0	0	1	0	5	13	1	1	0
1005	4	1	28	93	195	8	2	2	9	9	5	4	2	2	4	6	3	7	2
1006	13	3	20	163	137	4	8	1	8	7	5	3	1	1	2	4	3	7	2
1007	12	2	22	141	145	1	7	2	9	7	5	3	1	1	2	5	3	8	2
1008	8	2	33	191	178	9	6	5	9	11	6	11	3	1	3	5	4	6	2
1009	8	2	32	181	168	8	5	5	9	10	6	11	3	1	3	5	4	6	2
1010	9	3	39	160	118	3	5	16	1	8	2	3	1	3	3	7	3	4	3
1011	6	2	26	99	27	2	3	0	19	11	1	1	1	2	2	3	1	1	1
1012	12	6	64	313	78	9	3	0	3	6	2	2	2	2	5	11	3	4	2
1013	9	4	56	281	36	6	3	0	3	6	2	2	1	2	4	10	1	3	1
1014	7	2	14	338	109	44	4	5	7	7	4	3	2	2	5	5	2	5	2
1015	17	3	48	82	79	42	13	2	7	8	4	2	2	2	5	5	2	6	2
1016	14	2	39	61	65	35	12	2	6	6	4	2	2	1	4	4	1	5	1
1017	15	5	74	140	152	6	8	0	8	11	5	2	2	3	8	11	8	11	5
1018	10	3	71	111	108	4	6	0	7	10	4	2	2	3	7	9	5	9	3
1019	12	2	71	163	71	6	9	3	8	10	5	1	2	3	7	6	1	8	2
1020	9	1	69	123	62	3	7	0	8	10	5	1	2	3	6	6	1	8	2
1021	17	3	48	407	199	6	13	0	5	8	4	1	2	5	6	15	7	9	4
1022	8	2	29	219	88	1	6	0	3	4	3	1	1	3	3	8	3	4	2
1023	12	3	39	484	187	0	1	0	6	7	5	1	2	5	7	15	5	9	3
1024	7	2	0	273	105	0	3	0	3	4	3	0	1	3	4	8	3	4	2
1025	6	1	0	237	94	0	2	0	3	3	3	0	1	2	3	7	3	4	1
1026	13	3	34	434	221	6	8	0	5	7	4	1	2	1	8	16	8	14	4
1027	5	1	23	257	106	1	3	0	3	4	2	1	1	1	5	9	4	8	2
1028	16	5	31	186	157	6	8	0	8	9	5	1	2	2	10	11	8	11	4
1029	7	2	19	83	61	1	3	0	5	5	3	1	1	1	6	6	4	6	2
1030	14	3	6	459	182	8	8	0	11	9	7	1	2	1	5	9	8	12	4
1031	5	1	4	244	67	1	3	0	7	5	4	1	1	0	2	4	3	6	2
1032	6	2	35	99	293	7	3	0	10	12	6	2	3	4	6	12	11	12	6
1033	11	4	1	310	108	1	1	0	9	12	6	2	1	1	10	8	3	7	2

Desserts & Sweets

Food No.	Food Description & Amount	wt gm	wt oz	cal	% cal fat	prot gm	carbo gm	fiber gm
1034	Cake, cream (Include Italian rum-cream) [1/10 of 8" dia]	51	1.8	192	35%	3	29	0.3
1035	Cake, Dobos Torte (Include seven-layer cake) [1/12 of 8" dia]	123	4.3	496	50%	8	58	1.4
1036	Cake, frozen yogurt and cake layer, not chocolate, with icing [1/8 of cake]	148	5.2	429	26%	6	75	0.6
1037	Cake, frozen yogurt and cake layer, chocolate, with icing [1/8 of cake]	148	5.2	439	34%	6	71	1.5
1038	Cake, fruit cake, light or dark [1/12 of 7" dia]	113	4.0	366	25%	3	70	4.2
1039	Cake, German chocolate [1/12 of 2-layer, 8" dia]	109	3.8	396	46%	4	54	2.0
1040	Cake, gingerbread [1/10 of 8" dia]	69	2.4	213	30%	3	35	0.8
1041	Cake, graham cracker [1/10 of 9" dia]	45	1.6	159	39%	3	22	0.4
1042	Cake made with glutinous rice and dried beans [1 cubic inch]	21	0.7	38	2%	2	8	0.6
1043	Cake, ice box with fruit and whipped cream [1/10 of cake]	83	2.9	172	21%	4	31	0.4
1044	Cake, ice cream roll (or cake), chocolate [1/10 of roll]	34	1.2	101	44%	1	14	0.4
1045	Cake, ice cream roll (or cake), not chocolate [1/10 of roll]	34	1.2	92	40%	1	13	0.1
1046	Cake, jelly roll [1/10 of roll]	51	1.8	147	14%	3	29	0.2
1047	Cake, lemon, with icing [1/12 of 2-layer, 8" dia]	109	3.8	385	25%	3	71	0.6
1048	Cake, lemon, no icing [1/10 of 8" dia]	42	1.5	159	43%	2	21	0.2
1049	Cake, lemon, lowfat, no icing [1/10 of 1-layer, 8" dia]	42	1.5	132	23%	2	23	0.2
1050	Cake, lemon, lowfat, with icing [1/10 of 1-layer, 8" dia]	66	2.3	231	24%	2	43	0.2
1051	Cake, marble, with icing [1/12 of 2-layer, 8" dia]	109	3.8	377	31%	5	65	2.1
1052	Cake, marble, no icing [1/10 of 8" dia]	42	1.5	140	30%	2	24	0.7
1053	Cake, nut, with icing (Include butter pecan cake; pistachio cake) [1/12 of 2-layer, 8" dia]	109	3.8	420	42%	3	60	0.8
1054	Cake, nut, no icing (Include butter pecan cake; pistachio cake) [1/10 of 8" dia]	42	1.5	161	50%	2	19	0.5
1055	Cake, oatmeal [1/10 of cake]	78	2.8	282	34%	3	45	1.5
1056	Cake, oatmeal, with icing [1/10 of cake]	110	3.9	409	31%	3	70	1.4
1057	Cake, peanut butter, with icing [1/12 of 2-layer, 8" dia]	109	3.8	410	36%	6	62	1.3
1058	Cake, pineapple, very lowfat, no cholesterol, no icing [1 slice (3¾" x 2" x ½")]	28	1.0	69	1%	2	15	0.4
1059	Cake, plum pudding (Include date pudding) [1 piece]	42	1.5	131	39%	2	19	0.7
1060	Cake, Poor Man's (spice-type) [1/10 of 8" square]	48	1.7	154	23%	2	28	0.6
1061	Cake, poppyseed, no icing [1/12 of 10" dia]	90	3.2	356	46%	6	43	0.9
1062	Cake, pound, chocolate, with icing [1/10 of loaf]	91	3.2	386	47%	5	49	1.6
1063	Cake, pound, chocolate, very lowfat, no cholesterol [1 slice (3¼" x 2¾" x ½")]	28	1.0	77	4%	2	17	0.6
1064	Cake, pound, Puerto Rican style (Ponque) [1 slice (3½" x 3½" x 1")]	90	3.2	411	51%	6	45	0.4
1065	Cake, pound, very low fat, no cholesterol (Include Entenmann's Fat-Free, Cholesterol-Free Golden Loaf Cake) [1 slice (3¼" x 2¾" x 5/8")]	28	1.0	79	4%	2	17	0.3
1066	Cake, pound, with icing [1/10 of loaf]	123	4.3	483	35%	7	73	0.5
1067	Cake, pound, no icing (Include toasted cake, yogurt honey pound cake, butter rum cake, whiskey cake, lemon pound cake with glaze) [1/10 of loaf]	91	3.2	354	38%	6	49	0.5
1068	Cake, pound, reduced fat, no cholesterol [1 slice (3½" x 2" x ¾")]	28	1.0	86	20%	2	15	0.3
1069	Cake, pumpkin, no icing [1/10 of 8" square]	51	1.8	153	28%	2	26	0.8
1070	Cake, pumpkin, with icing [1/10 of 1-layer, 8" dia]	80	2.8	271	31%	2	46	0.9
1071	Cake, Quezadilla, El Salvadorian style [1/10 of cake]	150	5.3	526	42%	17	60	0.7
1072	Cake, raisin-nut, with icing [1/12 of 2 layer, 8" dia]	133	4.7	486	33%	6	78	1.9
1073	Cake, raisin-nut, no icing (Include prune cake; date-nut cake, raisin-nut cake) [1/10 of 8" dia]	59	2.1	220	35%	3	34	1.0
1074	Cake, Ravani (made with farina) [1/10 of cake]	56	2.0	176	23%	2	34	0.5
1075	Cake, rice flour (Include coconut mochiko, Filipino cake) [1 piece]	45	1.6	148	42%	2	20	1.0
1076	Cake, rum flavored (Sopa Borracha) [1 slice (4" x 3" x 1¾")]	185	6.5	494	7%	7	105	0.4
1077	Cake, shortcake, biscuit type, with fruit [1 biscuit (2" dia) with fruit]	65	2.3	146	33%	2	23	1.1
1078	Cake, shortcake, biscuit type, with whipped cream and fruit [1 biscuit (2" dia) with fruit and whipped cream]	74	2.6	173	41%	3	24	1.1
1079	Cake, shortcake, sponge type, with fruit [1 cake (3" dia) with fruit]	102	3.6	192	11%	4	40	1.2
1080	Cake, shortcake, sponge type, with whipped cream and fruit (Include strawberry shortcake) [1 cake (3" dia) with fruit and whipped cream]	118	4.2	212	22%	4	40	1.2

Food no.	fat gm	sat fat gm	choles mg	sodium mg	potas mg	vit A	vit E	vit C	thia	ribo	niac	vit B-6	fola	vit B-12	calc	phos	mag	iron	zinc
						% of Daily Value													
1034	8	4	57	90	41	9	1	0	8	7	5	1	1	1	6	5	1	8	2
1035	28	9	188	248	133	24	14	0	6	19	4	4	5	6	3	13	8	10	6
1036	13	4	34	456	181	6	5	1	13	16	8	3	2	5	17	15	4	12	4
1037	16	6	35	427	234	7	5	1	10	15	6	3	2	4	17	17	9	12	5
1038	10	1	6	305	173	2	16	1	4	7	4	3	1	1	4	6	5	13	2
1039	20	5	52	363	148	2	10	0	7	8	5	2	2	2	5	17	4	7	3
1040	7	2	24	316	167	1	4	0	9	8	5	1	2	1	5	12	3	13	2
1041	7	2	33	189	50	7	5	0	3	6	3	1	1	2	5	5	2	4	2
1042	0	0	0	200	47	0	0	0	2	1	2	1	2	0	1	2	2	1	1
1043	4	2	106	33	76	6	1	5	7	10	3	3	3	3	2	6	2	6	2
1044	5	2	15	45	57	2	1	0	3	4	2	1	1	1	4	4	2	3	2
1045	4	2	16	51	46	2	1	0	2	4	1	1	1	1	5	4	1	2	1
1046	2	1	93	30	44	4	1	2	5	9	3	2	2	3	1	5	1	5	2
1047	11	2	34	359	53	6	7	2	5	7	4	2	2	2	7	15	1	5	2
1048	8	1	34	221	27	2	8	0	2	4	2	1	1	1	3	11	1	2	1
1049	3	1	24	209	25	1	2	0	5	5	3	1	1	1	4	8	1	3	1
1050	6	1	24	238	30	4	4	0	5	5	3	1	1	1	4	9	1	3	1
1051	13	5	43	248	185	4	9	0	8	11	6	2	2	2	10	21	8	10	4
1052	5	1	23	126	65	1	4	0	4	5	3	1	1	1	4	9	2	4	1
1053	19	3	52	375	73	6	12	0	7	8	3	3	2	2	6	19	3	5	4
1054	9	1	29	190	38	1	6	0	4	4	2	1	1	1	3	11	2	3	2
1055	11	2	20	129	132	1	7	1	9	7	5	3	1	1	2	6	4	8	2
1056	14	3	21	167	142	4	9	1	12	7	6	3	1	1	2	6	4	11	2
1057	16	6	55	500	217	11	8	0	8	9	12	4	3	2	13	11	7	9	4
1058	0	0	0	65	33	0	0	0	4	5	2	1	1	0	2	3	1	2	1
1059	6	3	15	66	199	1	1	1	4	4	3	4	1	1	5	4	6	5	1
1060	4	1	3	125	21	0	0	0	7	5	5	0	1	0	2	3	1	5	1
1061	18	7	81	312	139	10	8	1	16	17	8	3	4	3	11	12	5	9	5
1062	20	6	69	242	123	18	11	0	10	12	6	2	3	3	4	10	7	9	4
1063	0	0	0	82	79	1	0	0	4	5	2	1	1	1	4	5	2	4	1
1064	23	14	173	243	69	24	3	0	13	14	8	2	3	4	2	8	2	13	3
1065	0	0	0	95	31	1	0	0	2	5	1	0	0	0	1	4	1	3	1
1066	19	4	121	280	91	21	12	0	16	17	10	3	4	4	7	10	2	15	4
1067	15	3	112	230	80	17	9	0	15	15	9	2	3	4	6	9	2	14	3
1068	2	0	0	117	41	0	2	0	4	5	2	0	1	0	5	6	1	3	1
1069	5	1	25	89	50	31	3	1	5	5	3	1	1	1	1	3	2	5	1
1070	9	2	26	118	63	39	6	1	6	6	4	1	2	1	2	4	2	5	1
1071	25	11	124	566	133	35	4	0	12	25	7	4	5	7	45	38	6	11	12
1072	18	4	56	316	252	4	12	1	12	14	7	5	4	2	10	27	8	11	4
1073	9	2	29	153	99	1	6	0	6	7	4	3	2	1	4	13	3	5	2
1074	5	1	19	108	30	5	3	2	4	4	3	1	1	1	4	3	1	4	1
1075	7	6	0	45	106	0	1	1	2	0	3	4	1	0	3	5	5	4	2
1076	4	1	148	63	107	7	2	0	7	17	4	3	4	5	3	9	3	8	4
1077	5	1	0	89	74	1	3	24	8	7	5	1	2	0	7	5	2	6	1
1078	8	3	9	101	89	3	4	23	8	7	5	1	2	1	8	6	2	6	2
1079	2	1	96	31	96	4	1	41	6	10	4	3	4	3	2	6	2	7	2
1080	5	2	109	48	114	7	2	45	3	10	2	3	5	4	3	6	2	5	2

Desserts & Sweets

Food No.	Food Description & Amount	wt gm	wt oz	cal	% cal fat	prot gm	carbo gm	fiber gm
1081	Cake, shortcake, with whipped topping and fruit, low calorie (Include Weight Watchers Strawberry Shortcake) [1 individual]	85	3.0	160	22%	3	30	1.2
1082	Cake, soybean [1/10 of 8" dia]	69	2.4	244	36%	6	37	3.2
1083	Cake, spice, with icing (Include walnut cake with whipped cream, Little Debbie Apple Spice, Stir-n-Frost Spice Cake) [1/12 of 2-layer, 8" dia]	109	3.8	368	29%	5	62	1.0
1084	Cake, spice, no icing [1/10 of 8" dia]	42	1.5	146	30%	2	24	0.5
1085	Cake, sponge, chocolate, with icing [1/12 of 10" dia]	92	3.2	292	22%	7	53	1.7
1086	Cake, sponge, chocolate, no icing [1/12 of 10" dia]	66	2.3	197	18%	5	36	1.0
1087	Cake, sponge, with icing [1/12 of 10" dia]	92	3.2	303	15%	3	62	0.3
1088	Cake, sponge, no icing (Include shortcake, sponge type, plain) [1/12 of 10" dia]	66	2.3	191	8%	4	40	0.4
1089	Cake, sweetpotato, with icing [1/10 of 8" dia]	76	2.7	277	40%	4	39	1.1
1090	Cake, torte, raspberry (Include fruit tortes) [1/12 of torte]	76	2.7	223	44%	3	29	0.9
1091	Cake, upside down, pineapple (Include all fruits) [1/12 of 9" dia]	121	4.3	387	34%	4	61	0.9
1092	Cake, white, pudding-type mix (oil, egg whites, and water added to dry mix), with icing (Include Pillsbury Plus, Duncan Hines, Betty Crocker Super Moist [1/12 of 2-layer, 8" dia]	109	3.8	400	33%	3	66	0.9
1093	Cake, white, pudding-type mix, no icing (Include Pillsbury Plus, Duncan Hines, Betty Crocker Super Moist [1/10 of 8" dia]	42	1.5	147	38%	2	22	0.2
1094	Cake, white, standard-type mix (egg whites and water added to mix), with icing (Include Jiffy, Washington) [1/12 of 2-layer, 8" dia]	109	3.8	393	24%	3	74	1.1
1095	Cake, white, standard-type mix (egg whites and water added to mix), no icing (Include Jiffy, Washington) [1/10 of 8" dia]	42	1.5	139	23%	2	25	0.3
1096	Cake, white, with icing, made from home recipe or purchased ready-to-eat (Include wedding cake) [1/12 of 2-layer, 8" dia]	109	3.8	420	31%	3	70	0.3
1097	Cake, white, no icing, made from home recipe or purchased ready-to-eat [1/10 of 8" dia]	42	1.5	155	38%	2	22	0.2
1098	Cake, white, eggless, lowfat [1/10 of 1-layer, 8" dia]	49	1.7	165	20%	2	31	0.4
1099	Cake, whole wheat, with fruit and nuts (Include apple nut loaf, whole wheat banana carob cake) [1/10 of loaf]	63	2.2	244	34%	3	40	2.4
1100	Cake, yellow, pudding-type mix (oil, eggs, and water added to dry mix), with icing (Include Pillsbury Plus, Duncan Hines, Betty Crocker Super Moist [1/12 of 2-layer, 8" dia]	109	3.8	401	34%	4	64	0.9
1101	Cake, yellow, pudding-type mix (oil, eggs, and water added to dry mix), no icing (Include Pillsbury Plus, Duncan Hines, Betty Crocker Super Moist [1/10 of 8" dia]	42	1.5	148	41%	2	20	0.2
1102	Cake, yellow, standard-type mix (eggs and water added to dry mix), with icing (Include Jiffy, Washington) [1/12 of 2-layer, 8" dia]	109	3.8	384	25%	3	70	1.1
1103	Cake, yellow, standard-type mix (eggs and water added to dry mix), no icing (Include Jiffy, Washington) [1/10 of 8" dia]	42	1.5	134	26%	2	23	0.3
1104	Cake, yellow, with icing, made from home recipe or purchased ready-to-eat [1/12 of 2-layer, 8" dia]	109	3.8	402	28%	4	70	1.0
1105	Cake, yellow, no icing, made from home recipe or purchased ready-to-eat [1/10 of 8" dia]	42	1.5	150	31%	2	24	0.2
1106	Cake, zucchini, with icing [1/12 of 2-layer, 8" dia]	133	4.7	552	45%	6	73	1.5
1107	Cake, zucchini, no icing [1/10 of 8" dia]	58	2.0	231	41%	2	32	0.7
1108	Cheesecake (Include cream cheese pie) [1/12 of 9" dia]	128	4.5	412	54%	11	37	0.4
1109	Cheesecake with cherries (Include other fruit) [1/12 of 9" dia]	142	5.0	389	45%	9	47	0.7
1110	Cheesecake, chocolate [1/12 of 9" dia]	128	4.5	505	57%	8	49	1.9
1111	Cheesecake, chocolate, reduced fat [1 piece (1/12 of 9" dia)]	128	4.5	334	42%	12	41	2.5
1112	Cheesecake, low calorie (Include Weight Watcher's) [1 individual cake (3½" x 3½" x 1")]	113	4.0	253	37%	6	34	0.9
1113	Cheesecake, low calorie, with fruit glaze (Include Weight Watcher's) [1 individual cake (3½" x 3½" x 1")]	113	4.0	242	36%	6	34	1.2
1114	Cheesecake-type dessert, made with yogurt, with fruit [1/10 of 8" dia]	64	2.3	131	21%	1	26	0.9

						% of Daily Value													
Food no.	fat gm	sat fat gm	choles mg	sodium mg	potas mg	vit A	vit E	vit C	thia	ribo	niac	vit B-6	fola	vit B-12	calc	phos	mag	iron	zinc
1081	4	1	7	16	201	0	4	22	8	7	5	1	3	1	7	11	3	6	2
1082	10	2	1	211	236	10	7	2	7	5	6	5	4	1	4	11	11	7	5
1083	12	3	50	281	136	4	10	0	9	11	6	2	2	2	8	21	3	8	2
1084	5	1	24	123	37	1	4	0	4	5	3	1	1	1	3	9	1	3	1
1085	7	3	155	58	150	8	2	2	7	15	4	3	4	5	4	12	8	12	6
1086	4	1	139	42	98	6	2	2	6	13	4	3	4	4	2	9	5	9	4
1087	5	1	62	189	66	6	3	0	10	10	6	2	2	3	5	9	2	9	2
1088	2	1	67	161	65	3	1	0	11	10	6	2	2	3	5	9	2	10	2
1089	12	2	40	204	133	19	8	9	6	7	4	5	3	1	6	12	5	6	3
1090	11	4	65	182	63	12	5	4	5	7	3	1	2	2	3	5	2	5	2
1091	15	4	27	388	140	7	7	3	12	11	7	2	2	2	14	10	4	10	3
1092	14	3	0	352	98	4	11	0	7	7	5	0	1	1	4	14	4	5	2
1093	6	1	0	185	26	0	5	0	4	4	3	0	0	0	2	7	1	2	0
1094	10	2	0	375	129	5	7	0	6	7	3	1	1	1	10	18	4	6	3
1095	4	1	0	221	43	0	3	0	4	4	2	0	1	1	6	11	1	3	1
1096	15	3	1	213	59	6	9	0	8	8	5	1	1	1	9	6	2	8	1
1097	7	1	1	107	36	0	4	0	6	5	4	0	1	0	6	4	1	5	1
1098	4	1	1	74	44	1	3	0	7	6	4	1	1	1	6	5	1	5	1
1099	9	2	22	9	168	1	5	1	6	6	5	4	2	1	2	7	7	6	3
1100	15	3	51	349	95	6	12	0	7	8	5	1	2	2	6	14	4	6	3
1101	7	1	31	182	25	1	5	0	4	5	3	1	1	1	3	8	1	3	1
1102	11	2	34	353	109	6	7	0	5	8	4	2	2	2	7	17	4	6	2
1103	4	1	23	199	30	1	3	0	3	5	2	1	1	1	4	10	1	3	1
1104	13	3	30	141	114	6	7	0	11	10	7	1	2	2	10	16	4	12	3
1105	5	1	19	57	36	1	3	0	7	5	4	1	1	1	6	9	1	6	1
1106	28	5	59	206	130	8	19	4	13	12	7	5	5	2	6	10	6	10	4
1107	11	1	30	90	48	2	9	2	6	6	4	1	2	1	3	4	2	5	1
1108	25	10	86	520	118	27	10	1	3	14	3	3	4	6	7	14	3	6	4
1109	19	8	67	406	124	23	8	2	3	12	3	3	3	4	6	11	3	7	3
1110	32	16	118	239	189	31	9	0	11	17	6	3	3	4	7	14	9	12	6
1111	16	9	112	290	405	22	2	0	3	22	2	4	5	7	14	23	13	15	9
1112	10	5	23	346	115	9	4	0	5	13	7	3	3	4	6	9	3	10	4
1113	10	5	20	304	122	8	3	14	5	11	6	3	5	4	5	8	3	10	4
1114	3	1	0	95	76	0	4	25	2	3	1	1	2	1	2	2	2	2	1

Desserts & Sweets

Food No.	Food Description & Amount	wt gm	wt oz	cal	% cal fat	prot gm	carbo gm	fiber gm
1115	Coffee cake, crumb or quick-bread type (Include cinnamon cake) [1/12 of 8" square]	50	1.8	163	28%	3	26	0.6
1116	Coffee cake, crumb or quick-bread type, reduced fat, no cholesterol (Include Dolly Madison Buttercrumb) [1 individual cake]	43	1.5	139	6%	1	32	1.2
1117	Coffee cake, crumb or quick-bread type, cheese-filled [1/12 of 8" square]	47	1.7	144	37%	4	18	0.4
1118	Coffee cake, crumb or quick-bread type, custard filled [1/12 of 8" square]	47	1.7	129	28%	3	21	0.5
1119	Coffee cake, crumb or quick-bread type, with fruit (Include apple pastry cake) [1/12 of 8" square]	47	1.7	158	25%	3	28	0.8
1120	Coffee cake, crumb or quick-bread type, with icing (Include with nuts) [1/12 of 8" square]	42	1.5	145	33%	2	23	0.6
1121	Coffee cake, yeast type (Include with or without nuts, coffee bread with icing) [1/8 of 8" dia]	41	1.4	153	40%	3	21	1.0
1122	Coffee cake, yeast type, made from home recipe or purchased at a bakery (Include with or without nuts, coffee bread with icing) [1/8 of 8" dia]	41	1.4	140	24%	3	23	0.8
1123	Coffee cake, yeast type, very lowfat, no cholesterol, with fruit [1 piece (5" x 7/8" x 1-1/8")]	33	1.2	94	2%	3	20	0.6
1124	Cupcake, not chocolate, with fruit and cream filling (Include Fruit & Creme Twinkies, all flavor varieties, prepackaged snack cakes) [1 cupcake]	43	1.5	144	28%	2	24	0.4
1125	Cupcake, chocolate, with icing or filling [1 cupcake (2¾" dia)]	46	1.6	173	35%	2	28	0.4
1126	Cupcake, chocolate, no icing or filling (Include chocolate crunch bar, with or without nuts) [1 cupcake (2¾" dia)]	33	1.2	102	27%	2	18	0.8
1127	Cupcake, chocolate, with/without icing, fruit filling or cream filling, very lowfat, no cholesterol (Include Nutri System) [1 cupcake]	39	1.4	118	7%	3	25	0.9
1128	Cupcake, chocolate, with/without icing, fruit filling or cream filling, very lowfat, no cholesterol (Include Hostess Lights Cake with Creamy Filling) [1 cupcake]	42	1.5	127	7%	4	27	1.0
1129	Cupcake, chocolate, with/without icing, fruit filling or cream filling, very lowfat, no cholesterol (Include Hostess Lights) [1 cupcake]	49	1.7	148	7%	4	32	1.2
1130	Cupcake, not chocolate, with icing or filling [1 cupcake (2¾" dia)]	48	1.7	175	28%	1	31	0.2
1131	Cupcake, not chocolate, no icing or filling [1 cupcake (2¾" dia)]	33	1.2	105	26%	2	18	0.3
1132	Cupcake, not chocolate, with icing, reduced fat, no cholesterol (Include Hostess Twinkies Lights) [1 cupcake]	35	1.2	118	15%	3	23	0.5
	Bars							
1150	Breakfast bar, cake-like (Include Carnation Breakfast Bars) [1 bar]	43	1.5	192	40%	6	23	0.4
1151	Breakfast bar, corn flake crust with fruit filling (Include Kelloggs Smart Start cereal bar) [1 bar]	42	1.5	155	18%	2	31	0.9
1152	Breakfast bar, date, with yogurt coating (Include Jenny's Cuisine) [1 bar]	45	1.6	150	30%	3	27	7.1
1153	Breakfast bar, diet meal type (Include Figurines, Slender Bars) [1 bar]	25	0.9	129	56%	5	9	0.3
1154	Brownie, butterscotch [1 brownie]	34	1.2	152	45%	2	20	0.3
1155	Brownie, carob and honey [1 brownie]	34	1.2	143	58%	2	16	2.0
1156	Brownie, chocolate, no icing (Include with nuts) [1 brownie]	34	1.2	129	32%	2	21	0.7
1157	Brownie, chocolate, with icing (Include with nuts) [1 brownie]	42	1.5	170	36%	2	27	0.9
1158	Brownie, chocolate, reduced fat, with icing [1 brownie]	40	1.4	140	18%	2	29	1.5
1159	Brownie, chocolate, fat free, no cholesterol, with icing [1 brownie (2" square)]	46	1.6	124	5%	2	30	1.9
1160	Brownie, chocolate, diet (Include Weight Watchers Chocolate Brownie; with nuts) [1 brownie]	34	1.2	131	26%	1	24	1.3
1161	Brownie, chocolate, with cream cheese filling, no icing (Include with nuts) [1 brownie]	42	1.5	171	43%	2	23	0.7
1162	Brownie, chocolate, with peanut butter fudge icing [1 brownie (2" square)]	30	1.1	121	38%	2	18	0.6
1163	Coconut bar [2 bars (2½" x 1¼")]	18	0.6	89	45%	1	12	0.7
1164	Cookie bar, with chocolate, nuts, and graham crackers (Include Magic Cookie Bars) [1 bar]	25	0.9	121	55%	1	13	0.5
1165	Date bar (Include date-nut bar, date macaroon, date pinwheel) [2 bars]	32	1.1	111	19%	1	23	1.5
1166	Fruit-filled bar (Include trail mix cookies, fruitcake cookies, Apple Newton, Blueberry Newton, Cherry Newton, Strawberry Newton) [2 bars]	32	1.1	130	28%	1	22	0.7

Food no.	fat gm	sat fat gm	choles mg	sodium mg	potas mg	% of Daily Value: vit A	vit E	vit C	thia	ribo	niac	vit B-6	fola	vit B-12	calc	phos	mag	iron	zinc
1115	5	1	48	215	43	2	4	0	6	6	4	1	2	2	6	11	2	4	2
1116	1	0	0	147	30	0	1	0	6	4	3	0	1	0	5	8	1	4	1
1117	6	2	42	162	49	4	3	0	4	6	3	1	2	2	8	10	2	3	3
1118	4	1	26	166	57	2	3	0	4	5	3	1	1	1	6	9	2	3	1
1119	4	1	40	182	83	2	3	0	5	5	3	2	2	1	5	10	2	5	2
1120	5	1	18	156	49	2	3	0	5	4	3	1	1	1	5	8	2	3	2
1121	7	2	27	157	46	3	5	1	9	6	5	2	2	1	3	3	2	4	2
1122	4	1	10	9	61	1	2	0	10	9	7	2	4	1	2	5	2	6	2
1123	0	0	0	53	59	1	0	1	6	7	4	1	3	0	2	3	1	4	1
1124	4	1	23	208	33	1	3	1	3	5	2	1	1	2	4	10	1	3	1
1125	7	1	8	196	56	0	4	0	7	8	6	1	1	1	3	4	5	9	2
1126	3	1	18	51	79	1	2	0	5	4	3	1	1	1	3	4	3	6	2
1127	1	0	0	143	130	0	0	0	6	8	4	1	1	1	5	7	4	7	2
1128	1	0	0	154	139	0	1	0	7	9	4	1	1	1	6	8	5	8	2
1129	1	0	1	180	163	0	1	0	8	11	5	1	1	1	6	9	5	9	3
1130	5	1	8	175	43	0	4	0	5	4	3	1	1	1	2	4	1	3	1
1131	3	1	18	156	24	1	2	0	3	4	2	1	1	1	3	8	1	2	1
1132	2	0	0	119	32	0	1	0	5	6	3	0	1	0	2	4	1	3	1
1150	9	6	0	258	76	6	1	13	13	13	13	13	13	13	13	13	13	12	3
1151	3	1	0	70	83	26	0	0	28	27	28	29	32	0	2	4	3	11	11
1152	5	1	0	5	199	0	8	1	9	3	5	4	4	0	2	8	9	6	5
1153	8	6	0	72	12	6	1	12	12	12	12	12	8	12	12	12	12	12	5
1154	8	1	21	90	72	7	4	0	4	4	3	1	1	1	2	3	2	4	1
1155	9	1	22	90	79	6	5	0	4	4	2	2	1	1	3	5	4	3	4
1156	5	1	12	14	61	0	2	0	5	4	3	1	1	0	1	3	3	6	2
1157	7	2	7	131	63	1	4	0	7	5	4	1	1	1	1	4	3	5	2
1158	3	1	9	103	141	0	2	0	6	6	4	1	1	1	2	5	6	9	3
1159	1	0	0	193	144	0	0	0	2	5	2	1	1	0	9	14	6	6	2
1160	4	2	0	32	107	0	3	0	2	3	2	0	0	0	0	2	1	3	0
1161	8	3	25	43	73	4	3	0	5	5	3	1	1	1	2	4	3	7	2
1162	5	1	8	25	74	0	2	0	4	3	5	1	2	0	1	4	4	5	2
1163	4	2	0	27	41	1	1	0	2	2	2	0	1	1	1	2	2	3	1
1164	7	3	4	56	80	3	3	0	2	3	1	1	1	1	4	4	3	2	2
1165	2	0	0	112	66	0	1	0	3	4	3	1	1	0	2	2	2	5	1
1166	4	1	3	134	36	0	1	0	5	5	4	2	0	0	0	4	1	4	1

Desserts & Sweets

Food No.	Food Description & Amount	wt gm	wt oz	cal	% cal fat	prot gm	carbo gm	fiber gm
1167	Fruit-filled bar, fat free (Include Newton bar) [1 bar (2" x 1½")]	19	0.7	62	1%	1	15	0.4
1168	Fruit-filled bar, fat free (Include Health Valley Apple Raisin) [1 bar]	25	0.9	82	1%	1	19	0.5
1169	Fruit-filled bar, fat free (Include Health Valley Apricot) [1 bar]	42	1.5	137	1%	2	32	0.9
1170	Fig bar (Include Fig Newton, Little Debbie Figaroos) [2 bars]	32	1.1	111	19%	1	23	1.5
1171	Fig bar, fat free (Include Newton) [2 bars]	38	1.3	127	2%	2	30	1.2
1172	Granola bar, oats, sugar, raisins, coconut (Include with chocolate chips, Nature Valley Chewy Granola Bars, Quaker Oats Chewy Granola Bars, New Trail Granola Bars) [1 bar]	43	1.5	195	35%	4	29	1.3
1173	Granola bar, peanuts, oats, sugar, wheat germ [1 bar]	43	1.5	206	40%	5	27	1.8
1174	Granola bar, oats, fruit and nuts, lowfat (Include Kelloggs) [1 bar]	21	0.7	80	15%	2	16	1.1
1175	Granola bar, oats, fruit and nuts, lowfat (Include Nature Valley) [1 bar]	28	1.0	106	15%	2	22	1.5
1176	Granola bar, oats, fruit and nuts, lowfat [1 bar]	24	0.8	91	15%	2	18	1.3
1177	Granola bar, nonfat [1 bar]	43	1.5	142	2%	3	33	3.2
1178	Granola bar, chocolate-coated (Include Quaker Oats Granola Dipps, Kudos Chocolate and Granola Snacks) [1 bar]	28	1.0	130	41%	2	19	1.0
1179	Granola bar, coated with non-chocolate coating (Include Quaker Oats Peanut Butter Whipps) [1 bar]	28	1.0	131	44%	2	17	0.8
1180	Granola bar, high fiber, coated with non-chocolate yogurt coating (Include lemon Fi-bar; raspberry Fi-bar) [1 bar]	28	1.0	96	27%	3	19	2.2
1181	Granola bar, with nougat (Include Nature Valley Granola Clusters) [1 bar or cluster]	34	1.2	138	30%	2	24	1.4
1182	Granola bar, with rice cereal (Include Kellogg's Rice Krispies Bar) [1 bar]	28	1.0	119	36%	2	18	1.1
1183	Granola bar with nuts, chocolate-coated (Include Kudos) [1 bar]	35	1.2	178	55%	3	19	1.3
1184	High protein bar, candy-like, soy and milk base (Include Hoffman's, Tiger's Milk) [1 bar]	50	1.8	223	29%	8	31	2.1
1185	High protein bar, cookie type, soy and milk base [2 cookies]	34	1.2	105	16%	14	10	0.2
1186	High protein bar, soy base (Include E.M.F. Meal in a Bar, Shaklee's Protein Bar) [1 bar]	71	2.5	324	37%	14	33	1.9
1187	Lemon bar [2 bars]	32	1.1	139	39%	2	20	0.3
1188	Meal replacement bar [1 bar]	34	1.2	140	38%	7	15	7.0
1189	PowerBar (fortified high energy bar) [1 bar]	65	2.3	229	7%	10	38	3.1
1190	Toffee bar [2 bars]	38	1.3	183	42%	2	25	0.9
	Cookies							
1200	Almond cookie [2 cookies]	20	0.7	103	55%	2	10	0.7
1201	Applesauce cookie (Include apple snacks, Dutch apple) [2 cookies]	26	0.9	96	30%	1	16	0.8
1202	Baby cookie (Include Gerber animal-shaped cookies) [5 cookies]	32	1.1	141	27%	4	22	0.1
1203	Batter cookie, raw, not chocolate [2 Tbs]	31	1.1	136	46%	2	17	0.3
1204	Biscotti [1 cookie]	32	1.1	146	40%	3	20	1.0
1205	Butter or sugar cookie (Include Pepperidge Farm Sugar, Bordeaux, Chessman, Pirouette) [4 cookies]	36	1.3	171	41%	2	24	0.3
1206	Butter or sugar cookie, with nuts and/or fruit (Include coconut) [2 cookies]	32	1.1	128	31%	2	21	0.3
1207	Butterscotch chip cookie [5 small cookies]	25	0.9	125	50%	1	15	0.3
1208	Caramel coated cookie, with nuts [2 cookies]	28	1.0	140	53%	1	16	0.7
1209	Carob cookie [2 cookies]	26	0.9	109	43%	3	15	2.7
1210	Chocolate cookie, rich with chocolate filling (Include walnut-fudge type Keebler Magic Middles, Archway Rocky Road Home Style Cookies) [2 cookies]	28	1.0	140	55%	1	15	0.8
1211	Chocolate and vanilla sandwich cookie [2 cookies (1" - 1½" dia)]	22	0.8	105	38%	1	16	0.5
1212	Chocolate chip cookie (Include with nuts) [2 cookies (2" dia)]	20	0.7	96	42%	1	13	0.5
1213	Chocolate chip sandwich [2 cookies (1" - 1½" dia)]	22	0.8	105	38%	1	16	0.5
1214	Chocolate chip cookie, bakery or made from home recipe (Include Toll House; made with M & M's; with nuts) [2 cookies (2" dia)]	20	0.7	98	52%	1	12	0.6
1215	Chocolate chip cookie, with raisins (Include date-nut chocolate chip bars) [2 cookies (2" dia)]	20	0.7	94	41%	1	14	0.5
1216	Chocolate chip cookie, reduced fat (Include Nabisco Chips Ahoy!) [2 cookies]	21	0.8	94	33%	1	15	0.5

						% of Daily Value													
Food no.	fat gm	sat fat gm	choles mg	sodium mg	potas mg	vit A	vit E	vit C	thia	ribo	niac	vit B-6	fola	vit B-12	calc	phos	mag	iron	zinc
1167	0	0	0	104	47	1	0	1	4	3	2	0	0	0	3	4	1	4	1
1168	0	0	0	136	61	1	0	1	5	4	3	1	1	1	4	5	1	5	1
1169	0	0	0	229	103	2	0	2	8	6	5	1	1	1	6	8	2	8	1
1170	2	0	0	112	66	0	1	0	3	4	3	1	1	0	2	2	2	5	1
1171	0	0	0	191	101	0	0	0	7	5	4	1	1	1	6	7	2	7	1
1172	8	5	0	120	140	0	1	1	8	3	4	8	9	0	3	12	11	8	5
1173	9	1	0	120	131	0	2	0	5	2	3	2	2	0	2	13	12	6	6
1174	1	0	0	53	50	4	0	0	7	5	5	8	8	0	1	5	4	6	3
1175	2	0	0	70	67	5	0	0	9	7	7	11	11	0	1	7	6	8	3
1176	2	0	0	60	57	4	0	0	8	6	6	10	10	0	1	6	5	7	3
1177	0	0	0	7	95	2	0	1	1	2	1	34	34	1	0	5	5	10	4
1178	6	3	3	50	86	2	2	1	4	4	2	2	2	1	3	6	4	3	2
1179	6	1	0	100	88	2	5	1	5	4	4	3	3	1	3	6	4	2	3
1180	3	1	0	6	107	0	3	0	8	3	4	2	2	0	2	11	9	4	4
1181	5	2	0	50	81	0	7	0	6	3	2	2	3	0	2	6	6	3	3
1182	5	1	0	138	59	5	3	6	9	7	8	7	7	0	1	5	4	4	3
1183	11	6	4	68	119	1	6	0	2	4	6	2	2	3	4	8	6	3	3
1184	7	3	0	337	195	0	6	0	32	36	3	46	22	3	15	15	9	31	13
1185	2	0	0	275	220	0	0	0	18	20	1	25	12	2	8	8	5	17	7
1186	13	2	0	444	257	23	6	45	45	45	45	45	29	45	45	15	20	32	18
1187	6	1	25	84	22	6	4	2	4	4	2	1	1	1	1	2	1	3	1
1188	6	2	0	100	160	18	1	35	35	35	35	35	20	35	10	10	10	35	35
1189	2	0	0	20	92	1	9	102	101	102	102	101	102	102	30	35	36	36	36
1190	9	3	0	120	51	0	5	0	6	6	5	1	1	0	1	4	3	6	2
1200	6	1	9	47	44	4	7	0	4	4	3	1	1	0	2	4	4	3	1
1201	3	1	6	56	54	3	2	0	3	2	1	1	1	0	2	3	2	3	1
1202	4	1	0	62	163	0	1	4	32	62	26	96	1	25	3	6	4	8	2
1203	7	1	15	100	32	7	5	0	6	4	3	1	1	1	2	2	1	3	1
1204	6	1	14	51	56	1	8	0	6	7	4	1	1	0	2	5	5	5	2
1205	8	2	18	150	37	4	4	0	6	5	5	1	1	1	2	4	1	4	1
1206	4	2	13	79	31	2	1	0	5	4	3	1	1	1	2	3	1	3	1
1207	7	2	11	92	37	5	4	0	4	3	2	1	1	1	1	2	1	3	1
1208	8	2	3	47	46	0	5	0	3	2	1	1	1	0	2	4	3	2	2
1209	5	1	19	64	135	1	3	0	3	6	3	3	2	2	8	7	4	3	3
1210	9	2	10	82	54	0	5	0	4	3	2	1	1	0	1	3	3	4	1
1211	4	1	0	105	29	0	3	0	2	3	3	0	0	0	1	2	2	4	1
1212	5	2	0	63	27	0	2	0	3	3	3	1	0	0	1	2	2	3	1
1213	4	1	0	105	29	0	3	0	2	3	3	0	0	0	1	2	2	4	1
1214	6	2	6	72	45	3	3	0	2	2	1	1	1	0	1	2	3	3	1
1215	4	1	0	59	35	0	2	0	3	3	3	1	0	0	1	2	2	3	1
1216	3	1	0	94	31	0	2	0	4	3	3	0	0	0	1	3	2	3	1

Desserts & Sweets

Food No.	Food Description & Amount	wt gm	wt oz	cal	% cal fat	prot gm	carbo gm	fiber gm
1217	Rich chocolate chip cookie, with chocolate filling (Include Keebler Magic Middles) [2 cookies]	28	1.0	140	55%	1	15	0.8
1218	Chocolate fudge cookie, with/without nuts (Include chocolate-jelly cookies; Peanut Butter'N Fudge Chocolate Chip Cookies (Duncan Hines)) [2 cookies (2" dia)]	26	0.9	113	30%	2	19	0.9
1219	Chocolate sandwich, chocolate covered (Include Fudge Covered Oreos, Nabisco Mystic Mint) [2 cookies]	40	1.4	192	49%	1	26	2.1
1220	Chocolate wafers (Include chocolate snaps) [2 cookies]	24	0.8	104	30%	2	17	0.8
1221	Chocolate cookie, chocolate covered or fudge sandwich [2 cookies (1" - 1½" dia)]	22	0.8	104	39%	1	15	0.7
1222	Chocolate cookie, with chocolate filling or coating, fat free (Include Snackwells) [2 cookies]	32	1.1	110	3%	2	26	0.9
1223	Cookie, chocolate, made with rice cereal (Include Little Debbie Star Crunch) [1 bar (2" square)]	30	1.1	128	44%	1	20	1.1
1224	Chocolate-covered marshmallow cookie (Include marshmallow puff, pinwheels) [2 cookies]	34	1.2	143	36%	1	23	0.7
1225	Chocolate-covered sugar wafer, creme-filled (Include Little Debbie Fudge Crispy Bar) [2 wafers]	30	1.1	151	46%	1	20	0.5
1226	Chocolate sandwich, with extra filling (Include Double Stuff Oreo) [2 cookies]	28	1.0	140	45%	1	19	0.6
1227	Chocolate sandwich, reduced fat (Include Oreo) [2 cookies]	21	0.8	86	14%	1	18	0.6
1228	Chocolate sandwich, reduced fat (Include Snackwells) [2 cookies]	23	0.8	92	14%	1	19	0.6
1229	Coconut cookie [2 cookies]	32	1.1	141	38%	1	21	0.3
1230	Coconut and nut cookie [2 cookies]	32	1.1	145	42%	1	21	0.4
1231	Cone shell, ice cream type [2 cones]	12	0.4	50	15%	1	9	0.4
1232	Cone shell, ice cream type, brown sugar [1 cone]	11	0.4	44	9%	1	9	0.2
1233	Dietetic cookie (Include coconut; thin diet wafers) [4 wafers]	24	0.8	115	55%	1	12	0.9
1234	Dietetic cookie, apple pastry [1 cookie]	24	0.8	115	55%	1	12	0.2
1235	Dietetic cookie, chocolate chip [4 cookies]	20	0.7	90	34%	1	15	0.3
1236	Dietetic cookie, chocolate flavored [4 cookies]	24	0.8	120	48%	1	15	0.5
1237	Dietetic cookie, fruit types [2 cookies]	22	0.8	102	46%	1	13	0.2
1238	Dietetic cookie, oatmeal with raisins [4 cookies]	28	1.0	126	36%	1	20	0.8
1239	Dietetic cookie, sandwich type [2 cookies]	22	0.8	101	43%	1	15	0.9
1240	Dietetic cookie, sugar or plain [4 cookies]	24	0.8	103	27%	1	18	0.2
1241	Fortune cookie [2 cookies]	16	0.6	60	6%	1	13	0.3
1242	Gingersnap cookie [2 cookies]	24	0.8	100	21%	1	18	0.5
1243	Graham cracker sandwich with chocolate and marshmallow filling [1 homemade S'mores (2-3/8" x 2-3/8")]	42	1.5	177	30%	2	30	0.8
1244	Granola cookie [2 cookies]	26	0.9	119	33%	2	17	1.1
1245	Japanese tea cookie (Include senbei, plain, ginger, or seaweed) [5 cookies]	25	0.9	96	1%	1	23	0.2
1246	Ladyfinger (Include anisette sponge, Stella D'Oro Egg Jumbo, Stella D'Oro Breakfast Treat) [2 ladyfingers]	28	1.0	102	22%	3	17	0.3
1247	Lebkuchen (Include honey nut bar) [2 cookies]	32	1.1	123	14%	2	25	0.9
1248	Lemon wafer, lowfat (Include NuSystem) [5 wafers]	5	0.2	20	9%	0	4	0.1
1249	Macaroon [2 cookies]	28	1.0	113	28%	1	20	0.5
1250	Marshmallow pie, chocolate covered (Include moon pies, sweetie pie, mallow pies, scooter pies, whoopie pie) [1 scooter pie]	34	1.2	143	36%	1	23	0.7
1251	Marshmallow cookie, with coconut [2 cookies]	36	1.3	152	36%	1	24	0.7
1252	Marshmallow cookie, with rice cereal (Include Rice Krispies bar cookie) [1 bar (2" sq)]	30	1.1	115	24%	1	22	0.2
1253	Meringue cookie (Include angel cup) [5 cookies]	20	0.7	72	0%	1	18	0.0
1254	Molasses cookie (Include hermits, gingerbread man) [2 cookies]	30	1.1	129	27%	2	22	0.3
1255	Multigrain cookie, high fiber (Include Fibbers High Fiber Cookies) [2 cookies]	48	1.7	194	39%	5	31	5.4
1256	Oat bran cookie, sweetened with fruit juice (Include Health Valley Fruit Jumbos, Honey Jumbos, Kathies) [2 cookies]	36	1.3	129	34%	4	22	3.7

Food no.	fat gm	sat fat gm	choles mg	sodium mg	potas mg	% of Daily Value: vit A	vit E	vit C	thia	ribo	niac	vit B-6	fola	vit B-12	calc	phos	mag	iron	zinc
1217	9	2	10	82	54	0	5	0	4	3	2	1	1	0	1	3	3	4	1
1218	4	1	1	151	55	0	2	0	4	4	4	0	1	0	1	3	3	6	2
1219	11	3	0	130	96	0	6	0	3	5	3	1	1	1	1	4	4	7	2
1220	3	1	0	139	50	0	2	0	3	4	3	0	1	0	1	3	3	5	2
1221	5	1	0	133	39	0	3	0	1	2	2	0	0	0	1	2	2	5	1
1222	0	0	0	62	83	0	0	0	7	4	4	0	1	0	1	4	3	8	2
1223	6	4	0	65	74	3	1	3	4	4	4	4	4	0	1	3	5	4	3
1224	6	2	0	57	62	0	3	1	2	4	1	1	0	1	2	3	3	5	1
1225	8	3	3	36	57	1	3	0	2	4	2	0	1	1	3	4	2	3	1
1226	7	1	0	138	34	0	5	0	1	2	2	0	0	0	1	3	2	4	1
1227	1	0	0	63	43	0	1	0	4	3	3	0	1	0	2	4	2	4	1
1228	1	0	0	68	46	0	1	0	5	4	3	0	1	0	2	5	2	4	1
1229	6	4	28	66	48	5	1	0	3	3	2	1	1	1	1	2	1	3	1
1230	7	4	28	65	51	5	1	0	4	3	2	1	1	1	1	2	2	3	1
1231	1	0	0	17	13	0	1	0	2	2	3	0	0	0	0	1	1	2	1
1232	0	0	0	35	16	0	0	0	4	3	3	0	0	0	0	1	1	3	1
1233	7	3	0	0	22	0	2	0	2	1	2	1	1	1	0	1	3	2	2
1234	7	2	0	0	22	0	7	0	2	1	2	0	1	0	0	1	2	2	0
1235	3	2	0	2	40	0	3	0	4	2	3	0	0	0	1	2	1	4	1
1236	6	2	0	3	20	0	6	0	3	2	2	1	1	1	1	1	2	2	1
1237	5	1	1	0	9	0	3	0	3	1	2	0	0	0	0	1	2	2	0
1238	5	2	0	3	49	0	4	0	6	3	3	1	1	0	1	4	2	5	1
1239	5	2	0	53	65	0	3	0	5	4	3	0	1	0	1	4	4	6	2
1240	3	1	0	1	25	0	2	0	6	3	4	0	0	0	1	2	1	5	1
1241	0	0	2	44	7	0	0	0	2	1	1	0	0	0	0	1	0	1	0
1242	2	0	0	157	83	0	2	0	3	4	4	2	0	0	2	2	3	9	1
1243	6	2	0	140	36	0	3	0	7	5	5	1	1	0	1	3	2	5	1
1244	4	3	0	86	94	0	0	0	10	4	2	5	5	0	2	9	7	4	3
1245	0	0	0	182	10	0	0	0	4	2	2	0	0	0	0	1	0	2	0
1246	3	1	102	41	32	5	1	2	5	7	3	2	3	4	1	5	1	6	2
1247	2	0	6	11	59	0	4	0	6	5	4	1	1	0	2	3	3	5	1
1248	0	0	0	16	7	0	0	0	2	1	1	0	0	0	0	1	0	1	0
1249	4	3	0	69	44	0	0	0	0	2	0	1	0	0	0	1	1	1	1
1250	6	2	0	57	62	0	3	1	2	4	1	1	0	1	2	3	3	5	1
1251	6	2	0	60	66	0	3	1	2	4	1	1	0	1	2	3	3	5	2
1252	3	1	0	131	12	9	2	7	7	7	7	7	7	0	0	1	1	3	1
1253	0	0	0	14	13	0	0	0	0	2	0	0	0	0	0	0	0	0	0
1254	4	1	0	138	104	0	3	0	7	5	5	4	1	0	2	3	4	11	1
1255	8	1	0	144	182	0	8	0	11	10	14	11	7	0	2	16	17	20	13
1256	5	1	0	221	164	1	5	2	9	3	6	4	2	0	1	12	11	7	5

Desserts & Sweets

Food No.	Food Description & Amount	wt gm	wt oz	cal	% cal fat	prot gm	carbo gm	fiber gm
1257	Oatmeal sandwich, with creme filling (Include Keebler Chipsies) [2 cookies (1" - 1½" dia)]	30	1.1	146	41%	1	20	0.6
1258	Oatmeal cookie[2 cookies (2½" dia)]	26	0.9	121	37%	1	18	0.7
1259	Oatmeal cookie, reduced fat, with raisins (Include Snackwells) [2 cookies]	27	1.0	103	13%	2	21	1.0
1260	Cookie, oatmeal, fat free, with raisins (Include Entenmanns, Health Valley) [2 cookies]	22	0.8	72	4%	1	17	1.6
1261	Oatmeal cookie, with chocolate and peanut butter [2 cookies]	68	2.4	281	38%	5	41	2.7
1262	Oatmeal cookie, with chocolate chips (Include with chocolate frosting; made with M&Ms) [2 cookies]	30	1.1	152	56%	2	16	0.8
1263	Oatmeal cookie, with fruit filling [1 cookie (2½" dia)]	27	1.0	115	35%	2	17	0.8
1264	Oatmeal cookie, with raisins (Include with dates, with nuts, Tastykake Oatmeal Raisin Bars) [2 cookies (2½" dia)]	26	0.9	117	36%	2	18	0.7
1265	Peanut cookie (Include chocolate peanut bars, peanut sandwich cookies, Nabisco Nutter Butter, Almost Home Peanut Butter Cream Sandwich) [2 cookies]	32	1.1	153	45%	3	19	0.6
1266	Peanut butter cookie (Include peanut butter wafers) [2 cookies]	32	1.1	153	45%	3	19	0.6
1267	Peanut butter cookie with rice cereal [2 bars (2" sq)]	48	1.7	195	32%	3	32	0.6
1268	Peanut butter cookie, with chocolate (Include Pepperidge Farm Nassau) [2 Nassau]	30	1.1	143	46%	3	18	0.7
1269	Peanut butter cookie, with oatmeal [2 cookies]	32	1.1	153	40%	3	21	0.6
1270	Peanut butter filled cookie, chocolate-coated (Include Girl Scout Tagalongs Peanut Butter Patties) [2 cookies]	26	0.9	132	51%	2	15	0.9
1271	Pfeffernusse [2 cookies]	26	0.9	104	22%	2	19	0.4
1272	Pizzelles (Italian style wafer) (Include rosettes) [2 wafers or rosettes]	28	1.0	138	40%	2	18	0.3
1273	Pumpkin cookie (Include carrot bars) [2 cookies]	22	0.8	85	43%	1	12	0.6
1274	Puerto Rican cookie (Mantecaditos polvorones) [2 cookies (2" x 2" x ¼")]	38	1.3	194	43%	2	25	0.6
1275	Raisin cookie(Include date-nut, raisin sugar cookie) [2 cookies]	32	1.1	128	31%	1	22	0.4
1276	Raisin sandwich cookie, cream-filled (Include Little Debbie Raisin Creme Pie) [1 cookie (3½" - 4" dia)]	30	1.1	135	41%	1	20	0.2
1277	Rugelach (Include cookie made with cottage cheese) [2 cookies]	28	1.0	119	53%	3	11	0.3
1278	Rum ball (Include bourbon balls) [2 balls]	22	0.8	87	29%	1	14	0.5
1279	Sandwich-type cookie, not chocolate or vanilla (Include banana cream-filled, Keebler Puddin' Cremes) [2 cookies (1" - 1½" dia)]	22	0.8	106	37%	1	16	0.3
1280	Shortbread cookie (Include Pecan Sandies, Greek cookies, Keebler Pecan Sandies, Pepperidge Farm Shortbread) [2 cookies]	30	1.1	151	43%	2	19	0.5
1281	Shortbread cookie, reduced fat [1 medium]	16	0.6	73	35%	1	11	0.2
1282	Shortbread cookie, with chocolate filling (Include Keebler Magic Middles) [2 cookies]	28	1.0	139	46%	2	18	0.7
1283	Sugar wafer [5 wafers]	35	1.2	179	43%	1	25	0.2
1284	Sugar cookie, iced (Include spice and other flavors) [2 cookies]	32	1.1	134	30%	1	23	0.2
1285	Sugar cookie, with chocolate frosting [2 cookies]	32	1.1	124	26%	1	22	0.3
1286	Vanilla cookie with caramel, coconut, and chocolate coating (Include Girl Scout Samoas) [2 cookies]	30	1.1	155	56%	1	18	0.7
1287	Vanilla sandwich, round (Include Pepperidge Farm Brussels Mint) [2 cookies]	22	0.8	106	37%	1	16	0.3
1288	Vanilla sandwich, reduced fat (Include Snackwells) [2 cookies]	24	0.9	100	14%	2	20	0.3
1289	Vanilla wafer (Include vanilla cookie) [5 wafers]	20	0.7	88	31%	1	15	0.4
1290	Vanilla wafer, reduced fat [1 cookie]	4	0.1	17	22%	0	3	0.0
1291	Vanilla waffle creme [2 cookies]	18	0.6	92	43%	1	13	0.1
1292	Whole wheat cookie, with dried fruit, nuts [2 cookies]	28	1.0	120	47%	2	16	1.2
	Pies and Cobblers							
1350	Apple cobbler [1 cup]	217	7.7	439	24%	5	81	2.6
1351	Apple pie (Include apple-peach, apple-berry) [1/8 of 9" dia]	150	5.3	356	42%	3	51	2.4
1352	Apple pie, individual size or tart [1 tart]	120	4.2	377	45%	4	49	1.7
1353	Apple pie, low calorie (Include Weight Watchers Apple Pie) [1 individual pie]	85	3.0	193	21%	2	38	1.7
1354	Apple pie, one crust (Include apple pie with crumb topping) [1/8 of 9" dia]	150	5.3	371	34%	3	60	2.0

Food no.	fat gm	sat fat gm	choles mg	sodium mg	potas mg	vit A	vit E	vit C	thia	ribo	niac	vit B-6	fola	vit B-12	calc	phos	mag	iron	zinc
						% of Daily Value													
1257	7	1	3	21	62	0	4	0	5	3	3	1	1	0	2	3	3	5	1
1258	5	1	0	65	26	0	3	0	6	2	3	0	1	0	2	4	2	5	1
1259	1	0	0	118	69	0	1	0	6	4	3	1	1	0	5	10	3	5	1
1260	0	0	0	66	47	0	0	0	2	3	1	1	0	0	1	2	2	3	1
1261	12	2	1	117	168	7	9	0	9	4	7	3	3	1	3	13	12	6	6
1262	10	2	7	80	60	3	5	0	4	3	2	1	1	0	1	3	4	4	2
1263	4	1	2	63	40	0	3	0	6	3	3	1	1	0	2	4	3	4	1
1264	5	1	0	100	37	0	3	0	5	4	3	1	0	0	1	4	2	4	1
1265	8	2	0	133	53	0	5	0	4	3	7	1	3	0	1	3	4	4	1
1266	8	2	0	133	53	0	5	0	4	3	7	1	3	0	1	3	4	4	1
1267	7	1	0	226	56	14	5	11	12	11	15	13	13	0	1	4	4	5	3
1268	7	2	0	106	59	0	4	0	3	3	6	1	2	0	1	3	4	4	1
1269	7	1	0	118	61	0	4	0	7	5	6	1	1	0	2	6	4	5	2
1270	7	1	0	60	76	0	9	0	5	4	5	1	1	0	1	3	3	4	2
1271	3	1	10	78	105	3	2	0	5	4	4	2	1	0	2	2	4	5	1
1272	6	1	36	126	27	7	4	0	6	6	3	1	1	1	4	4	1	4	1
1273	4	1	9	46	68	18	2	1	4	2	2	1	1	0	3	3	2	4	1
1274	9	4	9	1	24	0	1	0	9	6	6	0	1	0	0	2	1	6	1
1275	4	1	1	108	45	0	2	0	5	4	3	1	1	1	1	3	2	4	1
1276	6	1	0	70	29	0	3	0	3	3	2	1	0	0	1	2	1	3	0
1277	7	1	1	82	31	7	5	0	4	3	3	1	1	1	1	2	1	3	1
1278	3	0	0	57	95	0	1	0	3	2	2	2	0	0	2	2	4	4	2
1279	4	1	0	77	20	0	3	0	4	3	3	0	0	0	1	2	1	3	1
1280	7	2	6	137	30	0	4	0	7	6	5	0	1	0	1	3	1	5	1
1281	3	1	0	55	15	0	2	0	4	2	2	0	1	0	1	2	1	3	1
1282	7	2	4	103	43	0	3	0	5	5	4	0	1	0	1	3	3	4	1
1283	9	2	0	51	21	0	6	0	2	4	4	0	1	0	1	2	1	4	1
1284	4	1	9	63	17	3	2	0	2	3	2	0	0	0	1	2	1	2	0
1285	4	1	8	78	23	1	1	0	4	4	3	0	1	0	3	3	1	3	1
1286	10	4	2	46	74	0	4	0	1	2	1	1	0	0	2	3	3	2	2
1287	4	1	0	77	20	0	3	0	4	3	3	0	0	0	1	2	1	3	1
1288	2	0	0	77	38	0	1	0	5	4	3	0	1	1	4	5	1	3	1
1289	3	1	12	62	19	0	1	0	4	4	3	1	0	0	1	2	1	3	0
1290	0	0	0	10	4	0	0	0	1	1	1	0	0	0	0	0	0	1	0
1291	4	1	0	26	11	0	3	0	1	2	2	0	0	0	0	1	0	2	0
1292	6	1	15	67	111	4	3	0	3	2	2	3	1	1	2	5	5	4	2
1350	12	3	4	219	197	3	7	5	15	13	9	3	2	2	17	12	4	10	3
1351	17	3	0	399	98	5	11	8	3	2	2	3	2	0	2	4	3	4	2
1352	19	4	0	2	77	0	11	2	15	9	9	2	2	0	1	4	2	9	2
1353	5	1	0	245	61	0	5	0	7	5	4	1	1	0	1	2	1	5	1
1354	14	3	0	15	98	1	8	4	10	7	7	2	1	0	1	3	2	7	1

Desserts & Sweets

Food No.	Food Description & Amount	wt gm	wt oz	cal	% cal fat	prot gm	carbo gm	fiber gm
1355	Apple fried pie (Include McDonald's) [1 individual pie]	86	3.0	327	53%	3	37	1.2
1356	Apple-sour cream pie [1/8 of 9" dia]	159	5.6	339	40%	3	50	2.7
1357	Apricot cobbler [1 cup]	217	7.7	408	21%	6	78	4.5
1358	Apricot pie [1/8 of 9" dia]	150	5.3	419	41%	5	59	2.8
1359	Apricot pie, individual size or tart [1 tart]	120	4.2	359	43%	4	48	2.3
1360	Apricot fried pie [1 individual pie]	86	3.0	316	53%	3	35	1.7
1361	Banana cream pie [1/8 of 9" dia]	144	5.1	387	46%	6	47	1.0
1362	Banana cream pie, individual size or tart [1 tart]	117	4.1	280	41%	5	37	1.2
1363	Berry cobbler [1 cup]	217	7.7	507	24%	6	94	4.3
1364	Black bottom pie [1/8 of 9" dia]	99	3.5	274	53%	5	28	0.9
1365	Blackberry pie (Include boysenberry) [1/8 of 9" dia]	150	5.3	402	42%	4	56	4.7
1366	Blackberry pie, individual size or tart [1 tart]	117	4.1	339	44%	3	45	3.6
1367	Blueberry pie (Include huckleberry) [1/8 of 9" dia]	150	5.3	348	39%	3	52	1.5
1368	Blueberry pie filling [1 cup]	262	9.2	272	3%	2	68	3.7
1369	Blueberry pie, individual size or tart [1 tart]	120	4.2	349	44%	3	47	2.3
1370	Blueberry pie, one crust [1/8 of 9" dia]	137	4.8	293	37%	3	45	2.3
1371	Buttermilk pie [1/8 of 9" dia]	144	5.1	551	43%	6	75	0.6
1372	Cherry cobbler [1 cup]	217	7.7	426	24%	5	78	2.5
1373	Cherry pie [1/8 of 9" dia]	150	5.3	390	38%	3	60	1.2
1374	Cherry pie, individual size or tart [1 tart]	120	4.2	285	43%	3	39	1.7
1375	Cherry pie, one crust [1/8 of 9" dia]	137	4.8	313	34%	3	50	1.6
1376	Cherry pie, made with cream cheese and sour cream [1/8 of 9" dia]	159	5.6	454	42%	5	63	1.0
1377	Cherry fried pie (Include McDonald's) [1 individual pie]	86	3.0	287	51%	3	33	1.1
1378	Cherry pie filling [1 cup]	264	9.3	316	6%	2	76	2.3
1379	Cherry pie filling, low calorie [1 cup]	264	9.3	211	9%	2	51	1.6
1380	Chess pie (Include lemon chess pie) [1/8 of 9" dia]	89	3.1	367	44%	5	48	0.9
1381	Chiffon pie, chocolate [1/8 of 9" dia]	99	3.5	318	43%	6	41	1.3
1382	Chiffon pie, not chocolate [1/8 of 9" dia]	99	3.5	291	37%	7	40	0.5
1383	Chiffon pie, with liqueur (Include grasshopper pie) [1/8 of 9" dia]	99	3.5	342	51%	4	33	0.8
1384	Chocolate cream pie (Include chocolate Chocolate meringue, chocolate ice box dessert, chocolate pudding pie, Jello chocolate mousse pie) [1/8 of 9" dia]	144	5.1	388	44%	7	50	2.1
1385	Chocolate cream pie, individual size or tart [1 tart]	117	4.1	345	47%	6	42	1.7
1386	Chocolate-marshmallow pie[1/8 of 8" dia]	102	3.6	383	50%	5	47	1.6
1387	Coconut cream pie (Include coconut custard) [1/8 of 9" dia]	144	5.1	429	50%	3	54	1.9
1388	Coconut cream pie, individual size or tart [1 tart]	117	4.1	278	48%	6	30	0.9
1389	Cranberry pie, one crust (Include juneberry, gooseberry) [1/8 of 9" dia]	137	4.8	345	37%	2	54	3.8
1390	Custard pie (Include custard cream, egg pie) [1/8 of 9" dia]	136	4.8	286	50%	7	28	2.2
1391	Custard pie, individual size or tart (Include custard cream) [1 tart]	117	4.1	218	29%	7	31	0.6
1392	Frozen yogurt pie (Include all flavors) [1/8 of 9" dia]	144	5.1	361	50%	4	42	0.7
1393	Lemon cream pie (Include lemon ice box pie) [1/8 of 9" dia]	144	5.1	399	39%	7	56	0.6
1394	Lemon cream pie, individual size or tart [1 tart]	117	4.1	342	41%	6	46	0.6
1395	Lemon fried pie [1 individual pie]	85	3.0	284	51%	4	31	0.6
1396	Lemon pie (not cream or meringue) [1/8 of 9" dia]	99	3.5	384	36%	5	57	0.9
1397	Lemon pie (not cream or meringue), individual size or tart [1 tart]	120	4.2	478	38%	6	69	1.2
1398	Lemon meringue pie (Include key lime pie) [1/8 of 9" dia]	137	4.8	367	29%	2	65	1.6
1399	Lemon meringue pie, individual size or tart [1 tart]	117	4.1	301	41%	4	41	0.6
1400	Mince pie [1/8 of 9" dia]	150	5.3	434	34%	4	72	3.9
1401	Mince pie, individual size or tart [1 tart]	120	4.2	370	43%	4	51	2.3
1402	Oatmeal pie [1/8 of 9" dia]	114	4.0	447	36%	6	69	1.6
1403	Peach cobbler [1 cup]	217	7.7	425	21%	5	82	3.8
1404	Peach pie [1/8 of 9" dia]	150	5.3	335	40%	3	49	1.2
1405	Peach pie, individual size or tart [1 tart]	120	4.2	344	43%	4	47	2.0
1406	Peach pie, one crust [1/8 of 9" dia]	150	5.3	337	31%	3	57	2.7
1407	Peach fried pie [1 individual pie]	86	3.0	308	54%	3	34	1.5

Food no.	fat gm	sat fat gm	choles mg	sodium mg	potas mg	vit A	vit E	vit C	thia	ribo	niac	vit B-6	fola	vit B-12	calc	phos	mag	iron	zinc
						% of Daily Value													
1355	19	4	0	5	57	0	12	1	10	7	7	1	1	0	1	3	2	7	1
1356	15	5	8	17	218	4	7	6	10	8	6	3	1	0	4	5	4	8	2
1357	10	2	2	177	470	31	11	18	15	13	12	5	3	1	14	11	5	13	5
1358	19	4	0	2	244	17	14	10	16	11	12	3	3	0	2	5	4	12	3
1359	17	3	0	2	185	13	12	8	14	10	10	2	2	0	1	5	3	10	3
1360	18	4	0	3	136	8	13	5	10	7	7	1	1	0	1	3	2	7	2
1361	20	5	73	346	238	10	10	4	13	18	8	10	4	6	11	13	6	8	5
1362	13	3	50	38	199	4	7	4	10	14	6	9	3	3	7	9	5	7	3
1363	13	3	3	260	189	2	13	21	21	17	13	3	3	1	18	13	5	13	4
1364	16	7	90	162	169	16	5	1	3	11	2	3	2	4	8	10	6	7	4
1365	19	4	0	27	166	3	13	22	14	10	10	3	5	0	3	5	5	11	3
1366	17	3	0	19	127	2	11	16	13	9	9	2	4	0	2	4	4	9	2
1367	15	3	0	488	75	5	10	7	1	3	2	3	2	0	1	3	2	3	2
1368	1	0	0	68	97	2	11	4	5	8	1	4	1	0	1	3	3	5	1
1369	17	3	0	23	78	2	12	11	14	9	9	2	2	0	1	4	2	8	2
1370	12	2	0	5	67	1	12	2	11	9	7	2	1	0	1	4	2	8	2
1371	26	6	91	64	103	4	15	0	10	15	6	2	3	4	5	9	3	7	4
1372	12	3	2	223	197	11	7	4	15	14	10	4	3	1	15	11	5	20	3
1373	17	3	0	369	122	8	10	2	2	3	2	3	3	0	2	4	3	4	2
1374	14	3	0	16	110	2	8	2	10	8	7	2	1	0	1	4	3	7	1
1375	12	2	0	19	106	7	7	3	9	8	6	2	2	0	1	3	3	13	1
1376	21	10	78	98	138	20	7	2	7	13	4	3	3	3	6	8	3	10	3
1377	16	3	0	4	62	2	10	1	9	7	6	1	1	0	1	3	2	9	1
1378	2	0	0	39	201	17	3	7	2	6	2	4	4	0	2	2	3	16	1
1379	2	0	0	24	201	5	3	7	2	5	2	4	3	0	2	2	3	4	1
1380	18	8	129	205	53	13	13	0	7	12	4	2	4	4	2	7	2	6	3
1381	15	4	107	53	94	6	7	0	8	12	5	2	3	3	2	9	6	8	4
1382	12	3	139	44	71	6	7	8	8	14	5	3	4	4	2	8	2	7	3
1383	19	8	96	230	88	19	7	0	4	10	3	2	3	4	3	7	4	6	3
1384	19	7	77	44	233	7	8	1	13	17	8	3	4	5	11	17	11	11	7
1385	18	6	57	33	179	5	8	1	13	15	8	3	3	4	9	13	9	10	5
1386	21	10	10	218	202	10	8	1	5	11	4	2	2	4	10	12	7	6	5
1387	24	11	0	367	94	3	11	0	5	7	1	5	2	5	4	12	7	6	6
1388	15	5	74	54	157	6	7	1	10	16	6	3	3	4	9	12	4	7	4
1389	14	3	0	34	77	3	9	17	10	6	6	3	1	0	1	3	2	6	2
1390	16	4	45	326	144	7	7	1	4	17	2	3	7	10	11	15	4	4	5
1391	7	2	78	58	157	7	3	1	11	17	6	3	3	5	10	12	4	7	4
1392	20	10	3	252	166	12	8	10	4	10	4	2	3	5	10	10	4	4	4
1393	17	4	93	115	165	12	10	10	10	17	5	3	4	6	10	12	4	6	4
1394	16	4	68	84	127	9	9	7	9	14	5	3	3	5	7	10	3	6	3
1395	16	3	49	16	44	2	10	3	10	9	6	1	2	2	1	5	2	7	2
1396	16	3	76	47	67	5	9	10	12	13	7	2	3	2	2	6	2	8	3
1397	20	4	84	52	82	6	12	11	16	16	10	2	4	3	2	8	3	11	3
1398	12	2	62	200	122	7	9	7	6	17	4	2	3	3	8	14	5	5	4
1399	14	3	69	23	50	3	8	5	9	10	5	2	3	2	1	5	2	7	2
1400	16	4	0	381	305	0	13	15	15	9	9	5	2	0	3	6	5	12	2
1401	18	4	1	14	203	0	11	2	16	11	10	3	2	0	3	5	5	13	2
1402	18	4	87	154	85	10	11	0	13	12	5	3	3	3	2	11	6	9	5
1403	10	2	2	190	325	7	10	11	14	14	15	2	2	1	14	11	5	10	3
1404	15	3	0	405	188	3	12	3	6	3	2	2	2	0	1	4	2	4	1
1405	16	3	0	1	139	3	11	5	14	10	11	1	2	0	1	4	3	9	2
1406	12	2	0	1	210	5	10	9	10	8	11	1	2	0	1	4	3	7	2
1407	18	4	0	10	102	3	13	3	9	7	8	1	1	0	1	3	2	6	1

Desserts & Sweets

Food No.	Food Description & Amount	wt gm	wt oz	cal	% cal fat	prot gm	carbo gm	fiber gm
1408	Peanut butter cream pie [1/8 of 9" dia]	144	5.1	425	45%	12	49	1.8
1409	Pear cobbler [1 cup]	217	7.7	453	21%	5	89	4.3
1410	Pear pie [1/8 of 9" dia]	150	5.3	391	41%	4	56	2.6
1411	Pear pie, individual size or tart [1 tart]	120	4.2	342	44%	3	46	2.1
1412	Pecan pie (Include coconut-pecan pie, walnut pie) [1/8 of 9" dia]	114	4.0	456	42%	5	65	4.0
1413	Pecan pie, individual size or tart [1 tart]	85	3.0	363	49%	4	46	1.6
1414	Pie shell [1 tart shell]	29	1.0	149	57%	1	14	0.3
1415	Pie shell, chocolate wafer [1 pie shell (9" dia)]	210	7.4	1063	55%	11	114	3.2
1416	Pie shell, graham cracker [1 tart shell]	22	0.8	109	45%	1	14	0.3
1417	Pineapple cobbler [1 cup]	217	7.7	416	22%	4	80	1.7
1418	Pineapple pie [1/8 of 9" dia]	150	5.3	396	41%	4	56	1.4
1419	Pineapple pie, individual size or tart [1 tart]	120	4.2	342	44%	3	46	1.2
1420	Pineapple cream pie (Include millionaire's pie, Hawaiian pie, sunshine pie) [1/8 of 9" dia]	144	5.1	291	34%	5	43	0.8
1421	Plum cobbler [1 cup]	217	7.7	448	22%	5	86	3.0
1422	Plum pie [1/8 of 9" dia]	150	5.3	441	42%	4	61	1.9
1423	Praline mousse pie, with nuts [1 individual pie]	77	2.7	190	33%	5	27	0.3
1424	Prune pie [1/8 of 9" dia]	150	5.3	453	29%	6	77	3.5
1425	Pudding pie, chocolate, with chocolate coating, individual size [1 individual pie]	142	5.0	473	50%	5	55	1.7
1426	Pudding pie, flavors other than chocolate [1/8 of 9" dia]	144	5.1	322	45%	6	39	0.7
1427	Pudding pie, flavors other than chocolate, individual size or tart [1 tart]	120	4.2	404	53%	4	43	0.7
1428	Pudding pie, flavors other than chocolate, with chocolate coating, individual size [1 individual pie]	142	5.0	492	50%	5	58	1.2
1429	Pumpkin pie [1/8 of 9" dia]	154	5.4	323	41%	6	42	4.2
1430	Pumpkin pie, individual size or tart [1 tart]	117	4.1	272	53%	6	27	1.8
1431	Raisin pie [1/8 of 9" dia]	150	5.3	379	39%	4	56	1.8
1432	Raisin pie, individual size or tart [1 tart]	120	4.2	350	42%	4	49	1.6
1433	Raspberry pie [1/8 of 9" dia]	150	5.3	422	43%	4	58	5.4
1434	Raspberry pie, individual size or tart [1 tart]	120	4.2	377	45%	4	50	2.8
1435	Raspberry pie, one crust [1/8 of 9" dia]	137	4.8	328	36%	3	52	5.7
1436	Raspberry pie, two crust (Include cranberry, juneberry, gooseberry) [1/8 of 9" dia]	150	5.3	438	43%	4	60	3.6
1437	Raspberry cream pie [1/8 of 9" dia]	144	5.1	287	52%	3	33	3.5
1438	Rhubarb cobbler [1 cup]	217	7.7	545	24%	5	102	2.9
1439	Rhubarb pie [1/8 of 9" dia]	150	5.3	448	47%	5	56	2.3
1440	Rhubarb pie, individual size or tart [1 tart]	120	4.2	385	48%	4	46	1.9
1441	Rhubarb pie, one crust [1/8 of 9" dia]	137	4.8	338	39%	3	49	2.2
1442	Shoo-fly pie [1/8 of 9" dia]	114	4.0	397	29%	4	68	1.0
1443	Sour cream raisin pie [1/8 of 9" dia]	144	5.1	523	58%	8	50	2.1
1444	Squash pie [1/8 of 9" dia]	154	5.4	293	38%	6	40	2.1
1445	Strawberry pie, individual size or tart [1 tart]	120	4.2	319	43%	3	43	2.3
1446	Strawberry pie, one crust [1/8 of 9" dia]	168	5.9	385	38%	4	58	3.3
1447	Strawberry cream pie [1/8 of 9" dia]	144	5.1	294	48%	2	38	1.7
1448	Strawberry cream pie, individual size or tart [1 tart]	117	4.1	281	51%	2	33	1.4
1449	Strawberry-rhubarb pie [1/8 of 9" dia]	150	5.3	424	46%	5	54	2.6
1450	Sweetpotato pie [1/8 of 9" dia]	154	5.4	295	43%	6	36	1.5
1451	Tofu pie with fruit [1/8 of 9" dia]	144	5.1	311	52%	8	33	1.8
1452	Toll house pie [1/8 of 9" dia]	114	4.0	610	65%	7	52	2.4
1453	Vanilla cream pie (Include butterscotch pie) [1/8 of 9" dia]	144	5.1	400	47%	7	47	0.9
1454	Vanilla wafer dessert base [1 cup]	129	4.6	685	61%	5	65	0.1
	Frozen Desserts							
1500	Baked Alaska [1/8 of Baked Alaska]	103	3.6	254	35%	5	37	0.1
1501	Fruit juice bar with cream, frozen (Include Dole Fruit and Cream Bars) [1 bar]	65	2.3	86	14%	1	19	0.1

Food no.	fat gm	sat fat gm	choles mg	sodium mg	potas mg	% of Daily Value													
						vit A	vit E	vit C	thia	ribo	niac	vit B-6	fola	vit B-12	calc	phos	mag	iron	zinc
1408	21	5	66	143	296	7	14	1	14	20	19	7	7	6	12	20	12	10	8
1409	10	2	2	194	230	1	9	7	15	14	9	2	3	1	15	11	5	11	3
1410	18	4	0	2	113	0	12	4	14	10	9	1	2	0	1	4	3	9	2
1411	17	3	0	1	91	0	11	3	13	9	8	1	2	0	1	4	2	9	2
1412	21	4	36	483	84	5	13	2	7	8	1	1	2	2	2	9	5	7	4
1413	20	3	38	54	90	2	8	0	16	9	6	2	3	1	1	8	6	8	7
1414	10	3	0	188	32	0	7	0	5	6	4	1	1	0	1	2	1	4	1
1415	65	14	2	1411	353	46	49	0	22	26	22	0	0	1	6	22	21	35	11
1416	5	1	0	126	19	4	4	0	2	2	2	0	0	0	0	1	1	3	1
1417	10	2	2	211	172	1	6	10	19	12	10	5	2	1	15	10	7	12	3
1418	18	4	0	10	96	0	11	6	18	10	10	3	2	0	1	4	4	10	2
1419	17	3	0	8	77	0	10	4	16	9	9	2	2	0	1	4	4	9	2
1420	11	3	61	41	131	5	6	3	11	14	6	3	3	3	7	9	4	7	3
1421	11	2	2	194	290	5	9	16	17	18	12	6	2	1	14	11	5	10	3
1422	21	4	0	2	133	6	15	3	17	12	11	2	2	0	1	5	3	11	2
1423	7	1	5	180	26	0	4	1	2	2	1	0	1	0	6	1	1	10	1
1424	15	3	0	38	190	1	8	5	12	16	9	5	2	1	2	5	4	10	2
1425	26	9	7	498	198	2	16	1	14	21	9	4	2	3	8	11	8	11	4
1426	16	5	13	172	172	3	8	1	12	15	7	2	2	4	12	11	5	7	4
1427	24	8	6	519	146	1	16	1	14	19	8	3	2	3	7	8	5	9	3
1428	27	10	7	550	191	3	17	1	14	21	9	4	2	3	8	11	8	10	4
1429	15	3	31	434	237	74	11	4	6	14	1	4	6	10	9	11	6	7	5
1430	16	5	53	55	238	97	10	3	10	16	6	3	3	2	12	13	6	10	4
1431	17	3	0	6	191	0	10	2	15	10	9	3	2	0	2	6	4	11	2
1432	16	3	0	5	157	0	10	2	15	9	9	3	2	0	1	5	3	10	2
1433	20	4	0	28	132	3	13	24	15	12	12	3	4	0	2	5	5	11	4
1434	19	4	0	23	68	2	11	10	14	9	9	2	2	0	1	4	2	9	2
1435	13	3	0	32	131	3	9	28	9	9	8	3	4	0	2	3	5	8	3
1436	21	4	0	30	83	3	13	13	16	10	10	3	2	0	1	5	3	10	2
1437	17	7	35	14	124	11	7	14	7	7	6	3	3	1	3	4	4	6	2
1438	14	3	2	239	355	7	9	10	16	13	11	2	3	1	21	11	6	11	3
1439	23	5	0	3	107	0	14	3	20	13	12	2	3	0	12	6	5	13	3
1440	21	4	0	2	85	0	12	2	17	11	11	1	2	0	9	5	4	11	2
1441	15	3	0	3	105	1	9	4	13	9	8	1	2	0	15	4	5	9	2
1442	13	3	37	141	543	2	7	0	15	11	10	11	2	1	9	6	21	19	3
1443	34	12	81	87	329	17	15	2	17	19	10	5	4	4	10	14	6	13	4
1444	12	3	67	51	243	25	7	5	11	15	6	5	4	4	9	11	5	7	4
1445	15	3	0	2	132	0	9	51	13	10	8	2	3	0	1	4	3	9	2
1446	16	3	0	2	194	0	10	82	14	12	9	4	4	0	2	5	4	10	2
1447	16	7	33	11	129	10	5	55	6	7	4	2	3	1	3	4	3	5	2
1448	16	6	23	8	101	7	6	39	8	8	5	2	3	1	2	4	2	6	2
1449	22	4	0	3	134	0	13	33	18	13	12	2	3	0	6	6	5	12	3
1450	14	4	58	54	231	94	8	15	10	18	6	9	4	4	10	11	5	7	4
1451	18	4	31	240	180	15	10	23	5	9	3	4	4	1	9	11	19	23	5
1452	44	10	49	269	219	23	22	1	14	12	7	6	5	2	4	12	14	13	7
1453	21	6	89	374	181	12	9	1	13	18	7	4	4	7	13	15	5	8	5
1454	47	10	50	664	102	37	33	0	16	17	14	3	2	2	5	10	3	12	2
1500	10	4	59	126	146	11	3	1	6	15	3	2	2	5	8	8	3	5	3
1501	1	1	5	20	64	1	0	13	0	3	1	1	1	1	3	1	0	1	0

Desserts & Sweets

Food No.	Food Description & Amount	wt gm	wt oz	cal	% cal fat	prot gm	carbo gm	fiber gm
1502	Fruit juice bar, frozen, sweetened with low calorie sweetener, flavors other than orange (Include Dole) [1 bar]	54	1.9	24	1%	0	6	0.1
1503	Fruit juice bar, frozen, flavors other than orange (Include Dole Fruit 'N Juice Bar) [1 bar]	74	2.6	61	1%	1	15	0.0
1504	Fruit juice bar, frozen, orange flavor (Include Dole Fruit 'N Juice Bar) [1 bar]	74	2.6	68	0%	0	17	0.1
1505	Gelatin, frozen, whipped, on a stick (Include Jello Gelatin Pops) [1 pop]	53	1.9	31	0%	1	7	0.0
1506	Ices, fruit [1 cup]	193	6.8	151	0%	1	63	0.0
1507	Popsicle filled with ice cream, all flavors (Include Disney Cream Pop) [1 pop]	59	2.1	68	29%	1	12	0.0
1508	Popsicle [1 double stick]	128	4.5	92	0%	0	24	0.0
1509	Popsicle, sweetened with low-cal sweetener [1 double stick]	128	4.5	35	3%	1	5	0.0
1510	Rice dessert bar, frozen, flavors other than chocolate, non-dairy, carob covered [1 bar]	113	4.0	253	55%	3	31	4.3
1511	Rice, frozen dessert, nondairy, flavors other than chocolate (Include Rice Dream) [1 cup]	172	6.1	259	36%	3	40	2.1
1512	Snow cone, slurps [1 cup]	193	6.8	151	0%	1	63	0.0
1513	Sorbet, fruit, citrus [1 cup]	200	7.1	184	0%	1	46	0.2
1514	Sorbet, fruit, noncitrus [1 cup]	200	7.1	164	1%	2	40	0.0
1515	Tofu yogurt [1 cup]	262	9.2	254	17%	9	43	0.5
1516	Tofu, frozen dessert, chocolate (Include Tofutti) [1 cup]	193	6.8	423	61%	7	48	7.1
1517	Tofu, frozen dessert, flavors other than chocolate (Include Tofutti) [1 cup]	193	6.8	503	63%	9	45	1.4
	Puddings							
1550	Barfi or Burfi, Indian dessert, made from milk and/or cream and/or Ricotta cheese [1 cubic inch]	21	0.7	59	38%	1	8	0.1
1551	Basbousa (semolina dessert dish) [1 piece (3 x 2½")]	82	2.9	220	35%	4	33	0.6
1552	Chantilly Cream [1 cup]	120	4.2	380	83%	3	15	0.0
1553	Coconut custard, Puerto Rican style (Flan de coco) [1 cup]	245	8.6	695	34%	20	98	0.8
1554	Cornmeal coconut dessert, Puerto Rican style (Harina de maiz con coco) [1 cup]	262	9.2	768	63%	8	72	7.3
1555	Cornstarch coconut dessert, Puerto Rican style (Tembleque) [1 cup]	250	8.8	702	72%	5	52	5.3
1556	Custard [1 cup]	244	8.6	235	34%	12	27	0.0
1557	Danish dessert pudding [1 cup]	274	9.7	406	0%	0	103	1.2
1558	Diplomat pudding, Puerto Rican style (Budin Diplomatico) [1 cup]	256	9.0	731	29%	18	112	1.3
1559	Egg dessert, custard-like, made with water and sugar, Puerto Rican style (Tocino del cielo; Heaven's delight) [1 cup]	265	9.3	882	25%	15	155	0.0
1560	Fresh corn custard, Puerto Rican style (Mazamorra, Mundo Nuevo) [1 cup]	280	9.9	1114	56%	11	130	10.0
1561	Fruit dessert with cream and/or pudding and nuts (Include watergate salad) [1 cup]	178	6.3	360	44%	3	52	1.3
1562	Gelatin dessert with cream cheese [1 cup]	239	8.4	192	29%	4	31	0.0
1563	Gelatin dessert with bananas and grapes (Include other fruits) [1 cup]	240	8.5	159	3%	3	39	1.4
1564	Gelatin dessert with bananas and grapes (Include other fruits) and cream cheese [1 cup]	239	8.4	190	21%	3	37	1.4
1565	Gelatin dessert with strawberries, bananas, pineapple (Include other fruits) and sour cream [1 cup]	249	8.8	271	21%	3	54	2.5
1566	Gelatin dessert with apples, grapes, celery (Include other fruits and vegetables) [1 cup]	240	8.5	151	3%	2	37	1.7
1567	Gelatin dessert with bananas and grapes (Include other fruits) and whipped non-dairy topping [1 cup]	227	8.0	196	23%	2	38	1.3
1568	Gelatin dessert with bananas, grapes, walnuts (Include other fruits and nuts) and whipped non-dairy topping [1 cup]	227	8.0	235	35%	3	38	1.5
1569	Gelatin dessert with apples, grapes, celery, walnuts (Include other fruits, vegetables, nuts) [1 cup]	240	8.5	186	25%	3	34	1.6
1570	Gelatin dessert with sour cream [1 cup]	227	8.0	212	45%	4	27	0.0
1571	Gelatin dessert with whipped non-dairy topping [1 cup]	227	8.0	177	21%	3	33	0.0
1572	Gelatin dessert [1 cup]	240	8.5	142	0%	3	34	0.0
1573	Gelatin dessert, dietetic (low-cal sweetener) [1 cup]	240	8.5	18	0%	3	2	0.0

Food no.	fat gm	sat fat gm	choles mg	sodium mg	potas mg	% of Daily Value													
						vit A	vit E	vit C	thia	ribo	niac	vit B-6	fola	vit B-12	calc	phos	mag	iron	zinc
1502	0	0	0	2	9	0	0	31	0	1	0	1	0	0	0	0	1	0	0
1503	0	0	0	3	39	0	0	12	1	1	1	1	1	0	0	0	1	1	0
1504	0	0	0	6	74	2	0	32	0	1	1	1	4	0	1	1	1	2	0
1505	0	0	0	22	1	0	0	0	0	0	0	0	0	0	0	1	0	0	0
1506	0	0	0	42	6	0	0	3	0	0	0	0	0	0	0	0	0	2	0
1507	2	1	9	20	40	2	0	0	1	3	0	0	0	1	2	2	1	0	1
1508	0	0	0	15	5	0	0	0	0	0	0	0	0	0	0	0	0	0	0
1509	0	0	0	6	33	0	0	0	0	0	1	0	0	0	0	0	0	1	0
1510	15	7	0	100	110	0	17	0	7	5	10	9	3	0	4	9	10	3	4
1511	10	1	0	73	125	0	16	27	11	3	11	10	3	0	1	13	15	4	6
1512	0	0	0	42	6	0	0	3	0	0	0	0	0	0	0	0	0	2	0
1513	0	0	0	16	200	5	0	86	1	4	2	2	11	0	2	3	4	5	0
1514	0	0	0	8	106	1	0	32	1	2	2	3	3	0	1	1	2	2	1
1515	5	1	0	92	123	1	4	11	10	3	3	3	4	0	31	10	26	15	5
1516	29	6	0	478	527	0	19	0	3	5	2	3	4	0	5	19	29	24	11
1517	35	5	0	510	124	0	21	1	7	3	2	6	6	0	5	12	13	12	6
1550	3	1	8	11	27	2	1	0	0	2	0	0	0	1	3	3	1	0	1
1551	8	2	2	72	125	1	6	0	7	10	5	1	2	2	10	9	5	5	3
1552	35	22	130	57	91	40	3	1	1	10	0	1	1	3	6	6	2	0	1
1553	26	16	291	318	708	22	5	4	8	53	2	9	9	12	49	51	14	8	16
1554	54	47	0	35	642	1	8	8	16	7	15	7	10	0	4	25	24	28	12
1555	56	50	0	37	624	0	8	9	4	0	9	4	8	0	4	24	22	22	11
1556	9	4	202	160	380	18	3	2	5	32	1	6	6	13	28	28	8	4	9
1557	0	0	0	7	56	0	0	3	1	1	0	1	0	0	1	1	1	3	1
1558	24	7	423	345	393	32	13	6	15	45	8	10	10	17	24	33	9	20	12
1559	24	7	1001	65	100	46	11	0	7	34	0	15	21	32	11	39	2	16	17
1560	69	60	0	64	1125	3	10	22	21	6	21	8	22	0	5	41	39	31	17
1561	17	10	0	260	179	4	2	16	9	2	2	6	3	0	3	16	8	3	3
1562	6	4	19	145	23	8	1	0	0	2	0	1	1	1	2	7	1	2	1
1563	0	0	0	65	247	1	2	14	4	4	2	15	3	0	1	5	4	2	1
1564	4	3	12	95	248	6	2	14	4	5	2	14	3	1	2	6	4	2	1
1565	6	4	13	74	295	6	2	62	6	7	3	12	6	1	5	7	6	4	2
1566	0	0	0	76	165	1	2	13	4	2	1	4	2	0	2	5	2	2	1
1567	5	4	0	61	219	2	2	12	3	4	2	13	2	0	1	4	4	2	1
1568	9	4	0	60	247	2	3	12	5	4	2	14	3	0	2	6	7	2	2
1569	5	1	0	71	186	1	3	11	5	3	1	6	3	0	2	7	5	2	2
1570	11	7	22	101	74	10	1	1	1	5	0	1	1	2	6	8	2	0	1
1571	4	4	0	93	5	1	0	0	0	0	0	0	0	0	1	5	1	0	0
1572	0	0	0	101	2	0	0	0	0	0	0	0	0	0	0	5	1	0	0
1573	0	0	0	119	1	0	0	0	0	0	0	0	0	0	0	7	1	0	0

Desserts & Sweets

Food No.	Food Description & Amount	wt gm	wt oz	cal	% cal fat	prot gm	carbo gm	fiber gm
1574	Gelatin dessert, dietetic (low-cal sweetener), with cream cheese [1 cup]	239	8.4	128	79%	5	2	0.0
1575	Gelatin dessert, dietetic (low-cal sweetener), with bananas, grapes (Include other fruits) and cream cheese [1 cup]	239	8.4	128	31%	3	22	1.8
1576	Gelatin dessert, dietetic (low-cal sweetener), with strawberries, bananas, pineapple (Include other fruit) and sour cream [1 cup]	249	8.8	195	24%	14	26	2.6
1577	Gelatin dessert, dietetic (low-cal sweetener), with apples, grapes, walnuts (Include other fruits, vegetables, nuts) [1 cup]	240	8.5	120	43%	3	16	1.8
1578	Gelatin dessert, dietetic (low-cal sweetener), with bananas, grapes (Include other fruit) and whipped dietetic non-dairy topping [1 cup]	249	8.8	88	17%	2	20	1.4
1579	Gelatin dessert, dietetic (low-cal sweetener), with bananas, grapes (Include other fruit) [1 cup]	240	8.5	87	5%	3	20	1.6
1580	Gelatin dessert, dietetic (low-cal sweetener), with sour cream [1 cup]	227	8.0	105	74%	4	4	0.0
1581	Gelatin dessert, dietetic (low-cal sweetener), with whipped dietetic non-dairy topping [1 cup]	227	8.0	24	40%	2	3	0.0
1582	Gelatin powder, dietetic (low-cal sweetener), dry [2 Tbs]	18	0.6	62	0%	10	6	0.0
1583	Gelatin powder, sweetened with sugar, dry [2 Tbs]	24	0.8	91	0%	2	22	0.0
1584	Gelatin-vegetable (carrots, celery, green pepper, radishes) salad [1 cup]	243	8.6	126	1%	3	30	0.9
1585	Gelatin (dietetic) - vegetable (carrots, celery, green pepper, radishes) salad [1 cup]	243	8.6	14	8%	1	3	0.9
1586	Haupia (coconut pudding) [1 cup]	213	7.5	580	68%	4	50	4.2
1587	Lime souffle (Include other citrus fruits) [1 cup]	120	4.2	386	42%	10	49	1.3
1588	Milk dessert or milk candy, Puerto Rican style (Dulce de leche) [½ cup]	155	5.5	482	16%	8	96	0.0
1589	Mousse, chocolate [1 cup]	170	6.0	362	66%	7	27	1.0
1590	Mousse, chocolate, lowfat, made from dry mix, water added [1 cup]	216	7.6	770	19%	27	148	11.9
1591	Mousse, not chocolate (Include fruit mousse) [1 cup]	170	6.0	353	68%	2	29	1.4
1592	Pineapple custard, Puerto Rican style (Flan de pina) [1 cup]	260	9.2	413	25%	15	63	0.3
1593	Pudding pops, chocolate [1 pop]	57	2.0	87	28%	2	14	0.2
1594	Pudding pops, flavors other than chocolate [1 pop]	57	2.0	91	25%	2	15	0.0
1595	Pudding roll-up, chocolate [2 roll-ups]	28	1.0	107	28%	1	21	1.0
1596	Pudding roll-up, flavors other than chocolate [2 roll-ups]	28	1.0	110	26%	1	21	0.0
1597	Pudding, bread (Include with raisins) [1 cup]	200	7.1	311	28%	11	46	1.8
1598	Pudding, Mexican bread (Capirotada) [1 cup]	204	7.2	561	39%	8	80	2.6
1599	Pudding, chocolate, canned [1 cup]	261	9.2	347	27%	7	60	2.6
1600	Pudding, chocolate and non-chocolate flavors combined, canned [1 snack size]	113	4.0	149	26%	3	25	0.6
1601	Pudding, chocolate, canned, low calorie [1 cup]	250	8.8	164	21%	9	25	0.2
1602	Pudding, chocolate, home recipe made with whole milk [1 cup]	261	9.2	270	18%	8	49	0.8
1603	Pudding, chocolate, made from dry mix and whole milk [1 cup]	261	9.2	273	18%	8	50	0.9
1604	Pudding, chocolate, low calorie, made from dry mix and 2% fat milk (Include D-Zerta) [1 cup]	250	8.8	164	21%	9	25	0.2
1605	Pudding, chocolate, canned, fat free [1 cup]	261	9.2	227	3%	5	53	1.0
1606	Pudding, coconut [1 cup]	255	9.0	273	22%	8	47	0.4
1607	Pudding, flavors other than chocolate, canned[1 cup]	261	9.2	339	25%	6	57	0.3
1608	Pudding, flavors other than chocolate, canned, low calorie [1 cup]	250	8.8	157	19%	8	23	0.0
1609	Pudding, flavors other than chocolate, canned, fat free [1 cup]	261	9.2	230	1%	5	53	0.0
1610	Pudding, flavors other than chocolate, home recipe made with whole milk [1 cup]	261	9.2	264	16%	7	49	0.0
1611	Pudding, flavors other than chocolate, made from dry mix and whole milk [1 cup]	264	9.3	274	16%	8	51	0.0
1612	Pudding, flavors other than chocolate, low calorie, made from dry mix and 2% fat milk (Include D-Zerta) [1 cup]	260	9.2	163	19%	8	24	0.0
1613	Pudding, Indian [1 cup]	237	8.4	311	25%	10	48	1.5
1614	Pudding, pumpkin [1 cup]	265	9.3	244	21%	7	43	0.2
1615	Pudding, rice [1 cup]	225	7.9	303	12%	8	60	1.0
1616	Pudding, rice flour, with nuts (Indian dessert) [1 cup]	250	8.8	359	20%	9	63	0.6
1617	Pudding, cornstarch, with milk base (Include Diet Care) [1 cup]	255	9.0	138	3%	9	25	0.0
1618	Pudding, tapioca, canned [1 cup]	255	9.0	303	28%	5	49	0.3
1619	Pudding, canned, tapioca, fat free [1 cup]	255	9.0	222	1%	5	52	0.3

Food no.	fat gm	sat fat gm	choles mg	sodium mg	potas mg	% of Daily Value													
						vit A	vit E	vit C	thia	ribo	niac	vit B-6	fola	vit B-12	calc	phos	mag	iron	zinc
1574	11	7	35	198	39	14	1	0	0	4	0	1	1	2	3	9	1	2	2
1575	4	3	12	97	310	6	2	16	4	6	2	19	3	1	2	6	5	2	1
1576	5	4	2	479	340	1	2	61	6	8	3	12	7	2	6	32	7	5	2
1577	6	1	0	80	202	1	3	12	6	3	1	6	3	0	2	8	5	2	2
1578	2	1	0	94	242	1	2	14	4	4	2	14	2	0	1	6	4	1	1
1579	1	0	0	74	271	1	2	16	4	5	2	16	3	0	1	6	4	2	1
1580	9	7	3	109	84	0	0	1	1	5	0	1	2	3	6	9	2	0	2
1581	1	1	0	119	5	0	0	0	0	0	0	0	0	0	0	6	1	0	0
1582	0	0	0	390	3	0	0	0	0	1	0	0	1	0	0	23	0	0	0
1583	0	0	0	61	2	0	0	0	0	0	0	0	0	0	0	3	0	0	0
1584	0	0	0	97	113	28	1	26	2	2	1	3	3	0	1	5	2	1	1
1585	0	0	0	35	111	28	1	26	2	1	1	3	3	0	1	2	2	1	1
1586	44	39	0	29	481	0	6	9	3	0	7	3	7	0	3	19	17	17	8
1587	18	3	308	92	170	14	6	10	10	22	1	7	8	10	4	18	7	8	11
1588	9	5	34	125	354	6	1	2	3	22	1	2	2	2	30	24	7	2	6
1589	26	15	242	74	251	29	4	1	4	20	1	5	6	12	17	22	9	6	8
1590	16	5	11	312	1985	37	10	6	18	62	7	12	10	38	75	83	62	36	32
1591	27	16	98	29	220	31	3	31	2	7	2	8	3	2	5	6	4	1	2
1592	11	4	482	145	309	22	6	20	8	34	2	14	15	15	8	21	7	11	9
1593	3	1	1	94	128	2	0	0	1	6	0	1	0	5	8	6	3	1	1
1594	3	1	1	60	79	3	0	0	2	7	0	1	1	4	7	6	2	0	1
1595	3	1	1	43	99	0	3	0	1	3	0	1	1	2	3	3	3	3	2
1596	3	1	1	50	41	0	3	0	0	3	0	0	0	0	3	2	8	1	1
1597	10	4	127	294	445	15	5	2	12	27	7	7	6	7	23	22	9	12	7
1598	24	9	28	463	359	4	16	2	14	13	11	3	3	2	18	16	14	14	8
1599	10	2	8	337	470	3	1	8	5	24	5	4	2	0	23	21	14	7	7
1600	4	1	6	149	166	1	1	2	2	10	2	1	0	1	10	8	4	2	3
1601	4	2	13	477	623	13	1	2	5	23	1	4	2	8	29	42	13	5	7
1602	5	3	19	264	429	10	1	3	6	26	1	5	3	13	29	25	13	5	8
1603	6	3	19	508	441	11	1	4	6	24	1	5	3	14	28	44	13	5	8
1604	4	2	13	477	623	13	1	4	6	23	1	5	3	14	29	42	13	5	7
1605	1	0	3	553	290	7	0	1	2	11	1	2	1	4	15	15	8	4	5
1606	7	4	19	525	372	10	1	3	6	21	1	12	3	13	27	37	9	2	6
1607	9	1	18	352	295	2	1	0	4	21	3	1	0	4	23	18	5	2	4
1608	3	2	13	582	375	14	1	2	5	22	1	4	2	8	29	41	8	1	6
1609	0	0	3	579	230	8	0	1	2	12	1	2	1	5	17	14	4	1	4
1610	5	3	19	419	349	11	1	3	6	21	1	5	3	13	27	21	8	1	6
1611	5	3	19	594	356	11	1	3	5	21	1	4	2	11	28	38	8	1	6
1612	3	2	14	605	390	14	1	4	6	23	1	5	3	15	30	42	8	1	6
1613	9	5	89	129	709	10	2	1	12	28	7	14	5	6	30	24	24	13	8
1614	6	3	16	365	451	17	4	8	6	20	2	5	4	11	24	20	8	3	6
1615	4	2	15	93	416	9	1	3	6	18	3	7	2	6	23	21	9	4	7
1616	8	4	26	96	341	6	3	2	13	20	7	5	3	6	24	22	10	8	7
1617	1	0	5	260	467	12	0	4	7	23	1	6	3	17	33	27	8	1	7
1618	9	2	3	301	265	0	1	3	4	15	4	12	3	5	21	20	5	3	5
1619	0	0	3	566	224	8	0	1	2	12	1	2	2	5	17	14	4	3	4

Desserts & Sweets

Food No.	Food Description & Amount	wt gm	wt oz	cal	% cal fat	prot gm	carbo gm	fiber gm
1620	Pudding, tapioca, chocolate, made from dry mix and whole milk [1 cup]	165	5.8	175	18%	5	31	0.0
1621	Pudding, tapioca, vanilla, made from dry mix and whole milk [1 cup]	165	5.8	178	17%	5	33	0.0
1622	Pudding, tapioca, vanilla, made from home recipe [1 cup]	205	7.2	239	26%	10	35	0.0
1623	Pudding, with fruit and vanilla wafers [1 cup]	187	6.6	280	24%	6	49	1.6
1624	Puerto Rican bread pudding (Budin de pan) [1 cup]	175	6.2	473	31%	14	68	1.7
1625	Puerto Rican custard (Flan) [1 cup]	240	8.5	399	24%	12	65	0.0
1626	Puerto Rican pumpkin pudding (Flan de calabaza) [1 cup]	262	9.2	598	41%	13	78	1.0
1627	Rice dessert (rice, pineapple, marshmallows, whipped cream, sugar) (Include glorified rice) [1 cup]	155	5.5	277	47%	3	35	0.8
1628	Rice flour cream, Puerto Rican style (Majarete, manjar blanco) [1 cup]	250	8.8	395	19%	10	70	0.5
1629	Spanish custard, Puerto Rican style (Natilla Espanol) [1 cup]	243	8.6	448	34%	13	62	0.0
1630	Yookan, Japanese bean dessert [2 slices]	56	2.0	97	0%	1	24	0.4
1631	Zabaglione [1 cup]	60	2.1	157	31%	3	17	0.0
	Pastries							
1700	Air filled fritter or fried puff, without syrup, Puerto Rican style (Bunuelos de viento) (Include wheat flour turnover (Pastelillo de harina de trigo)) [2 puffs]	55	1.9	193	49%	3	22	0.3
1701	Blintz, cheese-filled [1 blintz]	70	2.5	136	39%	7	14	0.2
1702	Blintz, fruit-filled [1 blintz]	70	2.5	124	32%	4	17	0.5
1703	Baklava (Include Kadayif) [1 piece (2" x 2" x 1½")]	78	2.8	336	61%	5	29	1.8
1704	Breakfast tart (Include poptarts, toaster pastries) [1 poptart]	50	1.8	197	23%	2	36	1.0
1705	Breakfast tart, lowfat [1 Pop Tart]	52	1.8	193	14%	2	40	0.8
1706	Cheese puffs (Include cheese straws) [5 puffs/straws]	30	1.1	80	66%	3	4	0.1
1707	Churros (Include Mexican cruellers) [1 churro]	26	0.9	116	57%	1	12	0.2
1708	Cream puff, no filling or icing [1 cream puff]	27	1.0	98	64%	2	6	0.2
1709	Crepe suzette [1 crepe with sauce]	66	2.3	159	51%	4	16	0.4
1710	Crepe, dessert type, chocolate-filled [1 crepe]	78	2.8	119	34%	4	16	0.7
1711	Crepe, dessert type, blueberry-filled (Include other fruit) [1 crepe]	78	2.8	145	35%	4	21	1.0
1712	Crepe, dessert type, ice cream-filled [1 crepe]	78	2.8	161	43%	5	18	0.3
1713	Crisp, apple, apple dessert (Include apple betty) [1 cup]	246	8.7	402	20%	4	79	4.6
1714	Crisp, blueberry [1 cup]	246	8.7	632	36%	5	101	5.1
1715	Crisp, cherry [1 cup]	246	8.7	704	35%	6	113	2.8
1716	Crisp, peach [1 cup]	246	8.7	508	28%	4	92	4.1
1717	Crisp, rhubarb [1 cup]	246	8.7	556	26%	3	106	3.9
1718	Cruller [1 cruller (3¼" dia)]	49	1.7	206	49%	2	24	0.7
1719	Danish pastry (Include fruit and/or spice, pecan swirls, snail Danish, pastry with icing, Babka, bear claw) [1 pastry (5" dia)]	94	3.3	379	50%	7	42	1.2
1720	Danish pastry, with cheese [1 pastry (5" dia)]	112	4.0	419	53%	9	42	1.1
1721	Danish pastry, with cheese, very lowfat [1 slice (3¾ x 1¾ x ¾")]	32	1.1	95	2%	3	21	0.4
1722	Danish pastry, with fruit [1 pastry (4" dia)]	71	2.5	263	45%	4	34	1.3
1723	Danish pastry, with nuts [1 pastry (4" dia)]	65	2.3	280	53%	5	30	1.3
1724	Doughnut, cake type (Include coconut, sugar-coated, glazed, plain cruller) [1 doughnut (3" dia)]	42	1.5	177	49%	2	21	0.6
1725	Doughnut, cake type, chocolate (Include glazed) [1 doughnut (3" dia)]	42	1.5	175	43%	2	24	0.9
1726	Doughnut, cake type, chocolate covered [1 doughnut (3" dia)]	53	1.9	251	59%	3	25	1.1
1727	Doughnut, cake type, chocolate covered, dipped in peanuts (Include peanut stick) [1 doughnut (3" dia)]	53	1.9	214	48%	3	26	1.0
1728	Doughnut, cake type, chocolate, with chocolate icing [1 doughnut (3" dia)]	53	1.9	219	47%	3	28	1.1
1729	Doughnut, chocolate cream-filled [1 doughnut]	65	2.3	220	49%	4	25	0.8
1730	Doughnut, custard-filled (Include Long John, cream-filled) [1 doughnut]	65	2.3	235	61%	4	20	0.5
1731	Doughnut, custard-filled, with icing [1 doughnut]	70	2.5	245	36%	3	37	0.5
1732	Doughnut, eggless, carob-covered, raised or yeast [1 doughnut]	78	2.8	286	55%	5	33	6.7
1733	Doughnut, French cruller (Include sugar-coated, glazed) [1 cruller (3" dia)]	49	1.7	202	40%	2	29	0.6
1734	Doughnut, jelly [1 doughnut]	65	2.3	221	50%	4	25	0.6
1735	Doughnut, oriental (Include Okinawan) [2 doughnuts]	36	1.3	151	42%	2	20	0.4

Food no.	fat gm	sat fat gm	choles mg	sodium mg	potas mg	vit A	vit E	vit C	thia	ribo	niac	vit B-6	fola	vit B-12	calc	phos	mag	iron	zinc
						% of Daily Value													
1620	4	2	12	190	335	7	0	2	3	14	1	3	1	7	17	16	9	3	5
1621	3	2	13	263	242	7	1	2	4	15	1	3	2	8	19	15	5	1	4
1622	7	3	158	125	298	14	2	2	5	25	1	5	5	13	22	22	6	4	7
1623	7	3	83	216	369	6	3	8	7	19	5	18	5	6	12	14	8	5	4
1624	16	6	127	474	421	15	6	2	18	34	12	6	7	5	30	28	10	14	9
1625	11	5	256	146	279	14	3	1	3	29	1	5	6	8	21	24	6	5	8
1626	27	7	297	324	491	47	21	11	14	35	8	8	10	11	10	22	7	15	9
1627	15	9	53	21	104	16	1	13	9	4	5	5	2	1	3	5	4	5	3
1628	8	5	33	121	406	8	1	4	16	24	8	7	3	12	30	26	10	9	9
1629	17	8	430	124	370	25	6	3	8	33	1	10	11	24	31	36	8	7	12
1630	0	0	0	23	17	0	0	0	0	1	0	0	1	0	0	1	1	1	0
1631	5	2	221	10	44	10	2	0	2	7	0	3	6	9	3	9	1	4	4
1700	10	3	65	99	32	10	5	0	4	7	3	1	2	2	1	4	1	4	2
1701	6	2	68	223	75	8	3	0	5	10	3	2	3	6	7	10	2	4	3
1702	4	1	53	93	78	7	2	1	3	8	2	2	2	3	3	6	2	5	2
1703	23	9	36	293	144	12	9	2	13	9	7	2	3	0	3	9	9	10	3
1704	5	1	0	210	56	14	4	0	10	11	10	10	10	0	1	6	2	10	2
1705	3	1	0	131	34	5	3	3	10	17	10	10	10	0	2	5	6	10	1
1706	6	2	38	83	25	6	3	0	2	5	1	1	1	2	4	4	1	2	2
1707	7	2	2	7	8	1	5	0	3	2	2	0	0	0	0	1	0	2	0
1708	7	2	53	150	26	8	5	0	4	6	2	1	1	2	1	3	1	3	1
1709	9	4	83	74	85	8	3	5	6	10	3	2	3	4	5	7	2	4	2
1710	4	2	56	87	127	6	2	1	5	12	2	2	2	4	8	9	3	4	3
1711	6	1	61	72	89	8	5	7	5	9	3	2	2	3	4	6	2	4	2
1712	8	3	85	81	138	10	2	1	6	14	3	3	3	6	8	10	3	4	4
1713	9	2	0	343	239	7	6	9	14	10	10	5	3	0	7	6	4	10	3
1714	25	5	0	722	180	26	24	27	19	14	12	4	5	0	13	22	4	10	3
1715	27	5	2	836	219	25	20	5	14	15	10	7	4	2	15	32	5	19	2
1716	16	3	0	202	535	23	16	17	12	11	14	3	2	0	7	6	9	13	3
1717	16	3	0	202	323	17	12	9	11	9	8	3	3	0	28	5	9	12	2
1718	11	2	18	268	62	1	8	0	7	7	5	1	1	2	2	13	2	5	2
1719	21	5	28	349	118	1	13	0	19	15	13	2	8	3	7	10	4	10	5
1720	25	8	50	504	110	7	13	0	14	17	11	2	7	4	4	12	4	10	6
1721	0	0	0	88	39	0	0	0	6	6	4	1	2	1	1	3	1	3	1
1722	13	3	15	251	59	1	6	5	12	9	7	1	3	1	3	6	3	7	3
1723	16	4	30	236	62	1	8	2	10	9	7	3	4	2	6	7	5	7	4
1724	10	2	16	229	53	1	7	0	6	6	4	1	1	2	2	11	2	5	2
1725	8	2	24	143	50	1	5	0	1	2	1	1	2	1	9	7	4	5	2
1726	16	4	31	227	60	2	11	0	4	3	3	1	2	3	2	11	5	7	2
1727	11	2	15	218	85	1	7	0	6	6	5	2	2	2	2	13	4	5	3
1728	12	3	16	231	85	1	7	0	6	7	4	1	1	2	3	13	5	6	2
1729	12	3	5	188	78	1	7	0	13	8	7	2	3	1	4	6	3	6	3
1730	16	4	16	201	52	1	7	0	15	6	7	1	2	1	2	5	3	7	3
1731	10	3	4	161	61	1	6	0	10	6	6	1	2	1	3	5	3	5	2
1732	18	4	0	79	217	0	14	0	9	8	12	7	6	0	7	15	14	10	7
1733	9	2	5	169	38	0	6	0	6	7	4	1	1	1	1	6	1	4	1
1734	12	3	17	190	51	1	6	1	14	5	7	1	3	1	2	6	3	6	3
1735	7	2	25	77	31	1	5	0	6	6	4	1	1	1	5	4	1	5	1

Desserts & Sweets

Food No.	Food Description & Amount	wt gm	wt oz	cal	% cal fat	prot gm	carbo gm	fiber gm
1736	Doughnut, raised or yeast (Include glazed, doughboys, doughnut holes, honey dip, malasadas) [1 doughnut (3" dia)]	60	2.1	242	51%	4	27	0.7
1737	Doughnut, raised or yeast, chocolate covered [1 doughnut (3" dia)]	71	2.5	276	46%	4	36	1.1
1738	Doughnut, raised or yeast, chocolate [1 doughnut (3" dia)]	50	1.8	198	51%	3	22	1.5
1739	Doughnut, raised or yeast, chocolate, with chocolate icing [1 doughnut (3" dia)]	71	2.5	277	47%	4	36	2.4
1740	Doughnut, wheat (Include glazed) [1 doughnut]	42	1.5	151	48%	3	18	0.9
1741	Doughnut, wheat, chocolate covered [1 doughnut (3" dia)]	71	2.5	287	42%	4	39	2.2
1742	Eclair, custard-filled cream puff, chocolate icing [1 eclair (5" x 2" x 1¾")]	102	3.6	267	54%	7	25	0.6
1743	Eclair, custard-filled cream puff, no icing [1 eclair (5" x 2" x 1¾")]	90	3.2	232	54%	6	21	0.4
1744	Empanada, fruit-filled [1 cup]	142	5.0	590	49%	6	71	2.1
1745	Empanada, pumpkin (Include squash empanada, sweet potato empanada) [1 cup]	132	4.7	327	39%	5	46	2.6
1746	Fritter, apple [2 fritters]	48	1.7	174	57%	3	16	0.7
1747	Fritter, banana [2 fritters (2" long)]	68	2.4	223	56%	3	23	1.3
1748	Fritter, berry [2 fritters]	48	1.7	157	58%	3	14	0.9
1749	Fritter, wheat flour, no syrup [2 fritters]	44	1.6	198	78%	3	8	0.3
1750	Ladoo, round ball, Asian-Indian dessert [1 ball (1¾" dia)]	63	2.2	246	55%	4	26	3.2
1751	Meringues [2 meringues]	44	1.6	143	0%	3	33	0.0
1752	Pastry, Chinese, made with rice flour (Include nine-layer pudding) [1 piece]	56	2.0	135	22%	1	25	0.6
1753	Pastry, flour and water only, fried (Include Taco Bell Cinnamon Crispa) [3 crispas]	30	1.1	135	35%	2	20	1.0
1754	Pastry, cookie type, fried [1 pastry]	46	1.6	174	59%	3	16	0.4
1755	Pastry, fruit-filled (Include hamantaschen) [1 pastry]	78	2.8	265	51%	3	31	3.1
1756	Pastry, Italian, with cheese (Include cannoli) [1 pastry]	85	3.0	233	40%	8	27	0.7
1757	Pastry, Oriental, made with bean or lotus seed paste filling (baked) [1 Moon Cake]	138	4.9	459	11%	9	92	3.6
1758	Pastry, Oriental, made with bean paste and salted egg yolk filling (baked) [1 Moon Cake]	138	4.9	431	18%	10	77	3.0
1759	Pastry, puff (Include angel wings, flaky pastry, patty shell) [2 puffs]	22	0.8	123	62%	2	10	0.3
1760	Pastry, puff, custard or cream filled (Include cream horn, Napoleon) [2 puffs]	114	4.0	468	66%	6	34	1.0
1761	Sopaipilla with syrup or honey [2 sopaipillas (1½" square)]	24	0.8	86	39%	1	12	0.3
1762	Sopaipilla, no syrup or honey [2 sopaipillas (1½" square)]	20	0.7	73	49%	1	8	0.3
1763	Strudel, apple [2" square]	64	2.3	175	37%	2	26	1.4
1764	Strudel, berry [2" square]	64	2.3	161	23%	2	30	1.6
1765	Strudel, cheese and pineapple (Include other fruit) [2" square]	64	2.3	141	35%	4	19	0.6
1766	Strudel, cheese [2" square]	64	2.3	196	38%	6	24	0.4
1767	Strudel, cherry [2" square]	64	2.3	179	32%	3	29	1.1
1768	Strudel, peach [2" square]	64	2.3	127	22%	2	24	1.3
1769	Strudel, pineapple [2" square]	64	2.3	159	20%	2	31	0.8
1770	Tamale, sweet (Include with sugar and spices) [2 tamales]	68	2.4	176	44%	2	24	2.1
1771	Tamale, sweet, with bananas, pineapple, raisins [2 tamales]	98	3.5	198	38%	2	31	2.6
1772	Turnover or dumpling, apple [1 turnover]	82	2.9	290	46%	3	37	1.2
1773	Turnover or dumpling, berry [1 turnover]	78	2.8	279	45%	3	36	1.6
1774	Turnover or dumpling, cherry [1 turnover]	78	2.8	240	44%	3	31	1.0
1775	Turnover or dumpling, lemon [1 turnover]	78	2.8	238	47%	3	29	0.6
1776	Turnover or dumpling, peach [1 turnover]	78	2.8	256	44%	3	34	1.4
1777	Turnover, guava [1 turnover]	78	2.8	234	49%	2	28	2.6
1778	Turnover, pumpkin [1 turnover]	78	2.8	196	52%	4	20	1.3
	Sugar and Candy							
1800	Aspartame sweetener (Include Equal) [1 individual packet]	1	0.0	4	0%	0	1	0.0
1801	Aspartame-sugar blend, sugar substitute [1 individual packet (½ tsp)]	2	0.1	8	0%	0	2	0.0
1802	Bean paste, sweetened (Include Japanese red beans) [2 Tbs]	40	1.4	84	1%	2	19	2.1
1803	Cane and corn syrup blend [2 Tbs]	41	1.4	112	0%	0	30	0.0
1804	Carob syrup (carob powder in corn syrup) [2 Tbs]	37	1.3	79	1%	0	24	3.0
1805	Chocolate sauce (milk-based) [2 Tbs]	34	1.2	85	15%	1	18	0.5

Food no.	fat gm	sat fat gm	choles mg	sodium mg	potas mg	% of Daily Value: vit A	vit E	vit C	thia	ribo	niac	vit B-6	fola	vit B-12	calc	phos	mag	iron	zinc
1736	14	3	4	205	65	1	8	0	15	8	9	2	3	1	3	6	3	7	3
1737	14	4	4	184	94	2	7	0	13	8	7	2	3	1	3	7	6	7	4
1738	11	3	3	163	89	0	6	0	12	7	7	2	3	1	2	6	6	7	4
1739	14	4	3	179	138	1	7	0	12	8	8	2	3	1	3	9	10	9	5
1740	8	1	8	149	62	1	5	0	6	6	4	2	2	2	2	4	2	3	2
1741	13	4	19	103	128	1	9	0	8	7	7	3	2	2	5	10	8	7	4
1742	16	4	130	344	119	19	10	1	8	16	4	3	4	6	6	11	4	7	4
1743	14	3	121	307	104	18	9	0	7	15	4	3	3	5	6	10	3	6	4
1744	32	6	0	101	91	0	21	0	20	13	13	2	2	0	7	8	4	15	3
1745	14	3	34	10	184	107	10	3	16	13	11	3	4	1	4	7	6	16	3
1746	11	2	41	19	68	3	6	1	5	7	3	2	1	2	3	4	2	4	2
1747	14	3	40	32	193	4	8	5	6	9	4	12	2	2	3	5	4	4	2
1748	10	2	34	28	58	3	7	4	5	7	3	1	1	2	2	4	1	3	2
1749	17	4	70	110	35	11	10	0	5	8	3	1	2	2	1	4	1	4	2
1750	15	2	0	6	129	0	13	1	4	2	1	3	15	0	2	6	5	6	4
1751	0	0	0	49	44	0	0	0	0	8	0	0	0	1	0	0	1	0	0
1752	3	0	0	5	50	0	2	0	2	0	3	4	1	0	1	3	4	2	2
1753	5	1	0	135	38	0	4	0	10	5	5	1	1	0	4	4	2	6	1
1754	11	3	52	44	56	6	7	1	6	7	4	1	3	2	3	5	2	4	2
1755	15	2	15	6	148	2	7	2	11	8	6	5	2	0	1	6	5	8	4
1756	10	5	35	48	90	7	4	0	9	12	5	2	3	3	12	11	3	7	5
1757	6	1	69	117	153	3	4	1	24	19	14	3	16	2	2	11	7	16	5
1758	9	2	224	740	146	7	4	1	21	19	12	4	18	8	4	16	6	17	7
1759	8	1	0	56	14	0	2	0	5	3	4	0	0	0	0	1	1	3	1
1760	34	9	53	187	96	12	8	0	15	15	12	2	2	2	5	8	4	10	4
1761	4	1	0	28	13	0	2	0	4	3	3	0	0	0	2	2	1	3	1
1762	4	1	0	32	11	0	2	0	4	3	3	0	0	0	2	2	1	3	1
1763	7	2	18	172	62	1	5	2	2	1	1	1	1	2	1	2	1	1	1
1764	4	1	11	82	58	4	4	8	7	6	5	1	1	0	2	3	2	5	1
1765	5	3	28	61	88	6	2	4	6	7	3	2	2	1	7	6	3	4	3
1766	8	4	42	93	66	9	3	1	6	9	4	1	2	2	9	9	2	5	4
1767	6	1	9	74	104	7	3	5	7	5	4	3	2	0	2	4	4	5	2
1768	3	1	9	61	104	5	3	5	5	5	5	1	1	0	2	2	2	4	1
1769	4	1	10	63	59	4	3	5	7	5	4	2	1	0	1	2	2	4	1
1770	9	2	0	2	56	0	5	0	13	7	8	3	1	0	3	4	5	9	2
1771	8	2	0	2	136	0	5	3	14	8	8	7	1	0	4	4	7	9	2
1772	15	3	0	4	56	0	9	1	11	8	8	1	1	0	1	3	2	7	1
1773	14	3	0	3	55	0	9	5	12	8	8	1	1	0	1	3	2	7	2
1774	12	2	0	8	59	3	7	1	10	7	6	1	1	0	1	3	2	9	1
1775	12	3	48	13	32	3	7	3	9	7	5	1	2	2	1	4	1	6	2
1776	12	2	0	1	91	1	8	3	11	8	8	1	1	0	1	3	2	7	2
1777	13	3	0	13	120	3	9	80	10	7	7	3	2	0	1	3	2	6	2
1778	11	3	34	35	156	62	7	2	8	11	5	2	2	1	8	9	4	7	3
1800	0	0	0	0	0	0	0	0	0	0	0	0	0	0	0	0	0	0	0
1801	0	0	0	0	0	0	0	0	0	0	0	0	0	0	0	0	0	0	0
1802	0	0	0	1	150	0	0	0	3	1	1	2	6	0	1	3	3	4	2
1803	0	0	0	37	14	0	0	0	2	1	0	0	0	0	0	0	1	4	0
1804	0	0	0	3	62	0	0	0	0	2	1	1	1	0	3	1	1	1	1
1805	1	1	4	19	50	2	0	0	1	3	1	0	0	1	2	3	2	2	1

Desserts & Sweets

Food No.	Food Description & Amount	wt gm	wt oz	cal	% cal fat	prot gm	carbo gm	fiber gm
1806	Chocolate syrup, thin type [2 Tbs]	38	1.3	82	4%	1	22	0.7
1807	Corn syrup (Include Karo brand, light or dark) [2 Tbs]	41	1.4	116	0%	0	31	0.0
1808	Fructose sweetener [1 individual packet]	3	0.1	11	0%	0	3	0.0
1809	Apple butter (Include other fruit butters) [2 Tbs]	35	1.2	65	1%	0	17	0.5
1810	Fruit sauce (Include all fruits) [2 Tbs]	42	1.5	89	27%	0	17	0.1
1811	Fruit syrup (Include fruit-flavored pancake syrup) [2 Tbs]	39	1.4	105	0%	0	28	0.0
1812	Green papaya preserve, Puerto Rican style (Dulce de lechoza) [2 Tbs]	19	0.7	58	0%	0	15	0.3
1813	Guava paste [2 Tbs]	38	1.3	107	0%	0	28	0.4
1814	Hard sauce [2 Tbs]	21	0.7	96	48%	0	13	0.0
1815	Honey (Include pear honey, raw honey) [2 Tbs]	42	1.5	129	0%	0	35	0.1
1816	Icing, chocolate [2 Tbs]	34	1.2	136	25%	0	27	0.5
1817	Icing, white (Include creme filling) [2 Tbs]	40	1.4	163	24%	0	32	0.0
1818	Jam, preserves, all flavors [2 Tbs]	40	1.4	97	1%	0	26	0.5
1819	Jams, preserves, marmalades, low sugar (all flavors) [2 Tbs]	36	1.3	51	2%	0	13	0.6
1820	Jams, preserves, marmalades, dietetic, all flavors, sweetened with low-cal sweetener [2 Tbs]	40	1.4	4	25%	0	21	1.0
1821	Jams, preserves, marmalades, reduced sugar, all flavors (Include Polaner All Fruit) [2 Tbs]	40	1.4	73	3%	0	18	1.0
1822	Jellies, all flavors [2 Tbs]	38	1.3	102	0%	0	27	0.4
1823	Jellies, dietetic, all flavors, sweetened with low-cal sweetener [2 Tbs]	38	1.3	12	0%	0	22	0.3
1824	Jellies, reduced sugar, all flavors [2 Tbs]	38	1.3	67	0%	0	17	0.3
1825	Maple syrup (100% maple) (Include Maple Cream) [2 Tbs]	39	1.4	103	1%	0	26	0.0
1826	Marmalade, all flavors [2 Tbs]	40	1.4	98	0%	0	27	0.1
1827	Molasses [2 Tbs]	41	1.4	109	0%	0	28	0.0
1828	Plain dessert sauce (Include vanilla, rum sauce) [2 Tbs]	33	1.2	49	47%	0	6	0.0
1829	Raisin sauce [2 Tbs]	31	1.1	41	36%	0	7	0.2
1830	Saccharin (Include Necta Sweet) [1 tablet (½ grain)]	0	0.0	0	0%	0	0	0.0
1831	Saccharin-based liquid sweetener (Include Fasweet, Sweet n'Low, Sweet 10) [1 tsp]	5	0.2	0	0%	0	0	0.0
1832	**Sugar, brown** [2 Tbs]	28	1.0	103	0%	0	27	0.0
1833	Sugar, brown, liquid [2 Tbs]	42	1.5	109	0%	0	28	0.0
1834	Sugar, carmelized [2 Tbs]	30	1.1	113	0%	0	29	0.0
1835	Sugar, cinnamon [1 tsp]	4	0.1	16	0%	0	4	0.1
1836	Sugar, maple [2 Tbs]	18	0.6	64	1%	0	16	0.0
1837	Sugar, raw [2 Tbs]	24	0.9	92	0%	0	24	0.0
1838	Sugar, white, powdered, confectioner's [2 Tbs]	15	0.5	58	0%	0	15	0.0
1839	**Sugar, white**, granulated or lump (Include rock sugar, rock candy) [2 Tbs]	25	0.9	98	0%	0	25	0.0
1840	Sugar Twin [1 individual packet]	1	0.0	3	0%	0	1	0.0
1841	Sugar Twin, brown [1 tsp]	0	0.0	1	0%	0	0	0.0
1842	Sweet Magic [1 individual packet]	1	0.0	0	0%	0	1	0.0
1843	Sweet'ner, Sweet n' Low [1 individual packet]	1	0.0	4	0%	0	1	0.0
1844	Sweetpotato paste [1 cubic inch]	22	0.8	67	0%	0	17	0.1
1845	Syrup, brown sugar and water [2 Tbs]	30	1.1	37	0%	0	10	0.0
1846	Syrup, buttered blends (Include Mrs. Butterworth, Log Cabin with butter) [2 Tbs]	39	1.4	115	5%	0	30	0.0
1847	Syrup, corn and maple (2% maple) (Include pancake syrup, Log Cabin Brand) [2 Tbs]	39	1.4	104	0%	0	27	0.0
1848	Syrup, dietetic [2 Tbs]	30	1.1	12	0%	0	15	0.0
1849	Syrup, fruit flavored, used for milk beverages [2 Tbs]	40	1.4	106	0%	0	28	0.0
1850	Syrup, pancake [2 Tbs]	40	1.4	106	0%	0	28	0.0
1851	Syrup, reduced calorie [2 Tbs]	30	1.1	49	0%	0	13	0.0
1852	Syrup, sorghum [2 Tbs]	41	1.5	119	0%	0	31	0.0
1853	Syrup, white sugar and water syrup [2 Tbs]	30	1.1	38	0%	0	10	0.0
1854	Topping, butterscotch or caramel [2 Tbs]	42	1.5	122	7%	0	31	0.0
1855	Topping, chocolate, thick, fudge type [2 Tbs]	42	1.5	147	35%	2	25	0.5

Food no.	fat gm	sat fat gm	choles mg	sodium mg	potas mg	vit A	vit E	vit C	thia	ribo	niac	vit B-6	fola	vit B-12	calc	phos	mag	iron	zinc
						% of Daily Value													
1806	0	0	0	36	84	0	0	0	0	1	1	0	0	0	1	5	6	4	2
1807	0	0	0	50	2	0	0	0	0	0	0	0	0	0	0	0	0	0	0
1808	0	0	0	0	0	0	0	0	0	0	0	0	0	0	0	0	0	0	0
1809	0	0	0	0	32	0	0	1	0	0	0	1	0	0	0	0	0	0	0
1810	3	1	0	32	45	4	2	7	1	1	0	1	1	0	0	0	1	1	0
1811	0	0	0	15	7	0	0	2	0	0	0	0	0	0	0	0	0	0	0
1812	0	0	0	3	46	0	0	8	0	0	0	0	0	0	1	0	1	1	0
1813	0	0	0	1	26	0	0	28	0	0	0	1	0	0	0	0	0	0	0
1814	5	3	14	52	2	5	0	0	0	0	0	0	0	0	0	0	0	0	0
1815	0	0	0	2	22	0	0	0	0	1	0	1	0	0	0	0	0	1	1
1816	4	1	0	42	47	4	2	0	0	1	0	0	0	0	1	2	2	2	1
1817	4	1	0	51	7	4	3	0	0	0	0	0	0	0	1	0	0	0	0
1818	0	0	0	16	31	0	0	6	0	1	0	0	3	0	1	0	0	1	0
1819	0	0	0	0	38	0	0	17	0	1	0	1	1	0	0	0	1	1	0
1820	0	0	0	0	28	0	0	0	0	0	0	0	1	0	0	0	1	1	0
1821	0	0	0	10	205	0	0	25	1	2	1	3	1	0	1	2	3	3	1
1822	0	0	0	14	24	0	0	1	0	1	0	0	0	0	0	0	1	0	0
1823	0	0	0	0	25	0	0	0	0	0	0	1	0	0	0	0	0	0	0
1824	0	0	0	1	27	0	0	0	0	0	0	1	0	0	0	0	1	0	0
1825	0	0	0	4	80	0	0	0	0	0	0	0	0	0	3	0	1	3	11
1826	0	0	0	22	15	0	0	3	0	0	0	0	4	0	2	0	0	0	0
1827	0	0	0	15	600	0	0	0	1	0	2	14	0	0	8	1	25	11	1
1828	3	0	0	31	2	3	2	0	0	0	0	0	0	0	0	0	0	0	0
1829	2	0	0	20	27	2	1	0	0	0	0	0	0	0	0	0	0	1	0
1830	0	0	0	0	1	0	0	0	0	0	0	0	0	0	0	0	0	0	0
1831	0	0	0	1	5	0	0	0	0	0	0	0	0	0	0	0	0	0	0
1832	0	0	0	11	95	0	0	0	0	0	0	0	0	0	2	1	2	3	0
1833	0	0	0	11	100	0	0	0	0	0	0	0	0	0	2	1	2	3	0
1834	0	0	0	12	104	0	0	0	0	0	0	0	0	0	3	1	2	3	0
1835	0	0	0	0	1	0	0	0	0	0	0	0	0	0	0	0	0	1	0
1836	0	0	0	2	49	0	0	0	0	0	0	0	0	0	2	0	1	2	7
1837	0	0	0	10	84	0	0	0	0	0	0	0	0	0	2	1	2	3	0
1838	0	0	0	0	0	0	0	0	0	0	0	0	0	0	0	0	0	0	0
1839	0	0	0	0	1	0	0	0	0	0	0	0	0	0	0	0	0	0	0
1840	0	0	0	5	1	0	0	0	0	0	0	0	0	0	1	0	0	0	0
1841	0	0	0	2	0	0	0	0	0	0	0	0	0	0	0	0	0	0	0
1842	0	0	0	57	1	0	0	0	0	0	0	0	0	0	0	0	0	0	0
1843	0	0	0	4	45	0	0	0	0	0	0	0	0	0	0	0	0	0	0
1844	0	0	0	1	12	11	0	2	0	1	0	1	0	0	0	0	0	0	0
1845	0	0	0	5	34	0	0	0	0	0	0	0	0	0	1	0	1	1	0
1846	1	0	2	53	2	1	0	0	0	0	0	0	0	0	0	0	0	0	0
1847	0	0	0	24	2	0	0	0	0	0	0	0	0	0	0	0	0	0	1
1848	0	0	0	6	0	0	0	0	0	0	0	0	0	0	0	0	0	0	0
1849	0	0	0	1	0	0	0	0	0	0	0	0	0	0	0	0	0	0	0
1850	0	0	0	24	2	0	0	0	0	0	0	0	0	0	0	0	0	0	1
1851	0	0	0	60	1	0	0	0	0	0	0	0	0	0	0	1	0	0	0
1852	0	0	0	3	412	0	0	0	3	4	0	14	0	0	6	2	10	9	1
1853	0	0	0	1	0	0	0	0	0	0	0	0	0	0	0	0	0	0	0
1854	1	1	0	46	5	0	0	0	0	0	0	0	0	0	0	0	0	0	0
1855	6	2	5	55	91	1	0	0	1	5	0	1	0	2	4	7	5	3	2

Desserts & Sweets

Food No.	Food Description & Amount	wt gm	wt oz	cal	% cal fat	prot gm	carbo gm	fiber gm
1856	Topping, chocolate, hard coating [2 Tbs]	33	1.2	182	74%	2	16	2.7
1857	Topping, milk chocolate with cereal [2 Tbs]	35	1.2	217	71%	2	16	0.6
1858	Topping, chocolate flavor, fat free [2 Tbs]	40	1.4	102	5%	1	27	1.4
1859	Topping, chocolate, dietetic (apple juice and molasses base) [2 Tbs]	28	1.0	16	24%	1	4	0.9
1860	Topping, fruit (jam-type) [2 Tbs]	42	1.5	108	0%	0	28	0.4
1861	Topping, pineapple, unsweetened (Include Sorrell Ridge Brand) [2 Tbs]	40	1.4	24	1%	0	6	0.3
1862	Topping, marshmallow [2 Tbs]	38	1.3	118	1%	1	30	0.0
1863	Topping, walnuts in syrup (wet) [2 Tbs]	42	1.5	173	49%	2	23	0.7
1864	Topping, peanut butter, thick, fudge type [2 Tbs]	42	1.5	123	27%	3	24	1.8
1865	$100,000 Bar [1 bar]	43	1.5	200	35%	2	30	0.6
1866	3 Muskateer Bar [1 bar]	23	0.8	96	28%	1	18	0.4
1867	Almonds, chocolate covered [10 almonds]	30	1.1	169	73%	5	9	1.7
1868	Almonds, sugar-coated (Include Jordan almonds) [10 almonds]	35	1.2	160	37%	3	25	1.6
1869	Andes Mint Wafers [5 wafers]	25	0.9	135	54%	1	15	0.0
1870	Baby Ruth [1 bar]	34	1.2	164	40%	3	22	1.0
1871	Bar None [1 bar]	43	1.5	224	59%	4	22	1.4
1872	Butterfinger [1 bar]	45	1.6	216	35%	6	30	1.1
1873	Butterscotch hard candy [5 pieces]	30	1.1	119	8%	0	29	0.0
1874	Candy, dietetic or low calorie, chocolate covered (Include Dietetic Fruit and Nut Bar, Dietetic Milk Almond Bar, Dietetic Milk Chocolate Flavored Bar) [5 sections]	35	1.2	192	65%	4	15	2.5
1875	Candy corn [20 pieces]	20	0.7	72	0%	0	19	0.0
1876	Caramel, all flavors, sugar free [2 pieces]	35	1.2	149	30%	1	25	0.3
1877	Caramel with nuts, chocolate covered [2 turtles]	38	1.3	188	38%	4	24	1.6
1878	Chewing gum [1 piece]	3	0.1	9	1%	0	3	0.0
1879	Chewing gum, sugared (Include gum with natural sweeteners) [1 piece]	4	0.1	14	1%	0	4	0.0
1880	Chewing gum, uncoated, sugarless (Include chewing gum with non-nutritive sweeteners) [1 piece]	2	0.1	5	1%	0	2	0.0
1881	Chocolate chips, semi-sweet (Include Toll House morsels) [1 cup]	173	6.1	829	56%	7	109	10.2
1882	Chocolate with fondant and caramel [1 bar]	30	1.1	138	41%	2	21	0.7
1883	Espresso coffee beans, chocolate-covered [20 beans]	34	1.2	30	32%	1	4	0.1
1884	Fifth Avenue [1 bar]	32	1.1	149	41%	3	22	0.9
1885	Fruit Roll-Up [1 roll-up]	14	0.5	49	8%	0	12	0.5
1886	Fudge, brown sugar (penuche) [1 cubic inch]	21	0.7	84	25%	0	16	0.2
1887	Fudge, chocolate [1 cubic inch]	21	0.7	80	20%	0	17	0.2
1888	Fudge, chocolate, with nuts [1 cubic inch]	21	0.7	89	34%	1	15	0.3
1889	Fudge, divinity [2 pieces (1 cubic inch)]	12	0.4	48	17%	1	10	0.1
1890	Fudge, peanut butter (Include chocolate fudge with peanut butter) [1 cubic inch]	21	0.7	89	35%	1	14	0.3
1891	Gumdrops [10 gumdrops]	37	1.3	125	2%	0	31	0.0
1892	Gumdrops, dietetic or low calorie [5 pieces]	25	0.9	41	1%	0	22	4.5
1893	Halvah, plain [1 bar]	57	2.0	287	52%	6	32	2.6
1894	Hard candies, dietetic or low calorie [10 pieces]	30	1.1	113	0%	0	28	0.0
1895	Jellybeans [10 large]	28	1.0	104	1%	0	26	0.0
1896	Jujubes [1 box]	43	1.5	166	0%	0	43	0.0
1897	Licorice [1 shoestring (43" long)]	19	0.7	70	1%	0	18	0.0
1898	Lifesavers [1 piece]	3	0.1	8	0%	0	2	0.0
1899	M & M's Almond Chocolate Candies [1 cup]	195	6.9	1026	48%	16	118	6.2
1900	M & M's Plain Chocolate Candies [1 package]	48	1.7	236	39%	2	34	1.2
1901	M & M's Peanut Butter Chocolate Candies [1 package]	46	1.6	236	45%	5	28	1.2
1902	M & M's Peanut Chocolate Candies [1 package]	47	1.7	243	46%	4	28	1.6
1903	Mars Bar [2 pieces]	38	1.3	177	44%	3	24	0.8
1904	Marshmallow (Include Marshmallow creme, Marshmallow chicken) [2 regular or 20 tiny]	14	0.5	45	1%	0	11	0.0
1905	Milk Duds [1 box]	35	1.2	144	29%	2	26	0.6

Food no.	fat gm	sat fat gm	choles mg	sodium mg	potas mg	% of Daily Value: vit A	vit E	vit C	thia	ribo	niac	vit B-6	fola	vit B-12	calc	phos	mag	iron	zinc
1856	15	8	0	28	131	0	5	0	1	1	1	1	1	0	1	6	11	6	4
1857	17	6	5	36	85	0	10	0	1	4	1	1	1	2	4	5	3	1	2
1858	1	0	0	66	120	0	0	0	1	2	1	0	0	0	1	4	6	4	2
1859	0	0	0	2	114	0	0	0	0	1	0	1	0	0	1	2	5	3	1
1860	0	0	0	13	57	0	0	24	0	0	0	0	0	0	1	0	0	2	1
1861	0	0	0	0	49	0	0	6	3	0	1	1	0	0	1	0	1	1	0
1862	0	0	0	17	2	0	0	0	0	0	0	0	0	0	0	0	0	0	0
1863	9	1	0	18	89	0	2	1	5	3	1	4	2	0	2	5	7	2	3
1864	4	1	0	12	187	0	3	0	1	3	5	2	2	1	3	7	8	5	4
1865	8	5	8	89	97	1	1	0	8	11	7	7	7	2	5	6	4	1	3
1866	3	1	3	45	31	1	0	0	1	2	0	0	0	1	2	2	2	1	1
1867	14	3	2	9	192	0	20	0	3	10	3	1	2	1	7	13	16	5	5
1868	7	1	0	7	89	0	3	0	1	6	2	1	2	0	4	6	9	4	2
1869	8	5	5	23	72	0	3	0	1	4	1	1	1	3	5	4	1	0	1
1870	7	4	1	77	135	0	3	0	2	2	5	1	3	0	1	5	7	0	3
1871	15	9	7	45	168	1	3	0	2	7	3	1	3	3	6	9	8	3	4
1872	8	5	0	89	170	0	3	0	2	2	5	2	3	0	1	6	9	2	3
1873	1	0	3	13	1	1	0	0	0	0	0	0	0	0	0	0	0	0	0
1874	14	8	1	38	212	0	6	1	5	10	4	3	6	4	11	12	11	3	6
1875	0	0	0	8	3	0	0	0	0	0	0	0	0	0	0	0	0	0	0
1876	5	1	0	59	113	0	4	0	2	6	0	1	0	2	4	5	3	1	1
1877	8	2	0	9	169	0	6	1	1	4	9	3	9	0	3	6	8	4	5
1878	0	0	0	0	0	0	0	0	0	0	0	0	0	0	0	0	0	0	0
1879	0	0	0	0	0	0	0	0	0	0	0	0	0	0	0	0	0	0	0
1880	0	0	0	0	0	0	0	0	0	0	0	0	0	0	0	0	0	0	0
1881	52	31	0	19	631	0	9	0	6	9	4	3	1	0	6	23	50	30	19
1882	6	4	5	29	84	1	1	0	1	4	0	0	0	1	4	5	3	2	2
1883	1	1	1	9	448	0	0	0	0	1	7	0	0	0	2	1	10	3	1
1884	7	2	1	60	105	0	4	0	0	4	5	1	4	1	2	5	5	2	2
1885	0	0	0	9	41	0	0	1	0	0	0	2	0	0	0	0	1	1	0
1886	2	0	1	14	75	1	1	0	2	1	0	1	0	0	2	2	2	2	1
1887	2	1	3	13	22	1	0	0	0	1	0	0	0	0	1	1	1	1	1
1888	3	1	3	13	33	1	0	0	1	1	0	1	1	0	1	2	2	1	1
1889	1	0	0	6	10	0	0	0	0	1	0	0	0	0	0	1	1	0	0
1890	4	1	3	35	43	1	2	0	0	1	4	1	1	0	1	2	2	1	1
1891	0	0	0	13	2	0	0	0	0	0	0	0	0	0	0	0	0	1	0
1892	0	0	0	2	0	0	0	0	0	0	0	0	0	0	0	0	0	0	0
1893	17	3	0	9	91	0	10	0	11	1	5	2	5	0	3	17	19	10	15
1894	0	0	0	0	0	0	0	0	0	0	0	0	0	0	0	0	0	0	0
1895	0	0	0	7	11	0	0	0	0	0	0	0	0	0	0	0	0	2	0
1896	0	0	0	19	2	0	0	0	0	0	0	0	0	0	0	0	0	1	0
1897	0	0	0	5	7	0	0	0	0	0	0	0	0	0	0	0	0	1	0
1898	0	0	0	1	0	0	0	0	0	0	0	0	0	0	0	0	0	0	0
1899	54	19	14	209	739	4	60	3	5	41	12	5	7	4	27	49	56	21	20
1900	10	6	7	29	128	3	2	0	2	6	1	1	1	2	5	7	5	3	3
1901	12	4	6	58	179	0	7	1	2	4	9	4	6	3	5	13	9	3	5
1902	12	5	4	23	162	1	5	0	5	6	5	2	5	2	5	9	7	3	4
1903	9	2	3	65	124	2	1	1	1	7	2	1	1	2	6	9	7	2	3
1904	0	0	0	7	1	0	0	0	0	0	0	0	0	0	0	0	0	0	0
1905	5	3	4	73	89	1	1	0	1	4	0	1	0	1	5	5	2	1	2

Desserts & Sweets

Food No.	Food Description & Amount	wt gm	wt oz	cal	% cal fat	prot gm	carbo gm	fiber gm
1906	Milky Way Bar [1 bar]	54	1.9	228	34%	2	39	0.7
1907	Milky Way Dark Bar [1 bar]	50	1.8	224	33%	1	36	1.1
1908	Milky Way II [1 bar]	58	2.0	193	38%	2	43	0.9
1909	Mints, dietetic or low calorie [10 mints]	15	0.5	56	0%	0	14	0.0
1910	Mound [1 bar]	47	1.7	170	54%	2	27	1.5
1911	Mr. Goodbar [1 bar]	43	1.5	221	57%	5	22	1.8
1912	Nestle Bar [1 bar]	32	1.1	164	54%	2	19	1.1
1913	Nestle Bar with Almonds [1 bar]	41	1.4	216	59%	4	22	2.5
1914	Nougat, plain (Include Italian nougat candy) [2 pieces]	28	1.0	102	14%	1	22	0.1
1915	Nuts, carob-coated (Include peanuts, cashews, walnuts, almonds) [1 oz]	28	1.0	156	66%	4	10	1.6
1916	Peanut brittle [1 cubic inch]	20	0.7	91	38%	2	14	0.4
1917	Peanut butter chips [¼ cup]	42	1.5	209	54%	8	19	0.4
1918	Peanut Bar, chocolate covered [1 bar]	57	2.0	296	57%	7	29	1.9
1919	P.B. Max Peanut Butter Snack [1 bar]	42	1.5	238	58%	5	20	1.7
1920	Pecan roll [1 cubic inch]	19	0.7	87	45%	2	11	0.7
1921	Powerhouse [1 bar]	38	1.3	164	35%	4	25	1.3
1922	Pralines [1 cubic inch]	21	0.7	84	25%	0	16	0.2
1923	Raisinets [1 box]	35	1.2	137	34%	1	24	1.5
1924	Reese's Peanut Butter Cup [1 package]	45	1.6	222	58%	5	22	1.8
1925	Reese's Pieces [1 package]	50	1.8	235	40%	7	31	2.1
1926	Rolo [1 roll]	49	1.7	233	41%	2	34	0.3
1927	Skittles [1 bar]	35	1.2	142	10%	0	32	0.0
1928	Skor bar [1 bar]	40	1.4	169	31%	2	29	0.7
1929	Snickers Bar [1 bar]	57	2.0	273	46%	5	34	1.4
1930	Snickers Peanut Butter Bar [1 bar]	50	1.8	279	57%	6	23	2.0
1931	Special Dark [1 bar]	41	1.4	195	57%	2	25	2.3
1932	Starburst [1 package]	59	2.1	232	19%	1	49	0.1
1933	Sugar Daddy [1 sucker]	59	2.1	225	19%	3	45	0.7
1934	Take Five [1 bar]	40	1.4	205	51%	3	25	0.4
1935	Thin Mints [1 oz]	28	1.0	102	23%	1	22	0.3
1936	Tic Tacs [10 pieces]	5	0.2	19	0%	0	5	0.0
1937	Toblerone, milk chocolate with honey and almond nougat [1 package]	100	3.5	491	49%	6	62	2.9
1938	Toffee, chocolate-coated, with nuts (Include Almond Roca) [3 pieces]	33	1.2	145	38%	2	22	0.8
1939	Tootsie Roll [1 roll]	35	1.2	126	6%	1	31	0.3
1940	Twix Cookie Bars [1 package-2 bars]	54	1.9	269	44%	2	35	0.6
1941	Twix Chocolate Fudge Cookie Bars (Include Cookies-n-Creme Bars) [1 package]	45	1.6	248	54%	3	25	1.4
1942	Twix Peanut Butter Cookie Bars [1 package-2 bars]	54	1.9	286	55%	5	28	1.8
1943	Whatchamacallit [1 bar]	40	1.4	201	46%	4	24	1.2
1944	Wax candy, liquid filled [10 Pop Bottles]	42	1.5	53	0%	0	14	0.0
1945	Whoppers [1 pack]	57	2.0	283	48%	4	36	1.5
1946	Yogurt chips [1 oz]	28	1.0	147	49%	3	15	0.5
	Your Additions							

Food no.	fat gm	sat fat gm	choles mg	sodium mg	potas mg	% of Daily Value													
						vit A	vit E	vit C	thia	ribo	niac	vit B-6	fola	vit B-12	calc	phos	mag	iron	zinc
1906	9	4	8	130	130	3	2	1	1	7	1	1	1	4	7	9	5	2	3
1907	8	4	7	114	144	2	0	1	0	3	1	1	1	0	3	7	6	3	3
1908	8	7	12	153	152	1	2	0	2	5	1	1	1	3	6	7	5	3	3
1909	0	0	0	0	0	0	0	0	0	0	0	0	0	0	0	0	0	0	0
1910	10	5	0	59	99	0	4	0	1	2	0	1	0	0	1	6	8	10	3
1911	14	8	9	15	194	0	2	0	1	7	10	3	8	3	5	12	10	3	5
1912	10	6	7	26	123	2	2	0	2	6	1	1	1	2	6	7	5	2	3
1913	14	7	8	30	182	1	4	0	2	10	2	1	1	4	9	11	9	4	4
1914	2	1	0	59	9	0	0	0	1	1	1	1	0	0	0	0	0	1	0
1915	12	5	0	17	190	0	11	0	5	5	6	2	6	2	7	8	9	4	6
1916	4	1	3	90	42	1	1	0	3	1	3	1	4	0	1	2	3	2	1
1917	13	6	0	105	212	0	6	0	1	5	17	5	10	0	5	13	12	4	6
1918	19	5	7	109	228	3	3	0	4	6	16	2	6	1	6	10	10	3	5
1919	15	3	1	142	161	0	11	0	4	3	11	3	4	1	3	9	9	4	5
1920	4	1	2	45	60	0	3	0	1	1	5	1	2	0	1	4	4	1	3
1921	6	3	3	90	123	0	3	0	1	4	5	1	3	2	4	7	6	1	3
1922	2	0	1	14	75	1	1	0	2	1	0	1	0	0	2	2	2	2	1
1923	5	3	1	13	180	0	2	0	2	3	1	2	0	1	3	5	4	3	2
1924	14	6	5	131	180	1	3	0	1	6	9	2	3	3	4	11	10	3	4
1925	10	7	2	75	220	0	3	0	2	7	14	3	7	3	7	12	10	4	4
1926	11	5	11	83	127	1	2	1	2	7	0	2	1	6	7	8	4	1	2
1927	2	0	0	6	2	0	0	39	0	0	0	0	0	0	0	0	0	0	0
1928	6	4	4	81	105	1	1	0	1	5	1	1	1	1	6	6	3	1	2
1929	14	5	7	152	192	2	4	1	8	5	10	3	11	1	5	11	10	2	5
1930	18	4	3	134	201	1	0	1	4	4	15	4	9	1	5	10	11	3	5
1931	12	7	0	4	139	0	2	0	1	6	1	1	0	0	1	7	12	5	4
1932	5	1	0	63	19	0	3	39	0	2	0	0	0	0	1	1	1	1	0
1933	5	4	4	145	126	0	1	0	0	6	1	1	1	0	8	7	3	0	2
1934	12	7	8	40	123	1	1	1	2	6	1	1	0	4	7	7	4	2	3
1935	3	2	0	7	47	0	0	0	0	1	1	0	0	0	0	3	4	2	1
1936	0	0	0	2	0	0	0	0	0	0	0	0	0	0	0	0	0	0	0
1937	27	16	19	101	332	5	5	1	5	16	2	2	2	6	16	19	13	7	8
1938	6	3	3	59	103	1	2	0	2	4	2	1	2	1	5	6	4	2	2
1939	1	0	0	9	35	0	0	0	0	1	0	0	0	0	1	1	3	1	1
1940	13	5	3	104	109	1	3	0	6	7	3	1	1	2	5	6	4	2	3
1941	15	2	3	120	139	0	5	1	4	5	2	1	1	2	6	7	5	3	3
1942	17	6	3	147	192	1	3	1	3	5	11	4	3	1	4	10	10	3	5
1943	10	4	8	91	139	1	1	0	16	6	4	1	1	3	5	8	6	2	3
1944	0	0	0	1	0	0	0	0	0	0	0	0	0	0	0	0	0	0	0
1945	15	9	11	83	196	1	3	0	2	10	1	2	1	4	10	11	7	2	4
1946	8	2	1	13	63	0	5	0	8	7	5	1	1	1	4	5	2	5	2

Fruits and Vegetables

Fruits & Vegetables

Food No.	Food Description & Amount	wt gm	wt oz	cal	% cal fat	prot gm	carbo gm	fiber gm
	Fruits							
2000	Acerola, raw [1 fruit]	5	0.2	2	8%	0	0	0.1
2001	Ambrosia (oranges, bananas, coconut, sugar) [1 cup]	193	6.8	250	38%	3	41	6.4
2002	**Apple**, raw [1 apple (2¾" dia) (about 3 per lb)]	138	4.9	81	5%	0	21	3.7
2003	Apple, baked, unsweetened [1 apple with liquid]	161	5.7	102	5%	0	26	4.7
2004	Apple, baked, with sugar (Include scalloped apples) [1 apple with liquid]	171	6.0	173	3%	0	45	4.4
2005	Apple, cooked or canned, with syrup [1 cup, slices]	204	7.2	137	6%	0	34	4.1
2006	Apple, candied (caramel-covered, include caramel apples) [1 apple]	184	6.5	243	14%	2	54	4.3
2007	Apple-cabbage-mayonnaise salad [1 cup]	161	5.7	217	72%	1	17	3.6
2008	Apple chips [15 chips]	33	1.2	152	42%	0	24	3.2
2009	Apple, dried, cooked, unsweetened [1 cup]	255	9.0	145	1%	1	39	5.1
2010	Apple, dried, cooked, with sugar [1 cup]	280	9.9	244	1%	1	65	5.1
2011	Apple, dried, uncooked (Include dried diet snack, plain or flavored) [5 rings]	32	1.1	78	1%	0	21	2.8
2012	Apple, dried, uncooked, low sodium [5 rings]	32	1.1	78	1%	0	21	2.8
2013	Apple, fried (apples, margarine, sugar) [1 cup]	179	6.3	268	37%	0	46	4.5
2014	Apple, pickled (apples, sugar, vinegar; include spiced) [1 apple]	29	1.0	38	2%	0	10	0.5
2015	Apple rings, fried [4 rings]	76	2.7	97	40%	0	16	2.0
2016	Apple salad with dressing (Include Waldorf salad) [1 cup]	137	4.8	192	60%	2	21	3.2
2017	Applesauce, stewed apples, unsweetened or sweetened with low-cal sweetener [1 cup]	244	8.6	105	1%	0	28	2.9
2018	Applesauce, stewed apples, with sugar (Include apple pie filling) [1 cup]	255	9.0	194	2%	0	51	3.1
2019	Applesauce with other fruits [1 cup]	256	9.0	156	3%	1	40	2.8
2020	Apricot, raw [2 apricots]	70	2.5	34	7%	1	8	1.7
2021	Apricot, cooked or canned in heavy syrup, drained solids [2 whole apricots]	76	2.7	63	1%	0	16	1.7
2022	Apricot, cooked or canned, in heavy syrup (Include home canned) [2 whole apricots with liquid]	106	3.7	88	1%	1	23	1.7
2023	Apricot, cooked or canned, in light syrup [2 whole apricots with liquid]	106	3.7	67	1%	1	17	1.7
2024	Apricot, cooked or canned, juice pack [2 whole apricots with liquid]	90	3.2	43	1%	1	11	1.4
2025	Apricot, cooked or canned, unsweetened, water pack [2 whole apricots with liquid]	90	3.2	24	5%	1	6	1.4
2026	Apricot, dried, cooked, unsweetened [1 cup]	250	8.8	213	2%	3	55	8.0
2027	Apricot, dried, cooked, with sugar [1 cup]	270	9.5	304	1%	3	78	7.8
2028	Apricot, dried, uncooked [4 halves]	14	0.5	33	2%	1	9	1.3
2029	Avocado, raw [1 avocado, California (black skin)]	173	6.1	279	86%	3	13	8.7
2030	**Banana**, yellow, common, raw [1 fruit (9" long)]	114	4.0	105	5%	1	27	2.7
2031	Banana, yellow, boiled [1 fruit]	91	3.2	84	5%	1	21	2.2
2032	Banana, yellow, fried in margarine [1 fruit]	91	3.2	181	51%	1	24	2.4
2033	Banana, yellow, fried with cheese, Puerto Rican style (guineos nifios con queso) [1 banana (4" x 1½" x 1½")]	40	1.4	85	53%	1	10	1.0
2034	Banana, baked (banana, sugar, lemon juice) [1 banana (7" long)]	128	4.5	167	4%	1	43	3.4
2035	Banana, batter-dipped, fried (banana, pancake mix, soybean oil) [1 fruit]	136	4.8	341	59%	3	35	2.7
2036	Banana chips [1 cup]	92	3.2	338	16%	3	76	6.1
2037	Banana, chocolate-covered with peanuts [1 banana]	145	5.1	331	50%	7	43	5.1
2038	Banana flakes, dehydrated [1 cup]	100	3.5	346	5%	4	88	7.5
2039	Banana whip (bananas, egg white, sugar, lemon juice, salt) [1 cup]	130	4.6	179	2%	6	40	2.1
2040	Banana, apple ("apple-banana"), raw [1 fruit]	73	2.6	67	5%	1	17	1.8
2041	Banana, Chinese, raw (Include Cavendish, dwarf, finger) [1 fruit (5" long)]	63	2.2	58	5%	1	15	1.5
2042	Banana, green, cooked in salt water [1 fruit]	54	1.9	50	5%	1	13	1.3
2043	Banana, green, fried in corn oil [4 slices]	92	3.2	159	49%	1	22	2.3
2044	Banana, red, fried [1 fruit (7" long)]	94	3.3	194	53%	1	24	2.1
2045	Banana, red, ripe (guineo morado) [1 fruit (7" long)]	104	3.7	94	2%	1	24	2.1
2046	Banana, white, ripe (guineo blanco maduro) [1 fruit]	119	4.2	109	5%	1	28	2.9
2047	Blackberries, raw (Include dewberries, youngberries, marionberries) [1 cup]	144	5.1	75	7%	1	18	7.6

Food no.	fat gm	sat fat gm	choles mg	sodium mg	potas mg	% of Daily Value: vit A	vit E	vit C	thia	ribo	niac	vit B-6	fola	vit B-12	calc	phos	mag	iron	zinc
2000	0	0	0	0	7	0	0	140	0	0	0	0	0	0	0	0	0	0	0
2001	11	9	0	7	580	2	3	74	8	7	4	29	11	0	4	6	11	6	3
2002	0	0	0	0	159	1	2	13	2	1	1	3	1	0	1	1	2	1	0
2003	1	0	0	0	179	1	3	13	2	1	1	4	1	0	1	1	2	2	0
2004	1	0	0	0	170	1	2	12	1	2	1	4	1	0	1	1	2	2	0
2005	1	0	0	6	143	1	0	1	1	1	1	4	0	0	1	1	2	3	1
2006	4	3	3	102	253	1	3	14	2	6	1	4	2	0	7	6	4	2	2
2007	17	3	13	131	239	3	13	37	3	2	1	11	7	1	4	2	3	3	1
2008	7	1	0	32	150	0	11	1	1	2	1	3	0	0	0	1	1	3	1
2009	0	0	0	51	268	1	0	4	1	3	2	6	0	0	1	2	3	5	1
2010	0	0	0	51	268	1	0	4	1	3	2	6	0	0	1	2	3	5	1
2011	0	0	0	28	144	0	1	2	0	3	1	2	0	0	0	1	1	2	0
2012	0	0	0	0	144	0	0	2	0	3	1	2	0	0	0	1	1	2	0
2013	11	2	0	121	178	11	9	11	2	2	1	4	1	0	2	1	2	2	0
2014	0	0	0	0	28	0	0	2	0	0	0	0	0	0	0	0	1	0	0
2015	4	1	0	47	80	4	4	5	1	1	0	2	0	0	1	1	1	1	0
2016	13	2	5	153	208	2	6	11	4	2	1	6	4	1	3	5	6	3	2
2017	0	0	0	5	183	1	0	5	2	4	2	3	0	0	1	2	2	2	0
2018	0	0	0	8	156	0	0	7	2	4	2	3	0	0	1	2	2	5	1
2019	1	0	0	15	138	0	2	24	2	5	2	4	1	0	2	2	2	5	1
2020	0	0	0	1	207	18	3	12	1	2	2	2	2	0	1	1	1	2	1
2021	0	0	0	3	109	14	4	4	1	1	1	2	0	0	1	1	1	1	1
2022	0	0	0	4	148	13	4	5	1	1	2	3	0	0	1	1	2	2	1
2023	0	0	0	4	146	14	4	5	1	1	2	3	0	0	1	1	2	2	1
2024	0	0	0	4	149	15	4	7	1	1	2	2	0	0	1	2	2	2	1
2025	0	0	0	3	173	12	4	5	1	1	2	2	0	0	1	1	2	2	1
2026	0	0	0	8	1223	59	6	7	1	4	12	14	0	0	4	10	11	23	4
2027	0	0	0	8	1200	58	6	7	1	5	12	14	0	0	4	10	10	23	4
2028	0	0	0	1	193	10	0	1	0	1	2	1	0	0	1	2	2	4	1
2029	27	4	0	17	1036	11	11	23	12	12	17	24	27	0	2	7	17	10	5
2030	1	0	0	1	451	1	1	17	3	7	3	33	5	0	1	2	8	2	1
2031	0	0	0	1	324	1	1	10	2	5	2	24	2	0	1	2	7	2	1
2032	10	2	0	116	367	10	8	11	3	6	2	26	2	0	1	2	7	2	1
2033	5	1	3	38	156	1	4	4	1	3	1	11	1	1	3	3	3	1	1
2034	1	0	0	2	512	1	2	22	3	8	3	39	4	0	1	3	10	2	2
2035	22	3	3	160	347	1	21	10	10	13	8	24	3	1	2	13	8	8	2
2036	6	4	0	3	1212	3	0	9	10	12	11	18	3	0	2	6	22	5	3
2037	18	7	0	6	592	1	8	15	6	11	16	32	10	0	3	15	23	8	11
2038	2	1	0	3	1491	3	0	12	12	14	14	22	4	0	2	7	27	6	4
2039	0	0	0	83	387	1	1	16	2	18	2	24	3	1	1	2	8	2	1
2040	0	0	0	1	289	1	1	11	2	4	2	21	3	0	0	1	5	1	1
2041	0	0	0	1	249	1	1	10	2	4	2	18	3	0	0	1	5	1	1
2042	0	0	0	1	192	0	1	6	1	3	1	14	1	0	0	1	4	1	1
2043	9	1	0	1	335	1	9	10	2	5	2	24	2	0	1	2	7	2	1
2044	11	2	0	133	350	14	9	12	3	2	3	27	2	0	1	2	8	5	1
2045	0	0	0	1	385	4	1	17	3	2	3	30	5	0	1	2	8	5	1
2046	1	0	0	1	471	1	1	18	4	7	3	34	6	0	1	2	9	2	1
2047	1	0	0	0	282	2	5	50	3	3	3	4	12	0	5	3	7	5	3

Fruits & Vegetables

Food No.	Food Description & Amount	wt gm	wt oz	cal	% cal fat	prot gm	carbo gm	fiber gm
2048	Blackberries, cooked or canned, in heavy syrup (Include dewberries, youngberries, marionberries) [1 cup]	256	9.0	236	1%	3	59	8.7
2049	Blackberries, frozen [1 cup]	143	5.0	92	6%	2	22	7.2
2050	Blueberries, raw [1 cup]	145	5.1	81	6%	1	20	3.9
2051	Blueberries, cooked or canned, in heavy syrup (Include home canned) [1 cup]	256	9.0	225	3%	2	56	3.8
2052	Blueberries, cooked or canned, unsweetened, water pack [1 cup]	244	8.6	92	6%	1	23	4.4
2053	Blueberries, frozen [1 cup]	230	8.1	117	11%	1	28	6.2
2054	Blueberries, frozen, sweetened [1 cup]	230	8.1	186	1%	1	50	4.8
2055	Boysenberries, raw [1 cup]	144	5.1	75	7%	1	18	7.6
2056	Boysenberries, cooked or canned in heavy syrup [1 cup]	256	9.0	225	1%	3	57	6.7
2057	Boysenberries, frozen [1 cup]	143	5.0	72	5%	2	17	5.6
2058	Breadfruit, cooked, salt added (Include pana) [1 cup]	252	8.9	289	2%	3	76	13.8
2059	Breadfruit, fried in corn oil (tostones) [1 cup]	170	6.0	379	50%	2	52	9.4
2060	Calamondin, raw [4 fruit (1" dia)]	76	2.7	33	4%	0	9	1.7
2061	Cantaloupe (muskmelon), raw [¼ melon]	169	6.0	59	7%	1	14	1.4
2062	Cantaloupe, frozen (balls) [1 cup]	173	6.1	61	7%	2	14	1.4
2063	Carambola (starfruit), cooked with sugar [1 cup]	205	7.2	109	6%	1	27	5.9
2064	Cassaba melon, raw (Include crenshaw melon) [1 cup]	170	6.0	44	3%	2	11	1.4
2065	Cherries, sweet, raw (Queen Anne, Bing) [10 cherries]	68	2.4	49	12%	1	11	1.6
2066	Cherries, frozen [1 cup]	155	5.5	71	9%	1	17	2.5
2067	Cherries, maraschino [10 cherries]	43	1.5	50	2%	0	13	0.4
2068	Cherries, sour, red, cooked, unsweetened [1 cup, pitted]	244	8.6	88	3%	2	22	2.7
2069	Cherries, sour, red, raw [1 cup, pitted]	155	5.5	78	5%	2	19	2.5
2070	Cherries, sweet, cooked or canned, drained solids [1 cup, pitted]	179	6.3	149	2%	1	38	2.1
2071	Cherries, sweet, cooked or canned, in heavy syrup (Include home canned) [1 cup, pitted]	253	8.9	210	2%	2	54	3.8
2072	Cherries, sweet, cooked or canned, in light syrup [1 cup, pitted]	252	8.9	169	2%	2	44	3.8
2073	Cherries, sweet, cooked or canned, juice pack [1 cup, pitted]	250	8.8	135	0%	2	35	3.8
2074	Cherries, sweet, cooked, unsweetened, water pack [1 cup, pitted]	248	8.7	114	3%	2	29	3.7
2075	Carambola (starfruit), raw [1 medium (3-5/8" long)]	91	3.2	30	10%	0	7	2.5
2076	Cranberries, cooked or canned (Include cranberry sauce) [1 cup]	277	9.8	418	1%	1	108	2.8
2077	Cranberries, dried [1 cup]	110	3.9	363	3%	0	95	9.7
2078	Cranberries, raw [1 cup, chopped]	110	3.9	54	4%	0	14	4.6
2079	Cranberry salad (cranberry, pineapple, celery, walnuts, sugar, gelatin) [1 cup]	253	8.9	348	30%	5	61	4.5
2080	Cranberry-orange relish (cranberrry, orange, sugar), uncooked [1 cup]	275	9.7	470	1%	1	124	7.5
2081	Currants, dried [1 cup]	144	5.1	408	1%	6	107	9.8
2082	Currants, raw [1 cup]	112	4.0	63	3%	2	15	4.8
2083	Date [10 dates]	83	2.9	228	1%	2	61	6.2
2084	Dewberries, raw [1 cup]	144	5.1	75	7%	1	18	7.6
2085	Elderberries, cooked or canned in syrup [1 cup]	256	9.0	304	3%	1	78	13.1
2086	Elderberries, raw [1 cup]	145	5.1	106	6%	1	27	10.2
2087	Figs, raw [1 medium (2¼" dia)]	50	1.8	37	4%	0	10	1.7
2088	Figs, cooked or canned, in heavy syrup (Include home canned) [1 fig with liquid]	28	1.0	25	1%	0	6	0.6
2089	Figs, cooked or canned, in light syrup [1 cup]	252	8.9	174	1%	1	45	4.5
2090	Figs, cooked or canned, unsweetened, water pack [4 figs with liquid]	108	3.8	57	2%	0	15	2.4
2091	Figs, dried, cooked, unsweetened [1 cup]	259	9.1	280	4%	3	71	12.4
2092	Figs, dried, cooked, with sugar [1 cup]	270	9.5	358	3%	3	92	11.8
2093	Fruit cocktail or mix, raw, made with fresh fruit (no citrus fruits) [1 cup]	175	6.2	101	5%	1	26	3.5
2094	Fruit cocktail or mix, raw, made with fresh fruit (including citrus fruits) [1 cup]	175	6.2	99	5%	1	25	3.3
2095	Fruit cocktail or mix, frozen [1 cup]	215	7.6	112	7%	2	27	5.6
2096	Fruit cocktail, cooked or canned in heavy syrup, drained solids (Include fruit cocktail, mix, or salad of mixed cooked or canned fruits) [1 cup]	214	7.5	156	1%	1	40	3.9
2097	Fruit cocktail, cooked or canned, in heavy syrup (Include fruit cocktail, mix, or salad of mixed cooked or canned fruits) [1 cup]	248	8.7	181	1%	1	47	2.5

Food no.	fat gm	sat fat gm	choles mg	sodium mg	potas mg	vit A	vit E	vit C	thia	ribo	niac	vit B-6	fola	vit B-12	calc	phos	mag	iron	zinc
						% of Daily Value													
2048	0	0	0	8	253	6	8	12	5	6	4	5	17	0	5	4	11	9	3
2049	1	0	0	1	200	2	5	7	3	4	9	4	12	0	4	4	8	6	2
2050	1	0	0	9	129	1	7	31	5	4	3	3	2	0	1	1	2	1	1
2051	1	0	0	8	102	2	12	5	6	8	1	5	1	0	1	3	3	5	1
2052	1	0	0	12	131	1	7	18	4	4	3	3	1	0	1	2	2	2	1
2053	1	0	0	2	124	2	10	10	5	5	6	7	4	0	2	3	3	2	1
2054	0	0	0	2	138	1	7	4	3	7	3	7	4	0	1	2	1	5	1
2055	1	0	0	0	282	2	5	50	3	3	3	4	12	0	5	3	7	5	3
2056	0	0	0	8	230	1	8	26	4	4	3	5	22	0	5	3	7	6	3
2057	0	0	0	1	199	1	3	7	5	3	5	4	23	0	4	4	6	7	2
2058	1	0	0	5	1238	1	14	102	16	4	11	12	6	0	5	8	17	8	2
2059	21	3	0	4	847	1	29	65	11	3	8	9	3	0	3	6	12	6	2
2060	0	0	0	1	119	7	1	39	5	1	1	3	4	0	1	1	2	0	1
2061	0	0	0	15	522	54	1	119	4	2	5	10	7	0	2	3	5	2	2
2062	0	0	0	16	535	53	1	116	4	2	5	10	7	0	2	3	5	2	2
2063	1	0	0	4	320	9	4	62	3	3	4	10	5	0	1	4	5	3	2
2064	0	0	0	20	357	1	1	45	7	2	3	10	7	0	1	1	3	4	2
2065	1	0	0	0	152	1	0	8	2	2	1	1	1	0	1	1	2	1	0
2066	1	0	0	2	192	13	1	4	5	3	1	5	2	0	2	2	3	5	1
2067	0	0	0	21	54	0	0	0	0	0	0	0	0	0	1	1	0	1	0
2068	0	0	0	17	239	18	1	9	3	6	2	5	5	0	3	2	4	19	1
2069	0	0	0	5	268	20	1	26	3	4	3	3	3	0	2	2	3	3	1
2070	0	0	0	5	265	4	1	11	3	5	4	3	2	0	2	4	4	3	1
2071	0	0	0	8	367	4	1	15	4	6	5	4	3	0	2	5	6	5	2
2072	0	0	0	8	373	4	1	16	4	6	5	4	3	0	2	5	6	5	2
2073	0	0	0	8	328	3	1	10	3	4	5	4	3	0	4	6	8	8	2
2074	0	0	0	2	325	4	1	9	4	6	5	4	3	0	3	4	6	5	1
2075	0	0	0	2	148	4	2	32	2	1	2	5	3	0	0	1	2	1	1
2076	0	0	0	80	72	1	1	9	3	3	1	2	1	0	1	2	2	3	1
2077	1	0	0	3	96	0	3	1	1	6	0	3	0	0	2	1	2	3	1
2078	0	0	0	1	78	1	1	25	2	1	1	4	0	0	1	1	1	1	1
2079	12	1	0	30	300	1	3	28	12	5	3	12	6	0	5	8	13	6	5
2080	0	0	0	3	201	2	1	97	6	4	2	6	5	0	5	3	4	4	2
2081	0	0	0	12	1284	1	1	11	15	12	12	21	4	0	12	18	15	26	6
2082	0	0	0	1	308	1	1	77	3	3	1	4	2	0	4	5	4	6	2
2083	0	0	0	2	541	0	0	0	5	5	9	8	3	0	3	3	7	5	2
2084	1	0	0	0	282	2	5	50	3	3	3	4	12	0	5	3	7	5	3
2085	1	0	0	12	473	8	9	79	7	6	4	19	1	0	7	7	2	17	2
2086	1	0	0	9	406	9	7	87	7	5	4	17	2	0	6	6	2	13	1
2087	0	0	0	1	116	1	2	2	2	1	1	3	1	0	2	1	2	1	1
2088	0	0	0	0	28	0	1	0	0	1	1	1	0	0	1	0	1	0	0
2089	0	0	0	3	257	1	10	4	4	6	6	9	1	0	7	3	6	4	2
2090	0	0	0	1	111	0	4	2	2	2	2	4	1	0	3	1	3	2	1
2091	1	0	0	13	780	4	0	19	2	17	8	17	1	0	16	8	16	14	4
2092	1	0	0	13	742	4	0	18	2	16	8	16	1	0	15	7	15	13	3
2093	1	0	0	1	328	3	3	24	5	5	4	10	3	0	1	2	5	2	1
2094	1	0	0	1	309	1	3	49	4	4	2	12	4	0	2	2	4	2	1
2095	1	0	0	1	356	9	4	20	5	6	7	4	6	0	3	3	5	4	2
2096	0	0	0	13	193	7	4	7	3	3	4	5	2	0	1	3	3	3	1
2097	0	0	0	15	218	5	3	8	3	3	5	6	2	0	1	3	3	4	1

Fruits & Vegetables

Food No.	Food Description & Amount	wt gm	wt oz	cal	% cal fat	prot gm	carbo gm	fiber gm
2098	Fruit cocktail, cooked or canned, in light syrup (Include fruit cocktail, mix, or salad of mixed cooked or canned fruits) [1 cup]	242	8.5	138	1%	1	36	2.4
2099	Fruit cocktail, cooked or canned, juice pack (Include fruit cocktail, mix, or salad of mixed of cooked or canned fruits) [1 cup]	237	8.4	109	0%	1	28	2.4
2100	Fruit cocktail, cooked or canned, unsweetened, water pack (Include fruit cocktail, mix, or salad of mixed cooked or canned fruits) [1 cup]	245	8.6	78	1%	1	21	2.5
2101	Fruit mixture, dried (Include s three or more of: apples, apricots, dates, papaya, peaches, pears, pineapples, prunes, raisins) [1 cup]	136	4.8	330	2%	3	87	10.6
2102	Fruit salad, mixed, fresh, with dressing [1 cup]	188	6.6	117	16%	1	26	3.7
2103	Fruit salad (no citrus fruit) with cream substitute [1 cup]	175	6.2	148	20%	1	32	3.0
2104	Fruit salad (no citrus fruit) with cream [1 cup]	182	6.4	165	36%	1	28	3.3
2105	Fruit salad (no citrus fruit) with marshmallows [1 cup]	171	6.0	187	8%	1	46	2.7
2106	Fruit salad (no citrus fruit) with pudding [1 cup]	182	6.4	173	15%	3	35	0.8
2107	Fruit salad (no citrus fruit) with salad dressing or mayonnaise [1 cup]	188	6.6	184	40%	1	30	3.5
2108	Fruit salad (including citrus fruit) with cream [1 cup]	182	6.4	132	39%	1	21	2.7
2109	Fruit salad (including citrus fruit) with cream substitute [1 cup]	175	6.2	114	25%	1	22	2.6
2110	Fruit salad (including citrus fruit) with marshmallows [1 cup]	171	6.0	155	8%	1	37	2.4
2111	Fruit salad (including citrus fruit) with pudding [1 cup]	182	6.4	168	16%	3	34	1.1
2112	Fruit salad (including citrus fruit) with salad dressing or mayonnaise [1 cup]	188	6.6	152	47%	1	22	3.0
2113	Fruit salad, Puerto Rican style (Includes bananas, papayas, oranges, grapefruit, etc.) (Ensalada de frutas tropicales) [1 cup]	247	8.7	141	4%	2	36	3.8
2114	Genip, raw [10 small]	50	1.8	39	2%	1	10	2.1
2115	Gooseberries, cooked or canned [1 cup]	252	8.9	184	2%	2	47	6.0
2116	Gooseberries, raw [1 cup]	150	5.3	66	12%	1	15	6.5
2117	Grapefruit and orange sections, raw [1 cup]	217	7.7	84	3%	2	21	3.6
2118	Grapefruit and orange sections, cooked, canned, or frozen, in light syrup [1 cup]	254	9.0	152	1%	1	39	2.5
2119	Grapefruit and orange sections, cooked, canned, or frozen, unsweetened, water pack [1 cup]	244	8.6	65	3%	1	16	2.8
2120	Grapefruit, canned or frozen, in light syrup [1 cup]	254	9.0	152	2%	1	39	1.0
2121	Grapefruit, canned or frozen, unsweetened, water pack [1 cup]	244	8.6	88	3%	1	22	1.0
2122	Grapefruit, raw (Include chironja) [½ medium (about 4" dia)]	128	4.5	41	3%	1	10	1.4
2123	Grapes, American type, slip skin, raw (Include concord) [10 grapes]	24	0.8	15	5%	0	4	0.2
2124	Grapes, European type, adherent skin, raw (Include tokay, emperor, thompson, red flame grapes) [10 grapes]	50	1.8	36	7%	0	9	0.5
2125	Grapes, seedless, cooked or canned, in heavy syrup (Include home canned) [1 cup]	256	9.0	187	1%	1	50	1.0
2126	Grapes, seedless, cooked or canned, unsweetened, water pack [1 cup]	245	8.6	98	2%	1	25	2.5
2127	Guacamole with tomatoes (avocado, tomato, onion, garlic, parsley, lemon juice, salt) [1 cup]	233	8.2	273	80%	4	16	8.8
2128	Guacamole (avocado, onion, lemon juice, salt) (Include avocado dip) [1 cup]	233	8.2	369	85%	5	17	11.5
2129	Guava, canned in heavy syrup [1 cup]	310	10.9	300	4%	2	75	11.9
2130	Guava, raw [1 guava]	90	3.2	46	11%	1	11	4.9
2131	Honeydew melon, raw [1 wedge (1/8 of 6" to 7" dia melon)]	160	5.6	56	3%	1	15	1.0
2132	Honeydew, frozen (balls) [1 cup]	230	8.1	81	3%	1	21	1.4
2133	Huckleberries, raw [1 cup]	145	5.1	81	6%	1	20	3.9
2134	Jackfruit, cooked or canned [4 pieces]	88	3.1	83	3%	1	21	1.4
2135	Jackfruit, raw [1 cup, sliced]	165	5.8	155	3%	2	40	2.6
2136	Jobo, raw [1 fruit]	75	2.6	65	3%	1	17	1.1
2137	Juneberry, raw [1 cup]	165	5.8	92	6%	1	23	4.5
2138	Kiwi fruit, raw [1 fruit]	76	2.7	46	6%	1	11	2.6
2139	Kumquat, cooked or canned, in syrup [4 kumquats]	56	2.0	50	1%	0	13	2.4
2140	Kumquat, raw [4 kumquats]	76	2.7	48	1%	1	12	5.0
2141	Lemon, raw [1 fruit (2-1/8" dia)]	58	2.0	17	9%	1	5	1.6
2142	Lime, raw [1 fruit (2" dia)]	67	2.4	20	6%	0	7	1.9

Food no.	fat gm	sat fat gm	choles mg	sodium mg	potas mg	% of Daily Value: vit A	vit E	vit C	thia	ribo	niac	vit B-6	fola	vit B-12	calc	phos	mag	iron	zinc
2098	0	0	0	15	215	5	3	8	3	3	5	6	2	0	1	3	3	4	1
2099	0	0	0	9	225	7	2	11	2	2	5	6	1	0	2	3	4	3	1
2100	0	0	0	10	230	6	3	9	3	2	4	6	2	0	1	3	4	3	1
2101	1	0	0	24	1082	33	5	9	4	13	13	13	1	0	6	11	13	20	5
2102	2	1	5	3	327	5	3	28	5	5	4	9	4	0	2	3	5	2	1
2103	3	2	1	22	353	1	1	24	5	5	3	19	4	1	2	3	7	3	2
2104	7	4	18	7	359	6	2	25	6	6	3	19	4	0	2	3	7	3	1
2105	2	1	0	23	305	1	1	22	5	4	3	17	4	0	1	2	6	3	1
2106	3	2	11	283	199	4	1	4	3	9	2	4	2	5	10	20	4	2	3
2107	8	2	5	47	375	2	6	27	6	5	3	22	5	0	1	3	7	3	1
2108	6	4	15	18	260	5	2	82	8	4	3	5	5	0	4	3	5	2	1
2109	3	2	1	21	257	2	2	79	8	4	3	5	5	1	4	3	5	2	1
2110	1	1	0	23	218	1	1	72	7	3	3	5	4	0	3	2	4	2	1
2111	3	2	11	293	218	4	1	20	4	9	2	4	2	5	12	21	4	1	3
2112	8	2	5	51	274	2	6	95	8	3	3	8	7	0	4	2	5	2	1
2113	1	0	0	3	496	6	4	108	11	6	4	21	10	0	4	3	9	3	2
2114	0	0	0	3	117	0	1	4	2	1	2	3	2	0	1	1	2	2	0
2115	1	0	0	5	194	4	4	42	3	8	2	2	2	0	4	2	4	5	2
2116	1	0	0	2	297	4	3	69	4	3	2	6	2	0	4	4	4	3	1
2117	0	0	0	0	342	3	2	154	8	4	3	5	10	0	5	2	5	1	1
2118	0	0	0	4	316	2	2	116	8	3	3	4	7	0	5	2	5	3	1
2119	0	0	0	2	264	3	2	114	6	3	2	4	6	0	4	2	4	1	1
2120	0	0	0	5	328	0	3	90	6	3	3	3	5	0	4	3	6	6	1
2121	0	0	0	5	322	0	3	89	6	3	3	2	5	0	4	2	6	6	1
2122	0	0	0	0	178	2	1	73	3	2	2	3	3	0	2	1	3	1	1
2123	0	0	0	0	46	0	0	2	1	1	0	1	0	0	0	0	0	0	0
2124	0	0	0	1	93	0	2	9	3	2	1	3	0	0	1	1	1	1	0
2125	0	0	0	13	264	2	8	4	5	3	2	8	2	0	3	4	4	13	1
2126	0	0	0	15	262	2	8	4	5	3	2	8	2	0	2	4	4	13	1
2127	24	4	0	21	1096	13	11	47	14	13	17	25	27	0	2	8	17	11	5
2128	35	6	0	23	1374	14	14	32	16	16	22	32	36	0	3	9	22	13	6
2129	1	0	0	9	564	13	11	337	6	6	12	14	4	0	4	6	6	4	4
2130	1	0	0	3	256	7	5	275	3	3	5	6	3	0	2	2	2	2	1
2131	0	0	0	16	434	1	1	66	8	2	5	5	2	0	1	2	3	1	1
2132	0	0	0	23	623	1	2	95	12	2	7	7	3	0	1	2	4	1	1
2133	1	0	0	9	129	1	7	31	5	4	3	3	2	0	1	1	2	1	1
2134	0	0	0	3	240	2	1	7	1	5	2	4	2	0	3	3	8	3	2
2135	0	0	0	5	500	5	1	18	3	11	3	9	6	0	6	6	15	6	5
2136	0	0	0	2	203	3	2	61	5	2	2	4	3	0	1	3	2	4	1
2137	1	0	0	10	147	2	8	36	5	5	3	3	3	0	1	2	2	2	1
2138	0	0	0	4	252	1	4	124	1	2	2	3	7	0	2	3	6	2	1
2139	0	0	0	3	64	1	0	16	2	2	1	1	1	0	2	1	1	1	0
2140	0	0	0	5	148	2	1	47	4	4	2	2	3	0	3	1	2	2	0
2141	0	0	0	1	80	0	1	51	2	1	0	2	2	0	2	1	1	2	0
2142	0	0	0	1	68	0	1	32	1	1	1	1	1	0	2	1	1	2	0

Fruits & Vegetables

Food No.	Food Description & Amount	wt gm	wt oz	cal	% cal fat	prot gm	carbo gm	fiber gm
2143	Loganberries, cooked or canned in heavy syrup [1 cup]	256	9.0	225	1%	3	57	6.7
2144	Loganberries, frozen [1 cup]	147	5.2	81	5%	2	19	7.2
2145	Loganberries, raw [1 cup]	144	5.1	79	5%	2	19	7.1
2146	Loquats, raw [4 loquats]	64	2.3	30	4%	0	8	1.1
2147	Lychee, cooked or canned, in sugar or syrup [4 lychees with liquid]	84	3.0	76	3%	0	19	0.7
2148	Lychee, dried (lychee nuts) [4 nuts]	10	0.4	28	4%	0	7	0.5
2149	Lychee, raw (Include frozen) [1 lychee]	40	1.4	26	6%	0	7	0.5
2150	Mamey (mamea apple), raw [1 portion (¼ of fruit)]	212	7.5	108	9%	1	26	6.3
2151	Mango, raw [1 mango]	207	7.3	135	4%	1	35	3.7
2152	Mango, cooked [4 oz]	112	4.0	73	4%	1	19	2.0
2153	Mango, pickled [4 slices]	112	4.0	150	1%	0	39	1.4
2154	Mango, dried [10 strips (3¼" x 7/8" x 1/8")]	50	1.8	157	2%	1	41	2.6
2155	Mulberries, raw [1 cup]	140	4.9	60	8%	2	14	2.4
2156	Nectarine, cooked in heavy syrup [1 cup]	262	9.2	250	3%	2	63	3.0
2157	Nectarine, raw [1 fruit (2½" dia)]	136	4.8	67	8%	1	16	2.2
2158	Orange, raw [1 orange (2-5/8" dia)]	131	4.6	62	2%	1	15	3.1
2159	Orange peel [1 Tbs]	6	0.2	6	2%	0	2	0.6
2160	Orange, sections, canned, juice pack [1 cup]	204	7.2	92	3%	2	23	3.4
2161	Orange, mandarin, canned or frozen, drained [1 cup]	189	6.7	72	1%	2	18	2.3
2162	Orange, mandarin, canned or frozen, in light syrup [1 cup]	252	8.9	154	1%	1	41	1.8
2163	Orange, mandarin, canned or frozen, juice pack [1 cup]	249	8.8	92	1%	2	24	1.7
2164	Papaya, cooked or canned, in sugar or syrup [1 cup]	132	4.7	101	1%	1	26	1.6
2165	Papaya, raw [1 medium (5" long x 4" dia)]	288	10.2	112	3%	2	28	5.2
2166	Papaya, dried [4 strips]	92	3.2	238	3%	4	60	11.0
2167	Papaya, green, cooked [1 cup]	132	4.7	24	3%	1	6	1.6
2168	Passion fruit, raw [4 fruit]	72	2.5	70	6%	2	17	7.5
2169	Peach, raw [1 peach (2½" dia)]	98	3.5	42	2%	1	11	2.0
2170	Peach, cooked or canned in heavy syrup, drained solids [2 halves]	146	5.1	112	2%	1	29	2.5
2171	Peach, cooked or canned, in heavy syrup (Include home canned) [2 halves with liquid]	196	6.9	145	1%	1	39	2.5
2172	Peach, cooked or canned, in light or medium syrup [2 halves with liquid]	196	6.9	106	1%	1	29	2.5
2173	Peach, cooked or canned, juice pack [2 halves with liquid]	196	6.9	86	1%	1	23	2.5
2174	Peach, cooked or canned, unsweetened, water pack [2 halves with liquid]	196	6.9	47	2%	1	12	2.5
2175	Peach, dried, cooked, unsweetened [1 cup]	258	9.1	199	3%	3	51	7.0
2176	Peach, dried, cooked, with sugar [1 cup]	270	9.5	278	2%	3	72	6.5
2177	Peach, dried, uncooked [4 halves]	52	1.8	124	3%	2	32	4.3
2178	Peach, frozen, unsweetened [1 cup, sliced]	250	8.8	107	2%	2	28	5.0
2179	Peach, frozen, with sugar [1 cup, sliced]	250	8.8	235	1%	2	60	4.5
2180	Peach, pickled [1 fruit]	88	3.1	105	0%	0	27	1.2
2181	Peach, spiced [1 cup]	248	8.7	186	1%	1	50	3.2
2182	Pear, raw [1 pear (approx 2½ per lb)]	166	5.9	98	6%	1	25	4.0
2183	Pear, cooked or canned in heavy syrup, drained solids [1 half]	48	1.7	36	2%	0	9	1.2
2184	Pear, cooked or canned, in heavy syrup (Include home canned) [2 halves with liquid]	152	5.4	112	2%	0	29	2.4
2185	Pear, cooked or canned, in light syrup [2 halves with liquid]	152	5.4	87	0%	0	23	2.4
2186	Pear, cooked or canned, juice pack [2 halves with liquid]	152	5.4	76	1%	1	20	2.4
2187	Pear, cooked or canned, unsweetened, water pack [2 halves with liquid]	152	5.4	44	1%	0	12	2.4
2188	Pear, dried, cooked, unsweetened [1 cup]	255	9.0	324	2%	2	86	16.3
2189	Pear, dried, cooked, with sugar [1 cup]	280	9.9	392	2%	2	104	16.2
2190	Pear, dried, uncooked [4 halves]	72	2.5	189	2%	1	50	5.4
2191	Pear, Japanese, raw [1 fruit]	307	10.8	129	5%	2	33	11.1
2192	Pear salad with dressing [1 serving (lettuce, ½ pear, dressing)]	112	4.0	116	44%	1	18	2.2
2193	Pear, spiced, drained solids [1 pear]	45	1.6	42	4%	0	11	1.0
2194	Persimmon, raw [1 persimmon (2½" dia x 3½" high)]	168	5.9	118	2%	1	31	6.0

Food no.	fat gm	sat fat gm	choles mg	sodium mg	potas mg	% of Daily Value: vit A	vit E	vit C	thia	ribo	niac	vit B-6	fola	vit B-12	calc	phos	mag	iron	zinc
2143	0	0	0	8	230	1	8	26	4	4	3	5	22	0	5	3	7	6	3
2144	0	0	0	1	213	1	15	37	5	3	6	5	9	0	4	4	8	5	3
2145	0	0	0	1	209	1	14	37	5	3	6	5	9	0	4	4	8	5	3
2146	0	0	0	1	170	10	3	1	1	1	1	3	2	0	1	2	2	1	0
2147	0	0	0	1	84	0	2	45	0	2	1	2	1	0	0	2	1	1	0
2148	0	0	0	0	111	0	0	31	0	3	2	0	0	0	0	2	1	1	0
2149	0	0	0	0	68	0	1	48	0	2	1	2	1	0	0	1	1	1	0
2150	1	0	0	32	99	5	6	49	3	5	4	11	7	0	2	2	8	8	1
2151	1	0	0	4	323	81	11	96	8	7	6	14	7	0	2	2	5	1	1
2152	0	0	0	2	157	33	6	36	3	3	3	7	2	0	1	1	3	1	0
2153	0	0	0	2	140	28	4	33	3	3	2	5	3	0	1	1	3	1	0
2154	0	0	0	3	227	28	7	13	4	5	4	9	3	0	1	2	3	1	0
2155	1	0	0	14	272	0	3	85	3	8	4	4	2	0	5	5	6	14	1
2156	1	0	0	2	356	10	8	12	2	4	8	2	1	0	1	3	4	2	1
2157	1	0	0	0	288	10	6	12	2	3	7	2	1	0	1	2	3	1	1
2158	0	0	0	0	237	3	1	116	8	3	2	4	10	0	5	2	3	1	1
2159	0	0	0	0	13	0	0	14	0	0	0	1	0	0	1	0	0	0	0
2160	0	0	0	1	365	4	2	154	10	4	3	7	10	0	6	3	5	2	1
2161	0	0	0	9	255	25	6	107	11	3	4	4	2	0	2	2	5	3	7
2162	0	0	0	15	197	21	4	83	9	7	6	5	3	0	2	3	5	5	4
2163	0	0	0	12	331	21	6	142	14	4	6	5	3	0	3	2	7	4	8
2164	0	0	0	4	205	2	5	46	1	2	1	1	4	0	2	0	2	1	1
2165	0	0	0	9	740	8	15	297	5	5	5	3	27	0	7	1	7	2	1
2166	1	0	0	18	1566	9	31	126	8	10	9	5	29	0	15	3	15	3	3
2167	0	0	0	8	179	0	0	43	1	1	1	1	2	0	3	2	2	2	1
2168	1	0	0	20	251	5	4	36	0	6	5	4	3	0	1	5	5	6	0
2169	0	0	0	0	193	5	3	11	1	2	5	1	1	0	0	1	2	1	1
2170	0	0	0	9	137	7	8	7	1	2	4	1	1	0	0	2	2	2	1
2171	0	0	0	12	180	6	8	9	1	3	6	2	2	0	1	2	2	3	1
2172	0	0	0	10	190	7	8	8	1	3	6	2	2	0	1	2	2	4	1
2173	0	0	0	8	251	7	13	12	1	2	6	2	2	0	1	3	3	3	1
2174	0	0	0	6	194	10	8	9	1	2	5	2	2	0	0	2	2	3	1
2175	1	0	0	5	826	5	0	16	1	3	20	5	0	0	2	10	8	19	3
2176	1	0	0	5	788	5	0	15	1	3	19	5	0	0	2	9	8	18	3
2177	0	0	0	4	518	11	0	4	0	6	11	2	0	0	1	6	5	12	2
2178	0	0	0	0	443	13	8	394	3	6	12	2	2	0	1	3	4	2	2
2179	0	0	0	15	325	7	10	393	2	5	8	2	2	0	1	3	3	5	1
2180	0	0	0	0	134	3	2	6	1	2	3	1	0	0	0	1	2	1	1
2181	0	0	0	10	211	8	10	22	2	5	7	2	2	0	1	2	4	4	1
2182	1	0	0	0	208	0	4	11	2	4	1	1	3	0	2	2	2	2	1
2183	0	0	0	2	32	0	1	1	0	1	1	0	0	0	0	0	0	1	0
2184	0	0	0	8	99	0	3	3	1	2	2	1	0	0	1	1	2	2	1
2185	0	0	0	8	100	0	3	2	1	1	1	1	0	0	1	1	2	2	1
2186	0	0	0	6	146	0	3	4	1	1	2	1	0	0	1	2	3	2	1
2187	0	0	0	3	81	0	3	3	1	1	0	1	0	0	1	1	2	2	1
2188	1	0	0	8	658	1	0	17	1	3	4	4	0	0	4	7	10	14	3
2189	1	0	0	8	686	1	0	18	1	3	5	5	0	0	4	8	11	15	3
2190	0	0	0	4	384	0	0	8	0	6	5	3	0	0	2	4	6	8	2
2191	1	0	0	0	371	0	7	19	2	2	3	3	6	0	1	3	6	0	0
2192	6	1	4	114	123	2	5	6	1	2	1	1	3	1	1	2	2	2	1
2193	0	0	0	0	46	0	1	2	0	1	0	0	0	0	0	0	1	1	0
2194	0	0	0	2	270	36	5	21	3	2	1	8	3	0	1	3	4	1	1

Fruits & Vegetables

Food No.	Food Description & Amount	wt gm	wt oz	cal	% cal fat	prot gm	carbo gm	fiber gm
2195	Pineapple, raw [1 cup, diced]	155	5.5	76	8%	1	19	1.9
2196	Pineapple, cooked or canned, drained solids [2 slices (3" dia)]	70	2.5	42	2%	0	11	0.8
2197	Pineapple, cooked or canned, in heavy syrup (Include home canned) [2 slices (3" dia) with liquid]	98	3.5	76	1%	0	20	0.8
2198	Pineapple, cooked or canned, in light syrup [2 slices (3" dia) with liquid]	96	3.4	50	2%	0	13	0.8
2199	Pineapple, cooked or canned, juice pack [2 slices (3" dia) with liquid]	94	3.3	56	1%	0	15	0.8
2200	Pineapple, cooked or canned, unsweetened, waterpack [2 slices (3" dia) with liquid]	94	3.3	30	3%	0	8	0.8
2201	Pineapple, dehydrated [4 pieces]	112	4.0	280	8%	2	71	6.9
2202	Pineapple chunk, chocolate covered [4 pieces]	40	1.4	71	79%	0	4	0.8
2203	Pineapple salad with cream cheese [1 serving (lettuce, 1 slice of pineapple, cream cheese)]	66	2.3	89	54%	1	10	0.4
2204	Pineapple salad with dressing [1 serving (lettuce, 1 cup diced pineapple, dressing)]	184	6.5	141	38%	1	24	2.0
2205	Plantain, ripe, raw [1 fruit]	203	7.2	248	3%	3	65	4.7
2206	Plantain chips [2 oz]	56	2.0	291	58%	1	33	4.3
2207	Plantain, green, boiled (Include baked green plantain) [1 small]	152	5.4	176	1%	1	47	3.5
2208	Plantain, green, fried in corn oil, salted, Puerto Rican style (Tostones) [4 small tostones]	80	2.8	193	45%	1	29	2.1
2209	Plantain, ripe, boiled (Include baked ripe plantain) [1 small]	208	7.3	241	1%	2	65	4.8
2210	Plantain, ripe, fried in soybean oil, Puerto Rican style (Platano maduro frito) [½ plantain (2 slices, 4" x ¾")]	76	2.7	191	47%	1	27	2.0
2211	Plantain, ripe, fritters, Puerto Rican style (Pionono) [1 pionono (2"x 2½" x ¾")]	58	2.0	244	63%	7	17	1.4
2212	Plantain, ripe, rolled in flour, fried in soybean oil [2 pieces (2½" long)]	90	3.2	220	44%	2	33	2.2
2213	Plum, raw [2 plums (2½" dia)]	132	4.7	73	10%	1	17	2.0
2214	Plum, cooked or canned, heavy syrup, drained solids [2 plums]	62	2.2	55	1%	0	14	0.9
2215	Plum, cooked or canned, in heavy syrup (Include home canned) [2 plums with liquid]	92	3.2	82	1%	0	21	0.9
2216	Plum, cooked or canned, in light syrup [2 plums with liquid]	92	3.2	58	1%	0	15	0.9
2217	Plum, cooked or canned, juice pack [2 plums with liquid]	92	3.2	53	0%	0	14	0.9
2218	Plum, cooked or canned, unsweetened, water pack [2 plums with liquid]	92	3.2	38	0%	0	10	0.9
2219	Plum, dried, rock salt (Include plum seed, rock salt seed, dried Japanese plum/umeboshi) [4 plums]	12	0.4	41	2%	0	11	1.1
2220	Pomegranate, raw [1 pomegranate (3-3/8" dia)]	154	5.4	105	4%	1	26	0.9
2221	Prune, dried, cooked, unsweetened [4 prunes]	36	1.3	39	2%	0	10	2.4
2222	Prune, dried, cooked, with sugar (Include Ciruelas) [4 prunes]	36	1.3	45	2%	0	12	1.4
2223	Prune, dried, uncooked [4 prunes]	28	1.0	67	2%	1	18	2.0
2224	Prune whip (prunes, egg white, sugar, lemon juice, salt) [1 cup]	130	4.6	191	1%	6	44	5.9
2225	Quince, raw [1 quince]	92	3.2	52	2%	0	14	1.7
2226	Raisins (Include cinnamon-coated raisins) [1 cup]	145	5.1	435	1%	5	115	5.8
2227	Raisins, cooked [1 cup]	295	10.4	646	1%	4	169	5.5
2228	Raspberries, black, raw (Include black caps) [1 cup]	134	4.7	66	10%	1	16	9.1
2229	Raspberries, cooked or canned, in heavy syrup (Include home canned) [1 cup]	256	9.0	233	1%	2	60	8.4
2230	Raspberries, cooked or canned, unsweetened, water pack [1 cup]	243	8.6	80	10%	1	19	11.1
2231	Raspberries, frozen, unsweetened [1 cup]	250	8.8	123	10%	2	29	17.0
2232	Raspberries, frozen, with sugar [1 cup]	250	8.8	258	1%	2	65	11.0
2233	Raspberries, red, raw [1 cup]	123	4.3	60	10%	1	14	8.4
2234	Rhubarb, cooked or canned, drained solids [1 cup]	240	8.5	278	0%	1	75	4.8
2235	Rhubarb, cooked or canned, in heavy syrup (Include rhubarb sauce; rhubarb, home canned) [1 cup]	240	8.5	278	0%	1	75	4.8
2236	Rhubarb, cooked or canned, in light syrup [1 cup]	240	8.5	220	1%	1	56	3.5
2237	Rhubarb, cooked or canned, unsweetened [1 cup]	240	8.5	50	9%	2	11	4.3
2238	Rhubarb, frozen, with sugar [1 cup]	240	8.5	278	0%	1	75	4.8
2239	Rhubarb, raw [1 cup, diced]	122	4.3	26	9%	1	6	2.2

Food no.	fat gm	sat fat gm	choles mg	sodium mg	potas mg	% of Daily Value													
						vit A	vit E	vit C	thia	ribo	niac	vit B-6	fola	vit B-12	calc	phos	mag	iron	zinc
2195	1	0	0	2	175	0	1	40	10	3	3	7	4	0	1	1	5	3	1
2196	0	0	0	1	87	0	0	11	5	1	1	3	1	0	1	0	3	1	0
2197	0	0	0	1	102	0	0	12	6	1	1	4	1	0	1	1	4	2	1
2198	0	0	0	1	101	0	0	12	6	1	1	4	1	0	1	1	4	2	1
2199	0	0	0	1	115	0	0	15	6	1	1	3	1	0	1	1	3	1	1
2200	0	0	0	1	119	0	0	12	6	1	1	3	1	0	1	0	4	2	1
2201	2	0	0	6	646	1	3	29	25	11	11	22	8	0	4	4	20	12	3
2202	6	1	0	2	64	0	5	30	0	2	0	1	1	0	1	1	1	1	0
2203	5	3	17	46	74	7	1	6	3	3	1	2	2	1	2	2	2	2	1
2204	6	1	4	112	194	2	4	42	10	4	3	7	5	1	1	2	6	4	1
2205	1	0	0	8	1013	23	2	62	7	6	7	30	11	0	1	7	19	7	2
2206	19	16	0	3	300	0	14	6	3	1	2	7	2	0	1	3	11	4	3
2207	0	0	0	8	707	14	1	28	5	5	6	18	10	0	0	4	12	5	1
2208	10	1	0	5	409	8	10	20	3	3	3	12	3	0	0	3	9	3	1
2209	0	0	0	10	967	19	1	38	6	6	8	25	14	0	0	6	17	7	2
2210	10	1	0	3	386	7	10	18	2	2	3	12	2	0	0	3	8	3	1
2211	17	4	58	194	351	7	12	14	7	8	7	11	3	6	1	8	7	5	6
2212	11	1	0	4	411	8	10	19	5	4	4	12	3	0	0	4	9	4	1
2213	1	0	0	0	227	4	4	21	4	7	3	5	1	0	1	1	2	1	1
2214	0	0	0	12	58	2	3	0	1	1	1	1	0	0	1	1	1	3	0
2215	0	0	0	17	84	2	3	1	1	2	1	1	1	0	1	1	1	4	0
2216	0	0	0	18	86	2	3	1	1	2	1	1	1	0	1	1	1	4	0
2217	0	0	0	1	142	9	3	4	1	3	2	1	1	0	1	1	2	2	1
2218	0	0	0	1	116	8	3	4	1	2	2	1	1	0	1	1	1	1	0
2219	0	0	0	395	127	2	1	0	1	1	2	4	0	0	1	1	2	2	1
2220	0	0	0	5	399	0	4	16	3	3	2	8	2	0	0	1	1	3	1
2221	0	0	0	1	120	1	0	2	1	2	1	4	0	0	1	1	2	2	1
2222	0	0	0	1	112	1	0	2	1	2	1	4	0	0	1	1	2	2	1
2223	0	0	0	1	209	6	2	2	2	3	3	4	0	0	1	2	3	4	1
2224	0	0	0	80	347	2	0	9	1	17	3	10	0	1	2	4	6	6	2
2225	0	0	0	4	181	0	2	23	1	2	1	2	1	0	1	2	2	4	0
2226	1	0	0	17	1089	0	5	8	15	8	6	18	1	0	7	14	12	17	3
2227	1	0	0	24	929	0	4	5	11	7	5	15	1	0	7	13	12	16	3
2228	1	0	0	0	204	2	3	56	3	7	6	4	9	0	3	2	6	4	4
2229	0	0	0	8	241	1	5	37	3	5	6	5	7	0	3	2	8	6	3
2230	1	0	0	2	223	2	3	47	3	8	7	4	5	0	4	2	8	5	5
2231	1	0	0	0	342	3	5	73	5	13	11	7	15	0	5	3	11	8	8
2232	0	0	0	3	285	2	5	69	3	7	3	4	16	0	4	4	8	9	3
2233	1	0	0	0	187	2	3	51	2	7	6	4	8	0	3	1	6	4	4
2234	0	0	0	2	207	1	2	9	2	3	2	2	2	0	33	2	7	3	1
2235	0	0	0	2	230	2	2	13	3	3	2	2	3	0	35	2	7	3	1
2236	0	0	0	4	210	2	2	15	4	4	2	2	4	0	38	2	9	3	1
2237	0	0	0	10	622	2	2	22	3	4	3	3	2	0	20	3	7	3	2
2238	0	0	0	2	230	2	2	13	3	3	2	2	3	0	35	2	7	3	1
2239	0	0	0	5	351	1	1	16	2	2	2	1	2	0	10	2	4	1	1

Fruits & Vegetables

Food No.	Food Description & Amount	wt gm	wt oz	cal	% cal fat	prot gm	carbo gm	fiber gm
2240	Sapodilla, raw [1 sapodilla]	170	6.0	141	12%	1	34	9.0
2241	Soursop (annona muricata), raw [1 cup, pulp]	225	7.9	149	4%	2	38	7.4
2242	Strawberries, raw [4 medium (1¼" dia)]	128	4.5	38	11%	1	9	2.9
2243	Strawberries, cooked or canned, in syrup [1 cup]	254	9.0	234	3%	1	60	4.3
2244	Strawberries, cooked or canned, unsweetened, water pack [1 cup]	242	8.5	49	11%	1	11	3.7
2245	Strawberries, frozen, unsweetened [4 berries]	42	1.5	15	3%	0	4	0.9
2246	Strawberries, frozen, with sugar [1 cup]	255	9.0	222	1%	1	60	4.8
2247	Strawberries, raw, with sugar [1 cup, sliced]	174	6.1	83	7%	1	20	3.8
2248	Strawberry, chocolate covered [4 pieces]	76	2.7	136	79%	1	8	1.6
2249	Sweetsop (annona squamosa; "sugar-apple"), raw [1 fruit (2-7/8" dia)]	155	5.5	146	3%	3	37	6.8
2250	Tamarind pulp, dried, sweetened ("Pulpitas") [1 cup, pieces, without seeds]	220	7.8	558	2%	6	146	10.1
2251	Tamarind, raw [10 tamarind]	20	0.7	48	2%	1	13	1.0
2252	Tangelo, raw [1 fruit (2½" dia)]	95	3.4	45	2%	1	11	2.3
2253	Tangerine, raw (Include mandarin orange, satsuma) [1 fruit (2-3/8" dia)]	84	3.0	37	4%	1	9	1.9
2254	Watermelon, raw [1 cup, diced]	152	5.4	49	12%	1	11	0.8
2255	Watermelon, pickled [5 squares or cubes]	50	1.8	51	1%	1	13	0.6
2256	Wi-apple, raw [1 cup]	125	4.4	63	5%	1	16	2.5
2257	Youngberries, raw [1 cup]	144	5.1	75	7%	1	18	7.6
	Vegetables							
2350	Alfalfa sprouts, raw [1 cup]	33	1.2	10	21%	1	1	0.8
2351	Algae, dried (Include spirulina) [2 Tbs]	16	0.6	47	18%	7	6	0.7
2352	Artichoke salad (artichokes in olive oil) [1 cup]	130	4.6	155	64%	4	13	6.4
2353	Artichoke, globe (French), cooked, from canned [1 cup, hearts]	168	5.9	84	3%	6	19	9.0
2354	Artichoke, globe (French), cooked, from fresh [1 medium globe]	120	4.2	60	3%	4	13	6.5
2355	Artichoke, globe (French), cooked, from frozen [1 cup, hearts]	168	5.9	76	10%	5	15	7.7
2356	Artichokes, stuffed with mixture of breadcrumbs, celery, onion, parmesan cheese, olive oil, parsley, salt [1 stuffed globe]	251	8.9	400	33%	15	55	8.4
2357	Artichoke, Jerusalem, raw (Include sunchoke) [1 cup]	150	5.3	114	0%	3	26	2.4
2358	Arugula (Rocket, Roquette), raw [1 cup]	20	0.7	5	24%	1	1	0.3
2359	Asparagus, cooked, from canned [1 cup]	242	8.5	46	31%	5	6	3.9
2360	Asparagus, cooked, from fresh [1 cup]	180	6.3	43	12%	5	8	2.9
2361	Asparagus, cooked, from frozen [1 cup]	180	6.3	50	14%	5	9	2.9
2362	Asparagus, from canned, creamed or with cheese sauce [1 cup]	235	8.3	178	63%	10	9	2.8
2363	Asparagus, from fresh, creamed or with cheese sauce [1 cup]	235	8.3	216	60%	12	12	2.6
2364	Asparagus, from frozen, creamed or with cheese sauce [1 cup]	235	8.3	222	59%	13	13	2.6
2365	Asparagus, raw [1 cup]	134	4.7	31	8%	3	6	2.8
2366	Bamboo shoots, canned or cooked with salt [1 cup, slices]	120	4.2	33	10%	3	6	2.7
2367	Bamboo shoots, fried [1 cup]	156	5.5	100	51%	5	11	4.4
2368	Bean salad, yellow and/or green string beans (Include three bean salad) [1 cup]	150	5.3	140	49%	4	15	5.3
2369	Bean sprouts, cooked, from canned [1 cup]	125	4.4	15	5%	2	3	1.0
2370	Bean sprouts, cooked, from fresh [1 cup]	124	4.4	58	38%	6	6	1.0
2371	Bean sprouts, raw (soybean or mung) [1 cup]	104	3.7	31	5%	3	6	1.9
2372	Beans, lima and corn (succotash), cooked, with salt [1 cup]	192	6.8	179	9%	8	38	7.9
2373	Beet greens, cooked, with salt [1 cup]	144	5.1	39	7%	4	8	4.2
2374	Beet greens, raw [1 cup]	38	1.3	7	3%	1	2	1.4
2375	Beets with Harvard sauce (sugar, vinegar, margarine, cornstarch, salt) [1 cup]	246	8.7	291	25%	3	56	4.9
2376	Beets, cooked, from canned [1 cup, slices]	170	6.0	53	4%	2	12	2.9
2377	Beets, canned, low sodium [1 cup]	170	6.0	48	2%	1	11	2.0
2378	Beets, cooked, from fresh or frozen [1 cup, slices]	170	6.0	75	4%	3	17	4.8
2379	Beets, raw [1 cup]	136	4.8	58	4%	2	13	3.8
2380	Bittermelon, cooked (Include Balsam pear) [1 cup]	124	4.4	24	9%	1	5	2.5
2381	Bittermelon leaves, horseradish leaves, jute leaves, or radish leaves, cooked [1 cup]	123	4.3	51	8%	5	10	2.4
2382	Broccoflower, cooked [1 cup, fresh]	82	2.9	26	9%	2	5	2.7

Food no.	fat gm	sat fat gm	choles mg	sodium mg	potas mg	% of Daily Value													
						vit A	vit E	vit C	thia	ribo	niac	vit B-6	fola	vit B-12	calc	phos	mag	iron	zinc
2240	2	0	0	20	328	1	2	42	0	2	2	3	6	0	4	2	5	8	1
2241	1	0	0	32	626	0	4	77	11	7	10	7	8	0	3	6	12	8	2
2242	0	0	0	1	212	0	1	121	2	5	1	4	6	0	2	2	3	3	1
2243	1	0	0	10	218	1	2	134	4	5	1	6	18	0	3	3	5	7	2
2244	1	0	0	4	269	0	1	146	2	6	2	5	7	0	2	3	4	3	2
2245	0	0	0	1	63	0	1	29	1	1	1	1	2	0	1	1	1	2	0
2246	0	0	0	5	250	1	2	172	3	10	4	4	6	0	3	3	4	8	1
2247	1	0	0	2	275	0	1	156	2	7	2	5	7	0	2	3	4	4	1
2248	12	2	0	3	121	0	10	57	1	3	1	2	3	0	1	2	2	2	1
2249	0	0	0	14	383	0	4	94	11	10	7	16	5	0	4	5	8	5	1
2250	1	1	0	56	1244	0	6	2	40	16	17	6	3	0	15	22	46	31	1
2251	0	0	0	6	126	0	1	1	6	2	2	1	1	0	1	2	5	3	0
2252	0	0	0	0	172	2	1	84	6	2	1	3	7	0	4	1	2	1	0
2253	0	0	0	1	132	8	1	43	6	1	1	3	4	0	1	1	3	0	1
2254	1	0	0	3	176	6	1	24	8	2	2	11	1	0	1	1	4	1	1
2255	0	0	0	1	49	0	0	5	1	1	1	2	0	0	1	1	1	1	0
2256	0	0	0	3	198	8	6	105	4	1	8	6	4	0	1	3	4	2	0
2257	1	0	0	0	282	2	5	50	3	3	3	4	12	0	5	3	7	5	3
2350	0	0	0	2	26	1	0	5	2	2	1	1	3	0	1	2	2	2	2
2351	1	0	0	130	209	1	4	2	19	26	8	3	9	0	4	2	14	24	3
2352	11	1	0	113	422	2	7	20	5	5	6	7	15	0	5	10	18	9	4
2353	0	0	0	529	591	3	1	28	7	7	8	9	21	0	8	14	25	12	5
2354	0	0	0	114	425	2	1	20	5	5	6	7	15	0	5	10	18	9	4
2355	1	0	0	89	444	3	1	14	7	16	8	7	50	0	4	10	13	5	4
2356	15	4	7	753	645	5	9	29	28	20	23	11	20	1	31	26	26	29	11
2357	0	0	0	6	644	0	1	10	20	5	10	6	5	0	2	12	6	28	1
2358	0	0	0	5	74	5	0	5	1	1	0	1	5	0	3	1	2	2	1
2359	2	0	0	695	416	13	5	67	9	14	12	13	55	0	4	10	6	25	6
2360	1	0	0	20	288	10	3	32	15	13	10	11	66	0	4	10	5	7	5
2361	1	0	0	7	392	15	10	73	8	11	9	2	61	0	4	10	6	6	7
2362	12	6	24	771	382	18	6	48	9	19	9	11	40	4	22	22	7	19	10
2363	14	7	30	361	359	19	6	29	16	23	10	11	59	4	27	26	8	8	11
2364	15	7	30	350	449	23	13	64	10	21	9	3	54	4	28	26	9	7	12
2365	0	0	0	3	366	8	12	29	13	10	8	9	43	0	3	8	6	6	4
2366	0	0	0	5	593	0	6	7	10	5	3	13	2	0	2	7	1	3	9
2367	6	1	0	68	1078	5	13	11	18	8	6	23	3	0	3	12	2	6	15
2368	8	1	0	520	247	2	8	7	5	6	2	2	14	0	4	8	7	8	4
2369	0	0	0	175	34	0	0	1	2	5	1	2	3	0	2	4	3	3	2
2370	2	0	0	12	261	0	0	21	10	6	6	5	16	0	4	9	10	6	6
2371	0	0	0	6	155	0	0	23	6	8	4	5	16	0	1	6	5	5	3
2372	2	0	0	86	509	4	3	19	9	8	13	9	16	0	3	13	11	9	6
2373	0	0	0	347	1309	73	2	60	11	24	4	10	5	0	16	6	24	15	5
2374	0	0	0	76	208	23	3	19	3	5	1	2	1	0	5	2	7	7	1
2375	8	2	0	224	571	8	8	10	3	5	3	6	34	0	3	7	12	9	4
2376	0	0	0	330	252	0	2	11	1	4	1	5	12	0	3	3	7	17	2
2377	0	0	0	36	241	1	2	8	1	4	1	5	12	0	2	3	7	6	3
2378	0	0	0	131	519	1	2	10	3	4	3	6	34	0	3	6	10	7	4
2379	0	0	0	106	442	1	2	11	3	3	2	5	37	0	2	5	8	6	3
2380	0	0	0	7	396	1	4	68	4	4	2	3	16	0	1	4	5	3	6
2381	0	0	0	14	639	56	3	81	11	21	7	44	25	0	18	9	28	16	5
2382	0	0	0	18	228	1	0	99	4	5	3	8	8	0	3	5	4	3	3

Fruits & Vegetables

Food No.	Food Description & Amount	wt gm	wt oz	cal	% cal fat	prot gm	carbo gm	fiber gm
2383	Broccoflower, raw [1 cup]	64	2.3	20	9%	2	4	2.0
2384	Broccoli casserole (broccoli, noodles, and cream sauce) [1 cup]	228	8.0	312	47%	9	34	3.6
2385	Broccoli casserole (broccoli, rice, cheese, and mushroom sauce) [1 cup]	228	8.0	285	42%	12	31	2.4
2386	Broccoli salad with cauliflower, cheese, bacon bits, and dressing [1 cup]	154	5.4	428	79%	10	17	2.9
2387	Broccoli, batter-dipped and fried [1 cup]	85	3.0	122	65%	3	9	2.2
2388	Broccoli, cooked [1 cup]	184	6.5	52	11%	5	9	5.3
2389	Broccoli, cooked, from fresh, with cheese sauce [1 cup]	228	8.0	230	60%	13	13	4.3
2390	Broccoli, cooked, from fresh, with mushroom sauce [1 cup]	228	8.0	138	51%	6	14	3.6
2391	Broccoli, cooked, from frozen [1 cup, frozen, chopped]	184	6.5	52	4%	6	10	5.5
2392	Broccoli, cooked, from frozen, with cheese sauce [1 cup]	228	8.0	213	57%	13	13	4.7
2393	Broccoli, cooked, from frozen, with cream sauce [1 cup]	228	8.0	174	52%	8	16	4.3
2394	Broccoli, cooked, from frozen, with mushroom sauce [1 cup]	228	8.0	132	47%	6	14	4.0
2395	Broccoli, cooked, with cheese sauce [1 cup]	228	8.0	230	60%	13	13	4.3
2396	Broccoli, cooked, with cream sauce [1 cup]	228	8.0	174	52%	8	16	4.3
2397	Broccoli, cooked, with mushroom sauce [1 cup]	228	8.0	132	47%	6	14	4.0
2398	Broccoli, raw [1 cup, chopped]	88	3.1	25	11%	3	5	2.6
2399	Brussels sprouts, cooked, from fresh [1 cup]	155	5.5	60	12%	4	13	4.0
2400	Brussels sprouts, cooked, from frozen [1 cup]	155	5.5	65	8%	6	13	6.4
2401	Brussels sprouts, from fresh, creamed [1 cup]	228	8.0	198	52%	7	20	3.5
2402	Brussels sprouts, from frozen, creamed [1 cup]	228	8.0	203	50%	9	20	5.4
2403	Brussels sprouts, raw [1 cup]	88	3.1	38	6%	3	8	3.3
2404	Buckwheat sprouts, raw [1 cup]	140	4.9	277	6%	10	60	1.5
2405	Burdock, cooked (Include gobo) [1 cup]	125	4.4	110	1%	3	26	2.3
2406	Cabbage salad or coleslaw with apples, raisins, mayonnaise [1 cup]	132	4.7	255	71%	2	20	2.8
2407	Cabbage salad or coleslaw with pineapple, mayonnaise [1 cup]	132	4.7	133	49%	1	18	1.9
2408	Cabbage salad or coleslaw, "regular" [1 cup]	184	6.5	271	81%	2	14	3.5
2409	Cabbage, Chinese, cooked (Include bok choy) [1 cup]	170	6.0	24	12%	2	4	4.0
2410	Cabbage, Chinese, raw [1 cup]	76	2.7	10	14%	1	2	0.8
2411	Cabbage, Chinese, raw, with French dressing [1 cup]	76	2.7	66	74%	1	4	2.0
2412	Cabbage, creamed [1 cup]	200	7.1	158	58%	5	13	2.7
2413	Cabbage, green, cooked [1 cup]	150	5.3	33	18%	2	7	3.5
2414	Cabbage, raw [1 cup, chopped]	89	3.1	22	10%	1	5	2.0
2415	Cabbage, red, cooked [1 cup]	150	5.3	32	9%	2	7	3.0
2416	Cabbage, red, raw [1 cup, chopped]	89	3.1	24	9%	1	5	1.8
2417	Cabbage, savoy, cooked [1 cup]	145	5.1	39	3%	3	9	4.5
2418	Cactus, cooked (Include nopal) [1 cup]	149	5.3	22	3%	2	5	3.0
2419	Cactus, raw [1 cup]	118	4.2	19	7%	2	4	2.7
2420	Caesar salad (with romaine lettuce) [1 cup]	108	3.8	169	74%	5	6	1.4
2421	Calabasa (Spanish pumpkin), cooked [1 cup, cubed]	166	5.9	56	7%	2	13	4.8
2422	Plaintain, ripe, candied (margarine-sugar-wine syrup), Puerto Rican style (Platano en almibar) [½ plantain with syrup]	140	4.9	365	26%	1	70	1.8
2423	Carrot chips, dried [10 chips]	10	0.4	34	4%	1	8	2.4
2424	Carrot juice [1 cup]	236	8.3	94	3%	2	22	1.9
2425	Carrots in tomato sauce [1 cup]	176	6.2	209	45%	1	31	1.7
2426	Carrots, cooked, from canned, creamed [1 cup]	228	8.0	183	56%	5	16	2.1
2427	Carrots, cooked, from canned [1 cup, sliced]	146	5.1	34	7%	1	8	2.2
2428	Carrots, cooked, from canned, glazed [1 cup]	161	5.7	186	57%	1	21	2.1
2429	Carrots, cooked, from canned, low sodium [1 cup, sliced]	146	5.1	34	5%	1	8	2.6
2430	Carrots, cooked, from canned, with cheese sauce [1 cup]	228	8.0	230	61%	10	14	2.2
2431	Carrots, cooked, from fresh, creamed [1 cup]	228	8.0	206	48%	5	23	4.4
2432	Carrots, cooked, from fresh [1 cup, sliced]	156	5.5	70	4%	2	16	5.1
2433	Carrots, cooked, from fresh, glazed [1 cup]	161	5.7	217	49%	2	28	4.6
2434	Carrots, cooked, from fresh, with cheese sauce [1 cup]	228	8.0	255	53%	10	21	4.9
2435	Carrots, cooked, from frozen, creamed [1 cup]	228	8.0	199	51%	5	20	4.5

Food no.	fat gm	sat fat gm	choles mg	sodium mg	potas mg	% of Daily Value													
						vit A	vit E	vit C	thia	ribo	niac	vit B-6	fola	vit B-12	calc	phos	mag	iron	zinc
2383	0	0	0	15	192	1	0	94	3	4	2	7	9	0	2	4	3	3	3
2384	16	6	52	129	235	29	10	47	14	12	9	7	8	3	10	15	10	13	7
2385	13	6	23	667	437	23	10	76	13	21	10	11	10	5	27	28	11	10	11
2386	37	9	41	500	265	13	25	72	7	8	3	18	15	6	17	16	7	5	7
2387	9	1	15	64	242	10	13	89	5	8	4	5	9	1	7	7	5	5	3
2388	1	0	0	48	537	26	14	229	7	12	5	13	23	0	8	11	11	9	5
2389	15	7	31	404	537	31	15	180	8	22	5	12	20	5	32	28	12	9	11
2390	8	2	3	675	429	17	13	143	6	13	6	9	15	2	10	12	8	8	6
2391	0	0	0	44	331	35	11	123	7	9	4	12	20	0	9	10	9	6	4
2392	13	6	28	366	379	39	13	103	8	18	5	12	18	4	31	25	11	7	9
2393	10	3	6	359	388	31	14	92	9	16	5	11	16	4	18	17	10	6	5
2394	7	2	3	622	310	24	12	84	6	11	6	9	14	2	11	12	8	6	6
2395	15	7	31	404	537	31	15	180	8	22	5	12	20	5	32	28	12	9	11
2396	10	3	6	359	388	31	12	92	9	16	5	11	11	4	18	17	10	6	5
2397	7	2	3	622	310	24	10	84	6	11	6	9	10	2	11	12	8	6	6
2398	0	0	0	24	286	14	7	137	4	6	3	7	16	0	4	6	6	4	2
2399	1	0	0	33	491	11	6	160	11	7	5	14	23	0	6	9	8	10	3
2400	1	0	0	36	504	9	4	118	11	10	4	22	39	0	4	8	9	6	4
2401	11	3	7	386	559	15	11	132	14	17	6	13	20	5	17	17	10	10	6
2402	11	3	7	389	569	13	10	97	13	19	5	20	33	5	15	17	11	7	6
2403	0	0	0	22	342	8	4	125	8	5	3	10	13	0	4	6	5	7	2
2404	2	0	0	22	237	0	0	6	21	13	22	19	13	0	4	28	29	17	15
2405	0	0	0	5	450	0	1	5	3	4	2	17	6	0	6	12	12	5	3
2406	20	3	15	157	336	3	14	43	4	3	2	13	9	1	5	4	4	5	2
2407	7	1	5	160	211	3	4	41	5	2	2	5	8	1	4	2	4	3	1
2408	24	4	18	199	383	47	17	70	5	4	3	16	15	1	7	5	6	6	2
2409	0	0	0	36	497	31	1	67	4	6	3	16	20	0	14	5	5	6	2
2410	0	0	0	49	192	23	0	57	2	3	2	7	12	0	8	3	4	3	1
2411	5	1	0	183	160	9	5	28	2	2	1	7	13	0	5	2	2	1	1
2412	10	3	6	331	248	6	6	38	8	13	3	8	7	4	14	11	5	3	3
2413	1	0	0	12	146	2	1	50	6	5	2	8	8	0	5	2	3	1	1
2414	0	0	0	16	219	1	0	48	3	2	1	4	10	0	4	2	3	3	1
2415	0	0	0	12	210	0	1	86	3	2	2	11	5	0	6	4	4	3	2
2416	0	0	0	10	183	0	0	85	3	2	1	9	5	0	5	4	3	2	1
2417	0	0	0	39	300	13	1	60	6	2	2	12	20	0	5	5	10	3	2
2418	0	0	0	30	291	7	0	13	1	4	2	5	1	0	24	2	18	4	2
2419	0	0	0	26	376	5	0	26	1	3	3	4	1	0	19	2	17	4	2
2420	14	3	39	266	251	20	9	32	7	10	7	3	25	3	10	9	3	8	4
2421	0	0	0	8	342	366	8	12	3	5	3	5	5	0	4	6	10	13	2
2422	10	2	0	124	377	17	8	17	2	3	3	11	2	0	1	3	8	3	1
2423	0	0	0	28	254	106	2	2	4	2	3	5	1	0	2	3	3	2	1
2424	0	0	0	68	689	608	0	33	14	8	5	26	2	0	6	10	8	6	3
2425	10	1	0	176	239	80	12	49	3	2	3	8	3	0	2	3	6	6	1
2426	11	3	7	670	384	175	9	7	6	14	6	9	4	5	15	13	6	6	5
2427	0	0	0	353	261	201	3	6	2	3	4	8	3	0	4	4	3	5	3
2428	12	2	0	478	304	204	10	6	2	3	4	8	3	0	5	4	4	6	3
2429	0	0	0	50	231	141	3	5	2	2	3	8	3	0	5	3	3	4	3
2430	16	8	33	722	372	205	7	7	5	15	5	10	5	5	30	23	7	7	10
2431	11	3	7	443	445	316	9	6	8	15	5	18	6	5	16	14	8	6	5
2432	0	0	0	103	354	383	3	6	4	5	4	19	5	0	5	5	5	5	3
2433	12	2	0	232	371	354	10	5	3	5	4	17	5	0	6	5	6	6	3
2434	15	7	32	463	443	364	7	6	6	17	5	20	7	5	30	23	9	7	10
2435	11	3	7	445	358	223	9	7	7	14	5	10	5	5	16	13	7	5	5

Fruits & Vegetables

Food No.	Food Description & Amount	wt gm	wt oz	cal	% cal fat	prot gm	carbo gm	fiber gm
2436	Carrots, cooked, from frozen [1 cup, sliced]	146	5.1	53	3%	2	12	5.1
2437	Carrots, cooked, from frozen, glazed [1 cup]	161	5.7	205	51%	2	25	4.9
2438	Carrots, cooked, from frozen, with cheese sauce [1 cup]	228	8.0	249	56%	11	17	5.0
2439	Carrots, raw [1 medium (5½"x1")]	50	1.8	21	4%	1	5	1.5
2440	Carrots, raw, salad (Include carrot-raisin salad) [1 cup]	175	6.2	419	64%	3	40	4.3
2441	Casabe, cassava bread [1 piece (6" dia)]	100	3.5	228	3%	6	51	3.0
2442	Cassava (yuca blanca), cooked [4 pieces]	80	2.8	97	3%	3	22	1.3
2443	Cassava Pasteles, Puerto Rican style (Pasteles de yuca) [1 pastel (6" x 2" x ½")]	145	5.1	347	65%	11	21	1.6
2444	Cassava with creole sauce, Puerto Rican style (Yuca al mojo) [1 serving (2 pieces with sauce)]	230	8.1	253	29%	5	43	3.7
2445	Cauliflower, batter-dipped, fried (Include breaded, fried) [2 flowerets]	52	1.8	106	68%	2	7	1.0
2446	Cauliflower, cooked, from canned [1 cup]	180	6.3	41	18%	3	7	4.8
2447	Cauliflower, cooked, from fresh [1 cup, pieces]	125	4.4	29	18%	2	5	3.4
2448	Cauliflower, cooked, from frozen [1 cup]	180	6.3	34	10%	3	7	4.9
2449	Cauliflower, creamed (Include with cheese sauce) [1 cup]	228	8.0	249	64%	12	12	3.7
2450	Cauliflower, from canned, creamed [1 cup]	228	8.0	247	64%	12	12	3.7
2451	Cauliflower, from fresh, creamed [1 cup]	228	8.0	249	64%	12	12	3.7
2452	Cauliflower, from frozen, creamed [1 cup]	228	8.0	202	62%	10	11	4.2
2453	Cauliflower, raw [1 cup]	100	3.5	25	8%	2	5	2.5
2454	Celeriac, cooked (Include Puerto Rican apio) [1 cup, pieces]	155	5.5	64	7%	2	15	2.9
2455	Celery, cooked [1 cup, diced]	150	5.3	27	8%	1	6	2.4
2456	Celery, creamed [1 cup]	228	8.0	175	58%	5	14	2.2
2457	Celery, raw [2 small stalks (5" long)]	34	1.2	5	8%	0	1	0.6
2458	Celery, stuffed with cheese [1 small stalk (5" long)]	32	1.1	39	78%	1	1	0.4
2459	Chard, cooked [1 cup, stalk and leaves]	145	5.1	29	4%	3	6	3.0
2460	Chard, raw [1 cup]	36	1.3	7	9%	1	1	0.6
2461	Chives, dried or dehydrated [2 Tbs]	2	0.1	6	22%	1	1	0.5
2462	Chives, raw [2 Tbs]	6	0.2	2	22%	0	0	0.2
2463	Christophine, cooked (Include chayote) [1 cup]	160	5.6	42	11%	2	9	5.3
2464	Christophine, creamed, Puerto Rican style (Chayote a la crema) [½ chayote (4½" x 3½" x 1½"), without shell]	107	3.8	158	27%	3	27	2.6
2465	Cilantro, raw [1 cup]	16	0.6	4	18%	0	1	0.4
2466	Cress, cooked, from canned [1 cup]	135	4.8	31	23%	3	5	0.9
2467	Cobb salad with dressing [1 cup]	129	4.6	180	74%	8	5	2.3
2468	Collards, cooked, from canned [1 cup, canned]	162	5.7	43	6%	2	10	4.5
2469	Collards, cooked, from fresh [1 cup, fresh]	128	4.5	35	6%	2	8	3.6
2470	Collards, cooked, from frozen [1 cup, frozen]	170	6.0	61	10%	5	12	4.8
2471	Collards, raw [1 cup]	186	6.6	58	6%	3	13	6.7
2472	Corn fritter [1 cup]	107	3.8	405	50%	8	43	2.2
2473	Corn with cream sauce [1 cup]	228	8.0	291	42%	8	39	3.4
2474	Corn with peppers, red or green, cooked (Include Mexican style corn) [1 cup]	178	6.3	179	11%	6	42	4.7
2475	Corn, cooked, from canned, with cream sauce, made with milk [1 cup]	228	8.0	261	46%	7	32	2.5
2476	Corn, cooked, from fresh, with cream sauce, made with milk [1 cup]	228	8.0	291	42%	8	39	3.4
2477	Corn, cooked, from frozen, with cream sauce, made with milk [1 cup]	228	8.0	259	44%	8	33	2.9
2478	Corn, dried, cooked [2 oz]	56	2.0	75	45%	1	11	0.9
2479	Corn, raw [1 cup]	154	5.4	132	12%	5	29	4.2
2480	Corn, scalloped or pudding (Include corn souffle) [1 cup]	214	7.5	260	39%	10	34	3.3
2481	Corn, white, cooked, from canned [1 cup]	164	5.8	133	11%	4	30	3.3
2482	Corn, white, cooked, from fresh [1 medium ear (6¾" to 7½" long)]	100	3.5	108	11%	3	25	2.7
2483	Corn, white, cooked, from frozen [1 cup]	164	5.8	131	5%	5	32	3.9
2484	Corn, white, from canned, cream style [1 cup]	256	9.0	184	5%	4	46	3.1
2485	Corn, yellow, canned, low sodium (Include corn, canned, no salt added) [1 cup]	164	5.8	177	11%	5	41	4.6
2486	Corn, yellow, cooked, from canned [1 cup]	164	5.8	133	11%	4	30	3.3
2487	Corn, yellow, cooked, from fresh [1 medium ear (6¾" to 7½" long)]	100	3.5	108	11%	3	25	2.8

Food no.	fat gm	sat fat gm	choles mg	sodium mg	potas mg	% of Daily Value: vit A	vit E	vit C	thia	ribo	niac	vit B-6	fola	vit B-12	calc	phos	mag	iron	zinc
2436	0	0	0	86	231	258	3	7	3	3	3	9	4	0	4	4	4	4	2
2437	12	2	0	222	274	259	10	6	3	3	3	9	4	0	6	4	5	5	2
2438	16	7	33	465	343	260	7	7	6	16	4	11	6	5	31	23	8	6	10
2439	0	0	0	17	161	140	1	8	3	2	2	4	2	0	1	2	2	1	1
2440	30	4	22	249	600	265	23	22	10	5	6	22	5	2	5	9	7	8	2
2441	1	0	0	15	1452	0	2	115	26	11	13	27	8	0	17	13	31	38	3
2442	0	0	0	6	556	0	1	42	10	4	5	11	3	0	7	5	13	15	1
2443	25	5	35	367	733	6	15	67	22	12	13	17	5	5	9	15	15	17	10
2444	8	1	0	347	1108	10	8	107	19	9	11	25	8	0	13	11	24	28	4
2445	8	2	5	96	103	2	6	20	4	5	3	3	4	1	4	8	2	3	2
2446	1	0	0	563	254	0	0	132	5	6	4	15	20	0	3	6	4	3	2
2447	1	0	0	19	178	0	0	92	4	4	3	11	14	0	2	4	3	2	2
2448	0	0	0	32	250	0	0	94	4	6	3	8	18	0	3	4	4	4	2
2449	18	8	36	441	320	13	5	98	7	18	4	14	16	5	32	26	7	5	10
2450	18	8	36	832	319	13	5	98	7	18	4	13	16	5	31	26	7	5	10
2451	18	8	36	441	320	13	5	98	7	18	4	14	16	5	32	26	7	5	10
2452	14	7	29	361	316	10	4	80	7	16	3	8	17	4	26	21	7	5	8
2453	0	0	0	30	303	0	0	77	4	4	3	11	14	0	2	4	4	2	2
2454	0	0	0	155	441	0	3	14	4	5	5	12	2	0	7	17	8	6	3
2455	0	0	0	137	426	2	2	15	4	4	2	6	8	0	6	4	5	4	1
2456	11	3	7	480	515	7	8	14	8	15	4	7	8	5	17	13	7	5	4
2457	0	0	0	30	98	0	1	4	1	1	1	1	2	0	1	1	1	1	0
2458	3	2	10	85	77	4	1	3	1	2	0	1	2	1	3	4	1	1	1
2459	0	0	0	260	796	46	12	44	3	7	3	6	3	0	8	5	31	18	3
2460	0	0	0	77	136	12	3	18	1	2	1	2	1	0	2	2	7	4	1
2461	0	0	0	1	59	8	0	16	1	1	1	1	4	0	2	1	2	2	1
2462	0	0	0	0	18	3	0	6	0	0	0	0	2	0	1	0	1	1	0
2463	1	0	0	7	237	1	1	21	3	4	4	10	8	0	3	4	6	4	4
2464	5	1	47	90	182	5	3	12	4	7	3	6	6	3	6	7	4	4	3
2465	0	0	0	9	82	10	1	7	1	2	1	1	2	0	1	1	1	1	0
2466	1	0	0	380	473	103	4	51	5	13	5	11	12	0	8	6	9	6	1
2467	15	4	72	256	376	14	9	20	7	11	10	10	16	5	6	11	6	6	5
2468	0	0	0	459	211	44	6	32	2	5	2	4	2	0	4	1	3	1	1
2469	0	0	0	20	168	35	5	26	2	4	2	3	2	0	3	1	2	1	1
2470	1	0	0	85	427	102	4	75	5	12	5	10	32	0	36	5	13	11	3
2471	0	0	0	37	314	62	19	72	4	7	3	6	6	0	5	2	4	2	2
2472	23	5	72	318	203	6	13	6	18	20	14	3	8	3	13	16	6	16	5
2473	14	4	8	426	461	9	8	13	21	17	11	6	15	5	14	23	13	6	7
2474	2	0	0	28	429	5	1	37	24	7	13	7	19	0	0	17	13	6	5
2475	13	3	8	649	400	8	8	17	8	18	9	5	14	5	14	19	10	8	6
2476	14	4	8	426	461	9	8	13	21	17	11	6	15	5	14	23	13	6	7
2477	13	3	8	412	346	9	8	7	12	17	10	10	10	5	14	18	9	4	6
2478	4	1	0	138	98	4	2	7	1	3	3	1	6	0	1	3	2	2	1
2479	2	0	0	23	416	4	1	17	21	5	13	4	18	0	0	14	14	4	5
2480	11	3	155	140	420	16	6	11	9	21	11	15	13	7	9	21	9	6	7
2481	2	0	0	530	320	0	1	22	3	8	10	4	19	0	1	11	8	8	4
2482	1	0	0	17	249	0	0	10	14	4	8	3	12	0	0	10	8	3	3
2483	1	0	0	8	241	0	1	8	9	7	11	11	13	0	1	9	8	3	4
2484	1	0	0	730	343	0	1	19	4	8	12	8	27	0	1	13	11	5	9
2485	2	0	0	28	408	4	1	17	24	7	13	5	19	0	0	17	13	6	5
2486	2	0	0	351	320	3	1	22	3	8	10	4	19	0	1	11	8	8	4
2487	1	0	0	17	249	2	0	10	14	4	8	3	12	0	0	10	8	3	3

Fruits & Vegetables

Food No.	Food Description & Amount	wt gm	wt oz	cal	% cal fat	prot gm	carbo gm	fiber gm
2488	Corn, yellow, cooked, from frozen [1 cup]	164	5.8	131	5%	5	32	3.9
2489	Corn, yellow, from canned, cream style [1 cup]	256	9.0	184	5%	4	46	3.1
2490	Cowpeas with snap beans, cooked [1 cup]	138	4.9	126	4%	4	26	6.7
2491	Cress, cooked, from fresh [1 cup]	135	4.8	31	23%	3	5	0.9
2492	Cress, raw [1 cup]	50	1.8	16	20%	1	3	0.6
2493	Cucumber-carrot-mushroom namasu (marinade of vinegar, sugar, ginger root) [1 cup]	155	5.5	52	3%	1	13	1.3
2494	Cucumber salad without oil (cucumber, onions, vinegar, sugar) [1 cup]	159	5.6	48	3%	1	12	1.1
2495	Cucumber salad with oil (cucumber, onion, vinegar, soybean oil, sugar, salt) [1 cup]	159	5.6	179	78%	1	11	1.0
2496	Cucumber salad (cucumbers with sour cream) [1 cup]	133	4.7	68	74%	1	4	0.8
2497	Cucumber, cooked [1 cup]	180	6.3	29	9%	2	6	1.8
2498	Cucumber, raw [1 small (6-3/8" long)]	158	5.6	19	12%	1	4	1.1
2499	Dandelion greens, cooked [1 cup, chopped]	105	3.7	35	16%	2	7	3.0
2500	Dandelion greens, raw [1 cup]	55	1.9	25	14%	1	5	1.9
2501	Dasheen, boiled (Include malanga) [1 cup, pieces]	190	6.7	273	2%	4	67	10.4
2502	Dasheen, fried (Include malanga) [1 cup, pieces]	123	4.3	306	31%	1	52	7.7
2503	Eggplant in tomato sauce, cooked [1 cup]	231	8.1	67	6%	3	16	4.3
2504	Eggplant, batter-dipped, fried [1 cup]	220	7.8	329	65%	5	26	5.2
2505	Eggplant, cooked [1 eggplant]	538	19.0	151	7%	4	36	13.5
2506	Eggplant, raw [1 eggplant, peeled (yield from 1.25 lb)]	458	16.2	119	6%	5	28	11.5
2507	Endive, chicory, escarole, or romaine, raw [1 cup, mixed greens]	40	1.4	7	11%	1	1	1.2
2508	Escarole, cooked (Include endive) [1 cup]	130	4.6	29	11%	2	6	5.2
2509	Escarole, creamed [1 cup]	200	7.1	173	57%	6	14	5.1
2510	Fern shoots, cooked (Include fiddle heads) [1 cup]	142	5.0	57	2%	0	16	5.3
2511	Flowers or blossoms of sesbania, squash, or lily [1 cup]	104	3.7	16	5%	1	3	0.9
2512	Fried stuffed potatoes, Puerto Rican style (Rellenos de papas) [1 fritter (4"x2"x ¾")]	95	3.4	167	51%	5	16	1.3
2513	Garlic, cooked [4 cloves]	8	0.3	12	3%	1	3	0.2
2514	Garlic, raw [4 cloves]	12	0.4	18	3%	1	4	0.3
2515	Greek Salad [1 cup]	105	3.7	106	62%	7	3	1.0
2516	Green peppers and onions, cooked, fat added [1 cup]	144	5.1	80	38%	2	12	1.9
2517	Green plantain with cracklings, Puerto Rican style (Mofongo) [1 ball (3" dia)]	64	2.3	229	63%	6	17	1.2
2518	Greens, cooked, from canned [1 cup]	170	6.0	44	9%	2	9	4.7
2519	Greens, cooked, from fresh [1 cup]	146	5.1	38	9%	2	8	4.1
2520	Greens, cooked, from frozen [1 cup]	161	5.7	52	12%	5	9	4.5
2521	Hominy, cooked [1 cup]	165	5.8	119	11%	2	24	4.1
2522	Horseradish (marong-gay), pods, cooked [1 cup]	118	4.2	42	5%	2	10	5.0
2523	Jai, Monk's Food (mushrooms, lily roots, bean curd, water chestnuts) [1 cup]	188	6.6	179	23%	10	29	5.6
2524	Jicama, raw (Include yambean) [1 cup]	130	4.6	49	2%	1	11	6.4
2525	Kale, cooked, from canned [1 cup, canned]	163	5.7	52	11%	3	9	3.2
2526	Kale, cooked, from fresh [1 cup]	130	4.6	42	11%	2	7	2.6
2527	Kale, cooked, from frozen [1 cup]	130	4.6	39	15%	4	7	2.6
2528	Kohlrabi, cooked [1 cup]	165	5.8	48	3%	3	11	1.8
2529	Kohlrabi, creamed [1 cup]	187	6.6	149	52%	5	15	1.3
2530	Kohlrabi, raw [1 cup]	135	4.8	36	3%	2	8	4.9
2531	Lambsquarter, cooked [1 cup]	180	6.3	58	20%	6	9	3.8
2532	Leek, cooked [1 cup]	171	6.0	163	39%	3	24	3.1
2533	Leek, raw [1 leek]	89	3.1	54	4%	1	13	1.6
2534	Lettuce salad with egg, cheese, tomato, and/or carrots, with or without other vegetables, no dressing (Include McDonald's Garden Salad; McDonald's Side Salad) [1 salad]	236	8.3	122	56%	8	7	2.8
2535	Lettuce, Boston (Include deer tongue lettuce, native lettuce, red leaf lettuce) [1 cup, shredded or chopped]	55	1.9	7	15%	1	1	0.6

Food no.	fat gm	sat fat gm	choles mg	sodium mg	potas mg	% of Daily Value vit A	vit E	vit C	thia	ribo	niac	vit B-6	fola	vit B-12	calc	phos	mag	iron	zinc
2488	1	0	0	8	241	4	1	8	9	7	11	11	13	0	1	9	8	3	4
2489	1	0	0	730	343	3	1	19	4	8	12	8	27	0	1	13	11	5	9
2490	1	0	0	5	561	11	1	7	9	12	9	4	41	0	17	7	17	9	9
2491	1	0	0	11	477	104	4	52	5	13	5	11	12	0	8	6	9	6	1
2492	0	0	0	7	303	47	2	58	3	8	3	6	10	0	4	4	5	4	1
2493	0	0	0	8	221	46	1	11	3	4	4	3	4	0	2	4	5	2	2
2494	0	0	0	3	206	2	0	10	2	1	1	3	4	0	2	3	5	3	2
2495	15	2	0	329	186	2	14	10	2	1	1	3	4	0	2	3	5	3	1
2496	6	3	11	16	196	6	1	5	2	3	0	4	4	1	5	4	4	1	1
2497	0	0	0	4	288	4	1	16	3	3	2	4	5	0	3	4	6	3	3
2498	0	0	0	3	234	1	1	7	2	1	0	6	6	0	2	3	5	1	1
2499	1	0	0	46	244	123	12	32	9	11	3	8	3	0	15	4	6	11	2
2500	0	0	0	42	218	77	6	32	7	8	2	7	4	0	10	4	5	9	2
2501	1	0	0	27	1355	0	28	12	13	3	7	32	9	0	10	19	20	7	4
2502	11	2	0	23	726	0	9	10	9	2	4	24	5	0	3	11	11	6	3
2503	0	0	0	787	732	13	8	30	11	6	10	14	7	0	2	6	9	8	3
2504	24	5	36	66	465	2	15	4	13	12	10	9	8	2	6	10	8	9	4
2505	1	0	0	16	1334	3	1	12	27	6	16	23	19	0	3	12	17	10	5
2506	1	0	0	14	994	4	1	13	16	9	14	19	22	0	3	10	16	7	4
2507	0	0	0	10	137	12	2	12	2	2	1	1	13	0	3	2	2	2	1
2508	0	0	0	35	477	33	3	11	8	7	3	1	39	0	8	4	6	7	8
2509	11	3	7	386	605	36	9	12	12	18	5	3	38	5	20	14	9	9	11
2510	0	0	0	7	7	3	5	71	0	25	25	13	5	0	1	1	2	1	3
2511	0	0	0	6	110	18	0	9	1	2	2	3	11	0	4	4	7	5	1
2512	10	2	31	76	443	1	7	17	8	5	9	12	2	2	1	7	5	5	4
2513	0	0	0	1	32	0	0	3	1	0	0	5	0	0	1	1	1	1	1
2514	0	0	0	2	48	0	0	6	2	1	0	7	0	0	2	2	1	1	1
2515	7	3	119	410	181	13	4	10	5	18	5	8	11	10	12	12	5	6	6
2516	3	1	0	40	234	6	4	76	5	2	2	12	5	0	2	4	4	3	2
2517	16	4	15	276	326	5	8	12	9	4	8	10	2	5	0	8	6	3	4
2518	0	0	0	444	305	83	9	70	4	6	3	10	18	0	12	3	6	5	2
2519	0	0	0	32	264	72	8	61	4	5	3	8	16	0	11	3	5	5	2
2520	1	0	0	45	420	109	9	66	5	9	5	7	18	0	27	5	10	12	3
2521	1	0	0	347	15	0	0	0	0	1	0	0	0	0	2	6	7	6	12
2522	0	0	0	51	539	1	1	191	4	5	3	7	9	0	2	6	12	3	3
2523	5	1	0	28	641	1	1	19	11	19	17	19	12	0	10	18	31	29	17
2524	0	0	0	5	195	0	3	44	2	2	1	3	4	0	2	2	4	4	1
2525	1	0	0	500	369	120	6	111	6	7	4	11	5	0	12	5	7	8	3
2526	1	0	0	30	296	96	5	89	5	5	3	9	4	0	9	4	6	7	2
2527	1	0	0	20	417	83	1	55	4	9	4	6	5	0	18	4	6	7	2
2528	0	0	0	35	561	1	13	149	4	2	3	13	5	0	4	7	8	4	3
2529	9	2	6	308	487	5	13	97	7	10	4	10	4	4	12	13	8	4	4
2530	0	0	0	27	473	1	3	140	5	2	3	10	5	0	3	6	6	3	0
2531	1	0	0	52	518	175	11	111	12	28	8	16	6	0	46	8	10	7	4
2532	7	1	0	109	282	8	12	24	6	3	3	19	19	0	10	6	11	19	1
2533	0	0	0	18	160	1	4	18	4	2	2	10	14	0	5	3	6	10	1
2534	8	4	87	151	417	34	4	28	7	13	3	7	23	5	16	16	7	7	7
2535	0	0	0	3	141	5	1	7	2	2	1	1	10	0	2	1	2	1	1

Fruits & Vegetables

Food No.	Food Description & Amount	wt gm	wt oz	cal	% cal fat	prot gm	carbo gm	fiber gm
2536	Lettuce, cooked [1 cup]	81	2.9	10	14%	1	2	1.1
2537	Lettuce, manoa [1 cup]	50	1.8	7	14%	1	1	0.8
2538	Lettuce, iceberg, raw [1 cup, shredded or chopped]	55	1.9	7	14%	1	1	0.8
2539	Lettuce salad with assorted vegetables, no tomatoes, carrots, or dressing [1 cup]	74	2.6	11	10%	1	2	0.9
2540	Lettuce salad with assorted vegetables including tomatoes and/or carrots, no dressing (Include Burger King Side Salad, Hardee's Side Salad) [1 cup]	73	2.6	13	12%	1	3	1.1
2541	Lettuce salad with avocado, tomato, and/or carrots, with or without other vegetables, no dressing [1 cup]	87	3.1	45	63%	1	4	2.1
2542	Lettuce salad with cheese, tomato and/or carrots, with or without other vegetables, no dressing (Include Burger King Garden Salad) [1 cup]	77	2.7	79	64%	5	3	1.0
2543	Lettuce salad with egg, tomato, and/or carrots, with or without other vegetables, no dressing [1 cup]	88	3.1	47	47%	3	3	1.1
2544	Lettuce, wilted, with bacon dressing [1 cup]	125	4.4	103	76%	3	4	1.9
2545	Lima beans, canned, low sodium, no fat [1 cup]	174	6.1	124	4%	7	23	6.3
2546	Lima beans, cooked, from canned [1 cup]	174	6.1	213	2%	12	41	9.2
2547	Lima beans, cooked, from canned, with mushroom sauce [1 cup]	228	8.0	247	27%	10	36	6.5
2548	Lima beans, cooked, from fresh [1 cup]	170	6.0	209	2%	12	40	9.0
2549	Lima beans, cooked, from fresh, with mushroom sauce [1 cup]	228	8.0	248	27%	10	36	6.6
2550	Lima beans, cooked, from frozen [1 cup]	180	6.3	185	3%	11	34	10.6
2551	Lima beans, cooked, from frozen, with mushroom sauce [1 cup]	228	8.0	220	31%	9	30	7.2
2552	Lima beans, from canned, creamed or with cheese sauce [1 cup]	228	8.0	338	33%	18	39	7.9
2553	Lima beans, from fresh, creamed or with cheese sauce [1 cup]	228	8.0	340	33%	18	40	7.9
2554	Lima beans, from frozen, creamed or with cheese sauce [1 cup]	228	8.0	308	35%	18	33	8.9
2555	Lima beans, raw [1 cup]	156	5.5	176	7%	11	31	7.6
2556	Lotus root, cooked [1 cup]	120	4.2	79	1%	2	19	3.7
2557	Luffa (Chinese okra), cooked [1 cup]	178	6.3	57	5%	3	13	4.5
2558	Mixed salad greens, raw [1 cup, shredded or chopped]	55	1.9	9	13%	1	2	1.2
2559	Mixed vegetables (corn, lima beans, peas, green beans, and carrots), canned, low sodium [1 cup]	182	6.4	66	5%	3	13	5.6
2560	Mixed vegetables (corn, lima beans, peas, green beans, and carrots), cooked, from canned [1 cup]	182	6.4	86	5%	5	17	5.5
2561	Mixed vegetables (corn, lima beans, peas, green beans, and carrots), cooked, from frozen [1 cup]	182	6.4	107	2%	5	24	8.0
2562	Mixed vegetables (green beans, broccoli, onions, mushrooms), cooked [1 cup]	129	4.6	36	6%	2	8	3.4
2563	Mixed vegetables, stew type (including potatoes, carrots, onions, celery) cooked [1 cup]	160	5.6	77	2%	2	17	3.5
2564	Mushroom, Oriental, dried (Include shiitake) [1 cup]	145	5.1	80	4%	2	21	3.0
2565	Mushrooms, batter-dipped, fried [4 small]	32	1.1	71	68%	1	5	0.4
2566	Mushrooms, cooked, from canned [1 cup]	156	5.5	37	11%	3	8	3.7
2567	Mushrooms, cooked, from fresh or frozen [1 cup]	156	5.5	42	16%	3	8	3.4
2568	Mushrooms, from canned or frozen, creamed [1 cup]	217	7.7	171	56%	6	15	3.1
2569	Mushrooms, from fresh, creamed [1 cup]	217	7.7	174	56%	6	15	2.8
2570	Mushrooms, raw [1 cup, pieces]	70	2.5	18	15%	1	3	0.8
2571	Mushrooms, stuffed [2 stuffed caps]	48	1.7	138	48%	5	13	0.9
2572	Mustard cabbage, cooked [1 cup]	170	6.0	20	12%	3	3	2.7
2573	Mustard greens, cooked, from canned [1 cup, canned]	153	5.4	23	14%	3	3	3.0
2574	Mustard greens, cooked, from fresh [1 cup, fresh]	140	4.9	21	14%	3	3	2.8
2575	Mustard greens, cooked, from frozen [1 cup]	150	5.3	29	12%	3	5	4.2
2576	Mustard greens, raw [1 cup]	56	2.0	15	7%	2	3	1.8
2577	Okra, batter-dipped, fried in corn oil (Include cornmeal-dipped, fried) [1 cup]	92	3.2	178	63%	2	14	2.2
2578	Okra, cooked, from canned [1 cup]	167	5.9	53	5%	3	12	4.1
2579	Okra, cooked, from fresh [1 cup]	160	5.6	51	5%	3	12	4.0
2580	Okra, cooked, from frozen [1 cup]	184	6.5	68	7%	4	11	5.2
2581	Onion rings, batter-dipped, fried in corn oil [10 small rings (1½" dia)]	48	1.7	73	59%	1	7	0.8

Food no.	fat gm	sat fat gm	choles mg	sodium mg	potas mg	vit A	vit E	vit C	thia	ribo	niac	vit B-6	fola	vit B-12	calc	phos	mag	iron	zinc
						% of Daily Value													
2536	0	0	0	7	128	3	1	4	2	1	1	1	10	0	2	2	2	2	1
2537	0	0	0	4	121	7	1	11	2	2	1	1	10	0	2	1	1	2	1
2538	0	0	0	5	87	2	1	4	2	1	1	1	8	0	1	1	1	2	1
2539	0	0	0	15	132	1	1	5	2	1	1	2	6	0	2	2	2	1	1
2540	0	0	0	13	149	18	1	12	3	2	1	2	7	0	1	2	2	2	1
2541	3	1	0	15	263	35	2	14	4	3	3	5	9	0	1	3	4	3	1
2542	6	3	17	115	152	37	1	11	3	5	1	3	6	2	13	10	3	2	4
2543	2	1	91	42	176	38	2	12	3	8	2	4	8	4	2	5	2	3	2
2544	9	3	10	99	306	19	2	27	6	6	4	4	12	2	7	5	4	9	3
2545	1	0	0	7	496	3	2	25	3	4	5	5	7	0	5	12	15	16	7
2546	1	0	0	408	986	6	1	29	16	10	9	17	11	0	6	22	32	24	9
2547	7	2	3	896	767	5	5	21	13	12	9	12	9	2	9	20	24	18	10
2548	1	0	0	29	969	6	1	29	16	10	9	16	11	0	5	22	31	23	9
2549	7	2	3	638	770	5	5	21	13	12	9	12	9	2	9	20	24	18	10
2550	1	0	0	73	737	3	4	28	9	6	8	11	8	0	5	16	20	17	6
2551	7	2	3	681	577	3	6	27	8	10	9	8	7	2	7	13	12	11	7
2552	12	6	30	681	957	15	3	26	16	20	9	16	11	5	29	37	31	22	14
2553	12	6	30	358	961	15	3	26	16	20	9	16	11	5	29	37	31	22	14
2554	12	6	30	387	726	12	5	24	9	16	8	11	8	5	28	31	21	15	11
2555	1	0	0	12	729	5	5	61	23	9	11	16	13	0	5	21	23	27	8
2556	0	0	0	54	436	0	0	55	10	1	2	13	2	0	3	9	7	6	3
2557	0	0	0	9	573	10	6	48	16	6	8	17	20	0	11	10	25	4	7
2558	0	0	0	14	174	15	2	15	3	3	1	2	16	0	3	2	3	4	2
2559	0	0	0	47	251	92	2	12	4	4	4	7	8	0	4	7	7	7	6
2560	0	0	0	271	530	212	5	14	5	5	5	7	10	0	5	8	7	11	5
2561	0	0	0	64	308	78	3	10	9	13	8	7	9	0	5	9	10	8	6
2562	0	0	0	17	223	9	4	31	4	8	6	6	10	0	5	6	6	6	3
2563	0	0	0	66	366	103	2	16	7	3	6	12	5	0	3	4	4	6	2
2564	0	0	0	6	170	0	1	1	4	15	11	12	8	0	0	4	5	4	13
2565	5	1	1	51	71	0	5	1	3	7	5	1	1	0	1	5	1	3	1
2566	0	0	0	663	201	0	1	0	8	2	12	5	5	0	2	10	6	7	7
2567	1	0	0	3	555	0	1	10	8	28	35	7	7	0	1	14	5	15	9
2568	11	3	7	854	306	5	7	1	11	12	12	6	5	5	13	17	8	7	8
2569	11	3	7	344	579	5	7	9	10	32	29	8	7	5	12	20	7	13	10
2570	0	0	0	3	259	0	0	4	5	18	14	3	4	0	0	7	2	5	3
2571	7	2	6	298	209	5	4	5	10	15	13	3	3	2	10	11	4	8	5
2572	0	0	0	58	631	44	1	74	4	6	4	14	17	0	16	5	5	10	2
2573	0	0	0	428	307	46	14	64	4	6	3	7	28	0	11	6	6	6	1
2574	0	0	0	22	283	42	13	59	4	5	3	7	26	0	10	6	5	5	1
2575	0	0	0	38	209	67	12	35	4	5	2	8	26	0	15	4	5	9	2
2576	0	0	0	14	198	30	5	65	3	4	2	5	26	0	6	2	4	5	1
2577	13	2	2	122	190	4	14	17	12	8	7	6	10	1	6	12	9	7	3
2578	0	0	0	394	535	10	5	45	15	5	7	16	19	0	10	9	24	4	6
2579	0	0	0	8	515	9	5	43	14	5	7	15	18	0	10	9	23	4	6
2580	1	0	0	6	431	9	6	37	12	13	7	4	67	0	18	8	23	7	8
2581	5	1	1	46	61	0	5	3	3	3	2	2	1	0	1	4	1	2	1

Fruits & Vegetables

Food No.	Food Description & Amount	wt gm	wt oz	cal	% cal fat	prot gm	carbo gm	fiber gm
2582	Onion rings, from fresh, batter-dipped, baked or fried [10 medium rings (2½" dia)]	60	2.1	108	62%	1	9	1.0
2583	Onion rings, from frozen, batter-dipped, baked or fried [10 medium rings (2½" dia)]	60	2.1	108	63%	1	9	0.9
2584	Onion, dehydrated [2 Tbs]	7	0.2	23	1%	1	6	0.6
2585	Onions, creamed [1 cup]	228	8.0	188	45%	5	22	2.2
2586	Onions, from fresh, creamed [1 cup]	228	8.0	188	45%	5	22	2.2
2587	Onions, mature, cooked or sauteed, from fresh, fat added [1 cup]	215	7.6	126	30%	3	21	2.9
2588	Onions, mature, cooked or sauteed, from frozen, fat added [1 cup]	215	7.6	91	37%	2	14	3.4
2589	Onions, mature, cooked, from fresh [1 cup]	210	7.4	92	4%	3	21	2.9
2590	Onions, mature, cooked, from frozen [1 cup]	210	7.4	59	2%	2	14	3.4
2591	Onions, mature, raw (Include red onions) [1 cup, chopped]	160	5.6	61	4%	2	14	2.9
2592	Onions, pearl, cooked, from canned [1 cup]	185	6.5	81	4%	2	19	2.6
2593	Onions, pearl, cooked, from fresh [1 cup]	185	6.5	81	4%	3	19	2.6
2594	Onions, pearl, cooked, from frozen [1 cup]	185	6.5	52	2%	1	12	2.6
2595	Onions, young green, cooked, from fresh [1 cup]	219	7.7	74	5%	4	17	6.0
2596	Onions, young green, raw [1 cup, chopped]	100	3.5	32	5%	2	7	2.6
2597	Palm hearts, cooked [1 cup]	146	5.1	150	2%	4	39	2.2
2598	Parsley, cooked [10 sprigs]	12	0.4	4	20%	0	1	0.4
2599	Parsley, raw [1 cup]	60	2.1	22	20%	2	4	2.0
2600	Parsnips, cooked [1 cup, pieces]	156	5.5	126	3%	2	30	6.2
2601	Parsnips, creamed [1 cup]	228	8.0	252	40%	6	34	5.3
2602	Pea salad with cheese (peas, cheese, mayonnaise, egg, onion, pimento, salt [1 cup]	214	7.5	571	76%	19	18	5.6
2603	Pea salad (peas, mayonnaise, egg, onion, pimento, salt) [1 cup]	214	7.5	501	76%	11	21	6.9
2604	Peas and carrots, cooked, from canned [1 cup]	160	5.6	84	5%	5	16	5.0
2605	Peas and carrots, cooked, from canned, low sodium [1 cup]	160	5.6	61	6%	3	14	5.3
2606	Peas and carrots, cooked, from fresh [1 cup]	160	5.6	110	3%	6	22	7.4
2607	Peas and carrots, cooked, from frozen [1 cup]	160	5.6	77	8%	5	16	5.0
2608	Peas and carrots, from canned, creamed [1 cup]	244	8.6	229	46%	8	24	4.5
2609	Peas and carrots, from fresh, creamed [1 cup]	244	8.6	252	42%	9	28	6.5
2610	Peas and carrots, from frozen, creamed [1 cup]	244	8.6	223	48%	8	24	4.5
2611	Peas and corn, cooked [1 cup]	162	5.7	156	7%	7	33	6.7
2612	Peas and onions, cooked [1 cup]	180	6.3	81	4%	5	16	4.0
2613	Peas and potatoes, cooked [1 cup]	158	5.6	134	2%	6	28	6.0
2614	Peas with mushroom sauce [1 cup]	244	8.6	216	34%	9	28	7.1
2615	Peas with mushrooms, cooked [1 cup]	159	5.6	108	4%	7	20	7.7
2616	Peas, cooked, from canned, with mushroom sauce [1 cup]	244	8.6	196	37%	8	24	5.5
2617	Peas, cooked, from fresh, with mushroom sauce [1 cup]	244	8.6	216	34%	9	28	7.1
2618	Peas, cooked, from frozen, with mushroom sauce [1 cup]	244	8.6	208	35%	9	26	7.1
2619	Peas, cowpeas, field peas, or blackeye peas (not dried), cooked, from canned [1 cup]	180	6.3	173	4%	6	36	8.9
2620	Peas, cowpeas, field peas, or blackeye peas (not dried), cooked, from fresh [1 cup]	165	5.8	160	4%	5	34	8.3
2621	Peas, cowpeas, field peas, or blackeye peas (not dried), cooked, from frozen [1 cup]	170	6.0	224	5%	14	40	10.9
2622	Peas, from canned, creamed [1 cup]	244	8.6	249	42%	10	27	6.0
2623	Peas, from fresh, creamed [1 cup]	244	8.6	272	39%	11	31	7.7
2624	Peas, from frozen, creamed [1 cup]	244	8.6	264	40%	11	29	7.7
2625	Peas, green, canned, low sodium [1 cup]	170	6.0	90	5%	5	17	5.4
2626	Peas, green, cooked, from canned [1 cup]	170	6.0	117	5%	8	21	7.0
2627	Peas, green, cooked, from fresh [1 cup]	160	5.6	134	2%	9	25	8.8
2628	Peas, green, cooked, from frozen [1 cup]	160	5.6	125	3%	8	23	8.8
2629	Peas, green, raw [1 cup]	146	5.1	118	4%	8	21	7.4
2630	Pepper, banana, raw [1 medium (4½" long)]	46	1.6	12	15%	1	2	1.6

Food no.	fat gm	sat fat gm	choles mg	sodium mg	potas mg	% of Daily Value													
						vit A	vit E	vit C	thia	ribo	niac	vit B-6	fola	vit B-12	calc	phos	mag	iron	zinc
2582	7	1	1	71	72	0	7	3	4	4	3	2	2	0	2	6	1	3	1
2583	8	1	1	75	66	1	7	4	4	4	3	2	2	0	2	6	1	4	1
2584	0	0	0	1	114	0	0	9	2	0	0	6	3	0	2	2	2	1	1
2585	9	2	6	305	370	5	6	14	8	11	3	11	6	4	13	13	7	3	4
2586	9	2	6	305	370	5	6	14	8	11	3	11	6	4	13	13	7	3	4
2587	4	1	0	51	351	4	4	18	6	3	2	14	8	0	5	7	6	3	3
2588	4	1	0	63	222	4	4	13	3	3	1	7	7	0	5	2	4	4	1
2589	0	0	0	6	349	0	1	18	6	3	2	14	8	0	5	7	6	3	3
2590	0	0	0	21	220	1	2	13	3	3	1	7	7	0	4	2	4	4	1
2591	0	0	0	5	251	0	1	17	4	2	1	9	8	0	3	5	4	2	2
2592	0	0	0	514	305	0	1	16	5	3	2	12	7	0	4	6	5	2	3
2593	0	0	0	6	307	0	1	16	5	3	2	12	7	0	4	6	5	2	3
2594	0	0	0	15	187	0	1	16	2	2	1	6	6	0	5	0	4	3	1
2595	0	0	0	35	573	8	1	51	7	10	6	7	26	0	16	8	11	18	6
2596	0	0	0	16	276	4	1	31	4	5	3	3	16	0	7	4	5	8	3
2597	0	0	0	20	2637	1	3	17	4	15	6	53	7	0	3	20	4	14	36
2598	0	0	0	6	60	6	1	16	1	1	1	0	3	0	2	1	1	4	1
2599	0	0	0	34	332	31	5	133	3	3	4	3	23	0	8	3	8	21	4
2600	0	0	0	16	573	0	7	34	9	5	6	7	23	0	6	11	11	5	3
2601	11	3	7	372	623	6	12	29	12	15	7	8	20	5	17	19	13	6	5
2602	48	14	144	619	349	26	25	60	19	23	11	23	19	11	34	37	12	13	19
2603	42	7	125	450	381	17	30	74	22	17	13	27	21	6	5	20	12	14	13
2604	0	0	0	397	280	88	3	18	8	6	5	6	12	0	3	8	5	7	6
2605	0	0	0	6	160	92	3	17	7	5	5	7	7	0	4	7	6	7	6
2606	0	0	0	45	406	161	3	25	18	11	11	18	18	0	5	13	12	10	9
2607	1	0	0	109	253	124	2	22	24	6	9	7	10	0	4	8	6	8	5
2608	12	3	7	719	407	81	9	17	12	17	7	8	12	5	16	18	8	8	8
2609	12	3	8	419	514	142	9	23	20	21	12	18	16	5	17	22	14	11	11
2610	12	3	7	472	383	112	9	20	26	17	10	8	10	5	16	17	9	9	7
2611	1	0	0	16	421	7	2	27	26	10	15	11	22	0	2	18	14	10	9
2612	0	0	0	67	211	6	1	21	18	7	9	8	9	0	3	6	6	9	3
2613	0	0	0	190	473	5	2	29	19	8	13	19	14	0	3	12	12	8	8
2614	8	2	3	686	436	9	7	31	23	17	16	14	20	2	9	20	14	13	13
2615	0	0	0	112	326	9	1	23	26	13	16	9	20	0	3	14	10	14	10
2616	8	2	3	982	318	11	7	21	12	12	8	5	14	2	8	14	7	9	10
2617	8	2	3	686	436	9	7	31	23	17	16	14	20	2	9	20	14	13	13
2618	8	2	3	790	309	9	6	22	25	13	12	8	19	2	8	17	11	13	11
2619	1	0	0	511	747	14	2	7	12	16	13	6	57	0	23	9	23	11	12
2620	1	0	0	7	690	13	2	6	11	14	12	5	52	0	21	8	21	10	11
2621	1	0	0	9	638	1	3	7	29	6	6	8	60	0	4	21	21	20	16
2622	11	3	7	720	405	17	9	23	15	18	7	7	16	5	15	20	10	9	9
2623	12	3	7	383	538	14	9	34	29	24	16	17	23	5	16	27	17	14	14
2624	12	3	7	498	397	15	8	24	31	20	12	10	21	5	16	23	14	14	12
2625	1	0	0	15	170	6	3	28	13	7	7	6	12	0	3	9	7	10	8
2626	1	0	0	428	294	13	3	26	13	8	6	5	18	0	3	11	7	9	8
2627	0	0	0	5	434	10	3	38	28	14	16	17	25	0	4	19	16	14	13
2628	0	0	0	139	269	11	1	26	30	9	12	9	23	0	4	14	12	14	10
2629	1	0	0	7	356	9	3	97	26	11	15	12	24	0	4	16	12	12	12
2630	0	0	0	6	118	2	1	63	2	1	3	8	3	0	1	1	2	1	1

Fruits & Vegetables

Food No.	Food Description & Amount	wt gm	wt oz	cal	% cal fat	prot gm	carbo gm	fiber gm
2631	Pepper, Jalapeno [2 peppers]	90	3.2	36	5%	2	9	1.4
2632	Pepper, poblano, raw [1 pepper]	64	2.3	17	6%	1	4	1.2
2633	Pepper, Serrano, raw [4 peppers]	24	0.9	8	12%	0	2	0.9
2634	Pepper, sweet, green, raw [1 small]	74	2.6	20	6%	1	5	1.3
2635	Pepper, sweet, red, raw [1 small]	74	2.6	20	6%	1	5	1.5
2636	Peppers, green, cooked [1 cup]	136	4.8	38	6%	1	9	1.6
2637	Peppers, hot, cooked, from canned [1 cup, chopped]	136	4.8	57	4%	3	13	2.1
2638	Peppers, hot, cooked, from fresh [1 cup, chopped]	136	4.8	57	4%	3	13	2.1
2639	Peppers, hot, cooked, from frozen [1 cup, chopped]	136	4.8	57	4%	3	13	2.1
2640	Peppers, red, cooked [1 cup]	136	4.8	38	6%	1	9	1.6
2641	Pigeonpeas, cooked, from canned [1 cup]	153	5.4	169	11%	9	30	9.4
2642	Pigeonpeas, cooked, from fresh [1 cup]	153	5.4	170	11%	9	30	9.5
2643	Pimientos, cooked (no fat added in cooking) [1 cup]	184	6.5	52	12%	2	11	4.3
2644	Pinacbet (bitter melon, eggplant, tomato, onion, olive oil, garlic, oregano, salt) [1 cup]	214	7.5	156	64%	2	14	3.6
2645	Poi [1 cup]	240	8.5	269	1%	1	65	1.0
2646	Poke greens, cooked [1 cup]	155	5.5	31	18%	4	5	2.3
2647	Potato, baked, peel eaten [1 med (2½" dia, raw)]	122	4.3	133	1%	3	31	2.9
2648	Potato, boiled, with peel [1 med (2½" dia, raw)]	142	5.0	124	1%	3	29	2.6
2649	Potato, boiled, without peel, canned, low sodium [1 canned potato (1" dia)]	35	1.2	21	3%	0	5	0.8
2650	Potato, boiled, without peel (Include mashed, no fat or milk added) [1 med (2½" dia, raw)]	122	4.3	105	1%	2	24	2.2
2651	Potato chips (Include flavored potato chips except barbecued chips) [10 chips]	20	0.7	107	58%	1	11	0.9
2652	Potato chips, fat free [10 chips]	9	0.3	37	1%	1	8	0.7
2653	Potato chips, lowfat [10 chips]	17	0.6	80	40%	1	11	1.0
2654	Potato chips, restructured (Include Pringles, Hearty Potato Krunch Twists, Pringles Light) [10 chips]	20	0.7	112	62%	1	10	0.7
2655	Potato chips, restructured, baked [10 chips]	12	0.4	57	35%	1	9	0.6
2656	Potato chips, restructured, low fat and sodium [10 chips]	20	0.7	100	46%	1	13	0.7
2657	Potato chips, unsalted (Include barbecued, unsalted) [10 chips]	20	0.7	107	58%	1	11	1.0
2658	Potato chips, unsalted, reduced fat [10 chips]	14	0.5	66	40%	1	9	0.9
2659	Potato based snacks, reduced fat, low sodium, all flavors (Include Nutri/System Flavor Crisps) [20 crisps]	14	0.5	64	45%	1	8	0.6
2660	Potato, cooked, with cheese (Include au gratin) [1 cup]	244	8.6	342	45%	12	36	2.6
2661	Potato, dry, powdered [1 cup, dry flakes]	55	1.9	195	1%	5	45	3.8
2662	Potato, french fried, from fresh, deep fried (Include fried with skins) [10 strips (1" to 2")]	35	1.2	95	45%	1	12	1.1
2663	Potato, french fried, from frozen, deep fried (Include fast food orders) [10 strips (1" to 2")]	35	1.2	108	47%	1	13	1.1
2664	Potato, french fried, from frozen, oven baked [10 strips (1" to 2")]	35	1.2	70	34%	1	11	1.1
2665	Potato, french fries, breaded or battered [1 large fast food order]	179	6.3	336	48%	4	40	3.2
2666	Potato, french fries, breaded or battered [10 strips (2" to 3½")]	50	1.8	94	48%	1	11	0.9
2667	Potato, hash brown, from dry mix [1 cup]	156	5.5	340	47%	5	44	3.1
2668	Potato, hash brown, from fresh [1 small (2" dia, raw) yields]	87	3.1	182	60%	2	19	1.7
2669	Potato, hash brown, from frozen [1 cup]	145	5.1	316	47%	5	41	2.9
2670	Potato, home fries (Include fried raw; cottage style; German fried; potatoes O'Brien) [1 small (2" dia, raw) yields]	52	1.8	72	47%	1	9	0.9
2671	Potato, home fries, with green or red peppers and onions [1 cup]	145	5.1	127	13%	2	26	2.7
2672	Potato, mashed [1 small (2" dia, raw) yields]	92	3.2	79	1%	2	18	1.7
2673	Potato, mashed, made with milk [1 small (2" dia, raw) yields]	110	3.9	89	4%	2	20	1.7
2674	Potato, mashed, made with fat [1 small (2" dia, raw) yields]	110	3.9	129	31%	2	21	1.9
2675	Potato, mashed, made with milk and fat [1 small (2" dia, raw) yields]	110	3.9	119	32%	2	19	1.6
2676	Potato, mashed, made with milk, fat, and cheese [1 small (2" dia, raw) yields]	120	4.2	151	39%	4	20	1.6

Food no.	fat gm	sat fat gm	choles mg	sodium mg	potas mg	% of Daily Value vit A	vit E	vit C	thia	ribo	niac	vit B-6	fola	vit B-12	calc	phos	mag	iron	zinc
2631	0	0	0	6	306	52	3	364	5	5	4	13	5	0	2	4	6	6	2
2632	0	0	0	1	113	4	2	95	3	1	2	8	4	0	1	1	2	2	1
2633	0	0	0	2	74	2	1	18	1	1	2	6	1	0	0	1	1	1	0
2634	0	0	0	1	131	5	2	110	3	1	2	9	4	0	1	1	2	2	1
2635	0	0	0	1	131	42	2	234	3	1	2	9	4	0	1	1	2	2	1
2636	0	0	0	3	226	8	4	169	5	2	3	16	5	0	1	2	3	3	1
2637	0	0	0	10	482	10	4	487	8	7	6	18	7	0	3	7	9	9	3
2638	0	0	0	9	434	10	4	458	7	7	6	18	6	0	2	6	8	9	3
2639	0	0	0	9	434	10	4	458	7	7	6	18	6	0	2	6	8	9	3
2640	0	0	0	3	226	51	4	388	5	2	3	16	5	0	1	2	3	3	1
2641	2	1	0	377	693	2	1	71	35	15	16	4	38	0	6	18	15	13	8
2642	2	1	0	8	698	2	1	72	36	15	16	4	38	0	6	18	15	13	8
2643	1	0	0	32	356	60	7	319	3	8	7	24	3	0	1	4	3	21	3
2644	11	2	0	14	573	9	10	113	9	6	6	13	13	0	2	7	8	6	4
2645	0	0	0	29	439	0	2	16	21	6	13	33	13	0	4	9	14	12	4
2646	1	0	0	28	285	135	6	212	7	23	9	9	3	0	8	5	5	10	2
2647	0	0	0	10	510	0	0	26	9	2	10	21	3	0	1	7	8	9	3
2648	0	0	0	6	538	0	0	31	10	2	10	21	4	0	1	6	8	2	3
2649	0	0	0	2	80	0	0	3	2	0	2	3	0	0	0	1	1	2	1
2650	0	0	0	6	400	0	0	15	8	1	8	16	3	0	1	5	6	2	2
2651	7	2	0	119	255	0	4	10	2	2	4	7	2	0	0	3	3	2	1
2652	0	0	0	60	153	0	0	1	7	1	3	4	1	0	0	2	2	2	0
2653	4	1	0	84	296	0	2	7	2	3	6	6	1	0	0	3	4	1	0
2654	8	2	0	131	202	0	4	3	3	1	3	1	0	0	0	3	3	2	1
2655	2	0	0	110	87	0	1	0	3	0	2	3	0	0	2	3	1	1	0
2656	5	1	0	86	201	0	5	4	3	1	4	8	1	0	1	3	3	2	1
2657	7	2	0	2	255	0	4	10	2	2	4	7	2	0	0	3	3	2	1
2658	3	1	0	1	244	0	2	6	2	2	5	5	0	0	0	3	3	1	1
2659	3	0	1	75	152	0	7	3	3	1	2	0	1	0	1	2	2	8	1
2660	17	8	32	282	997	18	6	41	11	17	13	21	6	3	28	28	13	9	11
2661	0	0	0	59	596	0	1	77	38	4	17	21	6	0	1	8	9	4	2
2662	5	1	0	4	365	0	3	18	3	1	5	8	2	0	0	3	4	3	2
2663	6	2	0	57	249	0	0	3	3	1	4	5	3	1	1	5	3	3	1
2664	3	0	0	11	146	0	0	6	3	1	4	5	1	0	0	3	2	2	1
2665	18	3	3	480	447	1	15	16	16	11	15	18	4	1	3	18	8	9	4
2666	5	1	1	134	125	0	4	4	5	3	4	5	1	0	1	5	2	2	1
2667	18	7	0	53	680	0	1	16	12	2	19	10	3	0	2	11	7	13	3
2668	12	5	0	21	279	0	1	8	4	1	9	12	2	0	1	4	4	4	2
2669	17	7	0	49	632	0	1	15	11	2	18	9	2	0	2	10	6	12	3
2670	4	0	0	2	171	0	3	8	3	1	3	7	1	0	0	2	2	1	1
2671	2	0	0	26	442	3	2	37	8	2	8	19	4	0	2	6	7	3	2
2672	0	0	0	5	302	0	0	11	6	1	6	12	2	0	1	4	5	2	2
2673	0	0	1	13	333	1	0	12	7	3	6	13	2	1	3	5	5	2	2
2674	4	1	0	57	345	4	3	13	7	1	7	14	2	0	1	4	5	2	2
2675	4	1	1	57	321	5	3	11	6	3	6	12	2	1	3	5	5	2	2
2676	7	2	7	170	349	7	3	11	6	5	6	13	2	3	8	10	6	2	4

Fruits & Vegetables

Food No.	Food Description & Amount	wt gm	wt oz	cal	% cal fat	prot gm	carbo gm	fiber gm
2677	Potato, mashed, made with milk, fat, and egg (Include Pillsbury and Betty Crocker twice baked potatoes) [1 cup]	235	8.3	638	50%	17	66	5.2
2678	Potato, mashed, made with milk, fat, egg, and cheese (Include Betty Crocker Twice Baked Cheese & Potato Mix) [1 cup]	235	8.3	461	64%	19	25	3.7
2679	Potato, mashed, from complete mix, made with water [1 cup]	227	8.0	207	11%	2	44	3.6
2680	Potato, mashed, from dry, made with milk [1 cup]	210	7.4	116	9%	4	23	1.7
2681	Potato, mashed, made from 1 oz dry, with milk and fat	178	6.3	162	48%	3	19	1.4
2682	Potato, patty (Include potato croquettes) [1 cup]	196	6.9	374	57%	8	34	3.4
2683	Potato, puffs (Include Ore Ida Crispy Crowns) [1 cup]	128	4.5	284	44%	4	39	4.1
2684	Potato, raw (peel not eaten) [1 med (2½" dia, raw)]	122	4.3	96	1%	3	22	2.0
2685	Potato, roasted [1 med (2½" dia, raw)]	93	3.3	132	1%	3	30	2.7
2686	Potato, scalloped (Include white potato, creamed) [1 cup]	226	8.0	227	29%	7	35	2.5
2687	Potato, scalloped, with ham (Include with cheese) [1 cup]	232	8.2	253	29%	13	32	2.3
2688	Potatoes, stewed, Mexican style (Papas guisadas) [1 cup]	231	8.1	342	53%	4	37	3.8
2689	Potatoes, stewed, Puerto Rican style (Papas guisadas) [1 medium]	163	5.7	186	26%	4	30	2.9
2690	Potatoes, stewed with tomatoes [1 cup]	236	8.3	189	49%	3	23	2.7
2691	Potatoes, stewed with tomatoes, Mexican style (Papas guisadas con tomate) [1 cup]	231	8.1	200	48%	3	24	2.9
2692	Potato, sticks (Include french fry shaped) [20 sticks]	6	0.2	31	59%	0	3	0.2
2693	Potato, stuffed with ham, broccoli and cheese sauce, baked, peel eaten (Include Weight Watchers) [1 entree (11 oz)]	312	11.0	222	16%	16	31	3.4
2694	Potato, stuffed, baked, peel eaten, stuffed with bacon and cheese [1 long type (2-1/3" dia, 4¾" long, raw)]	264	9.3	419	33%	13	58	5.3
2695	Potato, stuffed, baked, peel eaten, stuffed with broccoli and cheese sauce [1 long type (2-1/3" x 4¾", raw)]	290	10.2	343	23%	9	60	6.5
2696	Potato, stuffed, baked, peel eaten, stuffed with cheese [1 long type (2-1/3" x 4¾", raw)]	254	9.0	375	28%	11	57	5.2
2697	Potato, stuffed, baked, peel eaten, stuffed with chicken, broccoli and cheese sauce (Include Weight Watchers) [1 entree (11 oz)]	312	11.0	399	23%	25	53	5.8
2698	Potato, stuffed, baked, peel eaten, stuffed with chili [1 long type (2-1/3" x 4¾", raw)]	350	12.3	421	21%	11	76	9.9
2699	Potato, stuffed, baked, peel eaten, stuffed with meat in cream sauce [1 long type (2-1/3" x 4¾", raw)]	274	9.7	360	27%	11	56	5.3
2700	Potato, stuffed, baked, peel eaten, stuffed with sour cream [1 long type (2-1/3" x 4¾", raw)]	284	10.0	405	38%	7	57	5.2
2701	Potato, stuffed, baked, peel not eaten, stuffed with bacon and cheese [1 long type (2-1/3" x 4¾", raw)]	215	7.6	340	41%	12	39	2.6
2702	Potato, stuffed, baked, peel not eaten, stuffed with broccoli and cheese sauce [1 long type (2-1/3" x 4¾", raw)]	241	8.5	262	30%	7	41	3.8
2703	Potato, stuffed, baked, peel not eaten, stuffed with cheese [1 long type (2-1/3" x 4¾", raw)]	206	7.3	296	36%	9	39	2.6
2704	Potato, stuffed, baked, peel not eaten, stuffed with chicken, broccoli and cheese sauce (Include Weight Watchers) [1 entree (11 oz)]	292	10.3	356	28%	25	39	3.6
2705	Potato, stuffed, baked, peel not eaten, stuffed with chili [1 long type (2-1/3" x 4¾", raw)]	295	10.4	329	27%	9	54	6.8
2706	Potato, stuffed, baked, peel not eaten, stuffed with meat in cream sauce [1 long type (2-1/3" x 4¾", raw)]	225	7.9	281	34%	9	38	2.7
2707	Potato, stuffed, baked, peel not eaten, stuffed with sour cream [1 long type (2-1/3" x 4¾", raw)]	236	8.3	327	48%	5	39	2.5
2708	Potato from Puerto Rican beef stew (with gravy) [1 medium]	160	5.6	119	11%	4	23	2.1
2709	Potato from Puerto Rican chicken fricassee (with sauce) [1 medium]	163	5.7	136	23%	3	24	2.1
2710	Potato from Puerto-Rican style stuffed pot roast (with gravy) [1 medium]	137	4.8	102	11%	3	20	1.8
2711	Potato only from Puerto Rican mixed dishes, gravy and other components reported separately [1 medium]	127	4.5	109	1%	2	25	2.3

Food no.	fat gm	sat fat gm	choles mg	sodium mg	potas mg	% of Daily Value													
						vit A	vit E	vit C	thia	ribo	niac	vit B-6	fola	vit B-12	calc	phos	mag	iron	zinc
2677	35	17	306	1874	1034	33	10	84	45	30	22	32	11	12	17	31	17	9	10
2678	33	17	229	910	463	29	11	26	14	26	6	5	9	14	41	38	11	7	14
2679	2	1	0	449	590	5	31	23	12	5	12	25	5	0	6	10	10	3	4
2680	1	1	4	57	354	2	0	36	19	6	8	11	3	2	7	9	6	2	3
2681	9	2	4	136	288	10	6	29	15	5	6	9	2	2	6	7	5	2	2
2682	24	6	148	467	489	9	14	15	13	16	11	19	7	5	6	14	8	8	6
2683	14	7	0	955	486	0	0	15	17	5	14	15	5	0	4	6	6	11	3
2684	0	0	0	7	662	0	0	40	7	3	9	16	4	0	1	6	6	5	3
2685	0	0	0	10	905	0	0	44	8	3	12	21	5	0	1	8	9	7	4
2686	7	2	8	115	953	10	4	39	10	13	12	19	5	2	12	16	11	8	6
2687	8	3	23	490	960	9	4	36	22	16	18	24	4	5	12	21	12	9	11
2688	20	5	9	12	979	0	11	40	8	4	13	24	5	0	2	10	10	8	5
2689	5	2	8	223	546	1	1	27	12	3	11	22	4	1	2	8	8	3	4
2690	10	1	0	14	672	4	11	42	7	4	9	15	5	0	2	7	8	6	3
2691	11	3	5	15	718	4	7	45	7	4	9	17	5	0	2	7	8	6	3
2692	2	1	0	15	74	0	1	5	0	0	1	1	1	0	0	1	1	1	0
2693	4	2	27	671	722	14	4	46	29	17	17	28	9	10	20	28	13	12	14
2694	15	7	26	545	1046	11	4	48	20	14	21	41	7	8	20	29	18	19	12
2695	9	3	9	178	1078	13	7	97	18	10	20	42	12	1	11	20	18	19	8
2696	12	6	20	430	1000	11	4	47	16	12	18	40	7	6	20	27	17	18	11
2697	10	3	55	200	1091	12	7	86	19	13	52	54	11	4	11	30	20	20	11
2698	10	3	14	510	1396	8	7	59	21	10	23	51	12	0	7	28	27	36	17
2699	11	3	21	233	997	6	6	45	18	10	23	39	7	11	5	20	16	21	13
2700	17	9	27	98	999	16	5	48	17	10	18	38	8	3	10	18	16	17	6
2701	15	7	26	540	794	11	4	37	16	12	15	29	5	8	19	25	14	5	11
2702	9	3	9	169	826	13	7	87	14	8	14	29	9	1	10	16	14	6	6
2703	12	6	20	424	753	11	4	36	12	10	12	28	4	6	19	23	13	5	9
2704	11	4	60	210	943	13	8	83	17	12	50	46	10	5	10	29	18	9	11
2705	10	3	14	507	1110	8	7	46	17	8	16	36	9	0	5	23	22	20	15
2706	11	3	21	222	752	6	6	34	14	8	17	27	5	11	3	16	12	8	11
2707	17	9	28	90	751	16	5	37	13	8	12	26	6	3	8	14	12	4	4
2708	1	1	2	327	383	0	0	13	8	2	9	14	3	1	1	6	5	4	6
2709	3	1	1	347	405	7	1	13	7	3	8	14	3	1	2	6	5	3	5
2710	1	1	1	280	328	0	0	11	7	2	7	12	2	1	1	5	5	3	5
2711	0	0	0	6	417	0	0	16	8	1	8	17	3	0	1	5	6	2	2

Fruits & Vegetables

Food No.	Food Description & Amount	wt gm	wt oz	cal	% cal fat	prot gm	carbo gm	fiber gm
2712	Potato pancake [2 pancakes (2¾" dia, 1/8" thick)]	44	1.6	85	48%	2	9	0.8
2713	Potato pudding [1 cup]	228	8.0	282	57%	8	25	2.4
2714	Potato puffs, cheese-filled [1 cup]	70	2.5	334	63%	6	27	1.8
2715	Potato salad [1 cup]	193	6.8	277	50%	3	34	3.1
2716	Potato skins, chips (Include Tato Skins baked potato, sour cream n' chives, and cheese n' bacon flavor) [10 chips]	20	0.7	112	62%	1	10	0.7
2717	Potato skins, with adhering flesh, baked [Skin from 1 med (2½" dia, raw)]	29	1.0	43	1%	1	10	1.4
2718	Potato skins, with adhering flesh, fried [Skin from 1 small (2" dia, raw)]	26	0.9	107	27%	2	18	2.6
2719	Potato skins, with adhering flesh, fried, with cheese and bacon [Skin from 1 small (2" raw dia)]	35	1.2	137	44%	4	15	2.1
2720	Potato skins, with adhering flesh, fried, with cheese [Skin from 1 small (2" dia, raw)]	21	0.7	85	37%	2	12	1.6
2721	Puerto Rican pasteles (Pasteles de masa) [1 pastel (5½" x 2¼" x ¼")]	149	5.3	312	55%	11	26	4.1
2722	Pumpkin fritters, Puerto Rican style [2 fritters (2" dia)]	70	2.5	170	34%	2	28	0.6
2723	Pumpkin, cooked, from canned [1 cup]	245	8.6	83	7%	3	20	7.1
2724	Pumpkin, cooked, from fresh or frozen [1 cup]	245	8.6	49	3%	2	12	2.7
2725	Radicchio, raw [1 cup, shredded]	40	1.4	9	10%	1	2	0.4
2726	Radish, Japanese (daikon), cooked [1 cup]	147	5.2	28	5%	1	6	2.5
2727	Radish, raw [4 small]	8	0.3	1	29%	0	0	0.1
2728	Ratatouille [1 cup]	214	7.5	152	72%	2	11	3.2
2729	Rutabaga, cooked [1 cup, pieces]	170	6.0	66	5%	2	15	3.1
2730	Rutabaga, raw [1 small]	192	6.8	69	5%	2	16	4.8
2731	Salsify (vegetable oyster), cooked [1 cup]	135	4.8	92	2%	4	21	4.2
2732	Sauerkraut, canned, low sodium [1 cup]	142	5.0	27	5%	1	6	3.6
2733	Sauerkraut, cooked [1 cup]	142	5.0	27	7%	1	6	3.6
2734	Seaweed, dried (Include sea moss, kelp) [½ cup]	8	0.3	22	12%	2	4	0.4
2735	Seaweed, prepared with soy sauce [1 cup]	96	3.4	41	9%	4	8	0.7
2736	Seaweed, raw (Include blanched) [1 cup]	80	2.8	31	6%	2	7	0.7
2737	Sequin (Portuguese squash), cooked [1 cup]	180	6.3	36	14%	2	8	2.5
2738	Seven-layer salad (lettuce salad made with a combination of onion, celery, green pepper, peas, mayonnaise, cheese, eggs, and/or bacon) [1 cup]	119	4.2	197	65%	5	13	1.6
2739	Snow peas, raw [1 cup]	145	5.1	61	4%	4	11	3.8
2740	Snowpea (pea pod), cooked, from fresh [1 cup]	160	5.6	67	5%	5	11	4.5
2741	Snowpea (pea pod), cooked, from frozen [1 cup]	160	5.6	83	7%	6	14	5.0
2742	Spinach and cheese casserole (Include spinach casserole) [1 cup]	200	7.1	271	48%	15	21	3.0
2743	Spinach and chickpeas, fat added [1 cup]	245	8.6	195	44%	10	21	8.5
2744	Spinach salad, no dressing [1 cup]	74	2.6	108	40%	5	11	1.6
2745	Spinach souffle [1 cup]	100	3.5	125	60%	5	7	0.9
2746	Spinach, raw [1 cup]	30	1.1	7	14%	1	1	0.8
2747	Spinach, cooked, from canned [1 cup, canned]	214	7.5	49	20%	6	7	5.1
2748	Spinach, cooked, from fresh [1 cup, fresh]	180	6.3	41	10%	5	7	4.3
2749	Spinach, cooked, from frozen [1 cup, frozen, chopped]	205	7.2	57	7%	6	11	6.2
2750	Spinach, cooked, from frozen [1 cup, frozen, leaf]	190	6.7	53	7%	6	10	5.7
2751	Spinach, cooked, from canned, with cheese sauce [1 cup]	200	7.1	157	59%	9	10	3.4
2752	Spinach, cooked, from fresh, with cheese sauce [1 cup]	200	7.1	170	58%	9	10	3.2
2753	Spinach, cooked, from frozen, with cheese sauce [1 cup]	200	7.1	172	55%	9	12	4.0
2754	Spinach, from canned, creamed [1 cup]	200	7.1	137	55%	6	11	3.2
2755	Spinach, from fresh, creamed [1 cup]	200	7.1	148	55%	7	12	3.0
2756	Spinach, from frozen, creamed [1 cup]	200	7.1	150	52%	7	14	3.8
2757	Sprouts (1:1 mix of alfalfa and mung sprouts) [1 cup]	56	2.0	16	15%	2	3	1.2
2758	Squash fritter or cake [2 fritters]	48	1.7	163	54%	3	16	1.2
2759	Squash, spaghetti, cooked [1 cup]	155	5.5	45	8%	1	10	2.2
2760	Squash, summer, and onions, cooked [1 cup]	185	6.5	53	8%	2	12	2.6
2761	Squash, summer, casserole, with tomato and cheese [1 cup]	217	7.7	148	65%	6	9	2.5

Food no.	fat gm	sat fat gm	choles mg	sodium mg	potas mg	vit A	vit E	vit C	thia	ribo	niac	vit B-6	fola	vit B-12	calc	phos	mag	iron	zinc
						% of Daily Value													
2712	4	1	31	12	250	1	3	12	3	3	4	6	2	1	1	4	3	3	2
2713	18	7	151	511	499	20	6	15	10	18	7	17	6	9	12	17	8	4	6
2714	23	7	12	604	545	4	12	7	7	9	8	5	1	1	13	23	9	4	6
2715	15	2	11	211	599	3	11	40	11	2	11	28	5	1	2	8	9	4	4
2716	8	2	0	131	202	0	4	3	3	1	3	1	0	0	0	3	3	2	1
2717	0	0	0	4	141	0	0	6	2	1	3	7	1	0	1	2	3	6	1
2718	3	1	0	7	258	0	2	9	3	2	6	12	2	0	1	4	5	11	1
2719	7	3	10	128	241	2	2	9	6	4	7	11	2	2	5	8	4	10	3
2720	3	1	5	31	168	1	2	6	2	2	4	8	1	0	4	5	3	7	2
2721	19	7	37	234	593	5	6	29	17	9	11	18	12	4	5	16	11	8	8
2722	6	2	6	1	199	8	3	6	6	6	4	2	2	0	1	4	2	5	2
2723	1	0	0	383	503	538	12	16	4	8	4	7	7	0	6	9	14	19	3
2724	0	0	0	2	564	26	12	19	5	11	5	5	5	0	4	7	6	8	4
2725	0	0	0	9	121	0	4	5	0	1	1	1	6	0	1	2	1	1	2
2726	0	0	0	31	319	0	0	40	2	2	1	3	8	0	4	3	6	3	1
2727	0	0	0	2	19	0	0	3	0	0	0	0	1	0	0	0	0	0	0
2728	12	2	0	79	474	6	8	32	7	4	5	10	7	0	4	6	8	5	2
2729	0	0	0	34	554	10	1	53	9	4	6	9	6	0	8	10	10	5	4
2730	0	0	0	38	647	11	3	80	12	5	7	10	10	0	9	11	11	6	4
2731	0	0	0	22	382	0	1	10	5	14	3	15	5	0	6	8	6	4	3
2732	0	0	0	437	241	0	1	35	2	2	1	6	9	0	4	3	5	12	2
2733	0	0	0	939	241	0	1	31	2	2	1	9	8	0	4	3	5	12	2
2734	0	0	0	43	93	0	2	1	6	9	2	1	6	0	3	1	9	10	2
2735	0	0	0	1061	147	15	4	12	4	14	7	3	24	0	10	6	16	11	5
2736	0	0	0	71	147	11	3	15	2	13	3	3	30	0	7	5	17	17	6
2737	1	0	0	2	346	5	1	17	5	4	5	6	9	0	5	7	11	4	5
2738	14	4	55	330	155	9	7	16	7	7	3	5	10	4	7	9	3	4	5
2739	0	0	0	6	290	2	3	145	15	7	4	12	15	0	6	8	9	17	3
2740	0	0	0	6	384	2	3	128	14	7	4	12	12	0	7	9	10	18	4
2741	1	0	0	8	347	3	2	59	7	11	5	14	14	0	9	9	11	21	5
2742	15	6	185	1032	442	67	7	20	12	30	7	10	21	8	30	26	16	18	12
2743	10	5	20	458	1034	164	10	32	15	29	6	27	81	0	28	18	47	44	14
2744	5	1	77	227	242	18	4	11	8	17	8	5	15	4	5	8	7	8	4
2745	8	2	98	128	174	30	6	6	5	14	2	4	10	6	10	10	6	5	4
2746	0	0	0	24	167	20	3	14	2	3	1	3	15	0	3	1	6	5	1
2747	1	0	0	58	740	188	13	48	2	17	4	11	50	0	27	9	41	27	7
2748	0	0	0	126	839	147	8	29	11	25	4	22	66	0	24	10	39	36	9
2749	0	0	0	176	611	159	9	42	8	20	4	15	55	0	30	10	35	17	10
2750	0	0	0	163	566	148	8	39	8	19	4	14	51	0	28	9	33	16	9
2751	10	4	16	297	562	125	11	31	4	19	4	8	33	3	32	17	28	19	8
2752	11	5	18	381	700	112	9	22	11	27	4	17	48	4	34	20	31	27	11
2753	11	4	18	394	489	108	9	27	8	22	4	11	36	4	35	18	25	13	10
2754	8	2	5	295	552	115	12	30	5	18	4	8	30	3	25	13	27	17	6
2755	9	2	6	373	678	101	10	20	11	25	5	16	44	4	26	15	29	25	8
2756	9	2	6	385	483	98	10	26	9	21	4	10	33	4	27	14	24	12	8
2757	0	0	0	3	61	1	0	10	3	4	2	2	6	0	1	4	3	3	3
2758	10	2	30	80	162	10	6	3	8	8	6	2	3	1	6	6	2	6	2
2759	0	0	0	28	181	2	1	9	4	2	6	8	3	0	3	2	4	3	2
2760	0	0	0	3	337	3	1	17	5	4	4	8	8	0	5	7	9	3	4
2761	11	4	13	417	560	19	6	33	8	9	5	10	7	2	16	15	11	6	6

Fruits & Vegetables

Food No.	Food Description & Amount	wt gm	wt oz	cal	% cal fat	prot gm	carbo gm	fiber gm
2762	Squash, summer, casserole, with cheese sauce [1 cup]	217	7.7	191	48%	7	19	2.4
2763	Squash, summer, casserole, with rice and tomato sauce [1 cup]	233	8.2	107	5%	3	24	2.8
2764	Squash, summer, cooked, from canned [1 cup, diced]	210	7.4	27	5%	1	6	2.9
2765	Squash, summer, cooked, from fresh [1 cup, diced]	210	7.4	42	14%	2	9	2.9
2766	Squash, summer, cooked, from frozen [1 cup, diced]	210	7.4	43	7%	3	9	2.8
2767	Squash, summer, creamed [1 cup]	217	7.7	156	57%	5	14	2.0
2768	Squash, summer, from canned, creamed [1 cup]	217	7.7	135	57%	4	11	2.1
2769	Squash, summer, from fresh, creamed [1 cup]	217	7.7	156	57%	5	14	2.0
2770	Squash, summer, from frozen, creamed [1 cup]	217	7.7	148	54%	5	14	2.0
2771	Squash, summer, souffle [1 cup]	136	4.8	169	64%	6	10	1.1
2772	Squash, summer, yellow or green, breaded or battered, fried (Include zucchini pancakes) [1 cup]	220	7.8	366	68%	4	26	2.6
2773	Squash, summer, yellow, raw [1 cup, sliced]	113	4.0	23	9%	1	5	2.1
2774	Squash, winter type, baked, fat and sugar added (Include acorn, butternut, hubbard) [1 cup, cubes]	214	7.5	158	28%	2	30	5.5
2775	Squash, winter type, baked (Include acorn, butternut, hubbard) [1 cup, cubes]	205	7.2	80	15%	2	18	5.7
2776	Squash, winter type, mashed (Include acorn, butternut, hubbard) [1 cup]	240	8.5	94	15%	2	21	6.7
2777	Squash, winter type, mashed, fat added (Include acorn, butternut, hubbard) [1 cup]	245	8.6	133	40%	2	21	6.7
2778	Squash, winter type, mashed, fat and sugar added (Include acorn, butternut, hubbard) [1 cup]	257	9.1	190	28%	2	36	6.6
2779	Squash, winter type, raw (Include pumpkin, acorn, butternut, hubbard) [1 cup cubes]	140	4.9	52	6%	2	12	2.1
2780	Squash, winter, baked with cheese [1 cup]	224	7.9	331	56%	7	32	5.4
2781	Squash, winter, souffle [1 cup]	157	5.5	127	27%	5	19	3.4
2782	Squash, summer, yellow or green, breaded or battered, baked [1 cup]	220	7.8	156	12%	5	30	3.0
2783	Starchy vegetables, Puerto Rican style, including green or ripe plantains, tannier, yam, white sweet potato (viandas) [1 cup]	195	6.9	239	2%	3	58	5.9
2784	Starchy vegetables, Puerto Rican style, including yam, white sweet potato, tannier, no plantain (viandas) [1 cup]	190	6.7	237	2%	4	56	6.1
2785	String beans, green, and potatoes, cooked, with onion, pork fat, salt [1 cup]	143	5.0	110	23%	2	20	3.3
2786	String beans, green, and potatoes, cooked, with salt [1 cup]	138	4.9	82	3%	2	19	3.6
2787	String beans, green, raw [1 cup]	110	3.9	34	3%	2	8	3.7
2788	String beans, green, cooked, from canned [1 cup, canned]	135	4.8	27	5%	2	6	2.6
2789	String beans, green, canned, low sodium (Include pole beans; Italian beans; snap beans; french cut beans) [1 cup]	135	4.8	27	5%	2	6	2.6
2790	String beans, green, cooked, from fresh [1 cup, fresh]	125	4.4	44	7%	2	10	4.0
2791	String beans, green, cooked, from frozen [1 cup, frozen]	135	4.8	38	5%	2	9	4.1
2792	String beans, green, from canned, creamed or with cheese sauce [1 cup]	228	8.0	235	62%	11	12	2.7
2793	String beans, green, from fresh, creamed or with cheese sauce [1 cup]	228	8.0	264	59%	12	17	4.4
2794	String beans, green, from frozen, creamed or with cheese sauce [1 cup]	228	8.0	246	60%	12	15	4.2
2795	String beans, green, cooked, from canned, with mushroom sauce [1 cup]	228	8.0	135	54%	4	13	2.3
2796	String beans, green, cooked, from fresh, with mushroom sauce [1 cup]	228	8.0	153	50%	4	17	3.5
2797	String beans, green, cooked, from frozen, with mushroom sauce [1 cup]	228	8.0	143	51%	4	15	3.5
2798	String beans, green, with almonds, cooked [1 cup]	122	4.3	194	68%	7	13	4.9
2799	String beans, green, with chickpeas, cooked [1 cup]	134	4.7	87	12%	5	16	5.8
2800	String beans, green, with mushroom sauce (Include green bean casserole) [1 cup]	228	8.0	143	51%	4	15	3.5
2801	String beans, green, with onions, cooked, with margarine [1 cup]	151	5.3	88	39%	2	13	3.5
2802	String beans, green, with onions, cooked [1 cup]	146	5.1	46	5%	2	10	3.9
2803	String beans, green, with pinto beans, cooked, with salt (Include with Shellie beans) [1 cup]	136	4.8	41	6%	2	8	4.6
2804	String beans, green, with spaetzel, cooked [1 cup]	147	5.2	80	9%	4	17	4.1
2805	String beans, green, with tomatoes or tomato-based sauce, cooked, with salt [1 cup]	148	5.2	49	7%	2	11	3.8

Food no.	fat gm	sat fat gm	choles mg	sodium mg	potas mg	% of Daily Value													
						vit A	vit E	vit C	thia	ribo	niac	vit B-6	fola	vit B-12	calc	phos	mag	iron	zinc
2762	10	4	15	343	391	10	5	14	12	14	8	7	9	4	20	18	12	8	8
2763	1	0	0	638	506	11	6	26	12	6	11	12	8	0	4	9	12	9	6
2764	0	0	0	11	202	3	1	9	2	3	4	4	5	0	3	4	7	8	4
2765	1	0	0	2	403	6	1	19	6	5	5	7	11	0	6	8	13	4	5
2766	0	0	0	8	465	7	3	18	5	5	4	7	5	0	4	7	10	6	4
2767	10	3	6	316	385	9	6	13	8	13	5	6	8	4	14	14	11	4	6
2768	9	2	6	288	256	6	6	7	5	11	4	4	4	4	11	11	7	7	5
2769	10	3	6	316	385	9	6	13	8	13	5	6	8	4	14	14	11	4	6
2770	9	2	6	294	427	9	7	13	7	12	4	6	4	4	12	12	9	5	5
2771	12	3	118	152	235	17	7	5	6	15	3	5	6	5	9	12	6	5	5
2772	28	4	5	265	392	6	25	16	18	17	13	7	7	1	5	24	10	13	4
2773	0	0	0	2	220	2	1	28	5	2	3	6	7	0	2	4	6	3	2
2774	5	1	0	50	905	73	4	31	11	3	7	7	14	0	4	4	5	5	4
2775	1	0	0	2	896	73	1	33	12	3	7	7	14	0	3	4	4	4	4
2776	2	0	0	2	1049	85	1	38	14	3	8	9	17	0	3	5	5	4	4
2777	6	1	0	54	1049	90	4	38	14	3	8	9	17	0	4	5	5	4	4
2778	6	1	0	60	1087	88	4	38	14	3	8	9	17	0	5	5	6	6	4
2779	0	0	0	6	490	57	1	29	9	2	6	6	8	0	4	4	7	5	1
2780	20	6	12	437	820	79	12	28	19	11	13	8	13	1	17	13	7	11	7
2781	4	1	119	43	564	47	2	18	10	12	5	6	11	4	5	9	4	6	5
2782	2	0	5	300	444	7	3	19	21	19	15	8	9	2	6	27	11	15	5
2783	0	0	0	17	1192	4	2	59	16	6	8	27	10	0	7	11	19	17	3
2784	0	0	0	19	1252	0	2	65	18	6	8	27	8	0	9	12	20	20	3
2785	3	1	2	175	419	3	1	19	8	4	6	12	7	0	3	5	7	5	3
2786	0	0	0	163	432	5	1	20	8	5	7	11	7	0	4	5	8	6	3
2787	0	0	0	7	230	7	2	30	6	7	4	4	10	0	4	4	7	6	2
2788	0	0	0	354	147	5	1	10	1	4	1	2	10	0	4	3	4	7	3
2789	0	0	0	3	147	5	1	11	1	4	1	2	11	0	4	3	4	7	3
2790	0	0	0	4	374	8	1	20	6	7	4	4	10	0	6	5	8	9	3
2791	0	0	0	12	170	5	1	9	3	7	3	4	8	0	7	4	8	7	4
2792	16	8	34	758	275	17	5	11	5	18	3	5	12	5	32	23	9	9	10
2793	17	8	36	423	527	22	5	22	10	21	6	6	13	5	35	27	13	12	11
2794	16	8	34	413	298	18	5	10	7	20	4	6	10	5	35	25	12	9	12
2795	8	2	3	969	218	5	5	9	3	10	4	3	9	2	8	8	5	8	6
2796	9	2	3	720	410	8	6	18	7	12	7	4	9	3	10	10	8	10	6
2797	8	2	3	702	236	5	5	9	4	12	5	4	7	2	11	9	8	8	7
2798	15	1	0	6	488	6	26	16	7	16	7	4	10	0	11	18	26	12	8
2799	1	0	0	13	226	4	1	7	4	7	3	5	13	0	6	8	10	9	7
2800	8	2	3	702	236	5	5	9	4	12	5	4	7	2	11	9	8	8	7
2801	4	1	0	45	350	9	3	19	6	6	3	7	9	0	5	6	7	7	3
2802	0	0	0	11	196	5	1	11	4	7	2	5	8	0	6	5	8	6	4
2803	0	0	0	454	148	3	0	7	3	4	1	3	6	0	4	4	5	7	2
2804	1	0	10	6	360	8	1	19	9	8	6	4	10	0	6	7	9	11	4
2805	0	0	0	324	481	12	4	27	7	7	6	7	9	0	5	5	8	9	3

Fruits & Vegetables

Food No.	Food Description & Amount	wt gm	wt oz	cal	% cal fat	prot gm	carbo gm	fiber gm
2806	String beans, yellow, cooked, from canned [1 cup]	135	4.8	27	5%	2	6	1.8
2807	String beans, yellow, cooked, from fresh [1 cup]	125	4.4	44	7%	2	10	4.1
2808	String beans, yellow, cooked, from frozen [1 cup]	135	4.8	38	5%	2	9	4.5
2809	String beans, yellow, from canned, creamed or with cheese sauce [1 cup]	228	8.0	235	62%	11	12	1.9
2810	String beans, yellow, from fresh, creamed or with cheese sauce [1 cup]	228	8.0	264	59%	12	17	4.5
2811	String beans, yellow, from frozen, creamed or with cheese sauce [1 cup]	228	8.0	246	60%	12	15	4.6
2812	Sweetpotato and pumpkin casserole, Puerto Rican style [1 cup]	266	9.4	631	27%	8	112	5.9
2813	Sweetpotato leaves, squash leaves, pumpkin leaves, chrysanthemum leaves, bean leaves, or swamp cabbage, cooked [1 cup leaves]	64	2.3	15	8%	1	3	1.4
2814	Sweetpotato, baked, peel eaten [1 small]	77	2.7	95	1%	2	22	3.1
2815	Sweetpotato, baked, peel not eaten [1 small]	60	2.1	62	1%	1	15	1.8
2816	Sweetpotato, boiled, with peel [1 small]	78	2.8	82	3%	1	19	1.4
2817	Sweetpotato, boiled, without peel [1 small]	76	2.7	80	3%	1	18	1.4
2818	Sweetpotato, candied [1 piece (½ medium potato)]	104	3.7	156	22%	1	30	2.6
2819	Sweetpotato, canned in syrup [1 cup, pieces]	196	6.9	174	2%	2	41	4.9
2820	Sweetpotato, canned without syrup [1 cup, pieces]	200	7.1	182	2%	3	42	3.6
2821	Sweetpotato, canned [1 cup, pieces]	196	6.9	174	2%	2	41	4.9
2822	Sweetpotato, casserole or mashed (Include sweetpotato pudding) [1 cup]	247	8.7	276	21%	5	51	3.6
2823	Sweetpotato, fried [1 cup]	205	7.2	417	39%	4	61	4.5
2824	Sweetpotato with fruit [1 cup]	254	9.0	288	2%	2	72	3.4
2825	Sweetpotato, Puerto Rican, yellow, cooked [1 cup]	140	4.9	147	3%	2	34	2.5
2826	Sweetpotato, Puerto Rican, boiled [1 cup, diced]	140	4.9	147	3%	2	34	2.5
2827	Sweetpotato, Puerto Rican, fried [1 small]	227	8.0	792	32%	7	129	19.0
2828	Sweetpotato, Puerto Rican, roasted or baked [1 cup]	200	7.1	255	23%	3	47	5.8
2829	Tannier, cooked (Include yautia) [1 cup]	190	6.7	280	2%	4	69	10.7
2830	Tannier fritters, Puerto Rican style (Frituras de yautia) [2 fritters (2½"x1½"x ½")]	40	1.4	93	44%	3	11	1.6
2831	Tannier fritters, stuffed, Puerto Rican style (Alcapurrias) [2 small (4"x1"x ½")]	48	1.7	188	69%	6	10	1.2
2832	Taro chips [10 chips]	23	0.8	115	45%	1	16	1.7
2833	Taro leaves, cooked [1 cup]	145	5.1	75	16%	9	12	6.6
2834	Taro, baked [1 cup]	132	4.7	184	2%	3	45	7.0
2835	Thistle leaves, cooked [1 cup]	180	6.3	41	23%	3	7	1.3
2836	Tomato and celery, cooked [1 cup]	244	8.6	46	6%	2	11	2.7
2837	Tomato and corn, cooked [1 cup]	242	8.5	107	10%	4	25	3.4
2838	Tomato and lima beans, cooked [1 cup]	242	8.5	150	3%	8	30	6.7
2839	Tomato and okra, cooked [1 cup]	217	7.7	53	5%	3	12	3.5
2840	Tomato and onion, cooked [1 cup]	237	8.4	73	11%	3	16	2.6
2841	Tomato and onion, cooked, fat added [1 cup]	242	8.5	108	40%	3	16	2.6
2842	Tomato aspic [1 cup]	227	8.0	64	2%	6	12	0.8
2843	Tomato paste [1 cup]	262	9.2	215	6%	10	51	10.7
2844	Tomato puree [1 cup]	250	8.8	100	4%	4	24	5.0
2845	Tomato with corn and okra, cooked [1 cup]	212	7.5	86	9%	4	20	3.6
2846	Tomato, green, pickled [1 tomato (2-3/8" dia)]	74	2.6	27	6%	1	6	0.9
2847	Tomatoes, broiled [1 cup]	240	8.5	63	14%	3	14	3.3
2848	Tomatoes, canned, low sodium [1 cup]	240	8.5	46	6%	2	10	2.4
2849	Tomatoes, from canned, stewed [1 cup]	255	9.0	71	4%	2	17	2.6
2850	Tomatoes, from fresh, broiled [1 medium]	105	3.7	28	14%	1	6	1.4
2851	Tomatoes, from fresh, scalloped [1 cup]	235	8.3	248	51%	4	28	2.8
2852	Tomatoes, from fresh, stewed [1 cup]	255	9.0	185	32%	5	29	3.0
2853	Tomatoes, green, fried [1 cup]	180	6.3	356	68%	6	24	1.8
2854	Tomatoes, green, raw [1 small]	91	3.2	22	8%	1	5	1.0
2855	Tomatoes, red, dried [1 cup]	54	1.9	139	10%	8	30	6.6
2856	Tomatoes red, raw (Include plum and Italian tomatoes) [1 small (2-2/5" dia)]	91	3.2	19	14%	1	4	1.0
2857	Tomatoes, red, fried [1 cup]	180	6.3	300	68%	5	21	1.9
2858	Tomatoes, red, from fresh, fried [1 medium]	101	3.6	169	68%	3	12	1.1

Food no.	fat gm	sat fat gm	choles mg	sodium mg	potas mg	% of Daily Value													
						vit A	vit E	vit C	thia	ribo	niac	vit B-6	fola	vit B-12	calc	phos	mag	iron	zinc
2806	0	0	0	339	147	1	2	10	1	4	1	2	10	0	4	3	4	7	3
2807	0	0	0	4	374	1	2	20	6	7	4	4	10	0	6	5	8	9	3
2808	0	0	0	12	170	1	1	9	3	7	3	4	8	0	7	4	8	7	4
2809	16	8	34	743	275	14	6	11	5	18	3	5	12	5	32	23	9	9	10
2810	17	8	36	423	527	14	6	22	10	21	6	6	13	5	35	27	13	12	11
2811	16	8	34	413	298	14	5	10	7	20	4	6	10	5	35	25	12	9	12
2812	19	10	100	138	832	274	16	57	12	29	11	24	11	3	8	18	12	17	9
2813	0	0	0	36	281	24	3	13	2	6	2	4	6	0	3	3	5	8	1
2814	0	0	0	10	306	131	1	28	4	6	4	12	4	0	2	5	5	8	2
2815	0	0	0	6	209	131	1	25	3	4	2	7	3	0	2	3	3	2	1
2816	0	0	0	10	144	133	1	22	3	6	2	10	2	0	2	2	2	2	1
2817	0	0	0	10	140	130	1	22	3	6	2	9	2	0	2	2	2	2	1
2818	4	1	0	90	222	62	3	17	2	3	2	3	2	0	3	3	4	6	1
2819	0	0	0	86	363	112	2	34	3	5	4	5	3	0	3	5	6	9	2
2820	0	0	0	106	624	160	2	88	5	7	7	19	8	0	4	10	11	10	2
2821	0	0	0	86	363	112	2	34	3	5	4	5	3	0	3	5	6	9	2
2822	6	2	3	105	434	348	6	58	8	20	7	25	6	3	9	9	6	6	5
2823	18	4	0	33	460	426	13	71	9	21	8	31	7	0	5	7	6	8	4
2824	0	0	0	74	279	186	2	31	4	10	4	15	3	0	4	4	4	6	3
2825	0	0	0	18	258	239	2	40	5	12	4	17	4	0	3	4	4	4	3
2826	0	0	0	18	258	239	2	40	5	12	4	17	4	0	3	4	4	4	3
2827	29	6	0	42	3780	0	20	106	28	8	12	64	20	0	8	25	24	14	7
2828	7	1	0	94	672	425	7	79	9	14	6	23	11	0	6	11	10	5	4
2829	1	0	0	27	1390	0	28	13	13	3	7	33	9	0	11	20	20	8	4
2830	5	1	30	92	242	2	7	2	2	3	1	6	2	1	8	8	4	2	2
2831	14	3	19	188	277	2	11	7	7	4	6	8	2	4	1	7	4	3	5
2832	6	1	0	79	174	0	5	2	3	0	1	5	1	0	1	3	5	2	1
2833	1	0	0	5	1044	82	16	93	21	46	12	12	37	0	18	10	19	21	5
2834	0	0	0	19	1014	0	19	10	10	2	5	23	8	0	7	14	14	5	3
2835	1	0	0	14	635	139	6	69	7	17	7	14	17	0	11	9	12	8	2
2836	0	0	0	337	566	13	4	52	7	5	8	11	6	0	8	5	7	7	3
2837	1	0	0	423	509	10	3	48	6	7	11	9	15	0	5	9	9	9	4
2838	1	0	0	227	885	12	3	50	14	8	10	16	9	0	7	16	23	18	7
2839	0	0	0	197	567	13	5	54	12	5	9	14	12	0	9	7	16	6	5
2840	1	0	0	22	601	14	3	74	10	7	7	12	8	0	2	8	8	6	2
2841	5	1	0	22	602	17	6	74	10	7	7	12	8	0	2	8	8	6	2
2842	0	0	0	644	414	10	7	70	6	4	6	10	10	0	2	4	5	6	2
2843	1	0	0	231	2455	64	51	185	27	29	42	50	15	0	9	21	33	28	14
2844	0	0	0	85	1065	32	29	43	12	8	21	19	7	0	4	10	15	17	4
2845	1	0	0	268	513	10	4	46	9	6	10	11	16	0	7	9	14	7	5
2846	0	0	0	92	133	6	1	35	2	1	1	3	1	0	1	2	2	2	0
2847	1	0	0	27	666	17	5	91	11	8	9	11	8	0	2	7	8	8	2
2848	0	0	0	24	545	14	4	57	7	4	9	11	5	0	7	5	7	7	3
2849	0	0	0	564	607	14	4	48	8	5	9	2	3	0	8	5	8	10	3
2850	0	0	0	12	291	7	2	40	5	4	4	5	3	0	1	3	4	3	1
2851	14	3	0	300	641	27	12	78	16	12	12	11	6	0	4	9	9	11	3
2852	7	1	0	219	757	22	8	91	18	12	14	12	7	0	5	10	11	13	3
2853	27	6	51	167	317	10	17	43	14	14	8	6	4	3	13	13	5	10	3
2854	0	0	0	12	186	6	2	35	4	2	2	4	2	0	1	3	2	3	0
2855	2	0	0	1131	1851	5	0	35	19	16	24	9	9	0	6	19	26	27	7
2856	0	0	0	8	202	6	2	29	4	3	3	4	3	0	0	2	3	2	1
2857	23	5	42	138	356	10	15	40	13	13	9	6	5	2	10	11	6	9	3
2858	13	3	24	78	200	6	8	22	7	7	5	4	3	1	6	6	3	5	2

Fruits & Vegetables

Food No.	Food Description & Amount	wt gm	wt oz	cal	% cal fat	prot gm	carbo gm	fiber gm
2859	Tomatoes, scalloped [1 cup]	235	8.3	231	53%	4	25	2.8
2860	Tomatoes, stewed [1 cup]	255	9.0	71	4%	2	17	2.6
2861	Turnip, cooked, from fresh [1 cup, pieces]	155	5.5	28	4%	1	8	3.1
2862	Turnip, cooked, from frozen [1 cup, pieces]	155	5.5	36	9%	2	7	3.1
2863	Turnip, raw [1 cup]	130	4.6	35	3%	1	8	2.3
2864	Turnip, creamed [1 cup]	226	8.0	170	57%	5	15	2.7
2865	Turnip greens with roots, cooked, from canned [1 cup]	163	5.7	31	7%	1	8	4.4
2866	Turnip greens with roots, cooked, from fresh [1 cup]	163	5.7	31	7%	1	8	4.4
2867	Turnip greens with roots, cooked, from frozen [1 cup]	163	5.7	28	8%	3	5	2.9
2868	Turnip greens, cooked, from canned [1 cup, canned]	159	5.6	32	10%	2	7	5.5
2869	Turnip greens, cooked, from canned, low sodium [1 cup]	159	5.6	22	19%	2	4	2.1
2870	Turnip greens, cooked, from fresh [1 cup, fresh]	144	5.1	29	10%	2	6	5.0
2871	Turnip greens, cooked, from frozen [1 cup, frozen]	165	5.8	50	13%	6	8	5.6
2872	Vegetable combinations (including carrots, broccoli, and/or dark-green leafy), cooked, with butter sauce [1 cup]	196	6.9	176	52%	4	19	4.1
2873	Vegetable combinations (including carrots, broccoli, and/or dark-green leafy), cooked, with cheese sauce [1 cup]	228	8.0	142	19%	8	24	6.7
2874	Vegetable combination (including carrots, broccoli, and/or dark-green leafy), cooked, with cream sauce [1 cup]	228	8.0	197	53%	7	18	4.3
2875	Vegetable combinations (including carrots, broccoli, and/or dark-green leafy), cooked, with pasta [1 cup]	137	4.8	107	5%	5	22	3.8
2876	Vegetable combinations (including carrots, broccoli, and/or dark-green leafy), cooked, with sauce and pasta (Include Birdseye New England Style Mixed Vegetables) [1 cup]	197	6.9	203	34%	6	29	4.9
2877	Vegetable combination (including carrots, broccoli, and/or dark-green leafy), cooked, with soy-based sauce (Include stir-fry vegetables) [1 cup]	185	6.5	85	5%	5	18	4.3
2878	Vegetable combination (broccoli, carrots, corn, cauliflower, etc.), cooked [1 cup]	141	5.0	56	4%	3	12	4.2
2879	Vegetable combinations (no carrots, broccoli, or dark-green leafy), cooked, with cheese sauce [1 cup]	228	8.0	177	17%	9	31	6.9
2880	Vegetable combination (no carrots, broccoli, or dark-green leafy), cooked, with cream sauce [1 cup]	228	8.0	259	42%	9	30	5.8
2881	Vegetable combination (no carrots, broccoli, or dark-green leafy), cooked, with soy-based sauce [1 cup]	185	6.5	117	5%	5	25	4.7
2882	Vegetable combinations (no carrots, broccoli, or dark-green leafy), cooked, with pasta [1 cup]	137	4.8	130	5%	5	27	3.9
2883	Vegetable combinations (no carrots, broccoli, or dark-green leafy), cooked, with sauce and pasta [1 cup]	197	6.9	223	30%	7	34	5.0
2884	Vegetable combinations, Oriental style, (broccoli, green pepper, chinese cabbage, water chestnuts, etc), cooked [1 cup]	127	4.5	49	5%	3	10	3.3
2885	Vegetable mixture, dried (Include Salad Crunchies) [2 Tbs]	12	0.4	45	26%	2	7	2.4
2886	Vegetable stew without meat [1 cup]	239	8.4	135	16%	6	23	3.8
2887	Vegetable sticks, breaded (including corn, carrots, and green beans) [1 cup]	116	4.1	240	35%	5	36	3.6
2888	Vegetable tempura [1 cup]	63	2.2	102	56%	3	9	1.0
2889	Water chestnut [1 cup]	158	5.6	79	1%	1	20	4.0
2890	Watercress, cooked [1 cup]	137	4.8	15	8%	3	2	2.1
2891	Watercress, raw [1 cup, chopped]	34	1.2	4	8%	1	0	0.5
2892	Winter melon, cooked (Include Chinese melon, Togan) [1 cup]	175	6.2	23	14%	1	5	1.8
2893	Yam buns, Puerto Rican style (Bunuelos de name) [1 cup]	153	5.4	468	56%	5	46	5.3
2894	Yam, Puerto Rican (Name), cooked [1 cup]	140	4.9	162	1%	2	39	5.5
2895	Zucchini, summer squash, raw (Include green squash) [1 cup, sliced]	113	4.0	16	9%	1	3	1.4
2896	Zucchini with tomato sauce, cooked (Include summer squash with tomato sauce or tomatoes, zucchini with tomatoes) [1 cup] (See also squash, summer)	233	8.2	40	4%	2	10	2.9
	Your Additions							

Food no.	fat gm	sat fat gm	choles mg	sodium mg	potas mg	% of Daily Value													
						vit A	vit E	vit C	thia	ribo	niac	vit B-6	fola	vit B-12	calc	phos	mag	iron	zinc
2859	14	3	0	596	516	25	12	49	13	9	12	10	5	0	10	7	8	11	3
2860	0	0	0	564	607	14	4	48	8	5	9	2	3	0	8	5	8	10	3
2861	0	0	0	78	209	0	0	30	3	2	2	5	4	0	3	3	3	2	2
2862	0	0	0	56	282	0	0	10	4	3	4	5	3	0	5	4	5	8	2
2863	0	0	0	87	248	0	0	46	3	2	3	6	5	0	4	4	4	2	2
2864	11	3	7	419	326	6	6	26	7	13	4	6	4	5	15	12	6	3	4
2865	0	0	0	466	272	43	6	52	4	4	3	10	25	0	13	4	6	5	2
2866	0	0	0	65	273	43	6	52	4	5	3	10	25	0	13	4	6	5	2
2867	0	0	0	24	101	84	2	26	3	7	2	5	9	0	15	3	5	12	1
2868	0	0	0	454	321	87	12	72	5	7	3	14	47	0	22	5	9	7	1
2869	0	0	0	46	224	57	10	39	1	6	3	3	15	0	19	3	8	13	2
2870	0	0	0	42	292	79	11	66	4	6	3	13	43	0	20	4	8	6	1
2871	1	0	0	25	370	132	22	60	6	7	4	6	16	0	25	6	11	18	5
2872	10	6	26	426	419	90	3	66	5	5	7	12	8	0	5	8	7	7	4
2873	3	1	7	291	535	119	6	107	16	14	10	15	18	2	14	17	12	10	7
2874	12	3	8	418	401	70	11	59	9	17	5	10	13	5	17	15	9	6	5
2875	1	0	0	38	256	56	3	52	13	7	8	8	10	0	3	8	7	8	4
2876	8	1	0	130	319	82	8	68	17	9	11	10	12	0	4	10	9	11	6
2877	0	0	0	1195	476	17	5	133	8	13	13	13	13	0	6	10	10	14	5
2878	0	0	0	42	227	85	5	47	5	5	4	9	12	0	4	6	5	4	3
2879	3	1	8	297	555	22	3	125	16	13	12	17	15	2	11	18	13	10	7
2880	12	3	8	441	464	11	8	18	15	18	9	10	12	5	16	19	12	10	8
2881	1	0	0	1012	426	13	2	94	10	9	12	14	12	0	3	11	9	9	4
2882	1	0	0	726	256	10	2	57	13	6	10	9	8	0	2	8	8	8	4
2883	7	1	0	1002	330	19	7	73	17	8	13	11	11	0	3	11	10	10	6
2884	0	0	0	14	358	12	6	78	7	9	7	10	10	0	4	7	6	7	4
2885	1	0	0	58	212	39	4	44	7	4	4	6	7	0	3	5	5	9	3
2886	2	1	3	538	608	62	2	37	11	6	11	13	7	1	3	10	8	9	10
2887	9	1	0	729	227	55	8	7	15	10	10	7	8	0	3	9	7	11	4
2888	6	1	41	20	111	15	8	4	6	7	4	2	4	1	1	4	2	4	2
2889	0	0	0	13	186	0	4	3	1	2	3	13	2	0	1	3	2	8	4
2890	0	0	0	56	452	61	6	69	7	9	1	8	2	0	16	8	7	2	1
2891	0	0	0	14	112	16	2	24	2	2	0	2	1	0	4	2	2	0	0
2892	0	0	0	187	9	0	3	31	4	0	3	3	2	0	3	3	4	4	7
2893	29	10	81	409	904	9	7	26	14	11	7	16	7	3	4	11	7	8	4
2894	0	0	0	11	938	0	1	28	9	2	4	16	6	0	2	7	6	4	2
2895	0	0	0	3	280	4	1	17	5	2	2	5	6	0	2	4	6	3	2
2896	0	0	0	142	560	9	2	33	7	5	6	10	8	0	5	7	10	6	3

Fruit & Vegetables

Food No.	Food Description & Amount	wt gm	wt oz	cal	% cal fat	prot gm	carbo gm	fiber gm
	Your Additions							

						% of Daily Value													
Food No.	fat gm	sat fat gm	choles mg	sodium mg	potas mg	vit A	vit E	vit C	thia	ribo	niac	vit B-6	fola	vit B-12	calc	phos	mag	iron	zinc

Grains, Beans, Nuts, and Seeds

Grains, Beans, Nuts, Seeds

Food No.	Food Description & Amount	wt gm	wt oz	cal	% cal fat	prot gm	carbo gm	fiber gm
	Breads							
3000	Anisette toast (Include almond toast) [3 pieces]	33	1.2	139	20%	4	24	1.1
3001	**Bagel** (Include water bagels, flavored bagels, egg bagels, bialy) [1 bagel (3" dia)]	55	1.9	151	5%	6	29	1.3
3002	Bagel, multigrain, with raisins [1 bagel (3" dia)]	55	1.9	147	4%	6	31	3.8
3003	Bagel, multigrain [1 bagel (3" dia)]	57	2.0	148	4%	6	30	4.2
3004	Bagel, oat bran [1 bagel (3" dia)]	55	1.9	140	4%	6	29	2.0
3005	Bagel, pumpernickel (Include rye) [1 bagel (3" dia)]	55	1.9	159	4%	5	33	2.6
3006	Bagel, wheat bran [1 bagel (3" dia)]	55	1.9	150	5%	6	31	2.9
3007	Bagel, whole wheat, less than 100% [1 bagel (3" dia)]	55	1.9	159	4%	6	32	2.4
3008	Bagel, whole wheat, less than 100%, with fruit and nuts (Include California Energy Bar) [1 bagel (3" dia)]	55	1.9	162	8%	5	33	2.5
3009	Bagel, whole wheat, less than 100%, with raisins [1 bagel (3" dia)]	55	1.9	153	4%	5	32	2.3
3010	Bagel, whole wheat, 100% [1 bagel (3" dia)]	55	1.9	145	5%	6	31	5.1
3011	Bagel, whole wheat, 100%, with raisins [1 bagel (3" dia)]	55	1.9	134	4%	5	30	4.4
3012	Bagel, with blueberries (Include fruit other than raisins) [1 bagel (3" dia)]	55	1.9	152	6%	5	30	1.3
3013	Bagel, with raisins [1 bagel (3" dia)]	55	1.9	151	6%	5	30	1.3
3014	Bagel chip (Include all flavors) [2 chips]	28	1.0	119	22%	2	21	1.7
3015	Biscuit dough, raw [1 cup]	170	6.0	437	16%	11	81	2.7
3016	Biscuit dough, fried [1 piece]	43	1.5	144	38%	3	20	0.7
3017	Biscuit mix, dry [1 cup]	120	4.2	514	32%	10	76	2.5
3018	Biscuit, baking powder or buttermilk type, made from home recipe [1 biscuit (2" dia)]	30	1.1	106	41%	2	13	0.5
3019	Biscuit, baking powder or buttermilk type, made from mix (Include heat 'n eat biscuits) [1 biscuit (2" dia)]	30	1.1	97	33%	2	14	0.4
3020	Biscuit, baking powder or buttermilk type, made from refrigerated dough [1 biscuit]	19	0.7	66	38%	1	9	0.3
3021	Biscuit, baking powder or buttermilk type, made from refrigerated dough, lowfat [1 biscuit (2" dia)]	21	0.7	63	16%	2	12	0.4
3022	Biscuit, baking powder or buttermilk type, commercially baked [1 medium]	51	1.8	186	41%	3	25	0.7
3023	Biscuit, baking powder or buttermilk type, commercially baked (Include Kentucky Fried Chicken's) [1 biscuit]	61	2.2	222	41%	4	30	0.8
3024	Biscuit, baking powder or buttermilk type, commercially baked (Include McDonald's) [1 biscuit]	72	2.5	262	41%	4	35	0.9
3025	Biscuit, baking powder or buttermilk type, commercially baked (Include Hardee's) [1 biscuit]	97	3.4	353	41%	6	47	1.3
3026	Biscuit, cheese [1 biscuit (2" dia)]	30	1.1	113	45%	3	13	0.4
3027	Biscuit, cinnamon-raisin [1 biscuit (3" dia)]	64	2.3	227	34%	4	35	1.1
3028	Biscuit, whole wheat [1 biscuit (2" dia)]	30	1.1	95	34%	3	14	2.2
3029	Bread stick, soft (Include "crazy bread") [1 stick (7" long)]	32	1.1	113	22%	3	18	0.7
3030	Bread stick, soft, prepared with garlic and parmesan cheese [1 medium stick or slice]	47	1.7	191	39%	5	24	0.9
3031	Bread stick, hard (Include sesame sticks) [4 sticks (5" long)]	40	1.4	165	21%	5	27	1.2
3032	Bread stick, hard, low sodium [4 sticks (7" long)]	40	1.4	170	27%	5	26	0.7
3033	Bread stick, hard, whole wheat [4 sticks (8" long)]	32	1.1	130	22%	4	22	2.5
3034	Bread stuffing (Include homemade) [1 cup, moist type]	200	7.1	355	44%	6	43	1.8
3035	Bread, barley [1 slice]	26	0.9	74	11%	2	14	1.5
3036	Bread, batter [1 slice]	33	1.2	93	21%	3	15	0.5
3037	Bread, black [1 slice]	26	0.9	65	11%	2	12	1.7
3038	Bread, Boston Brown [1 slice]	45	1.6	88	7%	2	19	2.1
3039	Bread, bran (Include Granola, Branola, Honey Bran) [1 slice]	36	1.3	89	12%	3	17	1.4
3040	Bread, bran, with raisins [1 slice]	36	1.3	91	11%	3	19	1.4
3041	Bread, buckwheat [1 slice]	27	1.0	72	13%	2	14	0.9
3042	Bread, caressed, Puerto Rican style (Pan sobao) [1 slice]	25	0.9	67	12%	2	12	0.6
3043	Bread, cheese (Include onion cheese) [1 slice]	26	0.9	71	17%	2	12	0.6

Food No.	fat gm	sat fat gm	choles mg	sodium mg	potas mg	vit A	vit E	vit C	thia	ribo	niac	vit B-6	fola	vit B-12	calc	phos	mag	iron	zinc
						% of Daily Value													
3000	3	1	7	73	135	0	1	3	5	5	2	2	3	0	1	3	2	2	1
3001	1	0	0	294	56	0	0	0	20	10	13	1	3	0	4	5	4	11	3
3002	1	0	0	5	231	0	1	0	12	9	11	6	8	0	2	11	9	10	5
3003	1	0	0	282	211	0	1	0	16	8	12	5	10	0	2	12	10	10	7
3004	1	0	0	279	112	0	1	0	12	11	8	6	6	0	1	9	8	9	8
3005	1	0	0	3	86	0	0	0	17	13	14	3	7	0	1	7	5	10	4
3006	1	0	0	370	123	0	1	5	21	18	20	8	8	6	1	12	9	12	6
3007	1	0	0	4	105	0	1	0	18	13	16	4	7	0	1	9	7	11	5
3008	1	0	0	5	131	0	1	0	16	12	15	4	7	0	1	9	7	10	4
3009	1	0	0	4	125	0	1	0	16	12	15	4	6	0	1	8	6	10	4
3010	1	0	0	296	190	0	2	0	11	8	14	8	8	0	2	16	14	10	8
3011	1	0	0	238	192	0	2	0	10	7	12	7	7	0	2	13	12	9	7
3012	1	0	14	6	64	1	1	1	17	14	14	2	6	0	2	5	3	10	3
3013	1	0	0	177	84	0	0	1	14	9	8	2	3	0	1	4	3	12	3
3014	3	1	0	168	67	0	3	0	4	3	3	3	5	0	0	6	4	3	2
3015	8	2	0	2122	270	0	7	0	51	22	28	2	3	0	3	68	6	25	4
3016	6	1	0	521	66	0	4	0	9	5	6	1	0	0	1	17	2	6	1
3017	18	4	1	1531	196	0	13	0	46	31	27	5	2	2	21	70	8	18	5
3018	5	1	1	174	36	1	3	0	7	5	4	1	1	0	7	5	1	5	1
3019	4	1	1	276	56	1	2	0	7	6	4	1	0	1	5	14	2	3	1
3020	3	1	0	228	30	0	2	0	4	2	3	0	0	0	0	7	1	3	0
3021	1	0	0	305	39	0	1	0	6	3	4	0	0	0	0	10	1	4	1
3022	8	1	1	537	114	0	7	0	15	9	9	1	1	1	2	22	2	9	2
3023	10	2	1	642	137	0	8	0	17	10	10	1	1	1	3	26	3	11	2
3024	12	2	1	757	161	0	9	0	20	12	12	2	1	2	4	31	3	13	2
3025	16	2	1	1020	217	0	13	0	28	17	16	2	2	2	5	42	4	18	3
3026	6	2	4	150	45	2	3	0	7	6	4	1	1	1	9	7	2	5	2
3027	9	2	2	166	116	1	5	1	12	9	7	2	1	1	12	9	3	9	2
3028	4	1	1	100	95	1	3	0	5	3	5	3	2	1	7	9	7	4	4
3029	3	1	0	142	34	0	2	0	11	8	9	1	3	0	1	3	2	7	2
3030	8	2	1	218	48	0	6	0	15	11	12	1	4	0	4	5	2	9	3
3031	4	1	0	263	50	0	3	0	16	13	11	1	3	0	1	5	3	10	2
3032	5	1	0	14	86	0	1	0	17	12	13	1	1	0	3	7	5	10	3
3033	3	1	0	185	92	0	2	0	11	7	10	3	4	0	1	9	8	8	5
3034	17	3	1	1085	148	15	12	0	18	13	15	4	9	1	6	8	6	12	4
3035	1	0	0	4	42	0	0	0	6	4	6	1	2	0	1	3	2	4	2
3036	2	1	13	11	50	1	1	0	8	8	5	1	3	1	2	4	2	5	2
3037	1	0	0	174	54	0	1	0	6	5	4	2	2	0	2	5	4	4	3
3038	1	0	0	284	143	0	1	0	0	3	3	2	1	0	3	5	7	5	2
3039	1	0	0	175	82	0	1	0	10	6	8	3	2	0	3	7	7	6	3
3040	1	0	0	155	100	0	1	0	9	6	7	3	2	0	3	6	7	6	3
3041	1	0	0	4	56	0	1	0	7	5	6	2	2	0	1	4	4	4	2
3042	1	0	0	135	30	0	0	0	8	5	5	1	2	0	2	2	2	4	1
3043	1	0	2	141	31	0	0	0	8	5	5	1	2	0	4	3	2	4	1

Grains, Beans, Nuts, Seeds

Food No.	Food Description & Amount	wt gm	wt oz	cal	% cal fat	prot gm	carbo gm	fiber gm
3044	Bread, cinnamon [1 slice]	26	0.9	69	12%	2	13	0.6
3045	Bread, corn and molasses (Include Anadama bread) [1 slice]	32	1.1	88	17%	2	16	0.7
3046	Bread, cottonseed, toasted [1 slice]	41	1.4	129	18%	5	21	0.7
3047	Bread, cracked wheat (Include Honey Wheat, Roman Meal, Wheatberry, crushed wheat) [1 slice]	26	0.9	68	14%	2	12	1.1
3048	Bread, cracked wheat, made from home recipe or purchased at bakery [1 slice]	30	1.1	86	18%	3	15	1.1
3049	Bread, cracked wheat, reduced calorie, high fiber (Include Roman Light Wheat, Less, Wonder Light Wheat, Arnold's Bakery Light Golden Wheat) [1 slice]	28	1.0	55	10%	3	12	3.4
3050	Bread, cracked wheat, with raisins [1 slice]	26	0.9	69	13%	2	13	1.1
3051	Bread, Cuban (Include Spanish, Portuguese) [1 slice]	20	0.7	55	10%	2	10	0.6
3052	Bread, dough, fried (Include Indian fried) [1 piece (7" dia)]	104	3.7	389	44%	7	47	1.6
3053	Bread, egg, Chalah [1 slice]	23	0.8	66	19%	2	11	0.5
3054	Bread, French or Vienna (Include Hawaiian sandwich bread) [1 slice (4¾" x 4" x ½")]	25	0.9	69	10%	2	13	0.8
3055	Bread, French or Vienna, whole wheat, less than 100%, made from home recipe or purchased at bakery [1 slice (4¾" x 4" x ½")]	25	0.9	69	10%	2	13	1.2
3056	Bread, banana nut (Include other fruit-nut breads) [1 slice]	56	2.0	217	41%	3	30	1.0
3057	Bread, banana (Include other fruit breads, Keebler Banana Elfin Loaves) [1 slice]	41	1.4	134	29%	2	22	0.5
3058	Bread, garlic [1 slice (4¾" x 4" x ½")]	29	1.0	96	35%	2	13	0.8
3059	Bread, low gluten [1 slice]	30	1.1	73	17%	3	13	1.5
3060	Bread, Irish soda [1 slice]	30	1.1	87	16%	2	17	0.8
3061	Bread, Italian, Grecian, Armenian (Include sesame bread) [1 slice]	20	0.7	54	12%	2	10	0.5
3062	Bread, Italian, reduced calorie and/or high fiber [1 slice]	20	0.7	39	14%	2	8	1.9
3063	Bread, lard, Puerto Rican style (Pan de manteca) [1 slice]	25	0.9	70	9%	2	14	0.5
3064	Bread, lowfat, 98% fat free (Include Bonnie) [1 slice]	24	0.8	65	12%	2	12	0.6
3065	Bread, milk and honey (Include Arnold's) [1 slice]	28	1.0	73	7%	2	15	0.5
3066	Bread, multigrain [1 slice]	26	0.9	65	14%	3	12	1.7
3067	Bread, multigrain, reduced calorie, high fiber [1 slice]	26	0.9	53	10%	2	12	3.1
3068	Bread, multigrain, with raisins [1 slice]	26	0.9	66	10%	2	13	1.5
3069	Bread, Native water, Puerto Rican style (Pan de agua) [1 slice or bun]	25	0.9	69	10%	2	13	0.8
3070	Bread, Native, Puerto Rican style (Pan Criollo) [1 slice]	25	0.9	69	10%	2	13	0.8
3071	Bread, nut [1 slice]	49	1.7	167	40%	4	22	0.7
3072	Bread, oat bran [1 slice]	26	0.9	68	17%	3	11	1.3
3073	Bread, oat bran, reduced calorie, high fiber [1 slice]	29	1.0	58	14%	2	12	3.5
3074	Bread, oatmeal [1 slice]	25	0.9	67	15%	2	12	1.0
3075	Bread, onion [1 slice]	26	0.9	66	12%	2	12	0.6
3076	Bread, pita (Include Greek, Syrian flat bread, Sahara, Arab, pocket) [1 pita (5" dia)]	45	1.6	124	4%	4	25	1.0
3077	Bread, pita, whole wheat, 100% (Include roti) [1 pita (5" dia)]	45	1.6	120	9%	4	25	3.3
3078	Bread, pita, whole wheat, less than 100% [1 pita (5" dia)]	45	1.6	123	5%	5	25	2.4
3079	Bread, potato [1 slice]	26	0.9	69	12%	2	13	0.6
3080	Bread, pumpernickel (Include with raisins) [1 slice]	26	0.9	65	11%	2	12	1.7
3081	Bread, pumpkin (Include with raisins and/or nuts) [1 slice]	60	2.1	179	21%	2	34	1.1
3082	Bread, puri or poori (Indian puffed bread) filled with coconut, fried [1 puri (5"	36	1.3	113	36%	3	16	1.9
3083	Bread, raisin (Include cinnamon-raisin, Weight Watcher's) [1 slice]	26	0.9	71	14%	2	14	1.1
3084	Bread, reduced calorie, high fiber, white (Include Fresh Horizons, New World, Less, Roman Light White Bread, Lite Loaf, Sunbeam Lite, Lite 'N Up, Wonder Light White) [1 slice]	29	1.0	60	11%	3	13	2.8
3085	Bread, reduced calorie, high fiber, white, with fruit and/or nuts (Include Less Raisin) [1 slice]	29	1.0	60	12%	2	13	2.2
3086	Bread, rice [1 slice]	25	0.9	61	17%	2	11	1.2
3087	Bread, rye (Include corn rye) (Include Less) [1 slice]	26	0.9	67	11%	2	13	1.5
3088	Bread, rye, reduced calorie, high fiber (Include Less) [1 slice]	26	0.9	53	13%	2	11	3.1
3089	Bread, marble rye and pumpernickel [1 slice]	26	0.9	66	11%	2	12	1.6

						% of Daily Value													
Food No.	fat gm	sat fat gm	choles mg	sodium mg	potas mg	vit A	vit E	vit C	thia	ribo	niac	vit B-6	fola	vit B-12	calc	phos	mag	iron	zinc
3044	1	0	0	140	31	0	0	0	8	5	5	1	2	0	3	2	2	4	1
3045	2	0	1	9	103	1	1	0	7	6	5	2	2	0	3	4	4	5	1
3046	3	1	2	12	123	1	1	0	16	10	9	2	4	1	4	10	9	9	5
3047	1	0	0	138	52	0	1	0	7	4	5	1	3	0	3	4	3	5	2
3048	2	0	0	10	103	0	2	0	6	6	5	2	2	0	3	5	5	5	2
3049	1	0	0	143	35	0	0	0	8	5	5	2	2	0	2	3	2	5	2
3050	1	0	0	122	66	0	1	0	7	4	5	1	2	0	3	4	3	5	2
3051	1	0	0	122	23	0	0	0	7	4	5	0	2	0	1	2	1	3	1
3052	19	4	3	20	125	2	11	0	26	19	16	2	5	1	5	10	4	15	4
3053	1	0	12	113	26	1	1	0	7	6	6	1	4	0	2	2	1	4	1
3054	1	0	0	152	28	0	0	0	9	5	6	1	2	0	2	3	2	4	1
3055	1	0	0	4	55	0	1	0	6	5	6	2	2	0	1	4	3	4	2
3056	10	2	28	104	98	1	5	2	8	7	5	6	2	1	6	6	4	6	2
3057	4	1	18	124	55	5	3	1	5	5	3	3	1	1	1	2	1	3	1
3058	4	1	0	188	33	3	2	0	9	5	6	1	2	0	2	3	2	4	1
3059	1	0	0	132	59	0	1	0	13	5	10	3	2	0	2	5	5	6	3
3060	2	0	5	119	80	2	1	0	6	5	4	1	1	0	2	3	2	4	1
3061	1	0	0	117	22	0	0	0	6	3	4	0	2	0	2	2	1	3	1
3062	1	0	0	117	15	0	1	0	5	3	3	1	1	0	2	2	1	3	1
3063	1	0	1	108	22	0	0	0	7	5	5	1	2	0	0	2	1	4	1
3064	1	0	0	140	26	0	0	0	8	4	5	1	2	0	3	2	2	4	1
3065	1	0	0	5	36	0	0	0	8	6	5	1	3	0	1	3	1	5	1
3066	1	0	0	127	53	0	1	0	7	5	6	4	3	0	2	5	3	5	2
3067	1	0	3	133	45	0	0	0	7	4	5	2	4	0	2	6	6	4	4
3068	1	0	0	1	79	0	1	0	5	3	4	2	2	0	2	4	3	4	2
3069	1	0	0	152	28	0	0	0	9	5	6	1	2	0	1	3	2	4	1
3070	1	0	0	152	28	0	0	0	9	5	6	1	2	0	1	3	2	4	1
3071	7	1	28	108	73	2	3	0	8	8	4	2	2	1	8	8	4	6	3
3072	1	0	0	118	32	0	1	0	10	6	7	1	2	0	2	3	2	5	2
3073	1	0	0	102	30	0	1	0	7	3	5	1	2	0	2	4	3	5	2
3074	1	0	0	150	36	0	0	0	7	4	4	1	2	0	2	3	2	4	2
3075	1	0	0	131	32	0	0	0	8	5	5	1	2	0	3	2	2	4	1
3076	1	0	0	241	54	0	0	0	18	9	10	1	3	0	4	4	3	7	3
3077	1	0	0	239	77	0	2	0	10	2	6	5	4	0	1	8	8	7	5
3078	1	0	0	188	96	0	1	0	13	10	13	3	6	0	1	8	6	9	4
3079	1	0	0	140	31	0	0	0	8	5	5	1	2	0	3	2	2	4	1
3080	1	0	0	174	54	0	1	0	6	5	4	2	2	0	2	5	4	4	3
3081	4	1	26	79	86	33	4	1	6	6	4	2	2	1	3	4	2	6	1
3082	5	2	0	2	68	0	3	0	7	4	6	2	2	0	1	5	5	6	3
3083	1	0	0	101	59	0	1	0	6	6	5	1	2	0	2	3	2	4	1
3084	1	0	0	131	22	0	0	0	8	5	5	1	2	1	3	4	2	5	3
3085	1	0	0	95	49	0	0	0	6	4	4	1	2	1	2	3	2	4	2
3086	1	0	0	110	49	0	1	0	11	4	9	3	2	0	2	4	4	5	2
3087	1	0	0	172	43	0	1	0	8	5	5	1	3	0	2	3	3	4	2
3088	1	0	0	105	25	0	0	0	6	4	3	0	1	0	2	2	1	4	1
3089	1	0	0	173	49	0	1	0	7	5	4	1	3	0	2	4	3	4	2

Grains, Beans, Nuts, Seeds

Food No.	Food Description & Amount	wt gm	wt oz	cal	% cal fat	prot gm	carbo gm	fiber gm
3090	Bread, salt-rising [1 slice]	24	0.8	64	8%	2	13	0.4
3091	Bread, sour dough [1 slice (4¾" x 4" x ½")]	25	0.9	69	10%	2	13	0.8
3092	Bread, soy [1 slice]	26	0.9	69	13%	3	12	0.9
3093	Bread, Spanish coffee (Include Mallorca) [1 piece]	85	3.0	293	23%	6	50	1.6
3094	Bread, sprouted wheat [1 slice]	26	0.9	68	14%	2	12	1.1
3095	Bread, sunflower meal (Include sunflower seed bread) [1 slice]	27	1.0	75	17%	3	12	0.5
3096	Bread, sweetpotato [1 slice]	25	0.9	74	19%	2	13	0.5
3097	Bread, triticale [1 slice]	25	0.9	63	13%	2	12	1.6
3098	Bread, very low sodium [1 slice]	26	0.9	69	12%	2	13	0.6
3099	Bread, walnut, whole wheat, (Include other nut breads) [1 slice]	49	1.7	163	42%	4	21	2.1
3100	Bread, wheat germ [1 slice]	28	1.0	73	10%	3	14	0.6
3101	Bread, white and whole wheat (Include half and half, Health Nut, Golden Meal, Country Grain) [1 slice]	26	0.9	67	14%	2	12	1.2
3102	**Bread, white** [1 slice]	26	0.9	69	12%	2	13	0.6
3103	Bread, white, made from home recipe or purchased at a bakery [1 slice]	32	1.1	91	18%	3	16	0.6
3104	Bread, whole wheat, 100% (Include dark bread, brown bread, Hollywood Dark, Honey Graham) [1 slice]	26	0.9	64	15%	3	12	1.8
3105	Bread, whole wheat, 100%, made from home recipe or purchased at bakery [1 slice]	30	1.1	82	21%	3	15	2.1
3106	Bread, whole wheat, 100%, with raisins [1 slice]	26	0.9	66	13%	2	13	1.7
3107	Bread, whole wheat, less than 100%, made from home recipe or purchased at bakery [1 slice]	30	1.1	83	17%	3	15	1.8
3108	Bread, zucchini (Include squash bread, carrot bread) [1 slice]	40	1.4	151	45%	2	19	0.6
3109	Brioche (Include Pan de Huevo) [1 piece]	77	2.7	269	35%	8	36	1.1
3110	Coffee cake, yeast type (Include with or without nuts, coffee bread with icing) [1/8 of 8" dia]	41	1.4	153	40%	3	21	1.0
3111	Coffee cake, yeast type, made from home recipe or purchased at a bakery (Include with or without nuts, coffee bread with icing) [1/8 of 8" dia]	41	1.4	140	24%	3	23	0.8
3112	Coffee cake, yeast type, very lowfat, no cholesterol, with fruit [1 piece (5" x 7/8" x 1-1/8")]	33	1.2	94	2%	3	20	0.6
3113	Corn flour patties or tarts, fried [2 patties]	20	0.7	44	19%	1	8	0.9
3114	Corn pone (Include hoecake) [1 piece (1/8 of 9" dia x ¾" pone)]	61	2.2	129	22%	2	24	2.2
3115	Corn pone, fried [1 piece]	61	2.2	152	38%	2	22	2.1
3116	Cornstarch, dry (Include hydrolyzed powder, Uniopro Carboplex) [1 cup]	128	4.5	488	0%	0	117	1.2
3117	Cornbread, made from mix [1 piece (2½" x 2½" x 1½")]	65	2.3	152	29%	4	23	1.9
3118	Cornbread, made from home recipe [1 piece (2½" x 2½" x 1½")]	65	2.3	184	30%	4	28	1.5
3119	Cornbread, made with egg substitute, made from home recipe [1 piece (2½" x 2½" x 1½")]	46	1.6	86	10%	3	16	1.4
3120	Cornbread, muffins, sticks, rounds, made from home recipe [1 muffin]	52	1.8	158	30%	4	24	1.3
3121	Cornbread muffins, sticks, rounds, made from mix [1 muffin]	52	1.8	159	25%	3	26	1.8
3122	Cornmeal bread, Dominican style (Arepa Dominicana) [1 piece (4" x 2" x 1¾")]	115	4.1	308	47%	7	35	4.1
3123	Cornbread stuffing [1 cup, moist type]	203	7.2	363	44%	6	44	5.9
3124	Croissant (Include Sara Lee Wheat 'n' Honey) [1 croissant]	56	2.0	227	47%	5	26	1.5
3125	Croissant, cheese [1 croissant]	42	1.5	174	45%	4	20	1.1
3126	Croissant, chocolate (Include Vie de France) [1 croissant]	56	2.0	234	53%	5	25	2.2
3127	Croissant, fruit (Include Sara Lee Apple, Strawberry, Cinnamon-Nut-Raisin) [1 croissant]	92	3.2	351	46%	7	40	2.4
3128	Croissant, nut (Include Vie de France) [1 croissant]	56	2.0	230	48%	5	25	1.5
3129	Croutons (Include seasoned bread crumbs) [1 cup]	30	1.1	140	35%	3	19	1.5
3130	Crumpet [1 medium (3¾" dia)]	45	1.6	80	5%	3	17	0.8
3131	Flour, white [1 cup]	125	4.4	455	2%	13	95	3.4
3132	Flour, whole wheat [1 cup]	120	4.2	407	5%	16	87	14.6
3133	Gordita/sope shell, plain, no filling, fried in oil [1 shell (3" dia)]	40	1.4	111	37%	2	16	2.0
3134	Gordita/sope shell, plain, no filling, grilled [1 shell (3" dia)]	42	1.5	88	9%	2	18	2.3

Food No.	fat gm	sat fat gm	choles mg	sodium mg	potas mg	% of Daily Value													
						vit A	vit E	vit C	thia	ribo	niac	vit B-6	fola	vit B-12	calc	phos	mag	iron	zinc
3090	1	0	0	64	16	0	1	0	6	3	4	1	2	0	2	2	1	4	1
3091	1	0	0	152	28	0	0	0	9	5	6	1	2	0	2	3	2	4	1
3092	1	0	1	6	107	0	0	0	7	5	5	1	3	0	2	4	3	5	2
3093	7	1	32	12	82	1	4	0	25	17	15	2	7	1	1	8	3	14	5
3094	1	0	0	138	52	0	1	0	7	4	5	1	3	0	3	4	3	5	2
3095	1	0	1	6	34	0	1	0	10	5	6	1	2	0	2	4	3	4	2
3096	2	0	14	20	41	5	1	1	6	6	4	1	3	0	1	3	1	4	1
3097	1	0	0	148	52	0	1	0	7	4	5	2	3	0	2	4	4	4	3
3098	1	0	0	7	31	0	0	0	8	5	5	1	2	0	3	2	2	4	1
3099	8	1	28	109	119	2	4	0	5	5	5	4	3	1	8	11	8	5	5
3100	1	0	0	155	71	0	1	0	7	6	6	1	4	0	2	5	2	5	3
3101	1	0	0	138	48	0	1	0	7	4	5	2	3	0	2	4	4	5	2
3102	1	0	0	140	31	0	0	0	8	5	5	1	2	0	3	2	2	4	1
3103	2	0	1	115	47	1	2	0	9	7	6	1	3	0	2	4	2	5	1
3104	1	0	0	137	66	0	1	0	6	3	5	2	3	0	2	6	6	5	3
3105	2	0	0	4	115	0	2	0	5	3	5	4	3	0	2	7	7	5	4
3106	1	0	0	122	78	0	1	0	6	3	5	2	3	0	2	6	5	5	3
3107	2	0	0	104	94	0	2	0	6	4	6	3	4	0	1	6	6	5	3
3108	8	1	26	78	46	1	6	1	5	5	3	1	2	1	3	3	1	5	1
3109	10	2	73	117	93	11	6	1	19	19	15	2	6	3	3	9	4	12	4
3110	7	2	27	157	46	3	5	1	9	6	5	2	2	1	3	3	2	4	2
3111	4	1	10	9	61	1	2	0	10	9	7	2	4	1	2	5	2	6	2
3112	0	0	0	53	59	1	0	1	6	7	4	1	3	0	2	3	1	4	1
3113	1	0	0	1	28	0	1	0	7	4	4	2	0	0	1	2	3	4	1
3114	3	1	0	133	87	0	2	0	6	3	5	4	1	0	7	10	10	7	4
3115	6	1	0	125	82	0	4	0	5	3	5	4	1	0	7	9	9	6	4
3116	0	0	0	12	4	0	0	0	0	0	0	0	0	0	0	2	1	3	1
3117	5	2	22	356	105	3	3	0	8	9	5	3	1	2	7	19	3	5	3
3118	6	1	26	188	91	3	5	0	13	11	7	3	3	2	13	10	4	9	3
3119	1	0	2	202	92	2	0	2	8	7	4	3	2	1	4	5	3	4	2
3120	5	1	23	161	78	3	4	0	11	10	6	2	2	1	11	9	3	7	2
3121	4	1	27	271	36	2	3	0	9	10	5	2	4	2	4	15	5	8	2
3122	16	11	64	147	241	8	5	2	17	16	10	7	6	3	9	14	9	14	6
3123	18	4	0	924	126	17	13	3	16	11	13	4	4	0	5	7	7	11	3
3124	12	7	42	417	66	8	1	0	14	8	6	2	4	3	2	6	2	6	3
3125	9	4	27	233	55	7	2	0	15	8	5	2	3	2	2	5	3	5	3
3126	14	8	38	376	106	7	1	0	13	8	6	2	4	3	2	8	6	8	4
3127	18	10	62	617	123	11	2	3	22	12	9	3	6	4	3	9	4	10	4
3128	12	6	41	404	77	7	3	0	14	8	6	2	4	3	2	7	3	6	3
3129	5	2	1	371	54	0	2	0	10	7	7	1	3	0	3	4	3	5	2
3130	0	0	0	324	37	0	0	0	5	1	2	1	1	0	5	7	2	3	2
3131	1	0	0	3	134	0	0	0	65	36	37	3	8	0	2	14	7	32	6
3132	2	0	0	6	486	0	7	0	36	15	38	20	13	0	4	42	41	26	23
3133	5	1	0	2	63	0	4	0	15	8	9	4	1	0	3	5	6	9	3
3134	1	0	0	2	72	0	0	0	18	10	11	4	1	0	3	5	7	10	3

Grains, Beans, Nuts, Seeds

Food No.	Food Description & Amount	wt gm	wt oz	cal	% cal fat	prot gm	carbo gm	fiber gm
3135	Hush puppies (Include fried cornbread) [2 hush puppies]	44	1.6	148	36%	3	20	1.2
3136	Injera (Ethiopian bread) [1 injera (12" dia)]	127	4.5	173	6%	6	38	1.3
3137	Johnnycake [1 piece]	49	1.7	135	24%	4	21	1.6
3138	Matzo, fritters [2 fritters]	30	1.1	109	57%	2	10	0.2
3139	Melba toast (Include flavors, Nutrisystem Crisp Toast, Bagel Chips) [5 slices]	25	0.9	98	7%	3	19	1.6
3140	Melba toast with wheat germ [5 slices]	25	0.9	97	11%	3	19	1.9
3141	Muffin, bran (Include with raisins and nuts) [1 muffin (2-5/8" dia)]	50	1.8	148	27%	3	26	3.9
3142	Muffin, bran with fruit, lowfat (Include Jenny's Cuisine) [1 muffin (2¾" dia)]	58	2.0	136	19%	3	31	6.2
3143	Muffin, bran with fruit, no fat, no cholesterol (Include McDonald's Apple Bran) [1 muffin]	75	2.6	191	3%	8	40	3.1
3144	Muffin, buckwheat [1 muffin (2-5/8"dia)]	47	1.7	143	35%	4	20	1.3
3145	Muffin, carrot (Include with raisins) [1 muffin (2-5/8" dia)]	58	2.0	177	34%	4	26	1.0
3146	Muffin, cheese [1 muffin (2-5/8" dia)]	58	2.0	180	37%	5	23	0.7
3147	Muffin, chocolate chip [1 muffin (2-5/8" dia)]	58	2.0	188	36%	4	27	1.0
3148	Muffin, English (Include sour dough) [1 muffin]	58	2.0	136	7%	4	27	1.6
3149	Muffin, English, bran (Include Branola) [1 muffin]	58	2.0	127	11%	5	25	2.8
3150	Muffin, English, bran, with raisins [1 muffin]	58	2.0	140	10%	5	29	2.9
3151	Muffin, English, cheese [1 muffin]	58	2.0	141	12%	5	25	1.5
3152	Muffin, English, multigrain [1 muffin]	58	2.0	136	7%	5	27	1.6
3153	Muffin, English, oat bran [1 muffin]	66	2.3	144	14%	6	29	3.0
3154	Muffin, English, oat bran, with raisins [1 muffin]	58	2.0	133	13%	5	28	2.6
3155	Muffin, English, pumpernickel [1 muffin]	58	2.0	130	12%	6	25	5.5
3156	Muffin, English, rye [1 muffin]	58	2.0	137	10%	5	26	2.5
3157	Muffin, English, cracked wheat (Include Roman Meal) [1 muffin]	58	2.0	129	8%	5	26	2.7
3158	Muffin, English, wheat or cracked wheat, with raisins [1 muffin]	58	2.0	146	9%	5	30	2.5
3159	Muffin, English, whole wheat, 100% [1 muffin]	58	2.0	118	9%	5	23	3.9
3160	Muffin, English, whole wheat, 100%, with raisins [1 muffin]	58	2.0	143	9%	5	30	4.4
3161	Muffin, English, whole wheat, less than 100% [1 muffin]	58	2.0	129	8%	5	26	2.7
3162	Muffin, English, whole wheat, less than 100%, with raisins [1 muffin]	58	2.0	146	9%	5	30	2.5
3163	Muffin, English, with fruit other than raisins [1 muffin]	58	2.0	146	7%	5	29	1.8
3164	Muffin, English, with raisins [1 muffin]	58	2.0	141	10%	4	28	1.7
3165	Muffin, fruit and/or nuts (Include blueberry, cranberry nut) [1 muffin (2-5/8" dia)]	58	2.0	161	21%	3	28	1.5
3166	Muffin, fruit, reduced fat, no cholesterol (Include Entenmann's) [1 muffin (2¾" dia)]	57	2.0	149	2%	4	34	1.9
3167	Muffin, multigrain, with fruit [1 muffin (2¾" dia)]	57	2.0	148	20%	5	27	3.8
3168	Muffin, multigrain, with nuts [1 muffin]	66	2.3	210	41%	6	28	4.0
3169	Muffin, oat bran with fruit and/or nuts [1 muffin (2¾" dia)]	57	2.0	165	30%	4	28	2.6
3170	Muffin, oat bran [1 muffin (2-5/8" dia)]	47	1.7	127	25%	3	23	2.2
3171	Muffin, oatmeal (Include Granola) [1 muffin (2-5/8" dia)]	47	1.7	112	23%	3	18	0.7
3172	Muffin, plain (Include Matzo Meal) [1 muffin (2-5/8" dia)]	47	1.7	144	32%	4	21	0.6
3173	Muffin, plain, no wheat, sugar free [1 muffin (2¾" dia)]	57	2.0	176	33%	4	26	1.9
3174	Muffin, pumpkin (Include with raisins, nuts) [1 muffin (2-5/8" dia)]	58	2.0	181	21%	3	34	1.1
3175	Muffin, wheat [1 muffin (2-5/8" dia)]	47	1.7	143	34%	4	21	1.5
3176	Muffin, whole wheat (Include graham) [1 muffin (2-5/8" dia)]	47	1.7	140	36%	4	20	2.5
3177	Muffin, zucchini (Include squash muffin; with nuts) [1 muffin (2-5/8" dia)]	58	2.0	219	45%	3	27	0.8
3178	Papad (Indian appetizer), grilled or broiled [4 papad]	36	1.3	125	8%	8	22	3.1
3179	Pannetone (Italian-style sweetbread) [1 slice]	27	1.0	87	23%	2	15	0.6
3180	Popovers (Include Dutch Baby, Yorkshire pudding) [1 popover]	31	1.1	68	31%	3	9	0.3
3181	Roll, cheese [1 roll]	41	1.4	125	25%	4	20	1.2
3182	Roll, diet [1 roll]	28	1.0	77	10%	2	15	0.8
3183	Roll, egg bread [1 roll]	28	1.0	86	19%	3	15	1.0
3184	Roll, French or Vienna [1 roll]	45	1.6	125	14%	4	23	1.4
3185	Roll, garlic [1 roll]	35	1.2	105	22%	3	18	1.0

Food No.	fat gm	sat fat gm	choles mg	sodium mg	potas mg	% of Daily Value													
						vit A	vit E	vit C	thia	ribo	niac	vit B-6	fola	vit B-12	calc	phos	mag	iron	zinc
3135	6	1	20	294	63	2	2	0	10	9	6	2	2	1	12	8	3	7	2
3136	1	0	0	254	72	0	0	0	8	6	8	4	9	0	7	14	3	205	3
3137	4	1	36	154	106	3	2	0	12	11	6	4	4	2	5	7	4	6	3
3138	7	1	43	75	19	2	4	0	2	4	1	1	1	1	1	2	1	3	1
3139	1	0	0	207	51	0	0	0	7	4	5	1	2	0	2	5	4	5	3
3140	1	0	0	202	60	0	1	0	3	3	3	2	2	0	3	6	4	3	3
3141	4	1	5	248	83	3	3	0	8	9	6	1	1	0	2	13	3	7	1
3142	3	0	8	165	129	0	2	0	8	6	6	3	1	1	7	11	7	7	3
3143	1	0	1	109	191	2	1	1	14	20	11	4	3	2	9	18	12	11	5
3144	6	1	20	111	107	2	3	0	7	7	6	3	2	1	9	9	8	6	3
3145	7	1	18	153	111	26	6	2	10	9	6	2	2	1	8	7	2	7	2
3146	7	2	27	193	87	4	3	0	11	12	7	2	2	2	13	11	3	8	3
3147	7	2	23	117	92	2	3	0	11	11	7	1	2	1	9	9	4	8	3
3148	1	0	0	269	76	0	0	0	17	10	11	1	5	0	10	8	3	8	3
3149	2	0	0	49	125	0	1	7	22	21	21	10	11	9	5	12	9	12	6
3150	2	0	0	46	166	0	1	7	21	20	20	10	10	8	5	12	9	12	5
3151	2	1	3	274	75	1	0	0	16	10	11	1	5	0	12	9	3	8	3
3152	1	0	0	241	90	0	3	0	17	11	10	3	5	0	11	9	6	10	4
3153	2	0	0	11	143	0	2	0	22	16	14	3	13	0	7	15	9	13	5
3154	2	0	0	10	156	0	1	0	18	13	12	3	10	0	6	12	8	11	4
3155	2	0	0	10	181	0	3	0	11	12	12	6	12	0	6	17	13	11	10
3156	1	0	0	10	103	0	1	0	15	13	13	3	11	0	5	7	4	9	4
3157	1	0	0	222	108	0	1	0	17	10	10	3	6	0	10	7	6	9	4
3158	1	0	0	10	161	0	1	0	15	13	14	4	10	0	5	9	6	10	4
3159	1	0	0	369	122	0	2	0	12	5	10	5	7	0	15	16	10	8	6
3160	1	0	0	11	215	0	2	0	10	10	13	7	10	0	5	14	12	9	7
3161	1	0	0	222	108	0	1	0	17	10	10	3	6	0	10	7	6	9	4
3162	1	0	0	10	161	0	1	0	15	13	14	4	10	0	5	9	6	10	4
3163	1	0	0	280	84	0	1	1	18	10	12	1	6	0	11	8	3	8	3
3164	2	0	0	259	121	0	0	0	15	10	10	2	5	0	9	4	2	8	4
3165	4	1	17	259	71	1	3	1	5	4	3	1	2	6	3	11	2	5	2
3166	0	0	0	245	58	1	0	1	12	9	8	1	2	1	9	13	2	8	2
3167	3	1	40	156	239	3	4	1	10	10	7	7	3	2	12	17	14	10	7
3168	10	2	42	165	325	3	8	1	11	11	7	10	4	2	14	19	20	12	8
3169	6	1	0	202	294	0	6	1	10	3	1	5	3	0	4	20	22	13	7
3170	3	0	0	185	238	0	5	0	8	3	1	4	2	0	3	18	18	11	6
3171	3	1	17	121	58	2	1	0	9	8	5	1	1	1	9	7	2	6	2
3172	5	1	21	105	64	2	3	0	10	9	6	1	2	1	8	7	2	7	2
3173	6	1	23	171	354	2	4	6	7	5	5	3	3	2	12	12	7	20	4
3174	4	1	27	80	87	33	4	1	7	6	4	2	2	1	3	4	2	6	1
3175	5	1	20	138	89	2	3	0	7	7	6	2	2	1	10	10	5	6	3
3176	6	1	20	140	119	2	4	0	5	5	6	4	2	1	10	12	8	5	5
3177	11	2	38	113	66	2	9	2	8	7	5	2	2	1	4	5	2	7	2
3178	1	0	0	752	409	0	0	0	3	1	7	3	18	0	3	16	19	19	8
3179	2	1	19	28	54	2	0	0	7	7	5	1	5	1	2	4	1	4	1
3180	2	1	36	64	51	3	2	0	5	7	3	1	1	2	3	4	1	3	2
3181	4	1	3	216	54	1	1	0	13	8	8	1	3	0	6	6	2	7	2
3182	1	0	0	171	32	0	0	0	10	5	7	1	2	0	2	3	2	4	2
3183	2	0	14	153	29	1	1	0	10	9	5	1	4	1	2	3	2	5	2
3184	2	0	0	274	51	0	1	0	16	8	10	1	4	0	4	4	2	7	2
3185	3	1	0	181	47	0	1	0	11	7	7	1	3	0	4	4	2	6	2

Grains, Beans, Nuts, Seeds

Food No.	Food Description & Amount	wt gm	wt oz	cal	% cal fat	prot gm	carbo gm	fiber gm
3186	Roll, hoagie, submarine, or sandwich (Include steak roll, torpedo roll) [1 roll]	100	3.5	286	16%	9	50	2.7
3187	Roll, Mexican, bolillo [1 medium]	117	4.1	307	5%	10	61	2.2
3188	Roll, multigrain [1 roll]	28	1.0	74	21%	3	12	1.1
3189	Roll, oat bran [1 medium]	36	1.3	85	18%	3	14	1.5
3190	Roll, oatmeal [1 roll]	36	1.3	105	21%	3	17	1.0
3191	Roll, pumpernickel [1 roll]	36	1.3	100	9%	4	19	1.9
3192	Roll, rye [1 roll]	36	1.3	103	11%	4	19	1.8
3193	Roll, sour dough [1 roll]	45	1.6	123	10%	4	23	1.4
3194	**Roll, sweet** (Include butterhorn; Portuguese sweet bread) [1 roll]	55	1.9	205	40%	3	28	1.3
3195	Roll, sweet, cinnamon bun, frosted [1 roll (2½" dia)]	55	1.9	209	36%	3	31	1.1
3196	Roll, sweet, cinnamon bun, no frosting [1 roll (2½" dia)]	55	1.9	205	40%	3	28	1.3
3197	Roll, sweet, with fruit, frosted (Include hot cross buns) [1 roll (2½" dia)]	55	1.9	206	34%	3	32	1.1
3198	Roll, sweet, with fruit, no frosting (Include with jelly, sweetbread, Mexican sweetbread, apple rolls, Kolaches, Lakvar, Kuchen) [1 roll (2½" dia)]	55	1.9	202	37%	3	29	1.4
3199	Roll, sweet, with fruit and nuts, frosted [1 roll (2½" dia)]	55	1.9	213	38%	3	31	1.1
3200	Roll, sweet, with fruit and nuts, no frosting [1 roll (2½" dia)]	39	1.4	149	42%	3	20	1.0
3201	Roll, sweet, with fruit, frosted, low calorie (Include Weight Watcher's Apple Sweet Roll) [1 roll (2½" dia)]	55	1.9	151	19%	3	28	1.1
3202	Roll, sweet, Mexican, Pan Dulce, crumb topping (Include Pan de Huevo, crumb topping; Pan de Huevo; Pan Dulce; Mexican sweet bread) [1 roll]	79	2.8	291	28%	5	48	1.1
3203	Roll, sweet, Mexican, Pan Dulce, no topping (Include Pan de Huevo, no topping) [1 roll]	69	2.4	214	18%	5	39	1.1
3204	Roll, sweet, Mexican, Pan Dulce, sugar topping (Include Pan de Huevo, sugar topping) [1 roll]	77	2.7	262	26%	5	44	1.0
3205	Roll, sweet, with nuts, frosted (Include caramel roll) [1 roll (2½" dia)]	39	1.4	147	38%	2	21	0.8
3206	Roll, sweet, with nuts, no frosting [1 roll (2½" dia)]	55	1.9	213	44%	3	27	1.5
3207	Roll, sweet, with raisins and icing, Mexican (Pan Dulce) [1 roll]	72	2.5	280	24%	5	49	1.2
3208	Roll, white, hard (Include Kaiser) [1 roll]	50	1.8	147	13%	5	26	1.2
3209	Roll, white, soft (Include potato roll; onion roll; roll made from mix; soft, seeded roll; brown 'n' serve; hamburger; frankfurter; crescent roll) [1 roll]	28	1.0	80	16%	2	14	0.8
3210	Roll, white, soft, made from home recipe or purchased at a bakery [1 roll]	36	1.3	114	21%	3	19	0.7
3211	Roll, white, soft, reduced calorie, high fiber (Include Less) [1 roll]	43	1.5	84	9%	4	18	2.7
3212	Roll, whole wheat, 100% [1 roll]	36	1.3	96	16%	3	18	2.7
3213	Roll, whole wheat, 100%, made from home recipe or purchased at bakery [1 roll]	36	1.3	103	24%	4	17	2.4
3214	Roll, whole wheat, less than 100% [1 roll]	36	1.3	98	21%	3	17	1.4
3215	Roll, whole wheat, less than 100%, made from home recipe or purchased at bakery [1 roll]	36	1.3	106	23%	3	17	1.3
3216	Scone [1 scone]	42	1.5	150	38%	4	19	0.6
3217	Scone, whole wheat [1 scone]	42	1.5	144	42%	5	18	2.7
3218	Scone, with fruit [1 scone]	42	1.5	150	34%	4	21	0.7
3219	Spoonbread [1 cup]	187	6.6	311	38%	13	34	2.4
3220	Taco shell (Include tostada shell) [2 shells (5" dia)]	26	0.9	122	43%	2	16	2.0
3221	Taco shell, flour (Include flour tostada shell; fried flour tortilla; taco salad shell) [1 shell (7" dia)]	34	1.2	173	47%	3	19	1.2
3222	Toaster muffin, fruit, toasted (Include apple spice) [1 muffin]	33	1.2	110	27%	2	19	0.6
3223	Tortilla, corn [2 tortillas (6" dia)]	38	1.3	84	10%	2	18	2.0
3224	Tortilla, flour [1 tortilla (8" dia)]	52	1.8	169	20%	5	29	1.7
3225	Tortilla, whole wheat (Include chapati and puri) [1 tortilla]	35	1.2	73	6%	3	20	1.9
3226	Whole wheat, cracked (Include home ground) [1 cup]	120	4.2	392	4%	15	85	14.6
3227	Zwieback (Include rusk) [5 pieces]	35	1.2	149	20%	4	26	0.9
	Crackers, Pretzels, Chips							
3250	Cheese puffs and twists, lowfat [10 pieces]	13	0.5	56	25%	1	9	1.4
3251	Corn cake, puffed (Include Quaker) [3 cakes]	33	1.2	128	6%	3	28	0.6
3252	Corn chips, salted (Include plain, flavored, or barbecued; Fritos) [10 chips]	18	0.6	97	56%	1	10	0.9

Food No.	fat gm	sat fat gm	choles mg	sodium mg	potas mg	vit A	vit E	vit C	thia	ribo	niac	vit B-6	fola	vit B-12	calc	phos	mag	iron	zinc
						% of Daily Value													
3186	5	1	0	560	141	0	2	0	32	18	20	2	7	0	14	9	5	18	4
3187	2	0	1	7	98	0	0	0	46	28	33	2	10	0	1	9	6	21	5
3188	2	0	0	128	42	0	1	0	9	5	6	1	2	0	3	3	3	6	2
3189	2	0	0	149	39	0	1	0	11	6	9	1	3	0	3	4	3	8	2
3190	2	1	7	7	52	1	1	0	10	7	6	1	3	0	1	5	3	5	3
3191	1	0	0	205	75	0	1	0	9	6	5	2	3	0	2	6	5	6	4
3192	1	0	0	321	65	0	1	0	9	6	7	1	2	0	1	6	5	5	2
3193	1	0	0	274	51	0	0	0	16	9	11	1	3	0	3	5	3	6	3
3194	9	2	36	211	61	4	7	2	12	9	7	3	3	1	4	4	2	5	2
3195	8	2	29	183	51	4	7	1	10	7	5	2	3	1	3	3	2	4	2
3196	9	2	36	211	61	4	7	2	12	9	7	3	3	1	4	4	2	5	2
3197	8	2	26	166	75	4	6	2	9	6	5	3	2	1	3	3	2	4	2
3198	8	2	34	196	86	3	7	2	11	8	6	3	3	1	4	4	2	5	2
3199	9	2	26	166	70	4	6	2	9	7	5	3	3	1	3	4	3	4	2
3200	7	2	23	136	62	2	5	1	8	6	4	3	2	1	3	3	2	4	2
3201	3	1	21	156	79	1	2	1	11	11	8	2	10	1	4	6	2	6	2
3202	9	2	26	75	57	7	6	0	15	13	10	1	5	1	1	6	2	10	2
3203	4	1	34	12	59	2	2	0	16	13	10	2	6	1	1	6	2	10	3
3204	8	2	33	55	79	5	5	0	15	13	10	2	5	1	2	6	3	11	3
3205	6	1	20	122	42	2	4	1	7	5	4	2	2	1	4	3	2	3	1
3206	11	2	34	199	69	3	7	2	13	8	6	3	3	1	4	5	3	5	3
3207	7	2	32	51	84	5	5	0	15	13	10	2	5	1	1	6	3	10	2
3208	2	0	0	272	54	0	0	0	16	10	11	1	2	0	5	5	3	9	3
3209	1	0	0	157	39	0	1	0	9	5	6	1	2	0	4	2	1	5	1
3210	3	1	13	149	55	3	2	0	9	9	6	1	4	1	2	5	2	6	2
3211	1	0	0	190	34	0	0	0	11	4	11	1	3	2	3	6	3	7	3
3212	2	0	0	172	98	0	2	0	6	3	7	4	3	0	4	8	8	5	5
3213	3	0	12	17	165	1	3	0	5	6	6	4	3	1	4	10	9	5	5
3214	2	1	0	122	48	0	2	0	10	6	7	2	1	0	6	4	4	7	2
3215	3	0	12	17	131	1	2	0	8	8	6	3	3	1	4	7	6	6	3
3216	6	2	49	171	49	7	3	0	10	10	6	1	2	2	8	7	2	7	2
3217	7	2	50	175	114	7	4	0	6	6	6	4	3	2	9	13	8	6	5
3218	6	2	44	153	78	6	3	0	9	9	6	2	2	2	7	7	2	7	2
3219	13	5	167	196	369	22	6	2	17	34	8	9	8	11	23	26	10	11	9
3220	6	1	0	95	47	1	4	0	4	1	2	5	0	0	4	6	7	4	2
3221	9	2	0	168	46	0	7	0	9	5	6	1	1	0	4	4	2	6	2
3222	3	1	2	168	29	2	1	0	4	5	3	0	1	0	0	6	1	1	1
3223	1	0	0	61	59	1	0	0	3	2	3	4	1	0	7	12	6	3	2
3224	4	1	0	249	68	0	3	0	18	9	9	1	2	0	7	6	3	10	2
3225	0	0	0	171	82	0	2	0	7	1	4	3	2	0	1	8	6	4	4
3226	2	0	0	2	414	0	8	0	24	7	30	16	8	0	3	33	38	20	21
3227	3	1	7	81	107	0	1	3	5	5	2	1	2	0	1	2	1	1	1
3250	2	0	0	167	37	5	6	5	5	5	5	5	5	5	5	5	1	1	2
3251	1	0	0	161	52	1	0	0	5	1	8	2	2	0	1	5	9	3	4
3252	6	1	0	113	26	0	1	0	0	2	1	2	1	0	2	3	3	1	2

Grains, Beans, Nuts, Seeds

Food No.	Food Description & Amount	wt gm	wt oz	cal	% cal fat	prot gm	carbo gm	fiber gm
3253	Corn chips, unsalted (Include plain, flavored, or barbecued) [10 chips]	18	0.6	97	53%	1	10	0.8
3254	Corn or corn-cheese puffs and twists (Include Cheetos, Cheez Doodles, Funyuns, Bugles, Diggers, Flings, Planter's Sour Cream & Onion Puffs, Pizza Crunchies) [10 pieces]	15	0.5	83	56%	1	8	0.2
3255	Corn nuts (Include Frito Lay Toasted Corn Nuggets) [10 nuts]	18	0.6	79	29%	2	13	1.2
3256	Cracker, animal (Include sweet crackers) [10 crackers]	30	1.1	134	28%	2	22	0.3
3257	Cracker, butter (Include flavored snack crackers, bacon chips, Ritz, Waverly Wafers, Nabisco Dip and Chip, Club, Escorts, Sociables, Quackers, Keebler Toasteds, sesame seed crackers, meal mates) [10 crackers]	30	1.1	151	45%	2	18	0.5
3258	Cracker, butter, low sodium [10 crackers]	30	1.1	151	45%	2	18	0.5
3259	Cracker, cheese, low sodium (Include low-salt Better Cheddars) [10 crackers (1½" dia)]	13	0.5	65	45%	1	8	0.3
3260	Cracker, cheese, reduced fat (Include Snackwell's) [1 cup]	48	1.7	199	16%	6	34	1.3
3261	Cracker, cheese, reduced fat (Include Cheez-its) [1 cup]	64	2.3	265	16%	9	46	1.7
3262	Cracker, cheese (Include cheese sticks, Cheeblers, Cheez-its, Cheese Ritz, Better Cheddar, Cheddar Jrs.) [10 crackers]	30	1.1	151	45%	3	17	0.7
3263	Cracker, corn (Include Stoned Corn Crackers) [1 cracker (1 square or 2 rectangular pieces)]	37	1.3	177	43%	3	23	1.7
3264	Cracker, Cuban [5 crackers]	25	0.9	100	15%	2	19	0.5
3265	Cracker, Cuca [1 cracker]	28	1.0	122	24%	3	20	0.8
3266	Cracker, cylindrical, peanut butter-filled (Include Combos) [10 combos]	29	1.0	151	54%	5	14	1.4
3267	Cracker, graham [2 large rectangular or 4 squares or 8 small rectangular pieces]	28	1.0	118	21%	2	22	0.8
3268	Cracker, graham, higher fat (Include Graham Bites) [1 cup,]	64	2.3	289	34%	4	45	1.2
3269	Cracker, graham, fat free [1 cup]	44	1.6	164	2%	4	37	1.7
3270	Cracker, graham, chocolate covered [2 crackers (2½" x 2" x ¼")]	26	0.9	126	43%	2	17	0.8
3271	Cracker, graham, sugar-honey coated, cinnamon crisps (Include Teddy Grahams honey or cinnamon flavor) [2 large rectangular or 4 squares or 8 small rectangular pieces]	28	1.0	118	21%	2	22	0.8
3272	Crackers, graham, sandwich-type, with filling [10 sandwich crackers]	23	0.8	101	31%	1	17	0.3
3273	Cracker, graham, with raisins [2 large rectangular or 4 squares or 8 small rectangular pieces]	30	1.1	122	18%	2	24	0.9
3274	Cracker, high fiber (Include Wasa fiber-plus crisp bread) [2 crackers (4½" x 2½" x 1/8")]	22	0.8	73	2%	2	18	5.0
3275	Cracker, matzo [1 matzo]	30	1.1	119	3%	3	25	0.9
3276	Cracker, matzo, low sodium (Include with wheat germ) [1 matzo]	30	1.1	118	5%	3	24	1.1
3277	Cracker, milk (Include Milk Lunch New England Biscuit, Royal Lunch cracker) [2 crackers]	22	0.8	100	31%	2	15	0.4
3278	Cracker, mixed grain, salt free (Include Venus corn wafer, wheat wafer, rye wafer, and cracked wheat wafer) [10 crackers]	30	1.1	138	36%	3	20	0.6
3279	Cracker, oat bran (Include Nabisco Oat Thin) [10 crackers]	20	0.7	87	27%	2	14	1.0
3280	Cracker, oatmeal [2 crackers]	22	0.8	103	34%	2	15	0.6
3281	Cracker, oyster (Include chowder cracker) [1 cup]	45	1.6	195	24%	4	32	1.4
3282	Cracker, rice (Include rice paper) [10 crackers]	30	1.1	117	13%	2	23	0.4
3283	Cracker, saltine (Include soda cracker, Sea Toast, Uneeda Biscuit) [10 crackers]	30	1.1	130	24%	3	21	0.9
3284	Cracker, saltine, low sodium (Include low-sodium soda, oyster, chowder crackers; unsalted top, low salt) [10 crackers]	30	1.1	130	24%	3	21	0.9
3285	Cracker, saltine, fat free, low sodium [10 crackers]	31	1.1	122	4%	3	26	0.8
3286	Cracker, saltine, whole wheat [1 cracker]	30	1.1	131	28%	3	21	1.8
3287	Cracker, sandwich-type, peanut butter or cheese-filled (Include rye-cheese) [4 crackers]	32	1.1	154	43%	4	18	0.9
3288	Cracker, snack, lowfat, low sodium [10 crackers]	23	0.8	102	26%	2	17	0.7
3289	Cracker, snack, reduced fat [10 crackers]	26	0.9	102	7%	2	21	0.4
3290	Cracker, snack, reduced fat (Include Ritz) [10 crackers]	30	1.1	117	7%	2	25	0.5
3291	Cracker, snack, fat free (Include Snackwell's) [10 crackers]	23	0.8	88	3%	2	19	0.4

Food No.	fat gm	sat fat gm	choles mg	sodium mg	potas mg	vit A	vit E	vit C	thia	ribo	niac	vit B-6	fola	vit B-12	calc	phos	mag	iron	zinc
						% of Daily Value													
3253	6	1	0	3	33	1	6	1	2	2	1	2	0	0	2	3	3	2	1
3254	5	1	1	158	25	1	3	0	3	3	2	1	5	0	1	2	1	2	0
3255	3	0	0	99	50	0	1	0	0	1	2	2	0	0	0	5	5	2	2
3256	4	1	0	118	30	0	2	0	7	6	5	0	1	0	1	3	1	5	1
3257	8	1	0	254	40	0	6	0	8	6	6	1	1	0	4	7	2	6	1
3258	8	1	0	112	107	0	6	0	8	6	6	1	1	0	4	7	2	6	1
3259	3	1	2	60	14	0	1	0	5	3	3	4	1	1	2	3	1	3	1
3260	4	1	0	545	72	2	2	2	20	13	15	1	4	0	5	8	4	12	4
3261	5	1	0	727	96	3	3	3	27	18	19	2	5	0	7	11	5	17	5
3262	8	3	4	299	44	1	1	0	11	8	7	8	2	2	5	7	3	8	2
3263	8	2	0	406	41	1	5	0	11	6	7	3	2	0	2	6	3	7	1
3264	2	0	0	60	64	0	1	0	1	0	1	1	1	0	2	2	3	2	1
3265	3	1	0	365	36	0	2	0	11	8	7	1	2	0	3	3	2	8	1
3266	9	1	1	225	97	0	7	0	10	5	10	2	6	0	2	5	6	7	3
3267	3	1	0	169	38	0	2	0	4	5	6	1	1	0	1	3	2	6	2
3268	11	3	0	321	173	0	2	0	3	16	8	2	2	0	6	21	4	12	3
3269	0	0	0	153	61	0	0	0	14	8	10	2	2	0	1	5	4	12	3
3270	6	3	0	76	54	0	2	0	2	3	3	1	1	0	2	3	4	5	2
3271	3	1	0	169	38	0	2	0	4	5	6	1	1	0	1	3	2	6	2
3272	3	1	0	90	45	1	1	0	1	4	2	0	1	0	2	5	1	3	1
3273	3	1	0	149	74	0	2	0	4	5	5	2	1	0	1	3	2	6	1
3274	0	0	0	175	109	0	2	0	6	4	2	3	2	0	1	7	7	7	4
3275	0	0	0	1	34	0	1	0	8	5	6	2	1	0	0	3	2	5	1
3276	1	0	0	1	52	0	2	0	10	6	6	3	3	0	0	5	4	6	4
3277	3	1	4	130	25	0	2	0	8	5	5	0	1	0	4	7	1	4	1
3278	6	1	0	3	65	0	1	0	10	6	7	2	2	0	1	6	4	7	2
3279	3	0	0	120	41	0	2	0	7	3	3	1	1	0	2	6	3	4	2
3280	4	1	0	62	53	0	3	0	6	3	3	1	1	0	1	3	3	4	1
3281	5	1	0	586	58	0	3	0	17	12	12	1	3	0	5	5	3	14	2
3282	2	0	0	1	33	0	2	0	1	1	2	2	1	0	1	3	2	1	2
3283	4	1	0	391	38	0	2	0	11	8	8	1	2	0	4	3	2	9	2
3284	4	1	0	191	217	0	2	0	11	8	8	1	2	0	4	3	2	9	2
3285	0	0	0	197	36	0	0	0	11	11	9	1	1	0	1	4	2	13	2
3286	4	1	0	311	64	0	3	0	10	6	8	2	2	0	1	6	5	7	3
3287	7	2	2	317	78	1	6	0	9	6	10	24	2	0	3	10	5	5	2
3288	3	0	0	67	31	0	2	0	7	3	5	1	1	0	2	5	2	6	1
3289	1	0	0	283	32	0	1	0	12	6	8	0	1	0	4	4	1	10	1
3290	1	0	0	326	37	0	1	0	14	7	9	1	1	0	5	4	1	12	1
3291	0	0	0	234	27	0	0	0	11	5	7	1	1	0	4	7	1	9	1

Food No.	Food Description & Amount	wt gm	wt oz	cal	% cal fat	prot gm	carbo gm	fiber gm
3292	Cracker, toast thin (rye, pumpernickel, white flour) (Include pizza thin, pumpernickel, onion toast, Won-Ton Chip) [10 crackers]	20	0.7	92	36%	2	14	0.4
3293	Cracker, toast thin (rye, wheat, white flour), low sodium (Include Low Salt Wheat Thin) [10 crackers]	20	0.7	92	36%	2	14	0.4
3294	Cracker, water biscuit [10 crackers]	40	1.4	166	27%	4	28	1.3
3295	Cracker, wheat (Include Wheatsworth, Euphrates, Wheatable, Wheat Thin, toasted wheat, cracked wheat, stoned wheat) [10 crackers]	40	1.4	189	39%	3	26	1.8
3296	Cracker, wheat, reduced fat [10 crackers]	14	0.5	60	25%	1	10	0.8
3297	Cracker, wheat, reduced fat (Include Wheat Thins) [10 crackers]	17	0.6	72	25%	2	12	1.0
3298	Cracker, 100% whole wheat (Include 100% stoned wheat, Triscuits, Wheatbury, Wheatmeal English Biscuits) [10 crackers]	40	1.4	177	35%	4	27	4.2
3299	Cracker, 100% whole wheat, low sodium (Include low sodium 100% stoned wheat wafers, Triscuits) [10 crackers]	40	1.4	177	35%	4	27	4.2
3300	Cracker, 100% whole wheat, reduced fat (Include Triscuit) [10 crackers]	39	1.4	158	23%	5	28	5.1
3301	Cracker, whole wheat and bran (Include Wheat 'N Bran Triscuit) [10 crackers]	40	1.4	176	35%	4	27	4.4
3302	Crispbread, rye (Include Ry Krisp, Wasa rye crispbread, Finn rye crisp, Norwegian flatbread) [5 crackers (3½" x 1-7/8" x ¼")]	35	1.2	128	3%	3	29	5.8
3303	Crispbread, rye, low sodium [5 crackers (3½" x 1-7/8" x ¼")]	35	1.2	128	3%	3	29	5.8
3304	Crispbread, wheat (Include Armenian cracker bread, Lavosh, hardtack) [5 crackers]	30	1.1	122	2%	3	26	0.9
3305	Crispbread, wheat, low sodium (Include Low Sodium French Crisp Toast) [3 crackers]	26	0.9	103	2%	3	22	0.8
3306	Crispbread, white or rye, fat ingredient added (Include Wasa Extra Crisp) [5 crackers (5" x 2")]	30	1.1	119	15%	3	22	2.1
3307	Multigrain, chips [10 chips]	21	0.7	109	45%	1	13	1.3
3308	Multigrain mixture, pretzels, chex cereal, nuts (Include Chex Party Mix) [1 cup]	45	1.6	193	28%	5	31	2.5
3309	Multigrain mixture, bread sticks, sesame nuggets, pretzels, rye chips [1 cup]	103	3.6	493	43%	9	61	2.5
3310	Onion-flavored rings [20 rings]	20	0.7	100	41%	2	13	0.8
3311	Oriental party mix, with peanuts, sesame sticks, chili rice crackers and fried green peas [1 cup]	112	4.0	610	42%	19	58	14.8
3312	Popcorn cake (Include Chicosan; puffed corn and rice cake) [3 cakes]	27	1.0	104	7%	3	22	0.8
3313	Popcorn, air-popped [2 cups]	16	0.6	61	10%	2	12	2.4
3314	Popcorn, air-popped, buttered [2 cups]	26	0.9	126	52%	2	14	2.7
3315	Popcorn, buttered [2 cups]	28	1.0	146	57%	2	14	2.5
3316	Popcorn, flavored (Include cheese-, butter-, barbecued-, sour cream and onion-flavored) [2 cups]	24	0.8	121	53%	2	12	2.4
3317	Popcorn, microwave, lowfat, low sodium (Include Orville Redenbacher's Light Microwave popcorn) [2 cups]	12	0.4	48	21%	1	8	1.6
3318	Popcorn, popped in oil (Include microwave popcorn) [2 cups]	28	1.0	140	51%	3	16	2.8
3319	Popcorn, popped in oil, unsalted [2 cups]	16	0.6	82	51%	1	9	1.6
3320	Popcorn, popped in oil, lowfat [2 cups]	15	0.5	62	21%	2	11	2.2
3321	Popcorn, sugar syrup or caramel-coated [1 cup]	35	1.2	151	27%	1	28	1.8
3322	Popcorn, sugar syrup or caramel-coated, fat free [1 cup]	33	1.2	117	4%	1	29	0.8
3323	Popcorn, sugar syrup or caramel-coated, with nuts [1 cup]	35	1.2	140	18%	2	28	1.3
3324	Popcorn, with cheese (Include with parmesan cheese) [1 cup]	26	0.9	129	51%	3	13	2.3
3325	Pretzel, hard, unsalted [20 sticks (2½" x 1/8")]	10	0.4	38	8%	1	8	0.3
3326	Pretzel, yogurt-covered [10 pretzels (1-5/8" x 1-1/8" x ¼")]	42	1.5	192	36%	4	28	0.4
3327	Pretzel, baby [5 pretzels]	30	1.1	119	5%	3	25	0.7
3328	Pretzel, cheese-filled (Include Combos) [10 combos]	30	1.1	129	34%	3	18	0.7
3329	Pretzel, chocolate-coated [2 pretzels]	22	0.8	92	24%	2	16	0.7
3330	Pretzel, hard (Include flavored) [20 sticks (2½" x 1/8")]	10	0.4	38	8%	1	8	0.3
3331	Pretzel, hard, oatbran [10 pretzels]	30	1.1	115	13%	4	22	1.2
3332	Pretzel, hard, multigrain [10 pretzels]	30	1.1	114	7%	4	24	2.9
3333	Pretzel, soft [1 pretzel]	55	1.9	190	8%	5	38	0.9

Food No.	fat gm	sat fat gm	choles mg	sodium mg	potas mg	% of Daily Value													
						vit A	vit E	vit C	thia	ribo	niac	vit B-6	fola	vit B-12	calc	phos	mag	iron	zinc
3292	4	1	0	171	43	0	1	0	6	4	5	1	1	0	1	4	3	4	1
3293	4	1	0	50	43	0	1	0	6	4	5	1	1	0	1	4	3	4	1
3294	5	1	4	188	56	0	5	0	3	1	4	1	1	0	5	3	2	4	2
3295	8	1	0	318	73	0	7	0	13	8	10	3	2	0	2	9	6	10	4
3296	2	0	0	99	31	0	2	0	4	2	4	1	1	0	1	4	2	4	1
3297	2	0	0	121	37	0	2	0	5	3	4	1	1	0	2	5	3	5	2
3298	7	1	0	264	119	0	7	0	5	2	9	4	3	0	2	12	10	7	6
3299	7	1	0	99	119	0	7	0	5	2	9	4	3	0	2	12	10	7	6
3300	4	1	0	165	152	0	5	0	9	4	11	6	3	0	1	13	13	8	7
3301	7	1	0	260	124	0	7	0	5	3	9	4	3	0	2	12	11	7	6
3302	0	0	0	92	112	0	2	0	6	3	2	4	2	0	1	9	7	5	6
3303	0	0	0	92	112	0	2	0	6	3	2	4	2	0	1	9	7	5	6
3304	0	0	0	1	36	0	0	0	14	9	9	1	2	0	1	4	2	9	2
3305	0	0	0	83	30	0	0	0	12	7	7	1	1	0	0	3	2	7	1
3306	2	0	0	191	84	0	2	0	8	6	5	2	1	1	2	6	3	5	3
3307	5	0	0	88	28	1	5	0	1	0	1	2	1	0	0	2	2	1	1
3308	6	1	1	419	131	1	3	20	26	10	29	24	24	21	3	12	10	41	7
3309	23	4	1	1258	113	0	28	0	36	25	24	3	10	0	2	12	6	22	5
3310	5	1	0	196	29	0	1	1	3	4	3	1	1	0	1	1	1	4	0
3311	29	4	0	463	367	0	13	1	23	10	17	4	11	0	6	29	33	15	20
3312	1	0	0	78	88	0	0	0	1	3	8	2	1	0	0	7	11	3	7
3313	1	0	0	1	48	0	0	0	2	3	2	2	1	0	0	5	5	2	4
3314	7	4	17	67	56	6	1	0	2	3	2	2	1	0	0	6	6	3	4
3315	9	3	6	246	58	2	0	0	2	2	2	3	1	0	0	6	7	4	4
3316	7	2	2	201	57	1	4	0	2	3	2	2	1	0	2	6	5	2	4
3317	1	0	0	57	28	0	1	0	3	1	1	1	0	0	0	3	4	1	3
3318	8	1	0	248	63	0	0	0	3	2	2	3	1	0	0	7	8	4	5
3319	5	1	0	0	37	0	4	0	1	1	1	2	1	0	0	4	4	3	3
3320	1	0	0	134	37	0	1	0	4	1	2	1	1	0	0	4	6	2	4
3321	4	1	2	72	38	0	2	0	2	1	4	0	0	0	2	3	3	3	1
3322	0	0	0	94	36	0	0	0	1	1	1	1	0	0	1	2	2	1	1
3323	3	0	0	103	124	0	2	0	1	3	3	3	1	0	2	4	7	8	3
3324	7	2	2	255	55	1	0	0	2	2	2	3	1	1	4	8	7	4	5
3325	0	0	0	29	15	0	0	0	3	4	3	1	2	0	0	1	1	2	1
3326	8	6	1	26	101	3	1	1	9	9	6	1	2	3	6	6	2	4	2
3327	1	0	0	81	41	0	0	2	9	6	5	1	2	0	1	3	2	6	2
3328	5	1	4	421	85	3	3	0	7	12	6	2	5	1	6	7	3	6	2
3329	2	1	1	277	47	0	0	0	5	7	4	1	3	0	2	3	2	4	1
3330	0	0	0	172	15	0	0	0	3	4	3	1	2	0	0	1	1	2	1
3331	2	0	0	219	58	0	2	0	4	3	3	1	6	0	1	6	4	3	2
3332	1	0	0	3	86	0	1	0	6	3	6	4	2	0	1	9	10	4	5
3333	2	0	2	772	48	0	0	0	15	9	12	1	2	0	1	4	3	12	3

Grains, Beans, Nuts, Seeds

Food No.	Food Description & Amount	wt gm	wt oz	cal	% cal fat	prot gm	carbo gm	fiber gm
3334	Rice cakes, puffed (Include Arden, Chico San, Quaker, Spiral, rice cakes with seeds and other grains) [3 cakes]	27	1.0	104	7%	2	22	1.1
3335	Puffed rice cake, without salt (Include with seeds and other grains) [3 cakes]	27	1.0	104	7%	2	22	1.1
3336	Puffed wheat cake (Include Quaker Wheat Cakes) [3 cakes]	27	1.0	98	5%	4	20	2.5
3337	Rice cake, cracker-type [10 mini rounds (1¾" dia)]	30	1.1	120	10%	2	25	1.3
3338	Rice paper [2 pieces (8-5/8" dia)]	28	1.0	93	3%	1	21	0.6
3339	Salty snacks, wheat-based, high fiber [1 bag (1.5 oz)]	43	1.5	165	29%	5	28	8.1
3340	Salty snack mix, mostly corn-based, with pretzels, without nuts [1 cup]	40	1.4	202	47%	3	25	1.4
3341	Shrimp chips (tapioca base) [1 cup]	40	1.4	224	58%	3	21	0.2
3342	Tortilla chips (Include flavored or barbecued, Tostitos, Doritos, Suncheros) [10 chips]	18	0.6	90	47%	1	11	1.2
3343	Tortilla chips, light (baked with less oil) (Include flavored; Doritos Light) [10 chips]	16	0.6	74	30%	1	11	0.9
3344	Tortilla chips, lowfat, baked without fat [10 chips]	14	0.5	54	13%	2	11	0.7
3345	Tortilla chips, lowfat, baked without fat, unsalted [10 chips]	14	0.5	54	13%	2	11	0.7
3346	Tortilla chips, unsalted (Include flavored or barbecued) [10 chips]	18	0.6	91	47%	1	11	1.2
3347	Tortilla chips, with oat bran [10 chips]	18	0.6	88	47%	1	11	1.3
3348	Wheat- and corn-based chips [10 chips]	22	0.8	108	40%	2	14	0.7
3349	Wheat sticks, 100% whole wheat (Include with sesame seeds) [1 cup]	55	1.9	298	61%	6	26	1.5
	Pancakes and Waffles							
3350	Bread fritters, Puerto Rican style (Torrejas, Galician fritters) [2 fritters with syrup (4" x 2½" x 3¼")]	110	3.9	291	28%	5	48	0.8
3351	Crepe, plain (Include French pancake) [1 crepe (7" dia)]	50	1.8	113	45%	4	11	0.3
3352	Flour and milk patty [2 pancakes]	56	2.0	139	19%	5	25	4.0
3353	Flour and water patty (Include Chinese pancake) [2 pancakes]	56	2.0	116	2%	2	25	0.4
3354	French toast sticks, plain [2 sticks]	44	1.6	160	51%	3	18	0.8
3355	French toast, plain (Include Roman Meal) [1 slice]	65	2.3	160	35%	6	20	0.8
3356	Funnel cake [1 cake (6" dia)]	90	3.2	278	47%	7	29	0.9
3357	Pancakes, buckwheat [1 pancake (5" dia)]	40	1.4	71	32%	3	10	1.0
3358	Pancakes, cornmeal [1 pancake (5" dia)]	40	1.4	81	27%	2	13	0.9
3359	Pancakes, made with rice flour and dried peas (Include Indian pancakes) [2 pancakes]	58	2.0	158	3%	5	33	3.9
3360	Pancake, Norwegian Lefse, potato and flour [1 lefse (6" dia)]	34	1.2	78	30%	1	12	0.7
3361	Pancakes, plain [1 pancake (5" dia)]	40	1.4	92	13%	2	17	0.7
3362	Pancakes, reduced calorie, high fiber [1 pancake (4" dia)]	32	1.1	59	17%	2	12	2.2
3363	Pancakes, rye [1 pancake (5" dia)]	40	1.4	120	31%	3	18	1.2
3364	Pancakes, sour dough [1 pancake (5" dia)]	40	1.4	88	26%	2	14	0.6
3365	Pancakes, whole wheat [1 pancake (5" dia)]	40	1.4	93	40%	3	12	1.5
3366	Pancakes, with fruit (Include blueberry pancakes) [1 pancake (5" dia)]	40	1.4	76	30%	3	11	0.8
3367	Rice paste (Japanese Mochi) [2 oz]	56	2.0	132	2%	3	29	1.4
3368	Waffle, oat bran (Include Eggo) [1 waffle (4" square)]	38	1.3	107	33%	3	15	2.1
3369	Waffle, 100% whole wheat or 100% whole grain [1 waffle (4" square)]	37	1.3	99	38%	3	12	0.9
3370	Waffle, cornmeal [1 waffle (4" square)]	37	1.3	102	32%	3	14	0.8
3371	Waffle, fruit (Include blueberry) [1 waffle (4" square)]	37	1.3	88	27%	2	14	0.9
3372	Waffle, nut and honey [1 waffle (4" square)]	46	1.6	153	42%	4	20	0.4
3373	Waffle, multi-bran [1 waffle (4" square)]	38	1.3	103	38%	3	14	1.0
3374	Waffle, plain [1 waffle (4" square)]	37	1.3	98	28%	2	15	0.9
3375	Waffle, plain, fat free [1 waffle (4" square)]	30	1.1	74	1%	3	15	0.4
3376	Waffle, wheat, bran, or mixed grain (Include Roman Meal; Nutri-Grain Raisin and Bran) [1 waffle (4" square)]	37	1.3	111	34%	3	17	1.8
	Cooked Cereals (salt not added when optional, unless specified)							
3400	Barley, cooked [1 cup]	162	5.7	199	3%	4	46	6.2
3401	Buckwheat groats, cooked (Include kasha) [1 cup]	168	5.9	155	6%	6	33	4.5
3402	Bulgur, cooked or canned (Include wheat pilaf) [1 cup]	135	4.8	112	3%	4	25	6.1

Food No.	fat gm	sat fat gm	choles mg	sodium mg	potas mg	vit A	vit E	vit C	thia	ribo	niac	vit B-6	fola	vit B-12	calc	phos	mag	iron	zinc
						% of Daily Value													
3334	1	0	0	88	78	0	1	0	1	3	11	2	1	0	0	10	9	2	5
3335	1	0	0	7	78	0	0	0	1	3	11	2	1	0	0	10	9	2	5
3336	1	0	0	126	97	0	1	0	7	4	16	2	2	2	1	9	9	7	5
3337	1	0	0	21	128	0	1	0	1	3	12	2	2	0	0	11	10	2	6
3338	0	0	0	88	19	0	0	0	2	0	3	5	0	0	0	2	2	1	1
3339	5	1	0	88	153	0	7	0	9	7	12	6	7	0	2	13	12	8	7
3340	11	2	1	386	65	1	4	0	5	8	5	4	7	0	4	6	5	5	2
3341	14	3	23	31	30	0	19	0	0	0	2	1	0	2	2	3	1	4	1
3342	5	1	0	95	35	0	1	0	1	2	1	3	0	0	3	4	4	2	2
3343	2	0	0	160	44	1	2	0	2	3	0	1	1	0	3	5	4	1	1
3344	1	0	0	57	37	1	2	0	2	2	0	1	1	0	2	4	3	1	1
3345	1	0	0	2	37	1	2	0	2	2	0	1	1	0	2	4	3	1	1
3346	5	1	0	44	34	1	3	1	1	2	1	2	0	0	3	4	4	2	1
3347	5	1	0	90	39	0	1	0	1	2	1	3	1	0	3	4	4	2	2
3348	5	1	1	202	36	0	4	0	7	5	5	1	1	0	1	3	2	5	1
3349	20	4	0	818	97	0	10	0	5	2	4	2	3	0	9	8	6	2	4
3350	9	2	49	183	97	3	5	0	8	11	6	2	3	3	6	7	3	5	3
3351	6	2	79	38	79	5	3	0	6	11	3	2	2	4	5	7	2	4	3
3352	3	1	2	14	170	1	4	0	8	6	9	5	3	1	4	14	12	7	7
3353	0	0	0	2	37	0	0	0	1	1	3	3	1	0	1	4	2	1	2
3354	9	1	23	156	40	0	6	0	5	5	5	4	10	0	2	4	2	5	2
3355	6	2	91	210	85	5	3	0	9	14	7	3	4	4	6	8	3	7	3
3356	14	3	63	117	155	6	11	1	16	19	9	3	3	4	13	14	4	10	4
3357	3	1	23	184	81	2	1	0	4	5	2	2	1	2	9	14	5	4	3
3358	2	1	16	99	40	3	1	0	6	5	4	2	1	1	5	4	2	4	1
3359	1	0	0	1	162	0	1	0	7	2	5	7	6	0	1	7	6	3	4
3360	3	1	2	46	89	1	1	3	5	3	4	3	1	0	1	2	2	3	1
3361	1	0	4	204	29	1	1	0	10	11	8	1	1	1	2	15	1	8	2
3362	1	0	9	206	59	1	1	0	5	5	3	1	1	2	9	12	2	3	2
3363	4	1	15	111	184	1	3	0	5	5	3	4	1	1	4	5	7	6	2
3364	3	1	16	100	32	1	3	0	8	7	5	1	3	1	1	3	1	5	1
3365	4	1	24	128	96	2	4	0	4	5	4	3	2	2	8	9	5	4	3
3366	3	1	24	169	73	2	2	2	5	6	2	2	1	2	7	10	2	2	2
3367	0	0	0	7	14	0	0	0	2	1	2	2	0	0	0	1	2	1	4
3368	4	1	0	214	189	6	3	0	4	4	4	2	4	4	1	13	10	4	4
3369	4	1	35	125	86	3	2	0	5	7	4	2	2	2	10	9	4	4	3
3370	4	1	35	78	61	3	3	0	7	8	4	2	2	2	6	6	2	5	2
3371	3	0	8	250	47	12	2	2	8	9	7	14	3	13	7	13	2	8	1
3372	7	1	10	295	56	18	2	0	12	12	12	12	12	12	2	18	2	12	2
3373	4	1	0	165	61	0	4	0	7	7	6	2	1	0	4	9	4	6	2
3374	3	1	9	291	47	13	1	0	9	10	8	17	3	15	9	16	2	9	1
3375	0	0	0	130	38	0	0	0	5	7	3	0	1	0	3	5	1	3	1
3376	4	1	25	167	112	6	3	4	9	10	7	5	5	6	11	11	7	8	5
3400	1	0	0	5	151	0	0	0	9	6	17	9	6	0	2	9	9	12	9
3401	1	0	0	7	148	0	2	0	4	4	8	6	6	0	1	12	21	7	7
3402	0	0	0	7	92	0	0	0	5	2	7	6	6	0	1	5	11	7	5

Grains, Beans, Nuts, Seeds

Food No.	Food Description & Amount	wt gm	wt oz	cal	% cal fat	prot gm	carbo gm	fiber gm
3403	Cornmeal dumpling, includes salt (Include boiled cornbread) [1 cup]	240	8.5	405	26%	14	60	4.8
3404	Cornmeal mush, cooked, fried [1 slice]	51	1.8	80	21%	2	14	1.3
3405	Cornmeal mush, made with whole milk, salted [1 cup]	240	8.5	333	20%	15	51	3.4
3406	Cornmeal mush, made with water (Include polenta) [1 cup]	240	8.5	223	4%	5	47	4.5
3407	Cornmeal sticks (cornmeal, coconut milk, molasses, anise seed), boiled (Include guanimes) [1 cup]	211	7.4	380	30%	5	63	4.6
3408	Cornmeal, lime-treated, cooked (Masa harina) (Include Fu Fu) [1 cup]	240	8.5	235	9%	6	49	6.2
3409	Cornmeal, made with milk, sugar, salt, Puerto Rican style (Harina de maiz con leche) [1 cup]	227	8.0	297	21%	8	51	1.8
3410	Couscous, cooked [1 cup]	146	5.1	164	1%	6	34	2.0
3411	Couscous, cooked with salt [1 cup]	162	5.7	237	29%	6	36	2.1
3412	Cream of rice, cooked [1 cup]	244	8.6	127	2%	2	28	0.2
3413	Cream of rice, made with evap. milk, sugar, salt, Puerto Rican style [1 cup]	245	8.6	304	25%	9	48	0.3
3414	Cream of wheat, cooked, instant (Include farina; with fruit, spices, maple and brown sugar) [1 cup]	241	8.5	134	3%	4	28	1.2
3415	Cream of wheat, cooked, quick, salt added in cooking (Include farina) [1 cup]	239	8.4	105	3%	3	22	0.8
3416	Cream of wheat, cooked, regular (Include farina) [1 cup]	251	8.9	110	4%	3	23	1.1
3417	Cream of wheat, cooked with milk, sugar, salt Puerto Rican style [1 cup]	245	8.6	307	26%	10	47	1.0
3418	Cream of wheat, cooked with milk, salt [1 cup]	243	8.6	215	25%	11	29	0.8
3419	Grits, corn or hominy, cooked, made with water (Include regular, quick, instant) [1 cup]	242	8.5	111	3%	3	24	0.5
3420	Grits, corn or hominy, cooked with whole milk, salt (Include regular, quick, instant) [1 cup]	242	8.5	239	22%	11	35	0.5
3421	Grits, corn or hominy, flavored, instant, cooked with water, salt (Include Quaker Instant Grits-Country Ham, Red Eye Gravy, and Country Bacon varieties) [1 cup]	242	8.5	169	14%	4	34	1.9
3422	Grits, corn or hominy, cooked with cheese, salt [1 cup]	247	8.7	194	35%	8	23	0.4
3423	Millet, cooked [1 cup]	131	4.6	156	8%	5	31	1.7
3424	Multigrain cereal, cooked (Include seven-grain cereals) [1 cup]	246	8.7	202	10%	7	40	3.9
3425	Muesli, prepared, instant, with salt [1 cup]	254	9.0	232	14%	15	42	7.2
3426	Nestum, Puerto Rican cereal [1 cup]	245	8.6	42	6%	1	8	1.5
3427	Oats, dry, raw [1 cup]	81	2.9	311	15%	13	54	8.6
3428	Oat bran cereal, cooked (Include Mother's Oat Bran) [1 cup]	242	8.5	81	26%	6	22	5.1
3429	Oat bran cereal, cooked with milk, salt [1 cup]	242	8.5	208	33%	14	33	4.9
3430	Oat bran cereal, multi-grain, cooked, instant (Include Nabisco Oat Bran) [1 cup]	254	9.0	138	18%	8	33	7.7
3431	Oatmeal with raisins, cooked [1 cup]	234	8.3	190	11%	6	38	4.5
3432	Oatmeal with maple flavor, cooked (Include Maypo) [1 cup]	240	8.5	170	13%	6	32	5.8
3433	Oatmeal, cooked with salt, instant (Include with spice, fruit) [1 cup]	234	8.3	226	15%	9	39	6.7
3434	Oatmeal, cooked, regular or quick [1 cup]	234	8.3	146	15%	6	25	4.0
3435	Oatmeal, fortified, cooked, instant, with salt (Include plain, or with spice or fruit; Total Instant Oatmeal) [1 cup]	234	8.3	285	12%	8	57	5.9
3436	Oatmeal, made with milk, sugar, salt, Puerto Rican style (Avena con leche) [1 cup]	210	7.4	263	30%	10	37	1.8
3437	Oatmeal, with oat bran, cooked, fortified, instant, with salt [1 packet]	152	5.4	142	15%	4	26	2.9
3438	Oatmeal, multigrain, cooked [1 cup, cooked]	234	8.3	148	7%	5	33	5.3
3439	Rye, cream of, cooked (rye flour, water) [1 cup]	251	8.9	109	3%	2	24	4.3
3440	Wheat cereal, chocolate flavored, cooked, with salt (Include cocoa wheat cereal, Chocolate Malt-O-Meal) [1 cup]	246	8.7	123	9%	4	27	4.3
3441	Wheat hearts, cooked, with salt [1 cup]	245	8.6	114	5%	4	25	3.2
3442	Wheat, rolled, cooked [1 cup]	242	8.5	114	5%	4	25	3.2
3443	Whole wheat cereal, cooked (Include Wheatena, Ralston, Zoom, Roman Meal, Branola, home ground cereal, Roman Meal with oats) [1 cup, cooked]	246	8.7	114	5%	4	25	3.2
3444	Whole wheat cereal, wheat and barley, cooked (Include Maltex, Malt-O-Meal) [1 cup]	249	8.8	179	5%	6	40	3.0

Food No.	fat gm	sat fat gm	choles mg	sodium mg	potas mg	% of Daily Value													
						vit A	vit E	vit C	thia	ribo	niac	vit B-6	fola	vit B-12	calc	phos	mag	iron	zinc
3403	12	3	189	352	249	16	7	1	31	34	18	11	10	9	21	24	10	22	8
3404	2	0	0	4	29	1	1	0	6	4	4	2	1	0	0	2	2	4	1
3405	8	4	28	163	576	17	2	4	25	40	12	11	7	16	39	35	15	11	11
3406	1	0	0	14	99	2	1	0	23	13	14	7	5	0	1	5	7	14	4
3407	13	11	0	22	712	2	2	2	20	10	14	18	6	0	8	10	30	25	5
3408	2	0	0	19	192	0	1	0	49	26	29	11	3	0	10	14	19	26	9
3409	7	4	26	99	307	6	1	2	11	22	6	4	3	1	23	20	8	7	6
3410	0	0	0	7	85	0	0	0	6	2	7	4	5	0	1	3	3	3	3
3411	8	1	0	94	92	7	5	0	6	3	8	4	6	0	1	4	3	3	3
3412	0	0	0	2	49	0	0	0	0	0	5	3	2	0	1	4	2	3	3
3413	8	5	32	119	357	6	1	3	11	21	7	5	2	2	29	25	8	7	8
3414	1	0	0	12	42	0	0	0	11	4	7	2	3	0	6	4	4	58	3
3415	0	0	0	121	36	0	0	0	8	3	5	1	2	0	5	8	3	44	2
3416	0	0	0	10	34	0	0	0	8	3	6	2	2	0	5	3	3	45	2
3417	9	5	33	123	367	6	1	3	10	23	6	4	3	2	33	25	9	39	7
3418	6	4	23	133	435	13	1	4	12	27	5	6	4	13	35	28	10	33	8
3419	0	0	0	8	39	0	0	0	10	6	7	2	0	0	1	2	3	6	1
3420	6	3	22	128	434	12	1	3	16	30	8	7	3	12	31	26	10	7	7
3421	3	1	1	868	79	0	1	0	14	8	10	4	2	2	3	4	5	74	3
3422	8	5	19	352	109	6	1	0	10	12	6	4	1	5	17	16	4	7	7
3423	1	0	0	3	81	0	1	0	9	6	9	7	6	0	0	13	14	5	8
3424	2	0	0	2	138	0	16	0	26	27	22	23	4	0	7	18	17	30	6
3425	4	1	4	349	671	47	32	28	28	30	30	31	31	31	38	34	32	31	32
3426	0	0	0	8	31	0	1	6	3	5	2	4	1	0	4	5	4	2	2
3427	5	1	0	3	284	1	3	0	39	7	3	5	6	0	4	38	30	19	17
3428	2	0	0	9	177	0	3	0	20	4	1	2	3	0	2	23	20	10	7
3429	8	4	22	127	564	12	3	3	26	27	2	7	6	12	32	46	27	10	13
3430	3	1	0	13	233	66	5	0	39	26	41	44	44	0	4	36	24	44	44
3431	2	0	0	10	253	0	2	1	16	4	2	4	2	0	3	18	15	10	8
3432	2	0	0	10	211	70	8	48	48	42	47	48	2	48	12	25	13	47	10
3433	4	1	0	624	217	98	2	0	68	35	56	80	81	0	36	29	23	76	13
3434	2	0	0	8	126	0	1	0	15	3	1	2	2	0	2	17	15	9	8
3435	4	1	0	547	248	76	2	0	51	28	42	58	63	1	35	27	20	80	12
3436	9	5	30	113	370	6	1	3	9	21	2	3	3	2	28	29	13	5	9
3437	2	0	0	146	120	147	180	96	98	98	98	98	98	98	20	11	9	98	98
3438	1	0	0	7	173	0	2	0	7	3	7	5	2	0	2	15	13	7	10
3439	0	0	0	7	66	0	1	0	5	1	1	3	1	0	1	5	6	3	4
3440	1	0	0	9	219	0	2	0	7	6	8	6	5	0	2	15	15	9	8
3441	1	0	0	8	123	0	2	0	7	5	7	6	5	0	2	12	11	6	6
3442	1	0	0	8	123	0	2	0	7	5	7	6	5	0	2	12	11	6	6
3443	1	0	0	8	124	0	2	0	7	5	7	6	5	0	2	12	11	6	6
3444	1	0	0	10	266	0	4	0	17	6	12	4	6	0	2	18	14	10	12

Grains, Beans, Nuts, Seeds

Food No.	Food Description & Amount	wt gm	wt oz	cal	% cal fat	prot gm	carbo gm	fiber gm
	Ready To Eat Cereals							
3500	40% Bran Flakes, Kellogg [1 cup]	39	1.4	125	6%	4	32	6.6
3501	40+ Bran Flakes [1 cup]	43	1.5	138	6%	4	35	7.2
3502	100% Bran [1 cup]	66	2.3	178	17%	8	48	19.5
3503	100% Natural Cereal, plain [1 cup]	104	3.7	462	33%	11	71	7.8
3504	100% Natural Cereal, with apples and cinnamon [1 cup]	104	3.7	477	37%	11	70	6.9
3505	100% Natural Cereal, with oats, honey and raisins, Quaker [1 cup]	107	3.8	458	30%	10	75	7.7
3506	100% Natural Cereal, with raisins and dates [1 cup]	110	3.9	496	37%	11	72	7.3
3507	100% Natural Wholegrain Cereal with raisins, lowfat, Quaker [1 cup]	87	3.1	337	14%	8	69	5.5
3508	All-Bran with Extra Fiber [1 cup]	57	2.0	100	16%	7	43	29.1
3509	All-Bran [1 cup]	61	2.2	160	12%	8	45	19.8
3510	Almond Delight [1 cup]	38	1.3	147	13%	3	31	2.0
3511	Alpen [1 cup]	113	4.0	398	8%	13	86	10.3
3512	Alpha-Bits [1 cup]	34	1.2	133	5%	3	29	1.5
3513	Alpha-bits with marshmallows [1 cup]	32	1.1	124	4%	2	28	1.0
3514	Amaranth Flakes [1 cup]	38	1.3	134	27%	4	27	3.6
3515	Apple Cinnamon Cheerios [1 cup]	38	1.3	149	12%	2	32	2.0
3516	Apple Cinnamon Oh's Cereal [1 cup]	28	1.0	114	10%	2	24	1.0
3517	Apple Cinnamon Rice Krispies [1 cup]	37	1.3	138	1%	2	33	0.8
3518	Apple Cinnamon Squares [1 cup]	57	2.0	189	5%	4	46	4.9
3519	Apple Jacks [1 cup]	28	1.0	106	3%	1	25	0.9
3520	Apple Raisin Crisp [1 cup]	56	2.0	188	2%	4	48	4.5
3521	Banana-Flavored Frosted Flakes [1 cup]	38	1.3	147	8%	1	34	0.0
3522	Banana Nut Crunch Cereal (Post) [1 cup]	72	2.5	305	23%	8	51	5.1
3523	Basic 4 [1 cup]	49	1.7	179	13%	4	37	3.0
3524	Batman Cereal [1 cup]	28	1.0	108	7%	1	25	0.3
3525	Bill & Ted's Excellent Cereal [1 cup]	28	1.0	109	8%	2	24	1.2
3526	Blueberry Morning, Post [1 cup]	55	1.9	223	14%	4	44	1.9
3527	Berry Berry Kix [1 cup]	31	1.1	124	9%	1	27	0.2
3528	Bigg Mixx [1 cup]	59	2.1	235	14%	4	49	2.6
3529	Body Buddies, natural fruit flavor [1 cup]	33	1.2	127	7%	2	28	1.0
3530	Booberry [1 cup]	33	1.2	128	4%	1	30	0.4
3531	Bran Buds [1 cup]	84	3.0	232	8%	8	67	33.5
3532	Bran Chex [1 cup]	49	1.7	156	8%	5	39	7.9
3533	Bran Muffin Crisp [1 cup]	60	2.1	197	7%	5	47	6.5
3534	Bran News [1 cup]	38	1.3	134	5%	3	31	4.0
3535	Branola [1 cup]	110	3.9	465	22%	24	69	9.4
3536	Breakfast with Barbie [1 cup]	32	1.1	124	6%	2	28	0.6
3537	Buc Wheats [1 cup]	39	1.4	151	8%	4	32	3.5
3538	Bunuelitos cereal [1 cup]	32	1.1	135	15%	1	27	0.3
3539	C-3PO's [1 cup]	33	1.2	128	2%	2	28	0.0
3540	C.W. Post, plain [1 cup]	97	3.4	421	27%	8	73	7.2
3541	C.W. Post, with raisins [1 cup]	103	3.6	446	30%	9	74	13.6
3542	Cabbage Patch [1 cup]	25	0.9	97	7%	2	21	0.2
3543	Cap'n Crunch [1 cup]	37	1.3	147	11%	2	32	1.2
3544	Cap'n Crunch's Choco Crunch [1 cup]	37	1.3	144	16%	1	30	0.7
3545	Cap'n Crunch's Crunch Berries [1 cup]	35	1.2	140	11%	2	30	0.8
3546	Cap'n Crunch's Deep Sea Crunch [1 cup]	32	1.1	129	13%	2	27	0.9
3547	Cap'n Crunch's Peanut Butter Crunch [1 cup]	35	1.2	148	21%	3	27	1.0
3548	Cheerios [1 cup]	28	1.0	103	15%	3	22	2.5
3549	Chex cereal [1 cup]	39	1.4	143	6%	4	32	3.5
3550	Christmas Crunch [1 cup]	38	1.3	151	11%	2	32	1.2
3551	Cinnamon Toast Crunch [1 cup]	38	1.3	157	22%	2	30	1.9
3552	Clusters [1 cup]	57	2.0	221	15%	6	45	4.4

Food No.	fat gm	sat fat gm	choles mg	sodium mg	potas mg	% of Daily Value													
						vit A	vit E	vit C	thia	ribo	niac	vit B-6	fola	vit B-12	calc	phos	mag	iron	zinc
3500	1	0	0	304	236	49	33	33	34	32	33	33	34	33	2	19	42	61	33
3501	1	0	0	335	260	54	36	36	37	35	36	37	38	36	2	21	46	67	36
3502	3	1	0	457	652	0	7	105	106	105	105	106	12	105	5	80	78	45	38
3503	17	8	1	28	457	0	5	1	24	10	9	9	7	2	10	32	27	17	17
3504	20	15	0	52	514	1	3	2	22	34	9	5	4	5	16	35	18	16	13
3505	15	7	1	24	448	0	5	1	20	11	8	8	6	2	8	31	25	19	15
3506	20	14	0	47	538	1	4	0	21	38	10	8	11	2	16	35	31	17	14
3507	5	1	0	164	383	0	2	1	19	7	8	8	4	1	7	24	20	14	13
3508	2	0	0	241	570	49	6	55	53	54	55	54	57	55	22	55	57	55	55
3509	2	0	0	560	695	46	5	51	53	50	51	52	54	51	22	60	65	51	51
3510	2	1	0	267	113	1	1	34	33	1	34	33	34	34	3	8	5	13	13
3511	4	1	0	241	642	0	2	16	30	27	12	16	8	2	17	42	27	19	23
3512	1	0	0	216	66	45	0	0	29	30	30	31	30	30	1	6	5	18	12
3513	1	0	0	172	53	42	1	0	28	28	28	28	28	28	1	5	5	17	4
3514	4	1	0	13	134	0	15	2	2	2	5	1	1	0	1	13	2	4	1
3515	2	0	0	190	76	29	2	32	32	32	32	32	32	0	4	8	6	32	32
3516	1	1	0	115	38	35	1	20	35	20	37	28	31	25	1	3	6	27	22
3517	0	0	0	275	38	29	1	32	32	33	32	31	28	0	0	3	2	13	3
3518	1	0	0	21	172	0	3	0	27	27	26	26	29	26	2	16	13	93	10
3519	0	0	0	125	30	21	0	23	24	23	23	24	25	0	0	3	2	23	23
3520	1	0	0	380	87	24	2	0	26	26	26	25	28	26	2	9	3	11	10
3521	1	1	0	241	33	51	1	34	34	34	34	33	34	0	0	1	1	13	1
3522	8	1	0	241	266	95	4	0	63	64	64	63	64	63	0	20	20	25	25
3523	3	0	0	288	144	33	3	22	22	22	22	22	22	0	28	21	9	22	22
3524	1	0	0	138	23	2	1	1	25	15	25	25	25	25	1	2	2	25	25
3525	1	0	0	158	54	37	1	25	25	25	25	25	25	25	2	4	2	25	15
3526	3	0	0	243	102	36	11	0	24	24	24	24	24	24	2	8	6	10	6
3527	1	0	0	191	24	23	1	26	26	26	26	26	26	0	7	4	1	26	26
3528	4	1	0	399	112	47	2	0	52	52	52	52	52	52	1	9	8	52	52
3529	1	0	0	317	29	25	0	28	28	28	28	28	27	28	5	5	2	50	28
3530	1	0	0	235	19	0	0	28	28	28	28	28	27	0	2	3	1	28	28
3531	2	0	0	559	755	63	6	70	73	69	70	71	63	0	6	47	58	70	120
3532	1	0	0	345	216	1	3	43	42	16	43	44	43	43	3	17	17	78	43
3533	2	0	0	439	401	79	6	2	53	53	53	53	2	53	9	29	29	53	12
3534	1	0	0	214	163	0	2	0	33	20	34	33	34	20	2	14	12	34	20
3535	11	2	0	47	543	0	12	0	24	5	21	10	8	5	19	40	33	24	17
3536	1	0	0	67	38	1	1	1	28	17	28	28	28	28	1	4	3	28	17
3537	1	0	0	371	146	94	42	62	62	62	62	96	3	62	5	11	11	62	5
3538	2	0	0	135	28	42	2	0	28	28	28	28	28	0	0	2	2	51	1
3539	0	0	0	186	23	44	1	29	29	30	29	29	29	0	1	6	5	12	12
3540	13	2	0	167	198	128	3	0	84	86	85	87	86	86	5	22	17	86	11
3541	15	11	0	161	261	136	3	0	89	91	91	93	91	91	5	23	19	91	11
3542	1	1	0	203	31	0	0	22	22	13	22	22	22	13	0	2	1	22	13
3543	2	1	0	286	47	0	1	0	34	34	34	34	34	0	1	4	3	34	34
3544	3	2	0	261	39	1	1	0	33	20	33	33	33	20	1	3	3	33	20
3545	2	0	0	256	49	1	1	0	34	34	34	34	34	0	1	4	3	34	36
3546	2	1	0	214	68	0	0	0	39	23	34	35	51	17	1	3	3	34	23
3547	4	1	0	271	63	0	1	0	34	34	34	34	34	0	1	5	4	34	34
3548	2	0	0	268	84	35	1	24	24	24	24	24	24	0	5	11	8	43	24
3549	1	0	0	261	147	0	1	34	34	8	34	35	34	34	2	15	12	62	7
3550	2	1	0	293	49	0	1	0	35	35	35	35	35	0	1	4	3	35	35
3551	4	1	0	266	56	29	2	32	32	32	32	32	32	0	5	9	4	32	32
3552	4	0	0	248	177	0	14	22	26	26	26	26	26	0	7	16	13	26	7

Grains, Beans, Nuts, Seeds

Food No.	Food Description & Amount	wt gm	wt oz	cal	% cal fat	prot gm	carbo gm	fiber gm
3553	Cocoa Krispies [1 cup]	36	1.3	140	6%	2	32	0.5
3554	Cocoa Pebbles [1 cup]	32	1.1	131	12%	2	27	0.5
3555	Cocoa Puffs [1 cup]	30	1.1	119	7%	1	27	0.2
3556	Common Sense Oat Bran, plain [1 cup]	43	1.5	156	10%	6	33	5.7
3557	Common Sense Oat Bran, with raisins [1 cup]	56	2.0	185	4%	6	44	5.2
3558	Cookie-Crisp (Include all flavors) [1 cup]	30	1.1	120	8%	2	26	0.4
3559	Corn Bran [1 cup]	36	1.3	120	9%	2	30	6.4
3560	Corn Chex [1 cup]	29	1.0	114	1%	2	25	0.5
3561	Corn flakes (Include Kellogg) [1 cup]	25	0.9	91	2%	2	21	1.0
3562	Corn flakes, low sodium [1 cup]	25	0.9	100	1%	2	22	0.3
3563	Corn Pops [1 cup]	31	1.1	117	1%	1	28	0.7
3564	Corn Puffs [1 cup]	19	0.7	72	5%	1	16	0.5
3565	Corn Total [1 cup]	33	1.2	123	4%	2	28	0.8
3566	Count Chocula [1 cup]	33	1.2	129	7%	2	29	0.5
3567	Cracker Jack Cereal [1 cup]	28	1.0	109	13%	1	25	0.6
3568	Cracklin' Oat Bran [1 cup]	60	2.1	245	33%	5	44	6.8
3569	Crisp Crunch [1 cup]	30	1.1	116	9%	1	26	0.8
3570	Crispix [1 cup]	31	1.1	116	2%	2	27	0.7
3571	Crispy Brown Rice Cereal [1 cup]	32	1.1	124	8%	2	28	2.3
3572	Crispy Rice [1 cup]	28	1.0	111	1%	2	25	0.3
3573	Crispy Wheats'n Raisins [1 cup]	43	1.5	150	4%	3	35	2.7
3574	Croonchy Stars [1 cup]	28	1.0	114	12%	2	23	0.5
3575	Dairy Crisp with Strawberry Bits [1 cup]	119	4.2	503	30%	13	80	6.3
3576	Dino Pebbles [1 cup]	35	1.2	136	8%	1	31	0.5
3577	Donkey Kong Junior [1 cup]	33	1.2	128	8%	2	29	0.6
3578	Donkey Kong [1 cup]	32	1.1	124	8%	1	28	0.6
3579	Donuts Cereal, chocolate flavored [1 cup]	33	1.2	140	23%	2	26	0.6
3580	Donuts Cereal, powdered [1 cup]	33	1.2	140	23%	2	26	0.6
3581	Double Chex [1 cup]	43	1.5	152	3%	3	36	3.8
3582	Double Dip Crunch, Kellogg's [1 cup]	38	1.3	145	1%	1	35	0.6
3583	E.T. [1 cup]	38	1.3	174	35%	4	25	0.7
3584	Familia [1 cup]	122	4.3	473	15%	12	90	10.4
3585	Fiber One [1 cup]	57	2.0	117	12%	5	46	27.1
3586	Frankenberry [1 cup]	34	1.2	133	4%	1	31	0.2
3587	Froot Loops [1 cup]	28	1.0	109	7%	1	25	0.5
3588	Frosted Flakes, Kellogg [1 cup]	35	1.2	132	1%	2	32	0.6
3589	Frosted Bran, Kellogg [1 cup]	38	1.3	128	3%	3	32	4.3
3590	Frosted Flakes, Ralston Purina [1 cup]	38	1.3	149	3%	2	34	0.8
3591	Frosted Mini-Wheats (Include all flavors) [1 cup]	60	2.1	203	4%	6	50	6.4
3592	Frosted oat cereal with marshmallows [1 cup]	28	1.0	109	8%	2	24	1.2
3593	Frosted Rice Krinkles [1 cup]	45	1.6	173	0%	2	41	0.3
3594	Frosted Rice Krispies [1 cup]	45	1.6	170	2%	2	41	0.5
3595	Frosted Wheat Bites [1 cup]	57	2.0	198	2%	5	49	5.4
3596	Frosty O's [1 cup]	34	1.2	133	12%	4	23	1.8
3597	Fruit Rings [1 cup]	34	1.2	132	8%	1	31	0.7
3598	Fruit Wheats (Include Strawberry, Raisin, Apple, and Blueberry Fruit Wheats) [1 cup]	57	2.0	201	5%	4	46	6.0
3599	Fruit Whirls [1 cup]	28	1.0	109	8%	1	25	0.6
3600	Fruit'N Fiber Harvest Medley [1 cup]	57	2.0	185	10%	6	44	8.5
3601	Fruit'N Fiber, with apples and cinnamon [1 cup]	57	2.0	180	5%	5	45	6.3
3602	Fruit'N Fiber, with dates, raisins, and walnuts [1 cup]	55	1.9	186	14%	5	42	7.4
3603	Fruit'N Fiber with peaches, raisins, almonds and oat clusters [1 cup]	53	1.9	181	15%	5	39	7.0
3604	Fruit'N Fiber, with tropical fruit (pineapple, bananas, and coconut) [1 cup]	59	2.1	209	14%	5	45	8.3
3605	Fruitful Bran [1 cup]	110	3.9	355	3%	10	87	13.0

Food No.	fat gm	sat fat gm	choles mg	sodium mg	potas mg	vit A	vit E	vit C	thia	ribo	niac	vit B-6	fola	vit B-12	calc	phos	mag	iron	zinc
						% of Daily Value													
3553	1	1	0	244	70	26	1	29	29	30	29	29	27	0	0	3	3	12	12
3554	2	1	0	180	53	42	0	0	28	28	28	29	28	28	1	2	3	11	11
3555	1	0	0	181	52	0	1	25	25	25	25	25	25	0	3	4	2	25	25
3556	2	1	0	387	172	32	2	0	37	35	36	37	32	36	2	22	17	67	36
3557	1	0	0	376	256	34	3	0	38	38	38	36	38	37	3	19	15	38	38
3558	1	1	0	207	29	0	0	0	26	16	26	27	26	27	1	2	2	27	21
3559	1	0	0	338	75	1	2	0	7	33	33	33	33	0	3	5	5	56	33
3560	0	0	0	317	23	1	0	26	25	4	26	26	26	26	0	1	1	46	1
3561	0	0	0	272	30	19	0	21	22	21	21	21	22	0	0	1	1	39	1
3562	0	0	0	3	18	1	0	0	0	3	1	1	0	0	1	1	1	3	0
3563	0	0	0	97	23	23	0	26	27	26	26	26	27	0	0	1	1	10	10
3564	0	0	0	167	26	24	0	16	16	16	16	16	16	0	3	3	1	29	16
3565	1	0	0	223	37	41	117	110	110	110	111	110	110	149	26	12	2	110	110
3566	1	0	0	230	69	0	1	28	28	28	28	28	27	0	3	4	3	28	28
3567	2	1	0	93	61	0	0	0	25	15	25	25	25	25	3	2	3	25	15
3568	9	4	0	197	267	25	2	27	28	28	27	27	42	0	3	20	21	12	12
3569	1	0	0	117	23	0	0	0	26	16	26	26	26	16	1	1	3	26	16
3570	0	0	0	257	38	24	1	27	27	27	27	26	23	0	0	3	2	11	11
3571	1	0	0	4	76	0	0	0	2	1	3	1	2	0	1	9	7	2	3
3572	0	0	0	206	27	37	0	25	35	35	35	35	35	1	1	3	3	4	3
3573	1	0	0	223	180	29	2	0	19	19	20	20	19	0	5	11	8	20	6
3574	1	1	0	77	41	37	1	0	25	25	25	25	25	25	1	5	3	25	9
3575	17	12	0	588	409	158	4	105	105	105	105	5	105	105	357	37	30	105	15
3576	1	0	0	185	19	46	0	0	31	31	31	31	31	31	0	2	3	12	12
3577	1	1	0	140	47	44	0	29	29	29	29	29	0	29	0	3	2	29	0
3578	1	1	0	147	56	43	0	28	28	28	28	28	0	28	1	4	3	28	23
3579	3	2	0	213	0	44	1	29	29	29	29	29	0	29	2	5	2	29	0
3580	3	2	0	213	0	44	1	29	29	29	29	29	0	29	2	5	2	29	0
3581	0	0	0	289	114	0	1	38	38	6	38	38	38	38	2	17	14	68	30
3582	0	0	0	223	27	30	0	33	33	34	33	32	29	0	0	2	2	13	13
3583	7	4	0	228	91	50	1	33	33	34	33	33	34	33	0	6	6	33	3
3584	8	1	0	61	603	0	4	1	26	39	11	6	5	6	21	41	97	19	16
3585	2	0	0	271	412	0	3	29	48	48	48	48	47	0	11	32	32	48	16
3586	1	0	0	236	18	0	0	28	28	28	28	28	28	0	3	3	1	28	28
3587	1	0	0	131	29	20	0	22	24	23	23	24	21	0	0	2	2	22	23
3588	0	0	0	237	23	26	0	29	30	29	29	30	31	0	0	1	1	29	1
3589	0	0	0	261	155	28	1	31	30	31	31	30	29	30	1	12	12	31	31
3590	1	0	0	247	24	50	0	34	33	34	33	34	1	34	0	1	1	5	5
3591	1	0	0	2	200	0	2	0	28	28	27	27	28	27	2	17	15	98	11
3592	1	0	0	158	58	37	1	25	25	25	25	25	25	25	2	4	2	25	15
3593	0	0	0	284	23	60	0	0	39	40	40	41	40	40	1	3	3	16	16
3594	0	0	0	329	35	39	0	43	42	42	43	43	45	0	0	4	3	17	4
3595	0	0	0	9	195	0	1	0	27	27	27	27	27	27	3	16	14	11	11
3596	2	0	0	368	121	45	1	30	29	30	30	31	2	30	6	16	12	30	6
3597	1	0	0	150	36	45	1	120	30	30	30	30	30	0	1	2	2	30	30
3598	1	0	0	23	211	45	3	2	50	50	50	50	50	50	2	12	12	20	20
3599	1	0	0	114	54	22	1	99	25	25	15	25	25	25	2	3	2	6	25
3600	2	0	0	385	404	75	6	0	50	50	50	50	50	50	4	29	30	50	20
3601	1	0	0	323	295	76	6	0	50	50	50	50	50	50	3	21	24	50	20
3602	3	0	0	260	323	70	6	0	48	49	49	48	49	48	3	21	20	54	19
3603	3	0	0	251	310	67	6	0	45	45	45	45	45	45	3	21	20	45	15
3604	3	2	0	278	355	75	6	2	52	52	52	52	52	52	2	22	22	52	21
3605	1	0	0	776	485	66	12	0	73	73	73	73	73	73	0	43	47	73	18

Grains, Beans, Nuts, Seeds

Food No.	Food Description & Amount	wt gm	wt oz	cal	% cal fat	prot gm	carbo gm	fiber gm
3606	Fruity Marshmallow Krispies (formerly called Marshmallow Krispies) [1 cup]	33	1.2	125	1%	2	30	0.3
3607	Fruity Pebbles [1 cup]	32	1.1	130	12%	1	28	0.4
3608	Fruity Yummy Mummy cereal [1 cup]	28	1.0	113	10%	2	24	0.6
3609	G-I Joe Action Stars [1 cup]	28	1.0	109	17%	2	24	0.5
3610	Golden Grahams [1 cup]	39	1.4	150	8%	2	33	1.2
3611	Golden Harvest Proteinola [1 cup]	84	3.0	386	37%	9	56	7.1
3612	Granola (Include store brands) (See also Heartland Natural Cereal, Nature Valley Granola, etc.) [1 cup]	111	3.9	518	47%	16	59	11.7
3613	Granola, homemade [1 cup]	122	4.3	570	47%	18	65	12.8
3614	Granola, lowfat, Kellogg [1 cup]	98	3.5	380	14%	8	79	5.8
3615	Granola with Raisins, lowfat, Kellogg [1 cup]	98	3.5	360	12%	8	78	5.9
3616	Grape-Nut Flakes [1 cup]	39	1.4	144	7%	4	32	3.9
3617	Grape-Nuts [1 cup]	109	3.8	389	1%	13	89	10.9
3618	Great Grains, Raisin, Date, and Pecan Whole Grain Cereal, Post [1 cup]	97	3.4	355	21%	8	71	8.2
3619	Great Grains Double Pecan Whole Grain Cereal, Post [1 cup]	93	3.3	393	23%	10	66	10.1
3620	Gremlins [1 cup]	28	1.0	109	16%	1	24	0.3
3621	Halfsies [1 cup]	33	1.2	132	9%	2	28	2.2
3622	Healthy Choice with multi-grains, raisins, crunchy oat clusters, and almonds, Kellogg [1 cup]	59	2.1	232	8%	5	50	5.0
3623	Healthy Choice Multi-Grain Squares, Kellogg [1 cup]	44	1.6	150	5%	4	36	4.5
3624	Heartland Natural Cereal, plain [1 cup]	115	4.1	499	32%	12	79	7.0
3625	Heartland Natural Cereal, with coconut [1 cup]	105	3.7	463	33%	11	71	7.5
3626	Heartland Natural Cereal, with raisins [1 cup]	110	3.9	468	30%	11	76	6.1
3627	Heartwise with fruit nuggets [1 cup]	42	1.5	118	5%	3	32	7.6
3628	Heartwise, plain [1 cup]	39	1.4	113	7%	4	31	8.6
3629	Hidden Treasures, General Mills [1 cup]	44	1.6	184	15%	2	38	0.9
3630	Honey Bran [1 cup]	35	1.2	119	6%	3	29	3.9
3631	Honey Bunches of Oats [1 cup]	43	1.5	173	12%	3	36	2.1
3632	Honey Bunches of Oats with Almonds, Post [1 cup]	51	1.8	208	21%	4	39	3.1
3633	Honey Graham Chex [1 cup]	43	1.5	167	4%	2	38	1.3
3634	Honey Nut Cheerios [1 cup]	33	1.2	126	10%	3	27	1.7
3635	Honey Smacks [1 cup]	38	1.3	144	5%	2	33	1.4
3636	Honeycomb, plain [1 cup]	22	0.8	86	4%	1	20	0.6
3637	Horizon [1 cup]	85	3.0	330	16%	6	66	12.6
3638	Hot Wheels [1 cup]	37	1.3	143	8%	3	31	1.6
3639	Jenny O's [1 cup]	28	1.0	101	6%	4	20	1.8
3640	Jetsons Cereal [1 cup]	35	1.2	135	8%	2	30	0.7
3641	Just Right [1 cup]	43	1.5	160	6%	3	36	2.2
3642	Just Right with raisins, dates, and nuts [1 cup]	55	1.9	193	7%	4	44	2.8
3643	Kaboom [1 cup]	34	1.2	133	9%	3	27	1.7
3644	Kashi, Puffed [1 cup]	24	0.8	83	6%	3	18	2.4
3645	Kenmei Rice Bran, plain, Kelloggs [1 cup]	37	1.3	139	6%	3	31	1.1
3646	King Vitamin [1 cup]	21	0.7	81	9%	2	18	0.8
3647	Kix [1 cup]	19	0.7	72	5%	1	16	0.5
3648	Life (plain and cinnamon) [1 cup]	44	1.6	165	10%	4	35	2.6
3649	Lucky Charms [1 cup]	32	1.1	124	8%	2	27	1.3
3650	Malt-O-Meal Crisp Rice [1 cup]	28	1.0	106	3%	2	24	0.5
3651	Malt-O-Meal Honey and Nut Toasty O's [1 cup]	38	1.3	146	10%	4	31	2.0
3652	Malt-O-Meal Puffed Rice [1 cup]	14	0.5	54	2%	1	12	0.2
3653	Malt-O-Meal Puffed Wheat [1 cup]	12	0.4	44	5%	2	9	1.1
3654	Malt-O-Meal Sugar Puffs [1 cup]	32	1.1	122	5%	2	28	1.2
3655	Malt-O-Meal Toasted Oat Cereal [1 cup]	22	0.8	80	15%	2	17	1.9
3656	Malt-O-meal Tootie Fruities [1 cup]	28	1.0	109	8%	1	25	0.6
3657	Millet, puffed [1 cup]	21	0.7	74	10%	2	14	0.6

Food No.	fat gm	sat fat gm	choles mg	sodium mg	potas mg	vit A	vit E	vit C	thia	ribo	niac	vit B-6	fola	vit B-12	calc	phos	mag	iron	zinc
						% of Daily Value													
3606	0	0	0	197	19	27	0	29	29	29	30	30	33	0	0	2	2	12	2
3607	2	1	0	178	24	42	0	0	28	28	28	29	28	28	0	2	2	11	11
3608	1	0	0	153	39	37	1	25	25	25	25	25	25	25	2	5	4	25	2
3609	2	2	0	80	49	1	0	0	25	15	25	25	25	15	1	2	3	25	15
3610	1	0	0	357	69	29	1	33	33	33	33	33	32	0	2	5	3	33	33
3611	16	12	0	42	415	0	1	1	18	27	8	4	3	4	13	28	14	13	11
3612	27	5	0	27	597	0	65	3	55	18	11	18	24	0	9	51	49	26	30
3613	30	6	0	29	656	0	71	3	60	20	13	20	26	0	10	56	54	28	33
3614	6	1	0	240	245	45	45	0	52	52	50	49	49	51	4	24	21	20	50
3615	5	2	0	221	277	37	45	0	39	40	41	39	49	41	4	23	20	19	41
3616	1	1	0	220	136	52	0	0	34	34	34	35	34	34	2	12	11	62	5
3617	0	0	0	758	364	144	1	0	94	96	96	98	96	96	1	27	18	173	16
3618	8	1	0	219	383	123	10	0	82	82	82	82	82	82	6	27	27	55	22
3619	10	1	0	246	328	123	10	0	82	82	82	82	82	82	3	33	33	49	26
3620	2	2	0	210	36	0	0	0	25	15	25	25	25	15	0	2	3	25	15
3621	1	1	0	272	46	0	1	0	32	24	37	38	40	22	1	3	3	38	20
3622	2	0	0	271	218	5	15	0	37	37	38	37	27	38	3	15	14	38	11
3623	1	0	0	0	154	4	11	0	28	28	28	28	20	28	1	16	12	28	8
3624	18	5	0	293	385	1	4	2	24	9	8	10	16	0	7	42	37	24	20
3625	17	6	0	213	384	1	3	2	23	9	9	8	14	0	7	38	34	30	18
3626	16	4	0	226	415	1	4	2	21	8	8	10	11	0	7	38	35	22	19
3627	1	0	0	139	290	25	0	0	28	28	27	28	27	28	3	13	11	28	11
3628	1	0	0	168	265	31	0	0	34	34	35	34	34	33	3	15	14	34	14
3629	3	0	0	261	31	58	2	38	38	38	38	39	38	0	0	3	12	38	5
3630	1	0	0	202	151	46	4	31	30	31	31	32	6	31	2	13	11	31	6
3631	2	1	0	272	77	84	1	0	37	43	42	52	49	61	1	7	6	34	5
3632	5	1	0	288	108	68	7	0	45	45	45	45	45	45	2	7	7	27	4
3633	1	0	0	303	61	0	1	38	38	9	38	38	38	38	2	3	12	15	7
3634	1	0	0	285	94	25	2	28	28	28	28	28	27	0	2	11	8	28	28
3635	1	0	0	93	53	29	1	32	33	31	32	32	34	0	0	5	5	13	3
3636	0	0	0	124	25	29	0	0	19	19	19	20	19	19	0	2	2	12	8
3637	6	4	0	195	598	113	3	0	75	75	75	75	75	75	5	12	12	75	30
3638	1	0	0	208	77	49	1	33	33	33	33	33	33	33	3	5	3	33	20
3639	1	0	0	88	53	0	0	0	10	5	6	2	2	0	1	6	4	6	2
3640	1	0	0	197	62	46	1	31	31	31	31	31	31	31	0	3	3	31	18
3641	1	0	0	264	95	29	8	0	20	20	20	19	20	19	1	8	7	70	5
3642	2	0	0	266	156	34	14	0	22	23	23	22	28	23	0	11	8	83	7
3643	1	0	0	312	68	26	1	28	28	28	28	28	28	0	6	10	5	51	28
3644	1	0	0	2	66	0	0	0	3	2	4	1	2	0	1	6	9	4	5
3645	1	0	0	303	99	29	1	0	33	33	33	33	32	33	7	16	11	4	13
3646	1	0	0	178	56	21	7	14	104	17	18	17	17	18	0	5	4	33	18
3647	0	0	0	167	26	24	0	16	16	16	16	16	16	0	3	3	1	29	16
3648	2	0	0	230	110	0	0	0	37	36	37	37	37	0	13	18	10	68	37
3649	1	0	0	217	58	24	1	27	27	27	27	27	27	0	3	8	5	27	27
3650	0	0	0	300	33	21	0	23	24	23	23	24	25	0	0	3	3	9	3
3651	2	0	0	328	108	29	2	32	32	32	32	32	32	0	3	13	9	32	32
3652	0	0	0	1	16	0	0	0	4	0	4	0	0	0	0	2	1	2	1
3653	0	0	0	1	44	0	0	0	3	2	7	1	1	1	0	4	4	3	2
3654	1	0	0	79	45	24	1	27	28	26	27	27	28	0	0	4	4	11	3
3655	1	0	0	208	65	28	1	18	18	18	18	18	18	0	4	8	6	33	18
3656	1	0	0	118	30	37	0	99	25	25	25	25	25	0	0	2	2	25	25
3657	1	0	0	1	38	0	0	0	5	3	5	4	4	0	0	6	6	3	2

Grains, Beans, Nuts, Seeds

Food No.	Food Description & Amount	wt gm	wt oz	cal	% cal fat	prot gm	carbo gm	fiber gm
3658	Mini Buns Cereal (cinnamon) [1 cup]	39	1.4	150	5%	2	35	0.9
3659	Morning Funnies Cereal [1 cup]	28	1.0	109	8%	1	25	0.3
3660	Most [1 cup]	52	1.8	175	3%	7	40	7.3
3661	Mr. T. [1 cup]	28	1.0	118	15%	1	23	0.5
3662	Muesli with raisins, peaches, and pecans [1 cup]	76	2.7	277	18%	7	55	5.5
3663	Muesli with raisins, dates, and almonds [1 cup]	85	3.0	289	13%	8	66	6.2
3664	Muesli with apples and almonds, Ralston Purina [1 cup]	69	2.4	251	12%	7	52	5.0
3665	Multi Bran Chex [1 cup]	49	1.7	155	4%	3	43	6.9
3666	Multi Grain Cheerios [1 cup]	28	1.0	104	9%	2	23	1.8
3667	Mueslix Bran Muesli Cereal [1 cup]	82	2.9	262	8%	8	63	12.3
3668	Mueslix Five Grain Muesli Cereal [1 cup]	82	2.9	289	15%	6	63	5.6
3669	Mueslix Golden Crunch [1 cup]	71	2.5	261	18%	7	54	7.3
3670	Mueslix with raisins, walnuts, and cranberries [1 cup]	78	2.8	285	18%	8	57	5.7
3671	Natural Bran Flakes, Post (was called 40% Bran Flakes, Post) [1 cup]	47	1.7	152	4%	5	37	9.2
3672	Natural Muesli, Jenny's Cuisine [1 cup]	76	2.7	285	16%	9	53	6.7
3673	Nature Valley Granola, toasted oat mixture [1 cup]	113	4.0	510	35%	12	74	7.2
3674	Nature Valley Granola, with cinnamon and raisins [1 cup]	113	4.0	484	29%	10	79	5.9
3675	Nature Valley Granola, with fruit and nuts [1 cup]	113	4.0	520	40%	12	70	6.9
3676	Nintendo Cereal System [1 cup]	28	1.0	109	8%	1	25	0.3
3677	Nu System Cuisine Toasted Grain Circles [1 cup]	44	1.6	161	15%	5	34	3.9
3678	Nut & Honey Crunch Biscuits Cereal [1 cup]	57	2.0	196	11%	5	43	5.1
3679	Nut and Honey Crunch (flakes) [1 cup]	43	1.5	174	10%	3	36	0.7
3680	Nutri-Grain Almond Raisin [1 cup]	51	1.8	187	14%	4	40	4.1
3681	Nutri-Grain Biscuits, Whole Grain Shredded Wheat Cereal [1 cup]	46	1.6	153	2%	7	36	5.8
3682	Nutri-Grain Corn [1 cup]	49	1.7	187	5%	4	41	3.0
3683	Nutri-Grain Raisin Bran [1 cup]	58	2.0	190	7%	6	45	7.3
3684	Nutri-Grain Wheat [1 cup]	40	1.4	144	3%	3	34	2.5
3685	Nutrific Oatmeal Flakes [1 cup]	43	1.5	144	16%	4	32	6.1
3686	Nutty Nuggets, Ralston Purina [1 cup]	113	4.0	399	0%	12	96	8.0
3687	O.J.'s [1 cup]	28	1.0	118	15%	2	23	0.6
3688	Oat bran, uncooked [1 cup]	98	3.5	241	26%	17	65	15.1
3689	Oat Bran Flakes, Health Valley [1 cup]	57	2.0	201	4%	6	45	7.4
3690	Oat Bran Options, flakes, with raisins, dates, and oat nuggets [1 cup]	66	2.3	209	7%	6	51	5.6
3691	Oat flakes, fortified [1 cup]	48	1.7	180	5%	8	36	1.4
3692	Oat Flakes, Post [1 cup]	43	1.5	162	5%	7	33	3.2
3693	Oatbake, Honey Bran [1 cup]	85	3.0	340	27%	7	63	6.8
3694	Oatbake, Raisin Nut [1 cup]	85	3.0	340	27%	7	63	6.8
3695	Oatmeal Crisp [1 cup]	60	2.1	232	16%	4	47	2.1
3696	Oatmeal Crisp with Apples [1 cup]	60	2.1	224	8%	5	50	4.9
3697	Oatmeal Raisin Crisp [1 cup]	57	2.0	211	11%	5	45	3.6
3698	Oh's, Crunchy Nut [1 cup]	28	1.0	129	28%	2	20	1.1
3699	Oh's, Honey Graham [1 cup]	28	1.0	116	16%	1	24	0.7
3700	Pop Tarts Crunch Cereal [1 cup]	36	1.3	143	6%	2	32	0.6
3701	Popeye [1 cup]	14	0.5	56	12%	1	12	0.4
3702	Product 19 [1 cup]	33	1.2	121	3%	3	27	1.1
3703	Quaker Oat Bran Cereal [1 cup]	37	1.3	138	14%	5	27	4.7
3704	Quaker Oat Squares [1 cup]	57	2.0	220	11%	7	44	4.3
3705	Quaker Rice Bran Cereal [1 cup]	43	1.5	190	7%	5	34	8.0
3706	Quisp [1 cup]	30	1.1	121	12%	1	26	0.8
3707	Rainbow Brite [1 cup]	28	1.0	109	8%	1	25	0.4
3708	Raisin Bran, Kellogg [1 cup]	56	2.0	171	5%	5	43	7.5
3709	Raisin Bran, Nutri System [1 single serving package]	35	1.2	110	8%	6	20	6.5
3710	Raisin Bran, Post [1 cup]	56	2.0	172	6%	5	42	7.9
3711	Raisin Bran, Ralston Purina [1 cup]	56	2.0	178	1%	4	46	7.5

						% of Daily Value													
Food No.	fat gm	sat fat gm	choles mg	sodium mg	potas mg	vit A	vit E	vit C	thia	ribo	niac	vit B-6	fola	vit B-12	calc	phos	mag	iron	zinc
3658	1	0	0	270	48	29	0	33	34	32	33	33	29	0	1	3	4	33	33
3659	1	0	0	69	23	0	0	0	25	15	25	25	25	25	0	2	2	25	15
3660	1	0	0	276	340	275	250	184	184	184	183	185	183	184	8	36	26	183	18
3661	2	1	0	227	30	0	0	0	20	20	15	30	2	25	1	2	3	15	2
3662	6	1	0	175	314	69	12	2	46	46	46	46	46	46	2	18	15	37	18
3663	4	1	0	196	413	78	42	0	52	52	52	52	52	52	0	21	17	41	21
3664	3	1	0	235	285	63	5	0	42	42	42	42	42	42	0	17	17	34	17
3665	1	0	0	345	216	1	3	43	43	7	43	43	43	43	2	17	17	78	43
3666	1	0	0	237	91	21	1	23	23	23	23	23	23	0	5	11	7	42	23
3667	2	0	0	205	467	75	41	1	50	50	49	50	49	41	6	37	33	80	50
3668	5	1	0	107	369	75	41	1	50	50	49	50	49	55	7	21	21	50	50
3669	5	1	0	362	251	48	28	0	53	53	54	54	53	37	4	19	18	54	43
3670	6	2	0	180	323	71	3	3	47	28	47	48	47	47	3	19	15	38	19
3671	1	0	0	431	251	62	2	0	41	41	41	42	41	42	2	30	25	75	17
3672	5	1	0	66	300	1	3	1	23	7	5	5	5	0	4	27	22	14	11
3673	20	3	0	183	375	0	36	0	23	7	6	8	4	0	8	33	27	20	15
3674	16	2	0	181	388	0	27	0	25	5	6	8	4	0	9	33	28	15	13
3675	23	4	0	158	398	0	55	0	26	11	7	7	5	0	9	32	29	19	15
3676	1	0	0	69	23	0	0	0	25	15	25	25	25	25	0	2	2	25	15
3677	3	0	0	417	130	55	1	37	37	37	37	37	37	0	8	17	12	66	37
3678	2	0	0	11	187	0	3	0	50	50	50	51	50	50	2	18	13	50	20
3679	2	0	0	289	47	18	0	20	20	20	20	19	22	0	0	3	1	20	2
3680	3	0	0	181	182	0	23	0	24	24	23	23	26	23	16	17	3	7	23
3681	0	0	0	1	190	0	1	0	40	41	40	41	40	41	2	17	17	11	41
3682	1	0	0	322	114	65	59	43	42	43	43	44	43	43	0	14	8	6	43
3683	1	0	0	292	365	0	67	0	37	15	37	37	37	37	29	37	22	15	37
3684	0	0	0	272	109	0	48	35	35	35	35	36	35	35	1	15	8	6	35
3685	2	0	0	243	256	23	35	0	26	26	26	26	26	26	3	15	17	26	26
3686	0	0	0	558	358	150	1	0	99	100	100	99	100	100	4	24	24	179	32
3687	2	0	0	133	39	37	0	99	25	25	25	25	25	0	0	2	2	10	10
3688	7	1	0	4	555	0	8	0	76	13	5	8	13	0	6	72	58	29	20
3689	1	0	0	21	183	0	6	0	20	13	19	3	7	0	2	29	24	16	10
3690	2	0	0	231	295	24	7	0	40	40	40	40	40	40	4	18	17	40	24
3691	1	0	0	220	228	64	2	0	42	42	42	43	42	42	7	18	14	76	17
3692	1	0	0	192	202	57	1	0	38	38	38	38	38	38	6	15	17	68	15
3693	10	2	0	527	272	68	9	75	75	75	77	75	74	0	4	22	22	75	75
3694	10	2	0	553	323	68	9	75	75	75	77	75	74	0	3	21	20	75	75
3695	4	1	0	380	169	79	2	53	53	53	53	53	53	0	8	13	8	53	2
3696	2	0	0	307	174	0	2	16	27	27	27	27	27	0	3	13	12	27	27
3697	3	0	0	232	219	23	6	0	26	26	26	26	26	0	4	12	12	26	26
3698	4	3	0	84	25	0	0	0	41	20	35	30	44	25	0	2	2	25	15
3699	2	1	0	185	47	35	1	19	29	24	41	39	40	26	1	3	2	35	23
3700	1	0	0	148	39	27	0	30	31	30	30	31	27	0	3	2	3	30	30
3701	1	0	0	101	19	0	0	0	13	13	13	13	13	0	0	2	2	13	13
3702	0	0	0	358	45	25	111	110	110	111	110	111	116	110	0	4	3	110	110
3703	2	0	0	139	167	22	12	13	17	17	17	17	17	0	2	22	17	58	17
3704	3	0	0	268	232	17	11	11	29	29	29	29	29	0	4	19	18	89	29
3705	2	0	0	399	82	0	12	0	26	30	53	42	75	27	4	6	5	73	33
3706	2	0	0	216	40	0	1	0	28	28	28	28	28	0	1	5	4	28	28
3707	1	1	0	69	25	1	1	1	25	15	25	25	25	25	1	2	2	25	15
3708	1	0	0	325	401	23	2	0	26	26	25	25	26	25	3	20	20	26	25
3709	1	0	0	88	150	39	4	25	32	29	30	55	15	27	2	16	14	28	8
3710	1	0	0	365	345	74	6	0	49	49	49	50	49	49	3	23	24	49	20
3711	0	0	0	486	287	56	6	3	37	36	37	36	37	37	3	25	21	152	11

Grains, Beans, Nuts, Seeds

Food No.	Food Description & Amount	wt gm	wt oz	cal	% cal fat	prot gm	carbo gm	fiber gm
3712	Raisin Bran, Total [1 cup]	52	1.8	168	5%	4	40	4.7
3713	Raisin Grapenuts [1 cup]	118	4.2	426	1%	12	97	6.5
3714	Raisin Life [1 cup]	56	2.0	207	5%	10	40	3.4
3715	Raisin Nut Bran [1 cup]	57	2.0	217	19%	5	43	5.2
3716	Raisin Squares [1 cup]	28	1.0	95	7%	2	22	2.6
3717	Raisin, Rice, and Rye [1 cup]	46	1.6	155	1%	3	39	2.6
3718	Reese's Peanut Butter Puffs Cereal [1 cup]	37	1.3	159	22%	3	28	0.5
3719	Rice Chex [1 cup]	33	1.2	130	1%	2	29	0.6
3720	Rice Krispies [1 cup]	27	1.0	102	3%	2	23	0.5
3721	Rice Krispies Treats Cereal (Kellogg) [1 cup]	37	1.3	148	12%	1	32	0.4
3722	Rice, puffed [1 cup]	14	0.5	54	2%	1	12	0.2
3723	Ripple Crisp Golden Corn [1 cup]	37	1.3	144	5%	2	31	1.3
3724	Rocky Road [1 cup]	43	1.5	182	23%	2	35	0.8
3725	S'mores Crunch [1 cup]	38	1.3	148	9%	2	32	1.1
3726	S.W. Graham [1 cup]	57	2.0	195	3%	5	47	5.2
3727	Shredded Wheat'N Bran [1 cup]	43	1.5	137	8%	5	35	6.1
3728	Shredded Wheat, 100% [1 cup spoon size biscuits]	50	1.8	179	4%	5	40	4.9
3729	Slimer! and The Real Ghost Busters [1 cup]	32	1.1	124	3%	2	29	0.4
3730	Shredded Wheat with Oat Bran [1 cup spoon size biscuits]	51	1.8	180	9%	5	40	7.2
3731	Smurf Magic Berries (was called Smurfberry Crunch) [1 cup]	33	1.2	132	7%	2	30	0.5
3732	Special K [1 cup]	23	0.8	85	2%	5	17	0.7
3733	Sprinkle Spangles [1 cup]	32	1.1	124	8%	1	28	0.6
3734	Strawberry Krispies [1 cup]	45	1.6	175	2%	2	39	0.0
3735	Strawberry Shortcake [1 cup]	28	1.0	118	3%	1	25	1.4
3736	Strawberry Squares [1 cup]	57	2.0	194	8%	5	45	5.2
3737	Sugar-Sparkled Flakes [1 cup]	38	1.3	146	0%	2	35	0.5
3738	Sugar-Sparkled Rice Krinkles [1 cup]	32	1.1	123	0%	2	29	0.2
3739	Sun Country 100% Natural Granola, with Almonds [1 cup]	104	3.7	486	35%	12	70	5.4
3740	Sun Flakes (Include Corn and Rice Sun Flakes; Wheat and Rice Sun Flakes) [1 cup]	28	1.0	109	8%	2	24	0.3
3741	Super Golden Crisp [1 cup]	33	1.2	123	2%	2	30	0.5
3742	Super Raisin Bran, New Morning [1 cup]	56	2.0	198	8%	6	41	6.9
3743	Tasteeos [1 cup]	24	0.8	94	6%	3	19	2.5
3744	Team [1 cup]	42	1.5	164	4%	3	36	0.5
3745	Teddy Grahams Breakfast Bears Cereal, chocolate flavor [1 cup]	85	3.0	360	23%	6	66	3.0
3746	Teenage Mutant Ninja Turtles Cereal [1 cup]	28	1.0	109	2%	1	26	0.6
3747	Toasted Oatmeal, Honey Nut (Quaker) [1 cup]	50	1.8	206	21%	5	38	3.5
3748	Tiny Toon Adventures Cereal [1 cup]	30	1.1	115	9%	2	25	1.1
3749	Toasties [1 cup]	23	0.8	89	0%	2	20	0.8
3750	Toasty O's [1 cup]	28	1.0	109	15%	4	19	2.0
3751	Total [1 cup]	33	1.2	116	6%	3	26	2.9
3752	Triples [1 cup]	33	1.2	128	8%	3	27	0.9
3753	Trix [1 cup]	28	1.0	114	13%	1	24	0.7
3754	Uncle Sam's Hi Fiber Cereal [1 cup]	110	3.9	427	10%	17	79	29.0
3755	Weetabix Whole Wheat Cereal [1 cup]	57	2.0	213	7%	7	44	6.5
3756	Wheat bran, unprocessed, dry [1 cup]	58	2.0	125	18%	9	37	24.8
3757	Wheat Chex [1 cup]	46	1.6	169	6%	5	38	4.1
3758	Wheat germ, plain [1 cup]	113	4.0	432	25%	33	56	14.6
3759	Wheat germ, with sugar and honey [1 cup]	113	4.0	420	19%	30	66	11.5
3760	Wheat'n Raisin Chex [1 cup]	54	1.9	185	2%	5	43	3.6
3761	Wheat, puffed, plain [1 cup]	12	0.4	44	5%	2	9	1.1
3762	Wheat, puffed, presweetened with sugar [1 cup]	38	1.3	143	3%	2	34	1.0
3763	Wheaties [1 cup]	29	1.0	106	8%	3	23	2.0
3764	Wheaties Honey Gold [1 cup]	41	1.4	145	4%	1	36	1.6

Food No.	fat gm	sat fat gm	choles mg	sodium mg	potas mg	% of Daily Value													
						vit A	vit E	vit C	thia	ribo	niac	vit B-6	fola	vit B-12	calc	phos	mag	iron	zinc
3712	1	0	0	227	271	35	97	0	95	95	95	95	95	100	23	24	11	95	95
3713	1	0	0	588	444	158	7	0	104	104	104	104	104	104	5	27	25	42	24
3714	1	0	0	292	250	1	2	0	82	75	74	3	12	0	20	30	4	82	12
3715	5	1	0	255	226	0	10	0	26	26	26	26	26	0	8	17	14	26	8
3716	1	0	0	2	132	0	1	0	13	13	13	13	14	13	1	8	6	48	5
3717	0	0	0	350	144	47	1	1	31	32	31	32	31	31	1	5	5	31	31
3718	4	1	0	219	76	28	3	31	31	31	31	31	31	0	3	5	5	31	31
3719	0	0	0	276	38	0	0	29	29	1	29	30	29	29	0	3	2	52	3
3720	0	0	0	289	32	20	0	23	23	22	23	23	24	0	0	3	3	9	3
3721	2	0	0	234	23	28	0	31	32	30	31	31	28	31	0	3	2	12	2
3722	0	0	0	1	16	0	0	0	4	0	4	0	0	0	0	2	1	2	1
3723	1	0	0	366	59	49	1	33	33	33	33	33	33	0	3	5	3	33	3
3724	5	3	0	182	76	57	1	38	38	38	38	38	38	0	3	4	3	38	2
3725	2	0	0	269	61	29	1	32	32	32	32	32	32	0	2	5	3	32	32
3726	1	0	0	385	185	0	0	0	50	50	50	51	50	50	2	13	11	9	20
3727	1	0	0	0	178	1	5	0	6	2	12	2	5	0	1	15	15	12	12
3728	1	0	0	3	172	0	1	0	9	8	12	6	6	0	2	18	19	10	10
3729	0	0	0	130	45	1	1	1	28	17	28	28	28	17	1	2	2	28	17
3730	2	0	0	5	234	3	3	2	11	4	11	6	6	0	2	18	14	11	11
3731	1	0	0	82	37	44	0	0	29	29	29	29	29	29	1	3	3	29	14
3732	0	0	0	185	40	17	0	18	26	26	26	26	17	0	0	4	3	35	19
3733	1	0	0	147	28	42	2	28	28	28	28	28	28	0	0	2	3	28	2
3734	0	0	0	317	32	60	0	40	40	40	40	40	40	0	0	4	3	16	3
3735	0	0	0	174	29	37	2	25	25	25	25	25	0	25	1	4	0	25	0
3736	2	0	0	17	194	0	1	0	30	30	29	29	29	29	2	18	17	103	11
3737	0	0	0	215	86	50	0	0	33	34	33	34	34	34	0	1	1	3	0
3738	0	0	0	202	16	42	0	0	28	28	28	29	28	28	0	2	2	11	11
3739	19	2	0	34	404	0	10	0	21	11	5	6	9	1	9	31	24	25	14
3740	1	1	0	237	30	37	0	25	25	25	25	25	25	25	0	2	1	10	1
3741	0	0	0	51	48	44	1	0	29	29	29	30	29	29	1	4	5	12	12
3742	2	0	0	10	349	1	6	2	16	4	20	10	24	0	2	2	22	20	12
3743	1	0	0	183	71	32	1	21	21	21	21	22	21	21	1	10	7	38	5
3744	1	0	0	260	71	56	0	37	36	37	37	38	2	37	1	7	3	67	4
3745	9	1	0	405	120	113	6	3	75	75	75	75	75	3	3	12	12	75	75
3746	0	0	0	191	21	1	0	25	25	7	25	25	25	25	0	2	2	10	2
3747	5	1	1	182	207	16	10	38	27	26	27	27	27	1	6	16	12	47	27
3748	1	0	0	209	36	27	1	18	27	30	44	45	23	15	1	5	6	48	29
3749	0	0	0	241	27	30	0	0	20	20	20	21	20	20	0	1	1	3	0
3750	2	0	0	237	89	37	1	25	25	25	25	25	25	25	4	10	10	44	6
3751	1	0	0	218	107	41	117	110	110	110	111	110	110	141	28	23	9	110	110
3752	1	0	0	211	34	41	1	28	28	28	28	28	27	0	5	4	2	50	28
3753	2	0	0	184	17	21	3	23	23	23	23	23	23	0	3	2	1	23	23
3754	5	1	0	251	518	0	7	0	175	163	116	7	21	0	8	42	34	23	20
3755	2	0	0	221	311	0	3	0	41	33	16	13	7	0	6	10	13	16	7
3756	2	0	0	1	686	0	6	0	20	20	39	38	11	0	4	59	89	34	28
3757	1	0	0	308	173	0	1	41	40	10	40	41	41	41	2	18	15	73	8
3758	12	2	0	5	1070	0	93	11	126	55	32	55	99	0	5	129	90	57	126
3759	9	2	0	12	1089	0	113	0	101	46	27	28	94	0	6	114	77	51	105
3760	0	0	0	306	227	0	1	3	36	35	36	35	36	36	2	16	13	43	8
3761	0	0	0	1	44	0	0	0	3	2	7	1	1	1	0	4	4	3	2
3762	1	0	0	76	54	39	1	16	33	32	33	33	34	17	1	5	5	13	8
3763	1	0	0	215	101	22	2	24	24	24	24	24	24	0	5	9	8	44	5
3764	1	0	0	289	80	54	1	36	36	36	36	36	36	0	1	6	6	36	3

Grains, Beans, Nuts, Seeds

Food No.	Food Description & Amount	wt gm	wt oz	cal	% cal fat	prot gm	carbo gm	fiber gm
	Rice and Noodles							
3800	Macaroni, cooked (Include lasagna noodles, orzo, ziti, rotini, shells, wagon wheels, cart wheels, manicotti, rigatoni, mostaccioli, cavatoni ricci bows, twirls, spirals) [1 cup]	140	4.9	197	4%	7	40	1.8
3801	Macaroni, spinach, cooked [1 cup]	140	4.9	191	4%	7	38	5.4
3802	Macaroni, vegetable, cooked [1 cup]	91	3.2	116	1%	4	24	3.9
3803	Macaroni, whole wheat, cooked [1 cup]	140	4.9	174	4%	7	37	3.9
3804	Noodles, chow mein, deep fried (Include canned) [1 cup]	45	1.6	237	53%	4	26	1.8
3805	Noodles, rice noodles (made from mung beans), cooked (Include transparent or cellophane noodles) [1 cup]	190	6.7	160	0%	0	39	0.2
3806	Noodles, rice noodles (chow fun), cooked [1 cup]	152	5.4	163	3%	3	36	1.1
3807	Noodles, egg, cooked, with margarine, salt (Include pastina, egg noodles, Noodle Roni, Mug-O-Lunch) [1 cup]	165	5.8	247	22%	8	40	1.8
3808	Noodles, egg, cooked (Include pastina, egg noodles) [1 cup]	160	5.6	213	10%	8	40	1.8
3809	Noodles, spinach, cooked [1 cup]	160	5.6	193	4%	7	39	5.5
3810	Noodles, whole wheat, cooked [1 cup]	160	5.6	198	4%	9	42	4.5
3811	Pasta, corn-based, cooked, no sauce (Include macaroni, noodles, spaghetti) [1 cup]	119	4.2	148	5%	3	33	4.5
3812	Rice, brown, cooked [1 cup]	195	6.9	216	7%	5	45	3.5
3813	Rice, brown, cooked, instant [1 cup]	212	7.5	235	7%	5	49	3.8
3814	Rice, brown and wild, cooked [1 cup]	151	5.3	149	6%	4	31	1.6
3815	**Rice, white, enriched** (check label), cooked (most white rice is enriched) [1 cup]	205	7.2	267	2%	6	58	0.8
3816	Rice, white, not enriched (check label), cooked (most white rice is enriched) [1 cup]	204	7.2	267	2%	6	58	0.8
3817	Rice, white, instant, cooked (Include Minute Rice, yellow rice) [1 cup]	165	5.8	162	1%	3	35	1.0
3818	Rice, white, converted, cooked (Include Uncle Ben's) [1 cup]	175	6.2	200	2%	4	43	0.7
3819	Rice, white, glutinous, cooked (Include sticky rice, Japanese-style plain rice) [1 cup]	174	6.1	169	2%	4	37	1.7
3820	Rice, white and wild, cooked [1 cup]	151	5.3	147	2%	3	32	0.8
3821	Rice, wild, cooked [1 cup]	130	4.6	131	3%	5	28	2.3
3822	Rice, sweet (Include Japanese mochi rice) [1 cup]	175	6.2	246	2%	4	55	0.7
3823	Rice bran, uncooked (Include Ener-G Pure Rice Bran) [1 cup]	118	4.2	373	59%	16	59	24.8
3824	Rice polishings [1 cup]	105	3.7	278	43%	13	61	7.4
3825	Rice, cooked with oil, Puerto Rican style (Arroz blanco) [1 cup]	155	5.5	337	24%	5	57	0.9
3826	Rice, cooked, with whole milk, salt [1 cup]	200	7.1	288	14%	10	50	0.7
3827	Spaghetti, cooked, no sauce (Include fides, linguini, vermicelli) [1 cup]	140	4.9	197	4%	7	40	2.4
3828	Spaghetti, high protein type, cooked, no sauce [1 cup]	140	4.9	230	1%	11	44	2.4
3829	Spaghetti, whole wheat, cooked, no sauce [1 cup]	140	4.9	174	4%	7	37	6.3
	Beans and Peas/Legumes (salt not added when optional)							
3850	Bean cake, made with flour, lima beans, oil, sugar [1 cake]	32	1.1	130	47%	2	16	0.9
3851	Black, brown, or Bayo beans, cooked with salt pork [1 cup]	177	6.2	294	37%	13	34	8.4
3852	Chickpeas, cooked (Include garbanzos) [1 cup]	164	5.8	297	15%	16	49	14.2
3853	Cowpeas, cooked (Include blackeye peas, field peas) [1 cup]	169	6.0	196	4%	13	35	11.0
3854	Curd cheese (soybean product) [1 cup]	225	7.9	304	54%	28	14	0.0
3855	Fava beans, cooked [1 cup]	170	6.0	187	3%	13	33	9.2
3856	Lentil loaf (lentils, onion, sunflower seeds, breadcrumbs, oil, soy sauce, vinegar) [1 slice]	47	1.7	83	38%	4	10	3.0
3857	Lentils, cooked, [1 cup]	191	6.7	222	3%	17	38	15.1
3858	Lima beans, cooked (Include butter beans) [1 cup]	184	6.5	212	3%	14	38	12.9
3859	Mongo beans [1 cup]	180	6.3	189	5%	14	33	11.5
3860	Mung beans, cooked [1 cup]	200	7.1	225	3%	15	41	10.6
3861	Pink beans, cooked [1 cup]	169	6.0	252	3%	15	47	9.0

Food No.	fat gm	sat fat gm	choles mg	sodium mg	potas mg	% of Daily Value: vit A	vit E	vit C	thia	ribo	niac	vit B-6	fola	vit B-12	calc	phos	mag	iron	zinc
3800	1	0	0	1	43	0	0	0	19	8	12	2	2	0	1	8	6	11	5
3801	1	0	0	12	58	2	0	0	8	4	8	7	4	0	3	14	19	5	10
3802	0	0	0	5	28	0	0	0	7	3	5	1	1	0	1	5	4	2	3
3803	1	0	0	4	62	0	1	0	10	4	5	6	2	0	2	12	11	8	8
3804	14	2	0	198	54	0	0	0	17	11	13	2	2	0	1	7	6	12	4
3805	0	0	0	8	3	0	0	0	3	0	0	1	0	0	1	1	1	5	1
3806	1	0	0	91	29	0	0	0	3	1	5	9	0	0	1	4	4	1	2
3807	6	1	53	56	47	5	3	0	20	8	12	3	3	2	2	11	8	14	7
3808	2	0	53	11	45	1	0	0	20	8	12	3	3	2	2	11	8	14	7
3809	1	0	0	13	59	2	0	0	8	5	8	7	4	0	3	15	19	5	10
3810	1	0	0	5	70	0	1	0	12	4	6	6	2	0	2	14	12	9	9
3811	1	0	0	4	121	1	2	0	6	2	5	4	3	0	0	10	12	2	5
3812	2	0	0	10	84	0	6	0	12	3	15	14	2	0	2	16	21	5	8
3813	2	0	0	11	91	0	7	0	14	3	16	15	2	0	2	18	23	5	9
3814	1	0	0	7	98	0	1	0	8	3	11	9	2	0	1	13	15	3	7
3815	1	0	0	2	72	0	0	0	22	2	15	10	2	0	2	9	6	14	7
3816	1	0	0	2	72	0	0	0	3	2	4	10	2	0	2	9	6	2	7
3817	0	0	0	5	7	0	0	0	8	4	7	1	2	0	1	2	2	6	3
3818	0	0	0	5	65	0	0	0	29	2	12	2	2	0	3	7	5	11	4
3819	0	0	0	9	17	0	0	0	2	1	3	2	0	0	0	1	2	1	5
3820	0	0	0	7	63	0	0	0	11	2	9	4	2	0	1	6	5	8	5
3821	0	0	0	4	131	0	1	0	5	7	8	9	8	0	0	11	10	4	12
3822	0	0	0	2	63	0	0	0	18	2	12	8	1	0	2	7	5	11	6
3823	25	5	0	6	1752	0	32	0	217	20	201	240	19	0	7	198	230	122	48
3824	13	2	0	0	750	0	29	0	129	11	148	22	29	0	7	116	158	63	57
3825	9	1	0	7	78	0	9	0	22	2	15	6	1	0	2	8	5	16	5
3826	5	3	17	103	367	10	1	2	19	20	12	7	3	7	26	25	10	12	9
3827	1	0	0	1	43	0	0	0	19	8	12	2	2	0	1	8	6	11	5
3828	0	0	0	7	59	0	0	0	28	13	13	4	4	0	1	7	11	6	5
3829	1	0	0	4	62	0	0	0	10	4	5	6	2	0	2	12	11	8	8
3850	7	1	0	1	58	0	6	0	5	3	3	1	2	0	0	2	2	4	1
3851	12	4	12	207	622	0	1	0	23	5	5	6	31	1	6	18	19	13	13
3852	5	1	0	21	500	1	3	4	12	8	4	12	40	0	8	25	18	23	17
3853	1	0	0	7	470	0	2	1	23	5	4	8	88	0	4	26	22	24	15
3854	18	3	0	45	448	1	6	0	0	19	6	8	12	0	42	50	128	70	26
3855	1	0	0	9	456	0	1	1	11	9	6	6	44	0	6	21	18	14	11
3856	4	0	0	44	156	0	10	1	10	3	3	4	15	0	2	9	7	8	4
3857	1	0	0	4	705	0	1	5	22	8	10	17	86	0	4	34	17	35	16
3858	1	0	0	4	935	0	2	0	20	6	4	15	38	0	3	20	20	24	12
3859	1	0	0	13	416	1	1	3	18	8	14	5	42	0	10	28	28	18	10
3860	1	0	0	13	567	1	2	3	16	6	5	8	46	0	8	20	23	20	10
3861	1	0	0	3	859	0	3	0	29	6	5	15	71	0	9	28	27	22	11

Grains, Beans, Nuts, Seeds

Food No.	Food Description & Amount	wt gm	wt oz	cal	% cal fat	prot gm	carbo gm	fiber gm
3862	Pinto, calico, and red Mexican beans, cooked (Include October beans, Shellie beans) [1 cup]	173	6.1	196	3%	12	36	14.0
3863	Red kidney beans, cooked [1 cup]	172	6.1	218	4%	15	39	12.7
3864	Soy nuts, unsalted (roasted soybean kernels) (Include pernuts) [1 package]	135	4.8	636	49%	48	45	23.9
3865	Soybean flour (Include soybean meal) [1 cup]	122	4.3	532	43%	42	43	11.7
3866	Soybeans, cooked [1 cup]	180	6.3	311	47%	30	18	10.8
3867	Split peas, green or yellow, cooked [1 cup]	196	6.9	230	3%	16	41	16.2
3868	Tofu (soybean curd) [1 cup (½" cubes)]	184	6.5	140	57%	15	3	2.2
3869	Tofu (soybean curd), breaded, fried [1 slice (2¾" x 1" x ½")]	29	1.0	47	58%	3	3	0.4
3870	Tofu (soybean curd), deep fried (Include aburage) [1 oz]	28	1.0	76	67%	5	3	1.1
3871	Vermicelli, made from soybeans, cooked [1 cup]	140	4.9	500	0%	0	123	5.5
3872	White beans, cooked (Include Navy (pea), Great Northern) [1 cup]	175	6.2	243	2%	17	44	11.0
	Nuts and Seeds							
3900	Almond butter [2 Tbs]	32	1.1	203	84%	5	7	1.2
3901	Almond paste (Marzipan paste) [1 cup]	227	8.0	1040	54%	20	109	10.9
3902	Almonds, dry roasted, salted [22 almonds]	28	1.0	164	79%	5	7	3.8
3903	Almonds, dry roasted, unsalted [22 almonds]	28	1.0	164	79%	5	7	3.8
3904	Almonds, honey-roasted [20 almonds]	28	1.0	163	79%	5	7	2.8
3905	Almonds, roasted, salted [22 almonds]	28	1.0	173	84%	6	4	3.1
3906	Almonds, unroasted, unsalted [1 cup, whole almonds]	145	5.1	854	80%	29	30	15.8
3907	Brazil nuts [1 cup, shelled (32 kernels)]	140	4.9	918	91%	20	18	7.6
3908	Breadnuts [1 cup]	160	5.6	587	4%	14	127	23.8
3909	Butternuts [1 cup]	120	4.2	734	84%	30	14	5.6
3910	Carob chips [1 cup]	173	6.1	934	52%	14	97	6.6
3911	Carob powder or flour [1 cup]	140	4.9	252	3%	6	124	55.7
3912	Cashew butter [2 Tbs]	32	1.1	188	76%	6	9	0.6
3913	Cashew nuts, dry roasted, salted [1 cup]	137	4.8	786	73%	21	45	4.1
3914	Cashew nuts, honey-roasted, salted [10 whole cashews]	16	0.6	86	69%	2	6	0.5
3915	Cashew nuts, roasted, salted [18 whole cashews]	28	1.0	161	75%	5	8	1.1
3916	Cashew nuts, roasted, unsalted [18 whole cashews]	28	1.0	161	75%	5	8	1.1
3917	Chestnuts, roasted, unsalted [10 chestnuts]	84	3.0	206	8%	3	44	4.3
3918	Coconut cream (liquid expressed from grated coconut meat), canned, sweetened (Include Coco Lopez) [1 cup]	296	10.4	568	83%	8	25	6.5
3919	Coconut meat, dried, sweetened (Include flaked or shredded) [1 cup, shredded]	93	3.3	441	61%	3	44	4.0
3920	Coconut meat, fresh [1 piece (2" x 2" x ½")]	45	1.6	159	85%	1	7	4.1
3921	Coconut milk (liquid expressed from grated coconut meat, water added) [1 cup]	240	8.5	552	93%	5	13	5.3
3922	Coconut water (liquid from coconuts) [1 cup]	240	8.5	46	9%	2	9	2.6
3923	Filberts, hazel nuts [1 cup, whole]	135	4.8	853	89%	18	21	8.2
3924	Flaxseeds [1 cup]	145	5.1	722	61%	26	54	24.5
3925	Ginkgo nuts [1 cup (78 kernels)]	155	5.5	172	13%	4	34	14.4
3926	Hickory nuts, unsalted [1 cup]	120	4.2	788	88%	15	22	7.7
3927	Macadamia nuts, roasted, salted [1 cup]	134	4.7	962	96%	10	17	12.5
3928	Macadamia nuts, unroasted, unsalted [1 cup, whole or halves]	134	4.7	941	95%	11	18	12.5
3929	Mixed nuts, dry roasted, salted [1 cup]	137	4.8	814	78%	24	35	12.3
3930	Mixed nuts, in shell, unsalted [1 cup, in shell, edible yield]	26	0.9	167	88%	4	4	1.5
3931	Mixed nuts, roasted, with peanuts, salted [1 cup]	142	5.0	876	82%	24	30	12.8
3932	Mixed nuts, honey-roasted, with peanuts [20 assorted nuts]	21	0.7	122	77%	3	6	1.7
3933	Mixed nuts, roasted, without peanuts, salted [1 cup]	144	5.1	886	82%	22	32	7.9
3934	Peanut butter [2 Tbs]	32	1.1	190	77%	8	6	1.9
3935	Peanut butter, low sodium (Include unsalted) [2 Tbs]	32	1.1	190	77%	8	6	1.9
3936	Peanut butter, reduced fat [2 Tbs]	36	1.3	187	59%	9	13	1.9
3937	Peanut butter, reduced sodium [2 Tbs]	32	1.1	188	76%	8	7	2.1
3938	Peanut spread (Include imitation peanut butter) [2 Tbs]	32	1.1	192	78%	6	7	2.2
3939	Peanuts, boiled, salted [1 cup, shelled]	180	6.3	572	62%	24	38	15.8

						% of Daily Value													
Food No.	fat gm	sat fat gm	choles mg	sodium mg	potas mg	vit A	vit E	vit C	thia	ribo	niac	vit B-6	fola	vit B-12	calc	phos	mag	iron	zinc
3862	1	0	0	9	573	0	1	5	14	6	3	9	36	0	6	22	19	16	9
3863	1	0	0	3	693	0	1	3	18	6	5	10	56	0	5	24	19	28	12
3864	34	5	0	220	1985	3	12	5	9	12	10	14	71	0	19	49	49	29	28
3865	25	4	0	16	3068	1	11	0	47	83	26	28	105	0	25	60	131	43	32
3866	16	2	0	2	927	0	16	5	19	30	4	21	24	0	18	44	39	51	14
3867	1	0	0	457	705	0	3	1	25	6	9	5	32	0	3	19	18	14	13
3868	9	1	0	13	223	2	0	0	10	6	2	4	7	0	19	18	47	55	10
3869	3	1	6	30	39	1	1	0	3	2	1	1	1	0	3	3	7	9	2
3870	6	1	0	4	41	0	0	0	3	1	0	1	2	0	10	8	4	8	4
3871	0	0	0	6	4	0	0	0	0	0	0	0	0	0	8	3	1	14	40
3872	1	0	0	11	982	0	2	0	14	5	1	8	35	0	16	20	28	36	16
3900	19	2	0	144	243	0	29	0	3	12	5	1	5	0	9	17	24	7	7
3901	63	6	0	20	713	0	209	2	12	55	16	5	41	0	39	59	74	20	22
3902	14	1	0	218	216	0	7	0	2	10	4	1	4	0	8	15	21	6	9
3903	14	1	0	3	216	0	7	0	2	10	4	1	4	0	8	15	21	6	9
3904	14	1	0	192	170	0	6	0	2	14	4	1	4	0	6	14	19	5	8
3905	16	2	0	218	191	0	7	0	2	16	5	1	4	0	7	15	21	6	9
3906	76	7	0	16	1061	0	158	1	20	66	24	8	21	0	39	75	107	29	28
3907	93	23	0	3	840	0	48	2	93	10	11	18	1	0	25	84	79	26	43
3908	3	1	0	85	3218	4	25	124	3	13	17	55	45	0	15	28	46	41	20
3909	68	2	0	1	505	1	19	6	31	10	6	34	20	0	6	54	71	27	25
3910	54	50	5	185	1095	1	18	1	12	18	9	11	12	29	52	22	16	12	41
3911	1	0	0	49	1158	0	4	0	5	38	13	26	10	0	49	11	19	23	9
3912	16	3	0	196	175	0	2	0	7	4	3	4	5	0	1	15	21	9	11
3913	63	13	0	877	774	0	4	0	18	16	10	18	24	0	6	67	89	46	51
3914	7	1	0	86	74	0	1	0	4	1	1	2	2	0	1	6	9	3	4
3915	13	3	0	175	148	0	2	0	8	3	3	4	5	0	1	12	18	6	9
3916	13	3	0	5	148	0	2	0	8	3	3	4	5	0	1	12	18	6	9
3917	2	0	0	2	497	0	5	36	14	9	6	21	15	0	2	9	7	4	3
3918	52	47	0	148	299	0	10	9	4	7	1	4	11	0	0	7	13	8	12
3919	30	27	0	238	294	0	3	0	2	1	1	12	2	0	1	9	11	9	11
3920	15	13	0	9	160	0	1	2	2	1	1	1	3	0	1	5	4	6	3
3921	57	51	0	36	631	0	8	11	4	0	9	4	10	0	4	24	22	22	11
3922	0	0	0	252	600	0	0	10	5	8	1	4	2	0	6	5	15	4	2
3923	85	6	0	4	601	1	147	2	45	9	8	41	24	0	25	42	96	25	22
3924	49	5	0	96	1901	0	33	3	16	14	10	55	109	0	39	67	183	91	74
3925	3	0	0	476	279	5	25	24	14	5	28	15	13	0	1	8	6	2	2
3926	77	8	0	1	523	2	28	4	69	9	5	12	12	0	7	40	52	14	34
3927	103	15	0	348	441	0	2	0	19	9	14	13	5	0	6	27	39	13	10
3928	99	15	0	7	493	0	2	0	31	9	14	13	5	0	9	18	39	18	15
3929	70	9	0	917	818	0	37	1	18	16	32	20	17	0	10	60	77	28	35
3930	16	2	0	2	138	0	9	1	11	3	2	5	3	0	4	11	13	4	6
3931	80	12	0	926	825	0	39	1	47	19	36	17	29	0	15	66	83	25	48
3932	10	2	0	120	109	0	5	0	6	2	5	2	4	0	2	9	11	3	6
3933	81	13	0	1008	783	0	39	1	48	41	14	13	20	0	15	65	90	21	45
3934	16	3	0	149	214	0	15	0	2	2	21	7	6	0	1	12	13	3	6
3935	16	3	0	5	214	0	15	0	2	2	21	7	6	0	1	12	13	3	6
3936	12	3	0	194	241	0	11	0	6	1	26	6	5	0	1	13	15	4	7
3937	16	3	0	65	239	0	15	0	3	2	22	7	7	0	1	10	13	3	6
3938	17	2	0	191	170	0	12	0	2	2	20	5	6	0	2	10	14	4	6
3939	40	5	0	1352	324	0	26	0	31	7	47	14	34	0	10	36	46	10	22

Grains, Beans, Nuts, Seeds

Food No.	Food Description & Amount	wt gm	wt oz	cal	% cal fat	prot gm	carbo gm	fiber gm
3940	Peanuts, dry roasted, salted [1 cup]	144	5.1	842	76%	34	31	11.5
3941	Peanuts, dry roasted, unsalted [1 cup]	144	5.1	842	76%	34	31	11.5
3942	Peanuts, honey-roasted, salted (Include beer nuts) [1 cup]	136	4.8	742	71%	31	37	10.9
3943	Peanuts, in shell (shell not eaten), salted [1 cup, in shell, edible portion]	51	1.8	296	76%	13	10	4.7
3944	Peanuts, roasted, salted [1 cup, halves and whole]	146	5.1	848	76%	38	28	13.4
3945	Peanuts, roasted, unsalted [1 cup, halves and whole]	146	5.1	848	76%	38	28	10.1
3946	Pecans, unsalted [1 cup]	108	3.8	720	91%	8	20	8.2
3947	Pine nuts (Pignolias), unsalted [1 cup]	171	6.0	968	81%	41	24	7.7
3948	Pistachio nuts, roasted, salted [1 cup, in shell, edible yield]	58	2.0	351	78%	9	16	6.3
3949	Pistachio nuts, roasted, unsalted [1 cup, in shell, edible yield]	58	2.0	351	78%	9	16	6.3
3950	Pistachio nuts, unroasted, unsalted [1 cup, shelled]	128	4.5	739	75%	26	32	13.8
3951	Psyllium seed, husks [1 cup, ground]	134	4.7	67	9%	4	108	96.5
3952	Pumpkin and/or squash seeds, hulled, roasted, salted [1 cup]	227	8.0	1185	73%	75	30	8.9
3953	Pumpkin and/or squash seeds, hulled, unroasted, unsalted [142 seeds]	28	1.0	151	76%	7	5	1.1
3954	Sesame butter (tahini) (made from kernels) [2 Tbs]	30	1.1	178	81%	5	6	1.4
3955	Sesame paste (sesame butter made from whole seeds) [2 Tbs]	32	1.1	190	77%	6	8	1.8
3956	Sesame sauce (sesame seeds, water, lemon juice, garlic, salt) [1 cup]	192	6.8	384	74%	12	21	7.8
3957	Sesame seeds, toasted, salted [1 cup]	150	5.3	851	76%	25	39	25.4
3958	Sesame seeds, whole seed, unsalted [1 cup]	144	5.1	825	78%	26	34	17.0
3959	Sunflower seeds, hulled, dry roasted, salted [¼ cup without hulls; ¾ cup with hulls, edible portion]	30	1.1	175	77%	6	7	2.7
3960	Sunflower seeds, hulled, roasted, salted [¼ cup without hulls; ¾ cup with hulls, edible portion]	30	1.1	185	84%	6	4	2.0
3961	Sunflower seeds, hulled, roasted, unsalted [¼ cup without hulls; ¾ cup with hulls, edible portion]	30	1.1	185	84%	6	4	2.0
3962	Sunflower seeds, hulled, unroasted, unsalted [¼ cup without hulls; ¾ cup with hulls, edible portion]	30	1.1	171	78%	7	6	3.2
3963	Trail mix (peanuts, raisins, sunflower seeds, cashews, walnuts, almonds) (Include gorp) [1 cup]	140	4.9	702	64%	22	55	9.5
3964	Walnuts, unsalted [1 cup, chopped]	120	4.2	770	87%	17	22	5.8
3965	Walnuts, honey-roasted [1 cup]	114	4.0	676	81%	14	31	4.7
	Your Additions							

Food No.	fat gm	sat fat gm	choles mg	sodium mg	potas mg	vit A	vit E	vit C	thia	ribo	niac	vit B-6	fola	vit B-12	calc	phos	mag	iron	zinc
						% of Daily Value													
3940	72	10	0	1171	948	0	49	0	42	8	97	18	52	0	8	52	63	18	32
3941	72	10	0	9	948	0	51	0	42	8	97	18	52	0	8	52	63	18	32
3942	58	8	0	514	818	0	40	0	20	8	85	15	37	0	11	61	55	12	53
3943	25	3	0	221	348	0	17	0	9	3	36	7	16	0	4	26	24	5	23
3944	72	10	0	632	996	0	49	0	25	9	104	19	46	0	13	75	68	15	65
3945	72	10	0	9	996	0	49	0	25	9	104	19	46	0	13	75	68	15	65
3946	73	6	0	1	423	1	15	4	61	8	5	10	11	0	4	31	35	13	39
3947	87	13	0	7	1024	1	27	5	92	19	31	9	24	0	4	87	100	87	48
3948	31	4	0	452	563	1	17	7	16	8	4	7	9	0	4	28	19	10	5
3949	31	4	0	3	563	1	14	7	16	8	4	7	9	0	4	28	19	10	5
3950	62	8	0	8	1399	3	30	15	70	13	7	16	19	0	17	64	51	48	11
3951	1	0	0	47	240	3	4	1	63	6	9	16	23	0	27	18	12	26	24
3952	96	18	0	1305	1830	9	10	7	32	43	20	10	33	0	10	266	303	188	113
3953	13	2	0	5	226	1	1	1	4	5	2	3	4	0	1	33	37	23	14
3954	16	2	0	11	138	0	3	2	32	2	8	2	7	0	4	24	7	7	9
3955	16	2	0	4	186	0	3	0	5	4	11	13	8	0	31	21	29	34	16
3956	32	4	0	11	377	0	7	41	30	9	14	27	14	0	63	41	57	52	34
3957	72	10	0	59	609	1	15	0	121	41	41	11	36	0	20	116	130	65	102
3958	72	10	0	16	674	0	15	0	76	21	33	57	35	0	140	91	126	116	74
3959	15	2	0	234	255	0	69	1	2	4	11	12	18	0	2	35	10	6	11
3960	17	2	0	181	145	0	55	1	6	5	6	12	18	0	2	34	10	11	10
3961	17	2	0	1	145	0	69	1	6	5	6	12	18	0	2	34	10	11	10
3962	15	2	0	1	207	0	69	1	46	4	7	12	17	0	3	21	27	11	10
3963	50	6	0	12	998	0	71	4	18	14	43	25	32	0	12	67	51	21	37
3964	74	7	0	12	602	1	14	6	31	10	6	33	20	0	11	38	51	16	22
3965	61	6	0	36	484	3	13	5	20	8	5	25	13	0	9	30	40	14	17

Meat, Poultry, and Fish

Meat, Poultry, Fish

Food No.	Food Description & Amount	wt gm	wt oz	cal	% cal fat	prot gm	carbo gm	fiber gm
	Beef and Veal (weight columns are for cooked, boneless portion)							
4000	Beef brisket, cooked, lean and fat eaten [1 slice (4½" x 2½" x ¼")]	42	1.5	144	69%	10	0	0.0
4001	Beef brisket, cooked, lean only eaten [1 slice (4½" x 2½" x ¼")]	42	1.5	97	45%	12	0	0.0
4002	Beef, cow head, cooked [2 oz, boneless, cooked]	57	2.0	163	60%	15	0	0.0
4003	Beef jerky [1 cup, pieces]	90	3.2	369	56%	30	10	1.6
4004	Beef liver, battered, fried [2 oz, cooked]	56	2.0	132	33%	14	8	0.1
4005	Beef liver, braised [2 oz, cooked]	56	2.0	120	24%	17	5	0.0
4006	Beef liver, breaded, fried (Include floured, fried) [2 oz, cooked]	56	2.0	130	30%	14	7	0.1
4007	Beef liver, fried or broiled, no coating [2 oz, cooked]	56	2.0	122	33%	15	4	0.0
4008	Beef steak, battered, fried, lean and fat eaten [1 medium steak]	243	8.6	765	58%	57	19	0.8
4009	Beef steak, battered, fried, lean only eaten [1 medium steak]	186	6.6	487	45%	49	15	0.6
4010	Beef steak, braised, lean and fat eaten [1 medium steak]	187	6.6	547	56%	56	0	0.0
4011	Beef steak, braised, lean only eaten [1 medium steak]	146	5.1	328	36%	49	0	0.0
4012	Beef steak, breaded or floured, baked or fried, lean and fat eaten [1 medium steak]	243	8.6	805	55%	59	27	0.9
4013	Beef steak, breaded or floured, baked or fried, lean only eaten [1 medium steak]	186	6.6	518	43%	50	21	0.7
4014	Beef steak, broiled or baked, lean and fat eaten [1 medium steak]	204	7.2	521	53%	57	0	0.0
4015	Beef steak, broiled or baked, lean only eaten [1 medium steak]	156	5.5	310	36%	46	0	0.0
4016	Beef steak, fried, lean and fat eaten [1 medium steak]	204	7.2	592	54%	63	0	0.0
4017	Beef steak, fried, lean only eaten [1 medium steak]	156	5.5	362	37%	53	0	0.0
4018	Beef, bacon, cooked [2 slices]	13	0.5	58	69%	4	0	0.0
4019	Beef, bacon, cooked, lean only eaten [2 slices]	12	0.4	21	20%	3	1	0.0
4020	Beef, bacon, formed, lean meat added, cooked (Include Sizzlean) [1 strip]	11	0.4	49	69%	3	0	0.0
4021	Beef, dried, chipped, cooked in fat [1 oz, cooked]	28	1.0	71	61%	7	0	0.0
4022	Beef, dried, chipped, uncooked [1 oz]	28	1.0	46	21%	8	0	0.0
4023	Beef, neckbones, cooked [5 oz, with bone, cooked]	55	1.9	183	65%	15	0	0.0
4024	Beef, oxtails, cooked [3 oz, with bone, cooked]	48	1.7	126	49%	15	0	0.0
4025	Beef, pastrami (beef, smoked, spiced) [2 slices]	56	2.0	195	75%	10	2	0.0
4026	Beef, pickled [2 oz, boneless]	56	2.0	141	68%	10	0	0.0
4027	Beef, pot roast, braised or boiled, lean and fat eaten (Include chuck roast, arm roast, blade roast, shoulder roast) [1 slice (4½" x 2½" x ¼")]	42	1.5	129	61%	12	0	0.0
4028	Beef, pot roast, braised or boiled, lean only eaten (Include chuck roast, arm roast, blade roast, shoulder roast) [1 slice (4½" x 2½" x ¼")]	42	1.5	99	43%	13	0	0.0
4029	Beef, roast, canned (Include beef, steak, canned) [2 oz, boneless]	56	2.0	125	52%	14	0	0.0
4030	Beef, roast, roasted, lean and fat eaten (Include prime ribs, rib roast) [1 slice (4½" x 2½" x ¼")]	42	1.5	112	59%	11	0	0.0
4031	Beef, roast, roasted, lean only eaten (Include prime ribs, rib roast) [1 slice (4½" x 2½" x ¼")]	42	1.5	83	39%	12	0	0.0
4032	Beef, sandwich steak (flaked, formed, thinly sliced) (Include Steak-umms) [1 steak]	41	1.4	105	58%	10	0	0.0
4033	Beef, shortribs, barbecued, with sauce, lean and fat eaten [1 medium rib]	66	2.3	251	77%	11	2	0.2
4034	Beef, shortribs, barbecued, with sauce, lean only eaten [1 medium rib]	51	1.8	108	50%	10	3	0.3
4035	Beef, shortribs, cooked, lean and fat eaten (Include beef rib tips) [1 medium rib]	66	2.3	311	80%	14	0	0.0
4036	Beef, shortribs, cooked, lean only eaten (Include beef rib tips) [1 medium rib]	51	1.8	150	55%	16	0	0.0
4037	Beef, stew meat, cooked, lean and fat eaten [2 oz, boneless, cooked]	56	2.0	172	61%	16	0	0.0
4038	Beef, stew meat, cooked, lean only eaten [2 oz, boneless, cooked]	56	2.0	132	43%	18	0	0.0
4039	Calves liver, braised [2 oz, cooked]	56	2.0	92	38%	12	2	0.0
4040	Calves liver, breaded, fried (Include floured, fried) [2 oz, cooked]	56	2.0	144	38%	16	5	0.1
4041	Calves liver, fried or broiled, no coating [2 oz, cooked]	56	2.0	137	42%	17	2	0.0
4042	Corned beef, canned, ready-to-eat [1 slice]	40	1.4	100	54%	11	0	0.0
4043	Corned beef, cooked, lean and fat eaten [1 slice (4½" x 2½" x ¼")]	42	1.5	105	68%	8	0	0.0
4044	Corned beef, cooked, lean only eaten [1 slice (4½" x 2½" x ¼")]	42	1.5	105	54%	11	0	0.0
4045	Ground beef or patty, breaded, cooked [1 medium patty (4 oz, raw)]	101	3.6	350	62%	17	15	0.5
4046	Ground beef with textured vegetable protein, cooked [1 medium patty]	84	3.0	219	58%	20	1	0.8

Food No.	fat gm	sat fat gm	choles mg	sodium mg	potas mg	% of Daily Value													
						vit A	vit E	vit C	thia	ribo	niac	vit B-6	fola	vit B-12	calc	phos	mag	iron	zinc
4000	11	4	39	26	102	0	0	0	2	5	7	5	1	16	0	8	2	6	15
4001	5	2	39	29	120	0	0	0	2	5	8	6	1	18	0	10	2	7	19
4002	11	4	50	35	181	0	0	0	3	7	10	9	1	23	1	12	3	8	23
4003	23	10	43	1992	537	0	2	0	9	8	8	8	30	15	2	37	11	27	49
4004	5	1	239	42	186	513	3	19	10	97	35	19	35	600	1	20	3	25	17
4005	3	1	296	27	121	658	3	23	9	75	24	18	34	578	0	19	2	19	20
4006	4	1	247	95	197	550	2	20	9	126	38	37	28	956	2	24	3	19	19
4007	4	1	270	59	204	601	2	21	8	136	40	40	31	1043	1	26	3	20	20
4008	49	17	190	361	810	1	9	0	26	45	46	43	6	107	5	61	15	45	73
4009	24	8	146	285	698	1	6	0	22	38	38	37	5	90	4	51	13	38	63
4010	34	13	183	105	507	0	2	0	9	27	29	25	3	80	2	40	10	33	83
4011	13	5	144	88	431	0	1	0	7	23	24	22	3	67	1	35	9	29	76
4012	49	16	182	455	861	1	12	0	29	41	47	43	6	105	12	50	18	48	73
4013	25	7	141	356	736	1	9	0	25	35	39	37	5	88	9	43	15	40	63
4014	31	12	170	124	744	0	2	0	13	26	47	40	4	83	2	43	13	30	70
4015	13	5	126	102	642	0	1	0	11	22	41	36	4	66	1	36	11	24	61
4016	36	13	199	142	905	0	2	0	15	33	46	52	5	112	2	52	16	36	66
4017	15	5	153	115	767	0	1	0	13	28	39	44	5	92	1	44	13	30	56
4018	4	2	15	293	54	0	0	0	1	2	4	2	0	7	0	3	1	2	6
4019	0	0	5	173	51	0	0	0	1	1	3	2	0	5	0	2	1	2	3
4020	4	2	13	248	45	0	0	0	1	2	4	2	0	6	0	3	1	2	5
4021	5	2	22	15	94	0	0	0	2	4	4	4	1	13	0	6	2	4	8
4022	1	0	12	972	124	0	0	0	2	3	8	5	1	12	0	5	2	7	10
4023	13	5	54	33	135	0	0	0	3	8	9	8	1	27	1	12	3	10	25
4024	7	3	51	34	126	0	0	0	3	8	6	7	1	20	1	11	3	10	33
4025	16	6	52	687	128	0	1	3	4	6	14	5	1	16	1	8	3	6	16
4026	11	4	55	635	81	0	0	0	1	6	8	6	1	15	0	7	2	6	17
4027	9	3	42	26	106	0	0	0	2	6	6	6	1	17	0	9	2	7	21
4028	5	2	43	28	116	0	0	0	2	7	7	6	1	18	0	10	2	8	25
4029	7	3	45	34	145	0	0	0	1	8	12	4	1	22	1	6	3	8	23
4030	7	3	33	26	143	0	0	0	2	5	8	7	1	17	0	9	2	5	16
4031	4	1	32	28	159	0	0	0	3	5	8	7	1	18	0	9	3	6	18
4032	7	3	33	29	128	0	0	0	2	6	10	6	1	14	0	7	2	5	15
4033	22	9	47	172	144	2	2	2	2	5	7	6	1	22	1	9	3	7	17
4034	6	2	29	203	136	2	1	3	2	4	6	5	1	18	1	8	3	7	16
4035	28	12	62	33	148	0	1	0	2	6	8	7	1	29	1	11	2	8	21
4036	9	4	47	30	160	0	0	0	2	6	8	7	1	29	1	12	3	10	27
4037	12	5	56	35	141	0	0	0	3	8	8	8	1	23	1	12	3	10	28
4038	6	2	57	37	155	0	0	0	3	9	9	9	1	25	1	14	3	11	33
4039	4	1	314	30	115	451	1	29	5	64	24	14	106	341	0	18	3	8	36
4040	6	2	169	108	235	289	1	19	10	102	45	22	41	547	2	23	4	17	27
4041	6	2	185	74	245	315	1	21	9	111	47	24	45	597	1	25	4	16	29
4042	6	2	34	402	54	0	0	1	1	3	5	3	1	11	0	4	1	5	10
4043	8	3	41	476	61	0	0	0	1	4	6	5	1	11	0	5	1	4	13
4044	6	3	36	423	57	0	0	1	1	4	5	3	1	11	1	5	1	5	10
4045	24	6	54	231	236	1	11	0	10	12	24	9	2	30	7	14	6	15	22
4046	14	5	59	145	232	0	2	0	12	14	26	19	5	35	1	17	4	11	26

Meat, Poultry, Fish

Food No.	Food Description & Amount	wt gm	wt oz	cal	% cal fat	prot gm	carbo gm	fiber gm
4047	Ground beef, extra lean, cooked (Include ground sirloin, ground round) [1 medium patty (4 oz, raw)]	96	3.4	246	57%	24	0	0.0
4048	Ground beef, lean, cooked (Include ground chuck) [1 medium patty (4 oz, raw)]	88	3.1	239	61%	22	0	0.0
4049	Ground beef, meatballs, meat only [2 medium]	56	2.0	158	57%	16	0	0.0
4050	Ground beef, raw [2 oz]	56	2.0	155	73%	10	0	0.0
4051	Ground beef, regular, cooked [1 medium patty (4 oz, raw)]	85	3.0	246	64%	20	0	0.0
4052	Veal chop, broiled, lean and fat eaten [1 medium (6.5 oz, with bone, raw)]	107	3.8	232	51%	27	0	0.0
4053	Veal chop, broiled, lean only eaten [1 medium (6.5 oz, with bone, raw)]	85	3.0	135	32%	22	0	0.0
4054	Veal chop, fried, lean and fat eaten (Include breaded) [1 medium (6.5 oz, with bone, raw)]	107	3.8	244	36%	29	11	0.3
4055	Veal chop, fried, lean only eaten (Include breaded) [1 medium (6.5 oz, with bone, raw)]	85	3.0	203	36%	25	7	0.2
4056	Veal cutlet or steak, broiled, lean and fat eaten [2 oz, boneless, cooked]	56	2.0	90	26%	16	0	0.0
4057	Veal cutlet or steak, broiled, lean only eaten [2 oz, boneless, cooked]	56	2.0	102	23%	19	0	0.0
4058	Veal cutlet or steak, fried, lean and fat eaten (Include breaded or floured) [2 oz, boneless, cooked]	56	2.0	128	36%	15	6	0.2
4059	Veal cutlet or steak, fried, lean only eaten (Include breaded or floured) [2 oz, boneless, cooked, lean only]	56	2.0	102	23%	19	0	0.0
4060	Veal loaf [2 slices]	56	2.0	172	77%	8	2	0.0
4061	Veal patty, breaded, cooked [1 medium patty (4 oz, raw)]	79	2.8	212	54%	16	7	0.2
4062	Veal, ground or patty, cooked [1 medium patty (4 oz, raw)]	67	2.4	115	40%	16	0	0.0
4063	Veal, roasted, lean and fat eaten [1 slice (4½" x 2½" x ¼")]	42	1.5	97	44%	13	0	0.0
4064	Veal, roasted, lean only eaten [1 slice (4½" x 2½" x ¼")]	42	1.5	67	32%	11	0	0.0
	Pork (weight columns are for cooked, boneless portion)							
4150	Bacon (pork), smoked or cured, cooked [2 slices]	16	0.6	92	77%	5	0	0.0
4151	Bacon (pork), smoked or cured, cooked, lean only eaten [2 slices]	12	0.4	22	41%	3	0	0.0
4152	Bacon (pork), smoked or cured, lower sodium [2 slices]	16	0.6	92	77%	5	0	0.0
4153	Bacon (pork), formed, lean meat added, cooked (Include breakfast strips; Sizzlean) [2 strips]	22	0.8	101	72%	6	0	0.0
4154	Bacon or side pork, fresh, cooked [1 slice (¼" thick)]	26	0.9	150	77%	8	0	0.0
4155	Canadian bacon, cooked [1 slice]	23	0.8	43	41%	6	0	0.0
4156	Fat back, cooked [1 oz, raw (yield after cooking)]	20	0.7	162	98%	1	0	0.0
4157	Pork, fried chunks, Puerto Rican style (Carne de cerdo frita, masitas fritas) [1 piece (2½" x 2" x 1")]	38	1.3	104	53%	11	0	0.0
4158	Pork jerky [1 cup, pieces]	126	4.4	519	45%	67	0	0.0
4159	Ham, breaded, fried, lean and fat eaten (Include smoked, cured, canned; chicken fried ham) [1 slice (4½" x 2½" x ¼")]	42	1.5	97	53%	8	3	0.1
4160	Ham, breaded, fried, lean only eaten (Include smoked, cured, canned; chicken fried ham) [1 slice (4½" x 2½" x ¼")]	42	1.5	87	42%	9	3	0.1
4161	Ham, fresh, cooked, lean and fat eaten [1 slice (4½" x 2½" x ¼")]	42	1.5	115	58%	11	0	0.0
4162	Ham, fresh, cooked, lean only eaten [1 slice (4½" x 2½" x ¼")]	42	1.5	89	40%	12	0	0.0
4163	Ham, fried, lean and fat eaten (Include smoked, cured, canned) [1 slice (4½" x 2½" x ¼")]	42	1.5	94	60%	9	0	0.0
4164	Ham, fried, lean only eaten (Include smoked, cured, canned) [1 slice (4½" x 2½" x ¼")]	42	1.5	81	48%	10	0	0.0
4165	Ham, luncheon meat, chopped, minced, pressed, spiced (Include Spam, Treet) [2 slices (4¼" x 4¼" x 1/16")]	42	1.5	102	70%	7	0	0.0
4166	Ham, luncheon meat, chopped, minced, pressed, spiced, lowfat [2 slices (4¼" x 4¼" x 1/16")]	42	1.5	55	34%	8	0	0.0
4167	Ham, prosciutto [2 oz, boneless]	56	2.0	109	38%	16	0	0.0
4168	Ham, sliced, extra lean, prepackaged or deli-sliced (Include 95% or more fat-free) [1 slice (6¼" x 4" x 1/16")]	56	2.0	73	34%	11	1	0.0
4169	Ham, sliced, low salt, prepackaged or deli-sliced (Include low salt boiled ham) [2 slices (6¼" x 4" x 1/16")]	56	2.0	92	42%	12	0	0.0

Food No.	fat gm	sat fat gm	choles mg	sodium mg	potas mg	vit A	vit E	vit C	thia	ribo	niac	vit B-6	fola	vit B-12	calc	phos	mag	iron	zinc
						% of Daily Value													
4047	16	6	81	67	300	0	1	0	4	15	24	13	2	35	1	15	5	13	35
4048	16	6	77	68	265	0	1	0	3	11	23	11	2	34	1	14	5	10	31
4049	10	4	56	50	193	0	1	0	2	8	17	9	1	27	1	10	3	8	23
4050	12	5	44	38	142	0	0	0	2	6	13	7	1	22	0	8	2	6	14
4051	18	7	77	71	248	0	1	0	2	10	25	11	2	42	1	14	4	12	29
4052	13	6	110	100	348	0	2	0	4	18	47	18	4	22	2	23	7	5	22
4053	5	2	115	92	264	0	1	0	4	16	34	11	3	27	2	18	5	5	26
4054	10	3	120	486	397	1	3	0	11	22	55	21	5	22	4	27	8	10	20
4055	8	2	93	220	274	0	3	0	7	17	42	14	4	17	3	20	6	7	18
4056	3	1	58	38	218	0	1	0	2	11	28	9	2	11	0	13	4	3	11
4057	3	1	60	43	248	0	1	0	3	12	35	14	2	14	0	16	4	3	13
4058	5	2	63	254	208	1	1	0	6	12	29	11	3	12	2	14	4	5	10
4059	3	1	60	43	248	0	1	0	3	12	35	14	2	14	0	16	4	3	13
4060	15	6	36	744	116	0	1	0	4	7	10	5	1	36	1	7	2	7	9
4061	13	4	80	142	227	1	5	0	6	13	29	14	3	12	4	15	5	6	13
4062	5	2	69	56	226	0	0	0	3	11	27	13	2	14	1	15	4	4	17
4063	5	2	48	37	137	0	1	0	2	8	17	7	2	11	1	10	3	3	13
4064	2	1	57	45	131	0	1	0	2	8	17	5	1	13	1	9	3	2	13
4150	8	3	14	255	78	0	0	0	7	3	6	2	0	5	0	5	1	1	3
4151	1	0	7	186	47	0	0	0	7	1	4	3	0	2	0	4	1	1	1
4152	8	3	14	165	78	0	0	0	7	3	6	2	0	5	0	5	1	1	3
4153	8	3	23	462	103	0	0	0	11	5	8	4	0	6	0	6	1	2	5
4154	13	5	22	415	126	0	1	0	12	4	10	4	0	8	0	9	2	2	6
4155	2	1	13	356	90	0	0	0	13	3	8	5	0	3	0	7	1	1	3
4156	18	6	10	2	12	0	1	0	1	1	1	0	0	0	0	1	0	0	1
4157	6	2	34	30	162	0	0	1	28	7	10	9	1	5	1	10	3	2	6
4158	26	9	113	3623	879	1	3	1	108	48	58	53	7	28	2	35	8	15	51
4159	6	2	27	464	127	0	2	0	19	7	10	7	1	4	1	9	2	4	6
4160	4	1	27	495	120	0	2	0	17	7	10	8	1	4	1	9	2	3	6
4161	7	3	39	25	148	0	0	0	18	8	10	8	1	5	1	11	2	2	8
4162	4	1	39	27	157	0	0	0	19	9	10	9	1	5	0	12	3	3	9
4163	6	2	22	504	135	0	2	0	20	6	10	7	0	5	0	9	2	3	7
4164	4	1	22	529	126	0	2	0	18	6	10	9	0	5	0	9	2	2	7
4165	8	3	24	557	128	0	0	0	18	5	8	7	0	6	0	6	2	2	5
4166	2	1	20	600	147	0	1	0	26	6	10	10	0	5	0	9	2	2	5
4167	5	2	39	1509	286	0	1	0	21	8	11	12	1	8	1	18	4	3	10
4168	3	1	26	800	196	0	1	0	35	7	14	13	1	7	0	12	2	2	7
4169	4	1	32	543	203	0	1	0	28	9	15	10	0	6	0	14	3	4	10

Meat, Poultry, Fish

Food No.	Food Description & Amount	wt gm	wt oz	cal	% cal fat	prot gm	carbo gm	fiber gm
4170	Ham, sliced, prepackaged or deli-sliced (Include boiled ham) [2 slices (6¼" x 4" x 1/16")]	56	2.0	91	47%	10	1	0.0
4171	Ham, smoked or cured, canned, lean and fat eaten [1 slice (4½" x 2½" x ¼")]	42	1.5	80	62%	7	0	0.0
4172	Ham, smoked or cured, canned, lean only eaten [1 slice (4½" x 2½" x ¼")]	42	1.5	50	34%	8	0	0.0
4173	Ham, smoked or cured, cooked, lean and fat eaten (Include country ham; cottage ham; picnic ham; ham) [1 slice (4½" x 2½" x ¼")]	42	1.5	72	44%	9	0	0.0
4174	Ham, smoked or cured, cooked, lean only eaten (Include country ham; cottage ham; picnic ham) [1 slice (4½" x 2½" x ¼")]	42	1.5	66	32%	11	0	0.0
4175	Ham, smoked or cured, ground patty [2 oz, cooked]	56	2.0	192	81%	7	1	0.0
4176	Ham, smoked or cured, low sodium, cooked, lean and fat eaten (Include canned) [1 slice (4½" x 2½" x ¼")]	42	1.5	72	43%	9	0	0.0
4177	Ham, smoked or cured, low sodium, cooked, lean only eaten (Include canned) [1 slice (4½" x 2½" x ¼")]	42	1.5	61	34%	9	1	0.0
4178	Pork chop, battered, fried, lean and fat eaten [1 medium (5.5 oz, with bone, raw)]	110	3.9	297	53%	26	7	0.2
4179	Pork chop, battered, fried, lean only eaten [1 medium (5.5 oz, with bone, raw)]	84	3.0	212	49%	21	5	0.2
4180	Pork chop, breaded, broiled or baked, lean and fat eaten (Include Shake-n-Bake) [1 medium (5.5 oz, with bone, raw)]	100	3.5	259	49%	25	6	0.2
4181	Pork chop, breaded, broiled or baked, lean only eaten (Include Shake-n-Bake) [1 medium (5.5 oz, with bone, raw)]	80	2.8	184	40%	21	5	0.2
4182	Pork chop, breaded, fried, lean and fat eaten [1 medium (5.5 oz, with bone, raw)]	110	3.9	345	53%	24	15	0.5
4183	Pork chop, breaded, fried, lean only eaten [1 medium (5.5 oz, with bone, raw)]	84	3.0	241	46%	19	12	0.4
4184	Pork chop, broiled or baked, lean and fat eaten (Include floured) [1 medium (5.5 oz, with bone, raw)]	85	3.0	206	52%	23	0	0.0
4185	Pork chop, broiled or baked, lean only eaten (Include floured) [1 medium (5.5 oz, with bone, raw)]	67	2.4	141	42%	19	0	0.0
4186	Pork chop, fried, lean and fat eaten (Include floured) [1 medium (5.5 oz, with bone, raw)]	92	3.2	249	57%	25	0	0.0
4187	Pork chop, fried, lean only eaten (Include floured) [1 medium (5.5 oz, with bone, raw)]	70	2.5	159	46%	20	0	0.0
4188	Pork chop, smoked or cured, cooked, lean and fat eaten [1 medium (5.5 oz, with bone, raw)]	84	3.0	235	69%	17	0	0.0
4189	Pork chop, smoked or cured, cooked, lean only eaten [1 medium (5.5 oz, with bone, raw)]	67	2.4	114	37%	17	0	0.0
4190	Pork chop, stewed, lean and fat eaten [1 medium (5.5 oz, with bone, raw)]	77	2.7	184	51%	21	0	0.0
4191	Pork chop, stewed, lean only eaten [1 medium (5.5 oz, with bone, raw)]	66	2.3	139	43%	19	0	0.0
4192	Pork ears, tail, head, snout, miscellaneous parts, cooked [1 ear]	111	3.9	327	73%	20	0	0.0
4193	Pork liver, braised [2 oz, cooked]	56	2.0	92	24%	15	2	0.0
4194	Pork liver, breaded, fried (Include floured, fried) [2 oz, cooked]	56	2.0	143	33%	17	6	0.1
4195	Pork roast, loin, cooked, lean and fat eaten [1 slice (4½" x 2½" x ¼")]	42	1.5	104	53%	11	0	0.0
4196	Pork roast, loin, cooked, lean only eaten [1 slice (4½" x 2½" x ¼")]	42	1.5	88	41%	12	0	0.0
4197	Pork roast, shoulder, cooked, lean and fat eaten [1 slice (3" dia x ¼")]	28	1.0	82	66%	7	0	0.0
4198	Pork roast, shoulder, cooked, lean only eaten [1 slice (3" dia x ¼")]	28	1.0	64	53%	7	0	0.0
4199	Pork roast, smoked or cured, cooked, lean and fat eaten [1 slice (4½" x 2½" x ¼")]	42	1.5	69	42%	9	0	0.0
4200	Pork roast, smoked or cured, cooked, lean only eaten [1 slice (4½" x 2½" x ¼")]	42	1.5	66	32%	11	0	0.0
4201	Pork roll, cured, fried [2 slices]	56	2.0	199	82%	7	1	0.0
4202	Pork skin, boiled [1 slice]	33	1.2	208	91%	4	0	0.0
4203	Pork skin, rinds, deep-fried (Include snack type) [10 rinds]	10	0.4	54	52%	6	0	0.0
4204	Pork steak or cutlet, battered, fried, lean and fat eaten [3 oz]	75	2.6	210	55%	17	5	0.1
4205	Pork steak or cutlet, battered, fried, lean only eaten [3 oz]	63	2.2	152	47%	15	4	0.1
4206	Pork steak or cutlet, breaded, broiled or baked, lean and fat eaten [3 oz]	75	2.6	203	50%	18	6	0.2
4207	Pork steak or cutlet, breaded, broiled or baked, lean only eaten [3 oz]	63	2.2	149	40%	16	5	0.2
4208	Pork steak or cutlet, breaded, fried, lean and fat eaten [3 oz]	75	2.6	210	51%	17	7	0.2
4209	Pork steak or cutlet, breaded, fried, lean only eaten [3 oz]	87	3.1	228	46%	21	9	0.3

Food No.	fat gm	sat fat gm	choles mg	sodium mg	potas mg	vit A	vit E	vit C	thia	ribo	niac	vit B-6	fola	vit B-12	calc	phos	mag	iron	zinc
						% of Daily Value													
4170	5	2	30	716	166	0	1	0	33	8	14	11	0	7	0	13	3	3	8
4171	5	2	16	521	133	0	0	0	27	6	7	10	1	5	0	7	1	2	5
4172	2	1	16	527	153	0	0	0	23	6	11	9	1	6	0	9	2	2	5
4173	4	1	24	606	162	0	0	0	21	8	12	7	0	5	0	11	2	3	7
4174	2	1	23	557	133	0	0	0	19	6	11	10	0	5	0	10	2	2	7
4175	17	6	40	595	137	0	1	0	13	6	9	4	0	7	1	6	1	5	7
4176	3	1	24	407	162	0	0	0	20	8	12	7	0	5	0	11	2	3	7
4177	2	1	22	407	121	0	0	0	21	5	8	8	0	5	0	8	1	3	8
4178	18	6	78	82	412	1	4	1	55	20	26	18	2	10	4	24	7	6	13
4179	11	3	58	63	324	1	3	1	44	16	20	15	1	8	3	19	5	5	10
4180	14	5	72	415	400	0	2	1	54	18	24	21	1	10	2	24	7	6	15
4181	8	3	57	333	331	0	2	1	45	15	20	18	1	9	2	20	6	5	12
4182	20	6	100	240	371	2	7	1	50	21	26	16	3	10	7	23	7	11	14
4183	12	3	76	190	293	2	5	1	40	17	20	13	2	8	5	18	6	9	11
4184	12	4	68	53	360	0	1	1	50	16	21	20	1	10	2	21	6	4	14
4185	7	2	53	43	293	0	1	1	41	13	18	16	1	8	1	17	5	3	11
4186	16	6	73	57	390	0	1	1	52	17	24	18	1	11	2	22	6	4	14
4187	8	3	55	46	312	0	1	1	43	14	19	15	1	9	1	17	5	3	12
4188	18	6	49	900	217	0	1	0	34	9	17	12	1	13	1	19	3	4	14
4189	5	2	32	825	196	0	1	0	32	9	16	12	1	12	1	16	3	4	13
4190	10	4	62	37	288	0	1	1	32	12	17	14	1	7	2	14	4	5	12
4191	7	2	53	37	242	0	1	1	30	10	15	12	1	6	1	11	3	4	12
4192	27	10	112	91	185	0	1	0	14	8	10	11	1	8	2	9	3	7	13
4193	2	1	199	27	84	302	1	22	10	72	24	16	23	174	1	13	2	56	25
4194	5	1	234	101	191	379	3	26	12	125	49	16	35	269	2	21	4	97	30
4195	6	2	34	25	171	0	0	0	28	8	12	11	1	5	1	10	3	2	6
4196	4	1	34	24	179	0	0	0	28	8	12	12	1	5	1	10	3	3	7
4197	6	2	25	19	92	0	0	0	11	5	6	4	0	4	1	6	1	2	7
4198	4	1	25	21	97	0	0	0	12	6	6	4	0	4	1	6	1	2	8
4199	3	1	24	582	152	0	0	0	21	7	11	7	0	5	0	10	2	3	7
4200	2	1	23	557	133	0	0	0	19	6	11	10	0	5	0	10	2	2	7
4201	18	6	39	581	133	0	2	0	13	6	9	4	0	6	0	6	1	5	7
4202	21	8	31	11	78	0	1	0	7	2	4	2	0	2	2	5	1	1	3
4203	3	1	9	184	13	0	0	0	1	2	1	0	0	1	0	1	0	0	0
4204	13	4	61	64	241	1	3	1	38	15	16	11	1	9	4	16	4	5	14
4205	8	2	49	51	205	1	2	0	31	13	14	9	1	8	3	13	4	5	13
4206	11	4	61	79	251	0	1	1	40	17	17	14	1	10	3	16	5	7	16
4207	7	2	51	69	221	0	1	1	36	15	15	13	1	9	2	14	4	6	15
4208	12	4	73	131	238	1	2	1	36	17	16	13	1	10	4	16	5	8	15
4209	12	3	83	157	281	1	4	1	44	20	19	16	2	12	4	19	6	9	19

Meat, Poultry, Fish

Food No.	Food Description & Amount	wt gm	wt oz	cal	% cal fat	prot gm	carbo gm	fiber gm
4210	Pork steak or cutlet, broiled or baked, lean and fat eaten (Include floured) [3 oz]	75	2.6	177	51%	20	0	0.0
4211	Pork steak or cutlet, broiled or baked, lean only eaten (Include floured) [3 oz]	72	2.5	153	44%	20	0	0.0
4212	Pork steak or cutlet, fried, lean and fat eaten (Include floured) [3 oz]	75	2.6	204	57%	21	0	0.0
4213	Pork steak or cutlet, fried, lean only eaten (Include floured) [3 oz]	63	2.2	144	47%	18	0	0.0
4214	Pork, cracklings, cooked [1 cup]	91	3.2	524	77%	28	1	0.0
4215	Pork, dehydrated, oriental style [1 cup]	22	0.8	135	91%	3	0	0.0
4216	Pork, ground or patty, breaded, cooked [2 oz, cooked]	56	2.0	196	61%	10	9	0.3
4217	Pork, ground or patty, cooked [2 oz, cooked]	56	2.0	166	63%	14	0	0.0
4218	Pork, neckbones, cooked (Include pork backbone) [1 neckbone]	47	1.7	98	41%	13	0	0.0
4219	Pork, pickled [2 boneless pieces (1 cubic inch]	36	1.3	73	72%	5	0	0.0
4220	Pork, pig's feet, cooked [1 foot]	87	3.1	169	58%	17	0	0.0
4221	Pork, pig's feet, pickled [1 foot]	87	3.1	177	72%	12	0	0.0
4222	Pork, pig's hocks, cooked (Include ham hocks) [1 ham hock]	51	1.8	168	64%	14	0	0.0
4223	Pork, spareribs, cooked, lean and fat eaten (Include flank end) [1 medium rib]	35	1.2	139	69%	10	0	0.0
4224	Pork, spareribs, cooked, lean only eaten (Include flank end) [1 medium rib]	26	0.9	54	41%	7	0	0.0
4225	Pork, spareribs, barbecued, with sauce, lean and fat eaten [2 oz, with bone, cooked]	42	1.5	130	65%	9	2	0.2
4226	Pork, spareribs, barbecued, with sauce, lean only eaten [2 oz, with bone, cooked]	32	1.1	71	48%	7	1	0.1
4227	Pork, tenderloin, baked [2 oz, boneless, cooked]	56	2.0	97	31%	16	0	0.0
4228	Pork, tenderloin, battered, fried [2 oz, boneless, cooked]	56	2.0	117	36%	14	4	0.1
4229	Pork, tenderloin, braised [2 oz, boneless, cooked]	56	2.0	114	40%	16	0	0.0
4230	Pork, tenderloin, breaded, fried (Include floured) [2 oz, boneless, cooked]	56	2.0	110	42%	11	4	0.1
4231	Salt pork or fat back, cooked (Include hog jowl) [1 slice (4" x 1¾" x ½")]	47	1.7	337	96%	3	0	0.0
	Lamb (weight columns are for cooked, boneless portion)							
4250	Lamb hocks, cooked (Include mutton hocks) [2 oz]	38	1.3	92	50%	11	0	0.0
4251	Lamb liver, cooked (Include mutton) [2 oz, cooked]	56	2.0	123	36%	17	1	0.0
4252	Lamb, ground or patty, cooked (Include mutton, ground or patty) [1 patty (4 oz, raw)]	77	2.7	218	62%	19	0	0.0
4253	Lamb, loin chop, cooked, lean and fat eaten (Include lamb steak, mutton loin chop, mutton steak) [1 medium (5 oz, with bone, raw)]	89	3.1	281	66%	22	0	0.0
4254	Lamb, loin chop, cooked, lean only eaten (Include lamb steak, mutton loin chop, mutton steak) [1 medium (5 oz, with bone, raw)]	62	2.2	134	41%	19	0	0.0
4255	Lamb, ribs, cooked, lean and fat eaten (Include mutton ribs) [1 rib]	46	1.6	166	74%	10	0	0.0
4256	Lamb, ribs, cooked, lean only eaten (Include mutton ribs) [2 ribs]	50	1.8	118	50%	14	0	0.0
4257	Lamb, roast, cooked, lean and fat eaten (Include mutton roast; lamb leg; mutton leg) [1 slice (3" dia x ¼")]	28	1.0	75	61%	7	0	0.0
4258	Lamb, roast, cooked, lean only eaten (Include mutton roast; lamb leg; mutton leg) [1 slice (3" dia x ¼")]	28	1.0	55	42%	7	0	0.0
4259	Lamb, shoulder chop, cooked, lean and fat eaten (Include mutton shoulder chop) [1 chop (7 oz, with bone, raw)]	127	4.5	351	65%	29	0	0.0
4260	Lamb, shoulder chop, cooked, lean only eaten (Include mutton shoulder chop) [1 chop (7 oz, with bone, raw)]	91	3.2	186	48%	23	0	0.0
4261	Lamb, shoulder, cooked, lean and fat eaten (Include mutton shoulder) [1 slice (3" dia x ¼")]	28	1.0	77	65%	6	0	0.0
4262	Lamb, shoulder, cooked, lean only eaten (Include mutton shoulder) [1 slice (3" dia x ¼")]	28	1.0	57	48%	7	0	0.0
	Chicken (weight columns are for cooked, boneless portion)							
4300	Chicken, back, battered, fried, skin eaten (Include extra crispy fried chicken) [1 back]	212	7.5	703	60%	47	22	0.7
4301	Chicken, back, battered, fried, skin not eaten (Include extra crispy fried chicken) [1 back]	119	4.2	344	48%	36	7	0.2
4302	Chicken, back, breaded, fried or baked with added fat, skin eaten (Include Shake-n-Bake) [1 back]	212	7.5	703	59%	58	11	0.3

						% of Daily Value													
Food No.	fat gm	sat fat gm	choles mg	sodium mg	potas mg	vit A	vit E	vit C	thia	ribo	niac	vit B-6	fola	vit B-12	calc	phos	mag	iron	zinc
4210	10	4	67	47	269	0	1	1	40	17	17	14	1	11	2	17	4	5	17
4211	8	3	64	49	279	0	1	1	45	17	17	16	1	12	2	17	5	6	17
4212	13	5	60	46	325	0	1	1	41	14	19	15	1	9	2	18	5	3	12
4213	8	3	49	41	280	0	1	1	36	13	17	13	1	8	1	16	4	3	11
4214	45	16	77	1452	442	0	2	0	42	15	33	12	1	27	1	31	5	8	20
4215	14	5	15	151	31	0	0	0	7	2	2	2	0	1	0	3	1	1	2
4216	13	3	31	125	154	0	6	0	20	7	10	7	1	3	4	10	3	6	8
4217	12	4	53	41	203	0	1	1	26	7	12	11	1	5	1	13	3	4	12
4218	5	2	38	313	164	0	1	0	21	8	13	9	1	7	0	11	2	4	12
4219	6	2	33	332	85	0	0	0	0	1	1	7	0	4	1	1	0	1	3
4220	11	4	87	26	127	0	1	0	1	3	2	4	0	3	4	4	1	2	6
4221	14	5	80	803	204	0	1	0	0	2	2	17	1	9	3	3	1	3	7
4222	12	4	56	45	188	0	1	0	18	9	13	9	1	6	1	11	2	5	14
4223	11	4	42	33	112	0	0	0	10	8	10	6	0	6	2	9	2	4	11
4224	2	1	18	11	105	0	0	0	11	4	7	4	0	2	1	5	1	1	4
4225	9	3	36	140	120	1	1	2	8	7	9	6	0	5	2	8	2	4	9
4226	4	1	27	103	113	1	1	1	11	5	5	4	0	4	1	4	2	3	9
4227	3	1	44	31	242	0	1	0	35	13	13	12	1	5	0	14	4	5	10
4228	5	1	42	42	218	1	2	0	31	13	12	10	1	5	2	13	4	5	9
4229	5	2	44	28	217	0	1	1	25	9	13	11	1	5	1	10	3	4	9
4230	5	1	42	74	165	1	4	1	24	10	10	9	1	6	2	11	4	5	7
4231	36	13	40	601	30	0	1	0	3	2	4	1	0	2	0	2	1	1	4
4250	5	2	40	27	98	0	0	0	1	4	10	2	2	14	1	6	2	5	19
4251	5	2	281	31	124	419	2	4	9	133	34	14	10	714	0	24	3	26	29
4252	15	6	75	62	261	0	1	0	5	11	26	5	4	33	2	15	5	8	24
4253	21	9	92	62	254	0	1	0	6	15	33	6	3	37	2	18	5	9	19
4254	6	2	59	52	233	0	0	0	5	10	21	5	4	26	1	14	4	7	17
4255	14	6	46	35	124	0	0	0	3	6	16	3	2	19	1	8	3	5	12
4256	6	2	46	43	157	0	0	0	3	7	16	4	3	22	1	11	4	6	18
4257	5	2	26	18	79	0	0	0	2	4	9	2	1	12	0	5	2	3	9
4258	3	1	25	19	84	0	0	0	2	5	8	2	2	12	0	6	2	3	10
4259	25	11	117	84	319	0	1	0	8	18	39	8	7	56	3	23	7	14	44
4260	10	4	79	62	241	0	1	0	5	14	26	7	6	41	2	18	6	11	37
4261	6	2	26	18	70	0	0	0	2	4	9	2	1	12	1	5	2	3	10
4262	3	1	24	19	74	0	0	0	2	4	8	2	2	13	1	6	2	3	11
4300	47	12	186	671	381	8	12	0	17	27	62	25	4	9	6	29	10	18	28
4301	18	5	111	118	299	3	3	0	9	18	46	21	3	6	3	21	7	11	22
4302	46	12	187	817	497	8	9	0	12	27	74	31	4	10	6	37	12	18	35

Meat, Poultry, Fish

Food No.	Food Description & Amount	wt gm	wt oz	cal	% cal fat	prot gm	carbo gm	fiber gm
4303	Chicken, back, breaded, fried or baked with added fat, skin not eaten (Include Shake-n-Bake) [1 back]	119	4.2	344	48%	36	7	0.2
4304	Chicken, back, broiled or grilled, skin eaten [1 back]	134	4.7	402	63%	35	0	0.0
4305	Chicken, back, broiled or grilled, skin not eaten [1 back]	112	4.0	268	50%	32	0	0.0
4306	Chicken, back, floured, seasoned, fried or baked with added fat, skin eaten [1 back]	128	4.5	424	56%	36	8	0.3
4307	Chicken, back, floured, seasoned, fried or baked with added fat, skin not eaten [1 back]	103	3.6	300	48%	31	6	0.2
4308	Chicken, back, fried, no coating, skin eaten [1 back]	128	4.5	416	62%	37	0	0.0
4309	Chicken, back, fried, no coating, skin not eaten [1 back]	103	3.6	289	52%	32	0	0.0
4310	Chicken, back, roasted, skin eaten [1 back]	94	3.3	282	63%	24	0	0.0
4311	Chicken, back, roasted, skin not eaten [1 back]	72	2.5	172	50%	20	0	0.0
4312	Chicken, back, stewed, skin eaten [1 back]	106	3.7	273	63%	24	0	0.0
4313	Chicken, back, stewed, skin not eaten [1 back]	75	2.6	157	48%	19	0	0.0
4314	Chicken, breast, battered, fried, skin eaten (Include extra crispy fried chicken) [½ breast]	140	4.9	364	46%	35	13	0.4
4315	Chicken, breast, battered, fried, skin not eaten (Include extra crispy fried chicken) [½ breast]	88	3.1	165	23%	29	0	0.0
4316	Chicken, breast, breaded, fried or baked with added fat, skin eaten (Include regular fried chicken, Shake-n-Bake) [½ breast]	140	4.9	328	37%	42	7	0.2
4317	Chicken, breast, breaded, fried or baked with added fat, skin not eaten (Include regular fried chicken, Shake-n-Bake) [½ breast]	88	3.1	165	23%	29	0	0.0
4318	Chicken, breast, broiled or grilled, skin eaten [½ breast]	92	3.2	181	36%	27	0	0.0
4319	Chicken, breast, broiled or grilled, skin not eaten [½ breast]	81	2.9	134	19%	25	0	0.0
4320	Chicken, breast, floured, seasoned, fried or baked with added fat, skin eaten [½ breast]	98	3.5	218	36%	31	2	0.1
4321	Chicken, breast, floured, fried or baked with added fat [½ breast]	86	3.0	161	23%	29	0	0.0
4322	Chicken, breast, fried, no coating, skin eaten (Include sauteed) [½ breast]	98	3.5	214	37%	32	0	0.0
4323	Chicken, breast, fried, no coating, skin not eaten (Include sauteed) [½ breast]	86	3.0	160	23%	29	0	0.0
4324	Chicken, breast, roasted, skin eaten [½ breast]	98	3.5	193	36%	29	0	0.0
4325	Chicken, breast, roasted, skin not eaten [½ breast]	86	3.0	142	19%	27	0	0.0
4326	Chicken, breast, skinless, battered, fried, batter eaten (Include Chicken Tenders) [1 tender (piece)]	12	0.4	28	37%	3	1	0.0
4327	Chicken, breast, skinless, breaded, cooked, breading eaten (Include Weaver Crispy Light Fried Chicken, Perdue Done It Chicken Breast Tenders) [½ breast]	124	4.4	282	31%	37	10	0.3
4328	Chicken, breast, stewed, skin eaten [½ breast]	110	3.9	202	36%	30	0	0.0
4329	Chicken, breast, stewed, skin not eaten [½ breast]	95	3.4	143	18%	28	0	0.0
4330	Chicken, canned, dark meat [1 can (5 oz), meat portion]	125	4.4	239	42%	32	0	0.0
4331	Chicken, canned, light and dark meat [1 can (5 oz), meat portion]	125	4.4	230	40%	32	1	0.0
4332	Chicken, canned, light meat [1 can (5 oz), meat portion]	125	4.4	198	23%	36	0	0.0
4333	Chicken, crackling, Puerto Rican style (Chicharron de pollo) [2 pieces (1½" x 1", boneless)]	50	1.8	196	56%	11	10	0.4
4334	Chicken, drumstick, battered, fried, skin eaten (Include extra crispy fried chicken) [1 drumstick]	72	2.5	193	53%	16	6	0.2
4335	Chicken, drumstick, battered, fried, skin not eaten (Include extra crispy fried chicken) [1 drumstick]	46	1.6	90	37%	13	0	0.0
4336	Chicken, drumstick, breaded, fried or baked with added fat, skin eaten (Include Shake-n-Bake) [1 drumstick]	72	2.5	184	49%	19	4	0.1
4337	Chicken, drumstick, breaded, fried or baked with added fat, skin not eaten (Include Shake-n-Bake) [1 drumstick]	46	1.6	90	37%	13	0	0.0
4338	Chicken, drumstick, floured, baked or fried, prepared skinless, coating eaten [1 drumstick]	42	1.5	77	32%	12	0	0.0
4339	Chicken, drumstick, broiled or grilled, skin eaten [1 drumstick]	52	1.8	112	46%	14	0	0.0
4340	Chicken, drumstick, broiled or grilled, skin not eaten [1 drumstick]	45	1.6	77	30%	13	0	0.0

Food No.	fat gm	sat fat gm	choles mg	sodium mg	potas mg	% of Daily Value													
						vit A	vit E	vit C	thia	ribo	niac	vit B-6	fola	vit B-12	calc	phos	mag	iron	zinc
4303	18	5	111	118	299	3	3	0	9	18	46	21	3	6	3	21	7	11	22
4304	28	8	118	117	281	13	2	0	5	15	45	18	2	6	3	21	7	11	20
4305	15	4	101	108	265	3	1	0	5	14	40	19	2	6	3	18	6	9	20
4306	27	7	114	116	290	5	4	0	9	18	47	19	2	6	3	21	7	12	21
4307	16	4	95	102	258	3	3	0	8	15	39	18	2	5	3	18	6	9	19
4308	29	7	123	125	304	5	5	0	6	17	48	20	2	7	3	22	7	11	22
4309	17	4	103	110	271	3	3	0	5	15	40	19	2	6	3	19	6	9	20
4310	20	5	83	82	197	9	1	0	4	11	32	13	1	4	2	14	5	7	14
4311	9	3	65	69	171	2	1	0	3	9	25	12	1	4	2	12	4	6	13
4312	19	5	83	68	154	9	1	0	3	9	23	8	1	3	2	13	4	7	14
4313	8	2	64	50	119	2	1	0	2	8	17	8	1	3	2	10	3	5	12
4314	18	5	120	385	282	3	6	0	11	12	74	30	2	7	3	26	9	10	9
4315	4	1	80	69	243	1	2	0	5	6	65	28	1	5	1	22	7	6	6
4316	13	4	117	513	359	2	4	0	8	10	90	38	2	7	3	32	10	10	10
4317	4	1	80	69	243	1	2	0	5	6	65	28	1	5	1	22	7	6	6
4318	7	2	77	65	225	2	1	0	4	6	58	26	1	5	1	20	6	5	6
4319	3	1	69	60	207	0	1	0	4	5	56	24	1	5	1	18	6	5	5
4320	9	2	88	74	253	1	2	0	5	7	67	28	1	6	2	23	7	7	7
4321	4	1	79	68	237	1	2	0	5	6	64	27	1	5	1	21	7	5	6
4322	9	2	90	76	257	1	2	0	5	7	68	29	1	6	2	23	7	6	7
4323	4	1	79	68	238	1	2	0	5	6	64	28	1	5	1	21	7	5	6
4324	8	2	82	70	240	3	1	0	4	7	62	27	1	5	1	21	7	6	7
4325	3	1	73	64	220	1	1	0	4	6	59	26	1	5	1	20	6	5	6
4326	1	0	10	36	25	0	1	0	1	1	7	3	0	1	0	2	1	1	1
4327	10	2	97	657	325	1	5	0	8	8	80	34	2	6	3	29	9	9	8
4328	8	2	83	68	196	3	1	0	3	7	43	16	1	4	1	17	6	6	7
4329	3	1	73	60	178	1	1	0	3	7	40	16	1	4	1	16	6	5	6
4330	11	3	110	238	226	3	2	0	5	15	30	13	2	5	2	18	6	9	22
4331	10	3	63	169	191	4	2	0	0	7	15	12	1	21	2	19	6	9	21
4332	5	1	96	226	224	1	2	0	4	9	49	21	1	5	2	20	7	6	10
4333	12	3	39	115	106	2	5	6	6	7	18	8	1	2	1	8	3	6	5
4334	11	3	62	194	134	2	4	0	5	9	18	10	2	3	1	11	4	5	11
4335	4	1	43	44	115	1	1	0	2	6	14	9	1	3	1	9	3	3	10
4336	10	3	61	273	165	2	3	0	4	9	21	12	1	4	1	13	4	5	13
4337	4	1	43	44	115	1	1	0	2	6	14	9	1	3	1	9	3	3	10
4338	3	1	40	41	106	1	1	0	2	6	13	8	1	2	1	8	3	3	9
4339	6	2	47	47	119	2	1	0	2	7	16	9	1	3	1	9	3	4	10
4340	3	1	42	43	111	1	1	0	2	6	14	9	1	3	1	8	3	3	10

Meat, Poultry, Fish

Food No.	Food Description & Amount	wt gm	wt oz	cal	% cal fat	prot gm	carbo gm	fiber gm
4341	Chicken, drumstick, floured, fried or baked with added fat, skin eaten [1 drumstick]	49	1.7	120	50%	13	1	0.0
4342	Chicken, drumstick, floured, fried or baked with added fat, skin not eaten [1 drumstick]	42	1.5	82	37%	12	0	0.0
4343	Chicken, drumstick, fried, no coating, skin eaten [1 drumstick]	49	1.7	119	52%	13	0	0.0
4344	Chicken, drumstick, fried, no coating, skin not eaten [1 drumstick]	42	1.5	82	37%	12	0	0.0
4345	Chicken, drumstick, roasted, skin eaten [1 drumstick]	52	1.8	112	46%	14	0	0.0
4346	Chicken, drumstick, roasted, skin not eaten [1 drumstick]	44	1.6	76	30%	12	0	0.0
4347	Chicken, drumstick, skinless, breaded, cooked, breading eaten (Include Weaver Crispy Light Fried Chicken) [1 drumstick]	64	2.3	151	40%	16	5	0.2
4348	Chicken, drumstick, stewed, skin eaten [1 drumstick]	57	2.0	116	47%	14	0	0.0
4349	Chicken, drumstick, stewed, skin not eaten [1 drumstick]	46	1.6	78	30%	13	0	0.0
4350	Chicken, feet, roasted [1 foot]	34	1.2	73	61%	7	0	0.0
4351	Chicken, ground [1 cup, cooked]	127	4.5	304	51%	35	0	0.0
4352	Chicken, leg (drumstick + thigh), battered, fried, skin eaten (Include extra crispy fried chicken) [1 leg]	158	5.6	430	53%	34	14	0.4
4353	Chicken, leg (drumstick + thigh), battered, fried, skin not eaten (Include extra crispy fried chicken) [1 leg]	102	3.6	212	40%	29	1	0.0
4354	Chicken, leg (drumstick + thigh), breaded, fried or baked with added fat, skin eaten (Include Shake-n-Bake) [1 leg]	158	5.6	416	51%	41	8	0.3
4355	Chicken, leg (drumstick + thigh), breaded, fried or baked with added fat, skin not eaten (Include Shake-n-Bake) [1 leg]	102	3.6	212	40%	29	1	0.0
4356	Chicken, leg (drumstick + thigh), broiled or grilled, skin eaten [1 leg]	109	3.8	253	52%	28	0	0.0
4357	Chicken, leg (drumstick + thigh), broiled or grilled, skin not eaten [1 leg]	97	3.4	185	40%	26	0	0.0
4358	Chicken, leg (drumstick + thigh), floured, fried or baked with added fat, skin eaten [1 leg]	112	4.0	285	51%	30	3	0.1
4359	Chicken, leg (drumstick + thigh), floured, fried or baked with added fat, skin not eaten [1 leg]	94	3.3	195	40%	27	1	0.0
4360	Chicken, leg (drumstick + thigh), fried, no coating, skin eaten [1 leg]	112	4.0	280	53%	31	0	0.0
4361	Chicken, leg (drumstick + thigh), fried, no coating, skin not eaten [1 leg]	94	3.3	194	41%	27	0	0.0
4362	Chicken, leg (drumstick + thigh), roasted, skin eaten [1 leg]	114	4.0	264	52%	30	0	0.0
4363	Chicken, leg (drumstick + thigh), roasted, skin not eaten [1 leg]	95	3.4	181	40%	26	0	0.0
4364	Chicken, leg (drumstick + thigh), stewed, skin eaten [1 leg]	125	4.4	275	53%	30	0	0.0
4365	Chicken, leg (drumstick + thigh), stewed, skin not eaten [1 leg]	101	3.6	187	39%	27	0	0.0
4366	Chicken, liver paste or pate [1 slice (1 oz)]	28	1.0	56	59%	4	2	0.0
4367	Chicken, liver, battered, fried [1 oz, cooked]	28	1.0	60	36%	6	3	0.1
4368	Chicken, liver, braised [1 oz, cooked]	28	1.0	44	31%	7	0	0.0
4369	Chicken, liver, breaded or floured, fried [1 oz, cooked]	28	1.0	78	35%	8	4	0.1
4370	Chicken, liver, fried or sauteed, no coating [1 oz, cooked]	28	1.0	71	40%	9	2	0.0
4371	Chicken, neck, breaded, baked or fried, skin eaten (Include Shake-n-Bake) [1 neck]	52	1.8	174	65%	12	3	0.1
4372	Chicken, neck, breaded, baked or fried, skin not eaten (Include Shake-n-Bake) [1 neck]	25	0.9	57	47%	7	0	0.0
4373	Chicken, neck, floured, salted, fried or baked with added fat, skin eaten [1 neck]	36	1.3	119	64%	9	2	0.1
4374	Chicken, neck, floured, fried or baked with added fat, skin not eaten [1 neck]	22	0.8	50	47%	6	0	0.0
4375	Chicken, neck, fried, no coating, skin eaten [1 neck]	36	1.3	118	68%	9	0	0.0
4376	Chicken, neck, fried, no coating, skin not eaten [1 neck]	22	0.8	49	49%	6	0	0.0
4377	Chicken, neck, roasted, skin eaten [1 neck]	36	1.3	108	69%	8	0	0.0
4378	Chicken, neck, roasted, skin not eaten [1 neck]	24	0.8	56	56%	6	0	0.0
4379	Chicken, neck, stewed, skin eaten [1 neck]	38	1.3	94	66%	7	0	0.0
4380	Chicken, neck, stewed, skin not eaten [1 neck]	18	0.6	32	41%	4	0	0.0
4381	Chicken, nuggets (Include Weaver mini drums; Tyson chicken sticks) [4 nuggets]	72	2.5	204	55%	12	11	0.3
4382	Chicken nuggets, lowfat [4 nuggets]	72	2.5	140	29%	14	10	0.5

Food No.	fat gm	sat fat gm	choles mg	sodium mg	potas mg	vit A	vit E	vit C	thia	ribo	niac	vit B-6	fola	vit B-12	calc	phos	mag	iron	zinc
						% of Daily Value													
4341	7	2	44	44	112	1	2	0	3	6	15	9	1	3	1	9	3	4	9
4342	3	1	40	41	105	1	1	0	2	6	13	8	1	2	0	8	3	3	9
4343	7	2	45	44	113	1	2	0	2	6	15	9	1	3	1	9	3	4	10
4344	3	1	40	41	105	1	1	0	2	6	13	8	1	2	0	8	3	3	9
4345	6	2	47	47	119	2	1	0	2	7	16	9	1	3	1	9	3	4	10
4346	2	1	41	42	108	1	1	0	2	6	13	9	1	2	1	8	3	3	9
4347	7	2	51	359	152	1	3	0	4	8	18	11	1	3	1	12	4	5	12
4348	6	2	47	43	105	2	1	0	2	6	12	5	1	2	1	8	3	4	10
4349	3	1	40	37	92	1	1	0	2	6	10	5	1	2	1	7	2	4	9
4350	5	1	29	23	11	1	0	0	1	4	1	0	7	3	3	3	0	2	2
4351	17	5	112	104	283	6	2	0	5	13	54	25	2	6	2	23	7	9	16
4352	25	6	142	441	300	4	8	0	12	21	43	21	4	7	3	24	8	12	23
4353	10	2	101	97	259	2	2	0	6	15	34	20	2	6	1	20	6	8	20
4354	23	6	141	599	371	4	5	0	9	21	49	25	3	8	3	29	9	13	27
4355	10	2	101	97	259	2	2	0	6	15	34	20	2	6	1	20	6	8	20
4356	15	4	100	95	245	4	1	0	5	14	34	18	2	5	1	19	6	8	19
4357	8	2	91	88	235	2	1	0	5	13	31	18	2	5	1	18	6	7	18
4358	16	4	106	99	261	3	3	0	7	16	37	19	2	6	1	20	7	9	20
4359	9	2	93	90	239	2	2	0	5	14	31	18	2	5	1	18	6	7	19
4360	17	4	109	102	266	3	3	0	5	15	37	19	2	6	1	21	7	9	20
4361	9	2	94	90	240	2	2	0	5	14	31	18	2	5	1	18	6	7	19
4362	15	4	105	99	257	4	1	0	5	14	35	19	2	6	1	20	7	8	20
4363	8	2	89	86	230	2	1	0	5	13	30	18	2	5	1	17	6	7	18
4364	16	4	105	91	220	5	2	0	5	14	29	11	2	4	1	17	6	9	20
4365	8	2	90	79	192	2	1	0	4	13	24	11	2	4	1	15	5	8	19
4366	4	1	109	108	27	6	1	5	1	23	11	4	22	38	0	5	1	14	4
4367	2	1	147	22	67	151	3	15	3	35	13	8	51	100	1	8	2	15	7
4368	2	1	177	14	39	138	2	7	3	29	6	8	54	90	0	9	1	13	8
4369	3	1	198	30	90	208	4	20	4	48	17	10	71	138	1	11	2	21	9
4370	3	1	210	32	93	221	4	22	3	50	18	11	75	147	1	12	2	22	10
4371	12	3	47	195	97	3	3	0	2	7	13	6	1	2	2	7	2	7	10
4372	3	1	26	25	53	1	1	0	1	5	6	4	0	1	1	3	1	4	7
4373	9	2	34	29	65	2	2	0	2	6	10	5	1	2	1	5	2	5	7
4374	3	1	23	22	47	1	1	0	1	4	6	4	0	1	1	3	1	4	6
4375	9	2	35	31	67	2	2	0	1	5	10	5	0	2	1	5	2	5	8
4376	3	1	24	22	48	1	1	0	1	4	6	4	0	1	1	3	1	4	6
4377	8	2	48	27	59	3	0	0	1	6	8	4	0	2	1	5	1	5	7
4378	4	1	26	22	45	1	0	0	1	4	5	4	0	1	1	3	1	4	6
4379	7	2	27	20	41	2	0	0	1	6	6	2	0	1	1	5	1	5	7
4380	1	0	14	12	25	1	0	0	1	3	4	1	0	1	1	2	1	3	5
4381	12	4	43	383	177	2	6	0	4	6	24	11	2	4	1	14	4	5	5
4382	5	1	35	342	116	1	1	0	3	3	27	11	1	2	1	11	4	4	4

Meat, Poultry, Fish

Food No.	Food Description & Amount	wt gm	wt oz	cal	% cal fat	prot gm	carbo gm	fiber gm
4383	Chicken, patty with cheese, breaded, cooked (Include Cheese Recipe Chicken Rondelets) [1 patty]	85	3.0	237	54%	13	14	0.5
4384	Chicken, patty, breaded, cooked (Include Chicken Rondelets) [1 patty]	75	2.6	213	55%	12	11	0.3
4385	Chicken roll, roasted, dark meat [2 slices]	56	2.0	114	43%	15	0	0.0
4386	Chicken roll, roasted, light and dark meat [2 slices]	56	2.0	106	35%	16	0	0.0
4387	Chicken roll, roasted, light meat [2 slices]	56	2.0	89	42%	11	1	0.0
4388	Chicken, skin, roasted [skin from ½ chicken]	56	2.0	254	81%	11	0	0.0
4389	Chicken, tail, roasted [1 tail]	7	0.2	27	76%	2	0	0.0
4390	Chicken, thigh, battered, fried, skin eaten (Include extra crispy fried chicken) [1 thigh]	86	3.0	237	54%	19	8	0.2
4391	Chicken, thigh, battered, fried, skin not eaten (Include extra crispy fried chicken) [1 thigh]	54	1.9	118	43%	15	1	0.0
4392	Chicken, thigh, battered, fried, prepared skinless, coating eaten [1 thigh]	63	2.2	160	48%	14	6	0.2
4393	Chicken, thigh, battered, fried, prepared skinless, coating not eaten [1 thigh]	52	1.8	113	43%	15	1	0.0
4394	Chicken, thigh, breaded, fried or baked with added fat, skin eaten (Include Shake-n-Bake) [1 thigh]	86	3.0	231	52%	22	4	0.1
4395	Chicken, thigh, breaded, fried or baked with added fat, skin not eaten (Include Shake-n-Bake) [1 thigh]	54	1.9	118	43%	15	1	0.0
4396	Chicken, thigh, broiled or grilled, skin eaten [1 thigh]	58	2.0	143	56%	15	0	0.0
4397	Chicken, thigh, broiled or grilled, skin not eaten [1 thigh]	52	1.8	109	47%	13	0	0.0
4398	Chicken, thigh, floured, fried or baked with added fat, skin eaten [1 thigh]	62	2.2	162	51%	17	2	0.1
4399	Chicken, thigh, floured, fried or baked with added fat, skin not eaten [1 thigh]	52	1.8	113	43%	15	1	0.0
4400	Chicken, thigh, fried, no coating, skin eaten [1 thigh]	62	2.2	159	55%	17	0	0.0
4401	Chicken, thigh, fried, no coating, skin not eaten [1 thigh]	52	1.8	112	44%	15	0	0.0
4402	Chicken, thigh, roasted, skin eaten [1 thigh]	62	2.2	153	56%	16	0	0.0
4403	Chicken, thigh, roasted, skin not eaten [1 thigh]	52	1.8	109	47%	13	0	0.0
4404	Chicken, thigh, skinless, breaded, cooked, breading eaten (Include Weaver Crispy Light Fried Chicken) [1 thigh]	78	2.8	206	51%	19	6	0.2
4405	Chicken, thigh, stewed, skin eaten [1 thigh]	68	2.4	158	57%	16	0	0.0
4406	Chicken, thigh, stewed, skin not eaten [1 thigh]	55	1.9	107	45%	14	0	0.0
4407	Chicken, wing, battered, fried, skin eaten (Include extra crispy fried chicken) [1 wing]	49	1.7	159	61%	10	5	0.2
4408	Chicken, wing, battered, fried, skin not eaten (Include extra crispy fried chicken) [1 wing]	22	0.8	46	39%	7	0	0.0
4409	Chicken, wing, breaded, fried or baked with added fat, skin eaten (Include Shake-n-Bake) [1 wing]	49	1.7	159	61%	12	3	0.1
4410	Chicken, wing, breaded, fried or baked with added fat, skin not eaten (Include Shake-n-Bake) [1 wing]	22	0.8	46	39%	7	0	0.0
4411	Chicken, wing, broiled or grilled, skin eaten [1 wing]	35	1.2	102	60%	9	0	0.0
4412	Chicken, wing, broiled or grilled, skin not eaten [1 wing]	20	0.7	41	36%	6	0	0.0
4413	Chicken, wing, floured, fried or baked with added fat, skin eaten [1 wing]	32	1.1	103	62%	8	1	0.0
4414	Chicken, wing, floured, fried or baked with added fat, skin not eaten [1 wing]	20	0.7	42	39%	6	0	0.0
4415	Chicken, wing, fried, no coating, skin eaten [1 wing]	32	1.1	102	65%	8	0	0.0
4416	Chicken, wing, fried, no coating, skin not eaten [1 wing]	20	0.7	42	39%	6	0	0.0
4417	Chicken, wing, roasted, skin eaten [1 wing]	34	1.2	99	60%	9	0	0.0
4418	Chicken, wing, roasted, skin not eaten [1 wing]	21	0.7	43	36%	6	0	0.0
4419	Chicken, wing, stewed, skin eaten [1 wing]	40	1.4	100	61%	9	0	0.0
4420	Chicken, wing, stewed, skin not eaten [1 wing]	24	0.8	43	36%	7	0	0.0
	Turkey and Other Poultry (weight columns are for cooked, boneless portion)							
4450	Cornish game hen, roasted, skin eaten [1 hen (1¼ lb, raw)]	306	10.8	796	63%	68	0	0.0
4451	Cornish game hen, roasted, skin not eaten [1 hen (1¼ lb, raw)]	249	8.8	334	26%	58	0	0.0
4452	Dove, roasted (Include squab, pigeon) [1 dove]	111	3.9	243	53%	27	0	0.0
4453	Dove, floured, fried (Include squab, pigeon) [1 dove]	111	3.9	258	54%	26	2	0.1
4454	Duck, battered, fried [1 leg (drumstick + thigh)]	70	2.5	156	45%	16	5	0.2

Food No.	fat gm	sat fat gm	choles mg	sodium mg	potas mg	% of Daily Value													
						vit A	vit E	vit C	thia	ribo	niac	vit B-6	fola	vit B-12	calc	phos	mag	iron	zinc
4383	14	4	33	588	122	4	8	0	9	9	17	7	2	2	12	17	4	9	8
4384	13	4	45	399	185	2	7	1	5	6	25	12	2	4	1	15	4	5	5
4385	5	1	52	141	134	1	1	0	3	7	18	10	1	3	1	10	3	4	10
4386	4	1	50	135	136	1	1	0	3	6	26	13	1	3	1	11	3	4	8
4387	4	1	28	327	128	1	1	0	2	4	15	6	0	1	2	9	3	3	3
4388	23	6	46	36	76	4	1	0	1	4	16	3	0	2	1	7	2	5	5
4389	2	1	6	5	12	1	0	0	0	1	2	1	0	0	0	1	0	0	1
4390	14	4	80	248	165	2	4	0	7	12	25	11	2	4	2	13	4	7	12
4391	6	2	55	51	140	1	1	0	3	8	19	10	1	3	1	11	3	4	10
4392	9	2	59	197	124	1	3	0	5	9	18	9	2	3	1	10	3	5	9
4393	5	1	53	49	135	1	1	0	3	8	19	10	1	3	1	10	3	4	10
4394	13	4	80	326	206	2	2	0	5	12	28	14	2	4	1	16	5	7	14
4395	6	2	55	51	140	1	1	0	3	8	19	10	1	3	1	11	3	4	10
4396	9	3	54	49	129	3	1	0	3	7	18	9	1	3	1	10	3	4	9
4397	6	2	49	46	124	1	1	0	3	7	17	9	1	3	1	10	3	4	9
4398	9	3	61	54	147	2	1	0	4	9	22	10	1	3	1	12	4	5	10
4399	5	1	53	49	135	1	1	0	3	8	19	10	1	3	1	10	3	4	10
4400	10	3	63	56	151	2	1	0	3	9	22	11	1	3	1	12	4	5	11
4401	5	1	54	50	136	1	1	0	3	8	19	10	1	3	1	10	3	4	10
4402	10	3	58	52	138	3	1	0	3	8	20	10	1	3	1	11	3	5	10
4403	6	2	49	46	124	1	1	0	3	7	17	9	1	3	1	10	3	4	9
4404	12	3	67	425	189	1	3	0	5	10	24	13	2	4	1	15	5	6	12
4405	10	3	57	48	116	3	1	0	3	8	17	6	1	2	1	9	3	5	10
4406	5	1	50	41	101	1	1	0	2	7	14	6	1	2	1	8	3	4	9
4407	11	3	39	157	68	2	3	0	3	4	13	7	1	2	1	6	2	4	5
4408	2	1	18	20	46	0	0	0	1	2	8	7	0	1	0	4	1	1	3
4409	11	3	37	181	89	2	2	0	2	4	16	10	0	2	1	8	2	3	6
4410	2	1	18	20	46	0	0	0	1	2	8	7	0	1	0	4	1	1	3
4411	7	2	29	29	64	2	0	0	1	3	12	7	0	2	1	5	2	2	4
4412	2	0	17	18	42	0	0	0	1	2	7	6	0	1	0	3	1	1	3
4413	7	2	26	25	57	1	1	0	1	3	11	7	0	1	0	5	2	2	4
4414	2	0	17	18	42	0	0	0	1	2	7	6	0	1	0	3	1	1	3
4415	7	2	26	25	58	1	1	0	1	2	11	7	0	2	0	5	2	2	4
4416	2	0	17	18	42	0	0	0	1	2	7	6	0	1	0	3	1	1	3
4417	7	2	29	28	63	2	0	0	1	3	11	7	0	2	1	5	2	2	4
4418	2	0	18	19	44	0	0	0	1	2	8	6	0	1	0	3	1	1	3
4419	7	2	28	27	56	2	0	0	1	2	9	4	0	1	0	5	2	3	4
4420	2	0	18	18	37	0	0	0	1	2	6	4	0	1	0	3	1	1	3
4450	56	15	401	196	750	10	4	3	14	36	90	47	2	14	4	45	14	15	30
4451	10	2	264	157	623	5	3	2	12	33	78	45	1	12	3	37	12	11	25
4452	14	4	129	63	284	3	0	5	21	23	42	32	2	8	2	37	7	36	28
4453	16	4	124	61	276	3	1	5	21	23	41	31	2	7	2	36	7	36	27
4454	8	2	74	50	186	2	4	6	16	21	19	11	4	4	1	14	3	12	11

Meat, Poultry, Fish

Food No.	Food Description & Amount	wt gm	wt oz	cal	% cal fat	prot gm	carbo gm	fiber gm
4455	Duck, pressed, Chinese [2 oz, cooked]	56	2.0	107	47%	4	11	0.5
4456	Duck, roasted, skin eaten [½ duck]	382	13.5	1287	76%	73	0	0.0
4457	Duck, roasted, skin not eaten [½ duck]	221	7.8	444	50%	52	0	0.0
4458	Goose, wild, roasted [3 oz, with bone, cooked]	57	2.0	174	65%	14	0	0.0
4459	Pheasant, cooked (Include grouse) [½ pheasant breast]	127	4.5	314	44%	41	0	0.0
4460	Quail, cooked (Include partridge) [1 quail]	76	2.7	178	54%	19	0	0.0
4461	Turkey, back, roasted [1 back]	524	18.5	1273	53%	139	0	0.0
4462	Turkey, bacon, cooked [2 slices]	22	0.8	84	66%	7	1	0.0
4463	Turkey, canned [1 can (5 oz)]	125	4.4	204	38%	30	0	0.0
4464	Turkey, dark meat, roasted, skin eaten [2 slices (3" x 2" x ¼")]	56	2.0	124	47%	15	0	0.0
4465	Turkey, dark meat, roasted, skin not eaten [2 slices (3" x 2" x ¼")]	56	2.0	105	35%	16	0	0.0
4466	Turkey, drumstick, roasted, skin eaten [1 drumstick (14-18 lb bird)]	204	7.2	424	42%	57	0	0.0
4467	Turkey, drumstick, roasted, skin not eaten [1 drumstick (14-18 lb bird)]	188	6.6	352	35%	54	0	0.0
4468	Turkey, drumstick, smoked, salted, skin eaten [1 drumstick (14-18 lb bird)]	204	7.2	424	42%	57	0	0.0
4469	Turkey, gizzard, cooked [1 gizzard]	67	2.4	103	22%	18	1	0.0
4470	Turkey, ground, cooked [1 patty (4 oz, raw)]	60	2.1	141	50%	16	0	0.0
4471	Turkey ham roll [2 slices]	56	2.0	72	36%	11	0	0.0
4472	Turkey, light and dark meat, roasted, skin eaten [2 slices (3" x 2" x ¼")]	56	2.0	116	42%	16	0	0.0
4473	Turkey, light and dark meat, roasted, skin not eaten [2 slices (3" x 2" x ¼")]	56	2.0	95	26%	16	0	0.0
4474	Turkey, light meat, breaded, fried or baked with added fat, skin eaten [2 slices (3" x 2" x ¼")]	56	2.0	125	41%	15	3	0.1
4475	Turkey, light meat, breaded, fried or baked with added fat, skin not eaten [2 slices (3" x 2" x ¼")]	56	2.0	93	23%	16	0	0.0
4476	Turkey, light meat, roasted, skin eaten [2 slices (3" x 2" x ¼")]	56	2.0	110	38%	16	0	0.0
4477	Turkey, light meat, roasted, skin not eaten [2 slices (3" x 2" x ¼")]	56	2.0	88	18%	17	0	0.0
4478	Turkey, light or dark meat, battered, fried, skin eaten [2 slices (3" x 2" x ¼")]	56	2.0	158	57%	8	9	0.3
4479	Turkey, light or dark meat, battered, fried, skin not eaten [2 slices (3" x 2" x ¼")]	56	2.0	104	30%	16	1	0.0
4480	Turkey, light or dark meat, smoked, cooked, skin eaten [2 slices (3" x 2" x ¼")]	56	2.0	116	42%	16	0	0.0
4481	Turkey, light or dark meat, smoked, cooked, skin not eaten [2 slices (3" x 2" x ¼")]	56	2.0	95	26%	16	0	0.0
4482	Turkey, light or dark meat, stewed, skin eaten [2 slices (3" x 2" x ¼")]	56	2.0	97	33%	15	0	0.0
4483	Turkey, light or dark meat, stewed, skin not eaten [2 slices (3" x 2" x ¼")]	56	2.0	98	34%	15	0	0.0
4484	Turkey, liver, cooked [2 oz]	56	2.0	95	32%	13	2	0.0
4485	Turkey, neck, cooked [1 neck]	152	5.4	274	36%	41	0	0.0
4486	Turkey, nuggets (breaded, fried) [4 nuggets]	72	2.5	186	41%	17	10	0.3
4487	Turkey, pastrami [2 slices]	56	2.0	79	40%	10	1	0.0
4488	Turkey, roll, light or dark meat, roasted, [2 slices]	56	2.0	87	34%	12	2	0.0
4489	Turkey, salami [2 slices]	56	2.0	110	63%	9	0	0.0
4490	Turkey, tail, cooked [1 tail]	58	2.0	199	72%	13	0	0.0
4491	Turkey, thigh, roasted, skin eaten [1 thigh (14-18 lb bird)]	297	10.5	618	42%	83	0	0.0
4492	Turkey, thigh, roasted, skin not eaten [1 thigh (14-18 lb bird)]	274	9.7	512	35%	78	0	0.0
4493	Turkey, wing, roasted, skin eaten [1 wing]	174	6.1	398	49%	48	0	0.0
4494	Turkey, wing, roasted, skin not eaten [1 wing]	146	5.1	238	19%	45	0	0.0
4495	Turkey, wing, smoked, salted, skin eaten [1 wing]	174	6.1	398	49%	48	0	0.0
	Other Meats and Sausages (weight columns are for cooked, boneless portion)							
4550	Armadillo, cooked [2 oz, boneless, cooked]	56	2.0	90	25%	16	0	0.0
4551	Bear, cooked [2 oz, boneless, cooked]	56	2.0	145	47%	18	0	0.0
4552	Beaver, cooked [2 oz, boneless, cooked]	56	2.0	119	30%	20	0	0.0
4553	Bison, cooked [1 cup]	134	4.7	192	15%	38	0	0.0
4554	Caribou, cooked [2 oz, boneless, cooked]	56	2.0	94	24%	17	0	0.0
4555	Frog legs [2 oz, boneless, cooked]	56	2.0	144	42%	10	11	0.4
4556	Frog legs, steamed [2 oz, boneless, cooked]	56	2.0	59	4%	13	0	0.0
4557	Goat, head, cooked [2 oz, boneless, cooked]	56	2.0	80	34%	12	0	0.0
4558	Goat, liver, fried or broiled, no coating [2 oz, cooked]	56	2.0	133	48%	14	2	0.0

Food No.	fat gm	sat fat gm	choles mg	sodium mg	potas mg	vit A	vit E	vit C	thia	ribo	niac	vit B-6	fola	vit B-12	calc	phos	mag	iron	zinc
						% of Daily Value													
4455	6	2	18	51	104	2	2	5	5	5	6	3	1	1	1	4	2	5	3
4456	108	37	321	225	779	24	12	0	44	60	92	34	6	19	4	60	15	57	47
4457	25	9	197	144	557	5	7	0	38	61	56	28	6	15	3	45	11	33	38
4458	12	4	52	40	188	1	5	0	3	11	12	11	0	4	1	15	3	9	10
4459	15	4	113	55	344	7	2	5	6	13	48	48	2	15	2	31	7	10	12
4460	11	3	65	40	164	5	2	3	11	13	30	24	1	5	1	21	4	19	16
4461	75	22	477	383	1362	0	14	0	19	69	90	79	10	30	17	99	29	64	137
4462	6	2	22	503	87	0	0	0	1	3	4	4	0	1	0	10	2	3	4
4463	9	3	83	584	280	0	2	4	1	13	41	21	2	6	2	20	6	13	20
4464	6	2	50	43	153	0	2	0	2	8	10	9	1	3	2	11	3	7	16
4465	4	1	48	44	162	0	2	0	2	8	10	10	1	3	2	11	3	7	17
4466	20	6	173	157	571	0	6	0	8	29	36	34	5	12	7	41	12	26	58
4467	14	5	160	149	545	0	5	0	8	27	34	34	4	12	6	38	11	24	56
4468	20	6	173	2032	571	0	6	0	8	29	36	34	5	12	7	41	12	26	58
4469	2	1	130	45	120	4	4	2	1	10	13	4	9	22	1	10	3	15	20
4470	8	2	61	64	162	0	1	0	2	6	14	12	1	3	2	12	4	6	11
4471	3	1	31	558	182	0	2	0	2	8	10	7	1	2	1	11	2	9	11
4472	5	2	46	38	157	0	1	0	2	6	14	11	1	3	1	11	4	6	11
4473	3	1	43	39	167	0	1	0	2	6	15	13	1	3	1	12	4	6	12
4474	6	2	38	198	154	0	1	0	3	4	16	12	1	3	1	11	3	5	7
4475	2	1	38	35	168	0	1	0	2	4	19	15	1	3	1	12	4	4	8
4476	5	1	43	35	160	0	0	0	2	4	18	13	1	3	1	12	4	4	8
4477	2	1	39	36	171	0	0	0	2	4	19	15	1	3	1	12	4	4	8
4478	10	3	35	448	154	1	6	0	4	6	6	6	1	2	1	15	2	7	5
4479	3	1	41	38	162	0	1	0	3	6	15	12	1	3	1	12	4	6	11
4480	5	2	46	558	157	0	1	0	2	6	14	11	1	3	1	11	4	6	11
4481	3	1	43	558	167	0	1	0	2	6	15	13	1	3	1	12	4	6	12
4482	4	1	48	34	108	0	1	0	2	6	9	8	1	2	1	9	3	6	11
4483	4	1	47	34	114	0	1	0	2	7	10	8	1	3	1	10	3	5	11
4484	3	1	351	36	109	209	7	2	2	47	17	15	93	443	1	15	2	24	12
4485	11	4	185	85	226	0	4	0	4	17	13	16	3	6	6	19	6	19	72
4486	9	2	40	610	188	0	4	0	4	7	16	12	1	3	2	14	4	7	11
4487	3	1	30	585	146	0	1	0	2	8	10	8	1	2	1	11	2	5	8
4488	3	1	30	381	167	0	1	0	2	5	18	8	1	14	0	14	3	5	9
4489	8	2	46	562	137	0	1	0	2	6	10	7	1	2	1	6	2	5	7
4490	16	5	54	36	128	0	2	0	2	6	8	7	1	3	2	9	3	6	13
4491	29	9	252	229	832	0	8	0	12	42	53	49	7	18	10	59	17	38	85
4492	20	7	233	216	795	0	8	0	12	40	50	49	6	17	9	56	16	35	81
4493	22	6	141	106	463	0	1	0	6	14	50	37	3	10	4	34	11	14	24
4494	5	2	149	114	298	0	1	0	3	14	30	43	3	10	4	25	8	14	37
4495	22	6	141	1733	463	0	1	0	6	13	50	37	3	10	4	34	11	14	24
4550	2	1	43	34	222	0	1	0	12	5	12	12	1	7	1	8	4	3	11
4551	7	2	55	40	147	0	1	0	4	27	9	8	1	23	0	10	3	33	38
4552	4	1	66	33	226	0	2	3	2	10	6	13	2	77	1	16	4	31	8
4553	3	1	110	76	484	0	1	0	9	21	25	27	3	64	1	28	9	25	33
4554	2	1	61	34	174	0	0	3	9	30	16	9	1	62	1	13	4	19	20
4555	7	2	74	159	162	3	6	3	9	12	7	4	3	4	5	10	4	9	5
4556	0	0	41	47	208	1	4	0	7	11	4	4	2	5	1	9	4	6	5
4557	3	1	406	57	190	0	1	4	4	16	10	1	1	36	1	14	1	10	15
4558	7	3	276	69	197	437	2	12	13	151	47	27	56	800	1	24	3	32	21

Meat, Poultry, Fish

Food No.	Food Description & Amount	wt gm	wt oz	cal	% cal fat	prot gm	carbo gm	fiber gm
4559	Goat, ribs, cooked [1 rib]	46	1.6	66	19%	12	0	0.0
4560	Goat, baked [2 oz, boneless, cooked]	56	2.0	80	19%	15	0	0.0
4561	Goat, boiled [2 oz, boneless, cooked]	56	2.0	80	19%	15	0	0.0
4562	Goat, fried [2 oz, boneless, cooked]	56	2.0	87	27%	15	0	0.0
4563	Ground hog, cooked [3 oz, with bone, cooked]	69	2.4	174	53%	19	0	0.0
4564	Mock chicken leg (veal, pork, flour, egg), cooked (Include city chicken, pork and veal on a stick) [2 oz, cooked]	56	2.0	131	53%	12	3	0.1
4565	Moose, cooked [2 oz, boneless, cooked]	56	2.0	75	7%	16	0	0.0
4566	Opossum, cooked [3 oz, with bone, cooked]	69	2.4	152	42%	21	0	0.0
4567	Rabbit, stewed [1 piece]	105	3.7	216	37%	32	0	0.0
4568	Rabbit, domestic, breaded, fried [2 oz, boneless, cooked]	56	2.0	137	42%	16	3	0.1
4569	Rabbit, wild, cooked [3 oz, with bone, cooked]	69	2.4	119	18%	23	0	0.0
4570	Raccoon, cooked [2 oz, boneless, cooked]	56	2.0	143	51%	16	0	0.0
4571	Snails, steamed or poached [5 snails]	25	0.9	69	3%	12	4	0.0
4572	Squirrel, cooked [3 oz, with bone, cooked]	69	2.4	119	24%	21	0	0.0
4573	Turtle (terrapin) steamed or poached [1 cup, cooked]	140	4.9	158	5%	35	0	0.0
4574	Udder, cooked (Include milk ducts) [1 cup, pieces]	140	4.9	144	36%	21	0	0.0
4575	Venison, bologna (Include deer bologna, venison or deer sausage, caribou sausage) [2 oz]	56	2.0	175	82%	7	0	0.0
4576	Venison, chop, fried (Include deer chop) [1 chop]	89	3.1	186	41%	26	0	0.0
4577	Venison, ribs, fried (Include deer ribs)[3 oz, with bone, cooked]	69	2.4	118	18%	23	0	0.0
4578	Venison jerky (Include deer) [2 strips (4" long)]	28	1.0	96	41%	10	4	0.0
4579	Venison, steak, battered, fried (Include deer)[1 steak]	101	3.6	210	33%	22	11	0.4
4580	Venison, steak, fried (Include ground venison or deer) [2 oz, boneless, cooked]	56	2.0	97	19%	18	0	0.0
4581	Venison, cured (Include deer) [2 oz, boneless, cooked]	56	2.0	97	19%	18	0	0.0
4582	Venison, roasted (Include antelope, deer) [2 oz, boneless]	56	2.0	96	18%	18	0	0.0
4583	Venison, stewed (Include deer) [2 oz, boneless, cooked]	56	2.0	96	18%	18	0	0.0
4584	Wild pig, smoked [2 oz, boneless]	56	2.0	90	25%	16	0	0.0
4585	Beef, pressed, luncheon meat (Include smoked) [2 slices]	56	2.0	99	20%	16	3	0.0
4586	Bockwurst [1 sausage (7 per lb)]	65	2.3	184	72%	12	0	0.0
4587	Bologna ring (pork and beef), smoked (Include Alderfers) [2 slices]	56	2.0	177	80%	7	2	0.0
4588	Bologna, beef (Include veal bologna) [2 slices]	56	2.0	175	82%	7	0	0.0
4589	Bologna, beef, lower sodium [2 slices]	56	2.0	175	82%	7	1	0.0
4590	Bologna, beef, lowfat [2 slices]	56	2.0	129	74%	7	2	0.0
4591	Bologna, beef and pork [2 slices]	56	2.0	172	81%	7	1	0.0
4592	Bologna, beef and pork, lowfat [2 slices]	56	2.0	129	76%	6	1	0.0
4593	Bologna, beef, chicken, and pork [2 slices]	56	2.0	155	78%	7	1	0.0
4594	Bologna, Lebanon [2 slices]	56	2.0	119	56%	11	2	0.0
4595	Bologna, pork [2 slices]	56	2.0	138	72%	9	0	0.0
4596	Bologna, turkey (Include chicken bologna) [2 slices]	56	2.0	111	69%	8	1	0.0
4597	Bologna, with cheese [2 slices]	56	2.0	178	79%	7	2	0.0
4598	Brains and scrambled eggs, cooked [1 cup]	243	8.6	355	74%	17	6	1.0
4599	Brains, cooked [1 cup]	140	4.9	226	66%	18	0	0.0
4600	Bratwurst, [1 stick]	85	3.0	256	77%	12	2	0.0
4601	Bratwurst, with cheese [1 stick]	85	3.0	260	76%	13	2	0.0
4602	Capicola [2 slices (4¼" x 4¼" x 1/16")]	42	1.5	55	34%	8	0	0.0
4603	Cervalat, soft [2 slices (4-1/8" dia x 1/8")]	46	1.6	154	79%	7	0	0.0
4604	Chicken or turkey loaf or roll, luncheon meat (Include pressed, smoked; chicken or turkey luncheon meat) [2 slices]	56	2.0	85	43%	11	1	0.0
4605	Chicken salad spread [1 can (7.5 oz)]	213	7.5	426	61%	25	16	0.0
4606	Chitterlings, cooked [1 cup]	125	4.4	379	85%	13	0	0.0
4607	Chorizos (Include Spanish sausage, lenguica, Portuguese sausage) [1 link (4" long)]	60	2.1	273	76%	14	1	0.0
4608	Corned beef spread [1 can (5.5 oz)]	156	5.5	390	54%	42	0	0.0

Food No.	fat gm	sat fat gm	choles mg	sodium mg	potas mg	vit A	vit E	vit C	thia	ribo	niac	vit B-6	fola	vit B-12	calc	phos	mag	iron	zinc
						% of Daily Value													
4559	1	0	35	40	186	0	0	0	3	17	9	0	1	9	1	9	0	10	16
4560	2	1	42	48	227	0	0	0	3	20	11	0	1	11	1	11	0	12	20
4561	2	1	42	48	227	0	0	0	3	20	11	0	1	11	1	11	0	12	20
4562	3	1	41	47	223	0	1	0	3	20	11	0	1	11	1	11	0	11	19
4563	10	4	59	39	250	0	1	0	39	13	17	14	1	9	2	16	4	4	12
4564	8	2	49	40	160	0	3	0	10	10	14	8	1	10	1	11	3	3	13
4565	1	0	44	39	187	0	1	5	2	11	15	10	1	59	0	10	3	13	14
4566	7	1	89	40	302	0	2	0	5	15	29	16	2	95	1	19	6	18	10
4567	9	3	90	39	315	0	4	0	4	11	38	18	2	114	2	24	5	14	17
4568	6	2	48	58	163	0	4	0	4	5	18	9	1	53	2	12	3	10	8
4569	2	1	85	31	237	0	2	0	1	3	22	12	1	75	1	17	5	19	11
4570	8	2	54	44	223	0	2	0	22	17	13	13	2	77	1	15	4	22	8
4571	0	0	33	88	121	1	0	3	1	2	2	7	1	45	3	5	9	13	5
4572	3	1	83	82	243	0	2	0	3	12	16	13	2	75	0	15	5	26	8
4573	1	0	89	108	326	5	4	0	12	13	8	9	5	24	21	26	8	13	12
4574	6	3	140	68	398	0	1	7	1	14	0	2	1	28	1	12	3	16	24
4575	16	7	32	549	88	0	0	0	2	4	7	4	1	13	1	5	2	5	8
4576	8	2	96	49	305	0	4	0	12	29	29	13	1	95	1	21	6	20	16
4577	2	1	83	43	250	0	1	0	8	26	23	9	1	72	0	17	5	19	14
4578	4	2	38	820	106	0	1	0	3	11	10	4	0	30	0	7	2	8	6
4579	8	2	103	181	274	1	5	0	15	27	27	11	2	73	4	19	6	21	14
4580	2	1	68	34	202	0	1	0	6	21	19	7	1	59	0	14	4	15	11
4581	2	1	68	34	202	0	1	0	6	21	19	7	1	59	0	14	4	15	11
4582	2	1	68	35	203	0	1	0	6	21	19	7	1	59	0	14	4	15	11
4583	2	1	68	22	139	0	1	0	5	19	14	5	1	50	0	10	3	15	11
4584	2	1	43	34	222	0	1	0	12	5	12	12	1	7	1	8	4	3	11
4585	2	1	23	806	240	0	0	0	3	6	15	10	2	24	1	9	3	8	15
4586	15	5	43	728	202	0	0	0	16	7	14	6	0	8	1	10	3	2	7
4587	16	6	31	571	101	0	1	0	6	5	7	5	1	12	1	5	2	5	7
4588	16	7	32	549	88	0	0	0	2	4	7	4	1	13	1	5	2	5	8
4589	16	7	31	382	87	0	0	0	2	4	7	5	1	13	1	5	1	4	7
4590	11	4	21	632	82	0	0	1	2	3	7	4	1	13	1	10	2	3	7
4591	16	6	32	566	111	0	1	0	13	5	8	5	0	11	1	5	2	3	6
4592	11	4	22	620	87	0	1	0	6	4	7	5	1	12	1	10	2	2	6
4593	13	5	39	545	104	0	1	0	5	5	8	5	1	9	2	6	2	5	7
4594	7	3	39	749	168	0	0	0	2	6	12	7	0	24	1	8	2	8	15
4595	11	4	33	663	157	0	1	0	20	5	11	8	1	9	1	8	2	2	8
4596	9	3	55	492	111	0	1	0	2	5	10	6	1	3	5	7	2	5	6
4597	16	6	32	582	105	1	1	0	6	5	7	5	1	12	4	7	2	4	8
4598	29	6	2351	280	511	20	22	30	10	24	14	18	7	151	4	47	7	19	12
4599	17	4	3001	83	259	0	10	37	12	16	18	11	1	196	1	32	4	13	13
4600	22	8	51	473	180	0	1	1	29	9	14	9	0	13	4	13	3	6	13
4601	22	9	52	547	186	3	1	1	25	11	12	9	1	14	10	17	4	6	14
4602	2	1	20	600	147	0	1	0	26	6	10	10	0	5	0	9	2	2	5
4603	14	6	35	571	125	0	0	0	5	9	10	6	0	42	1	5	2	6	8
4604	4	1	28	310	140	0	1	0	3	7	16	7	1	2	2	9	2	4	5
4605	29	7	64	803	390	9	21	4	3	9	18	12	3	13	2	7	5	7	15
4606	36	13	179	49	10	0	1	0	0	6	1	1	1	21	3	6	3	26	42
4607	23	9	53	741	239	0	1	0	25	11	15	16	0	20	0	9	3	5	14
4608	23	10	134	1569	212	0	1	4	2	13	19	10	4	42	2	17	5	18	37

Meat, Poultry, Fish

Food No.	Food Description & Amount	wt gm	wt oz	cal	% cal fat	prot gm	carbo gm	fiber gm
4609	Corned beef, pressed [2 slices]	56	2.0	140	54%	15	0	0.0
4610	Giblets, excluding liver, cooked [2 giblets]	46	1.6	70	22%	12	1	0.0
4611	Ham and cheese loaf [2 slices]	56	2.0	145	70%	9	1	0.0
4612	Ham loaf, luncheon meat (Include ham sausage, hamettes) [2 slices (4¼" x 4¼" x 1/16")]	42	1.5	140	82%	5	1	0.0
4613	Ham salad spread [1 can (7.5 oz)]	213	7.5	460	65%	18	23	0.0
4614	Ham, deviled or potted [1 can (3 oz)]	85	3.0	284	82%	11	2	0.0
4615	Head cheese (Include jellied pork) [2 slices (4" x 4" x 3/32")]	56	2.0	119	67%	9	0	0.0
4616	Heart, boiled or simmered (Include beef, pork, veal, lamb, venison, chicken) [2 oz, cooked]	56	2.0	98	29%	16	0	0.0
4617	Heart, braised (Include beef, pork, veal, lamb, venison, chicken) [2 oz, cooked]	56	2.0	98	29%	16	0	0.0
4618	Heart, fried (Include beef, pork, veal, lamb, venison, chicken) [2 oz, cooked]	56	2.0	139	44%	14	5	0.2
4619	Hog lights (lungs), cooked [1 cup]	140	4.9	139	28%	23	0	0.0
4620	Hog maws (stomach), cooked [1 cup]	140	4.9	349	55%	37	0	0.0
4621	Honey loaf [2 slices]	56	2.0	72	31%	9	3	0.0
4622	Kidney, braised (Include beef, pork, veal, lamb, venison) [1 kidney, cooked, beef]	227	8.0	327	22%	58	2	0.0
4623	Kidney, breaded, fried (Include floured; beef, pork, veal, lamb, venison) [1 kidney, cooked, beef]	414	14.6	1127	38%	126	42	1.2
4624	Kidney, broiled or simmered (Include beef, pork, veal, lamb, venison) [1 kidney, cooked, beef]	227	8.0	327	22%	58	2	0.0
4625	Knockwurst (Include Knoblauch) [1 link (4" x 1-1/8")]	68	2.4	209	81%	8	1	0.0
4626	Liver, raw (Include all types) [2 oz]	56	2.0	77	25%	11	3	0.0
4627	Liverwurst (Include liver cheese, Braunschweiger, liver sausage, liver loaf, liver pudding, liver bacon, goose bacon, goose liver sausage) [2 slices (3-1/8" dia x ¼")]	56	2.0	201	80%	8	2	0.0
4628	Luncheon loaf (olive, pickle, or pimiento) [2 slices (1 oz) (4" x 4" x 3/32")]	56	2.0	139	68%	7	4	0.0
4629	Luncheon meat (Include tavern loaf, breakfast loaf, macaroni loaf, luxury loaf) [2 slices (4¼" x 4¼" x 1/16")]	42	1.5	148	82%	5	1	0.0
4630	Luncheon meat, ham and chicken, chopped, minced, pressed, spiced, canned [1 slice (½" thick)]	57	2.0	149	72%	8	2	0.0
4631	Luncheon meat, turkey ham, sliced, extra lean, prepackaged or deli [1 slice (4-1/8" x 4-1/8" x 1/8")]	42	1.5	50	29%	8	1	0.0
4632	Luncheon meat, turkey or chicken breast, (Include pressed, smoked) [2 slices]	56	2.0	62	13%	13	0	0.0
4633	Meat spread or potted meat [1 can (5.5 oz)]	156	5.5	521	82%	20	3	0.0
4634	Mettwurst [2 oz]	56	2.0	174	79%	7	1	0.0
4635	Mortadella [4 slices (15 per 8 oz pkg)]	60	2.1	187	73%	10	2	0.0
4636	Pepperoni [10 slices (1-3/8" dia x 1/8")]	60	2.1	298	80%	13	2	0.0
4637	Roast beef spread [1 can (5.5 oz)]	156	5.5	367	66%	12	19	0.3
4638	Salami (Include cotto salami) [2 slices (4" dia x 1/8")]	46	1.6	115	72%	6	1	0.0
4639	Salami, beef (Include kosher salami) [2 slices (4" dia x 1/8") (10 per 8 oz pkg)]	46	1.6	121	71%	7	1	0.0
4640	Salami, dry or hard (Include Italian salami, Goteborg) [2 slices (1¾" dia x 1/8")]	40	1.4	167	74%	9	1	0.0
4641	Salami, soft, cooked (Include beer bologna, beer sausage, beerwurst) [2 slices (4" dia x 1/8")]	46	1.6	115	72%	6	1	0.0
4642	Sandwich loaf, luncheon meat (Include old fashioned loaf, Dutch loaf, pepperloaf, praski) [2 slices]	56	2.0	109	56%	9	3	0.0
4643	Sausage, beef [1 patty (raw dimensions: 4" dia x ¼")]	27	1.0	85	81%	3	0	0.0
4644	Sausage, beef, brown and serve, links, cooked [2 links (2 oz, raw)]	26	0.9	85	81%	3	0	0.0
4645	Sausage, beef, fresh, bulk, patty or link, cooked [2 links]	26	0.9	87	71%	6	0	0.0
4646	Sausage, beef, smoked (Include Eckrich, Hillshire Farms) [2 links (2" x ¾")]	32	1.1	100	81%	4	1	0.0
4647	Sausage, beef, smoked, stick (Include beef jerky) [2 sticks]	20	0.7	108	82%	4	1	0.0
4648	Sausage, beef, with cheese, smoked (Include Hillshire Farms) [1 link]	86	3.0	275	81%	11	1	0.0
4649	Sausage, blood (Include blutwurst, blood pudding) [4 slices (2¼" dia x 1/8")]	32	1.1	121	82%	5	0	0.0
4650	Sausage, chicken and beef, smoked [1 sausage (5" x 7/8")]	57	2.0	169	73%	11	0	0.0
4651	Sausage, Italian (Include hot links) [1 link (5" long)]	68	2.4	220	72%	14	1	0.0

Food No.	fat gm	sat fat gm	choles mg	sodium mg	potas mg	% of Daily Value													
						vit A	vit E	vit C	thia	ribo	niac	vit B-6	fola	vit B-12	calc	phos	mag	iron	zinc
4609	8	3	48	563	76	0	0	1	1	5	7	4	1	15	1	6	2	6	13
4610	2	0	89	31	82	3	2	1	1	7	9	3	6	15	0	7	2	11	13
4611	11	4	32	752	165	1	1	0	22	6	10	7	0	8	3	14	2	3	7
4612	13	5	26	541	90	0	0	1	10	5	7	4	1	6	0	3	1	2	4
4613	33	11	79	1943	320	0	17	0	62	15	22	16	1	27	2	26	5	7	16
4614	26	9	53	1096	183	0	1	1	21	10	13	9	1	13	1	7	2	3	8
4615	9	3	45	704	17	0	1	0	1	6	3	5	0	10	1	3	1	4	5
4616	3	1	108	35	130	0	2	1	5	51	11	6	0	133	0	14	4	23	12
4617	3	1	108	35	130	0	2	1	5	51	11	6	0	133	0	14	4	23	12
4618	7	1	88	29	113	0	5	1	7	43	11	5	0	109	0	12	3	21	10
4619	4	2	542	113	211	0	2	18	7	27	10	6	1	47	1	26	4	128	23
4620	21	8	429	52	201	0	3	0	8	8	22	2	1	22	2	24	3	16	27
4621	3	1	19	739	192	0	1	0	18	8	9	9	1	10	1	8	2	4	9
4622	8	2	878	304	406	85	2	3	29	542	68	59	56	1941	4	69	10	92	64
4623	47	12	2761	1569	1861	52	20	51	132	774	227	86	36	2852	19	172	31	151	104
4624	8	2	878	304	406	85	2	3	29	542	68	59	56	1941	4	69	10	92	64
4625	19	7	39	687	135	0	2	0	16	6	9	6	0	13	1	7	2	3	8
4626	2	1	211	42	167	523	2	24	8	84	33	25	53	529	0	17	3	23	14
4627	18	6	87	640	111	236	1	0	9	50	23	9	6	188	1	9	2	29	10
4628	11	4	21	804	178	1	1	0	11	8	5	6	0	11	6	7	3	2	5
4629	14	5	23	543	85	0	0	0	9	4	6	4	1	9	0	4	1	2	5
4630	12	4	44	563	108	1	0	0	12	5	10	8	1	6	3	7	2	4	6
4631	2	1	28	436	126	0	1	0	1	6	7	5	1	2	0	13	2	3	7
4632	1	0	23	801	156	0	0	0	1	4	23	10	1	19	0	13	3	1	4
4633	47	17	97	2011	335	0	2	3	38	18	24	16	2	23	1	13	4	6	15
4634	15	6	38	603	152	0	1	0	9	7	8	5	1	15	2	8	2	5	8
4635	15	6	34	748	98	0	1	0	5	5	8	4	0	15	1	6	2	5	8
4636	26	10	47	1224	208	0	1	0	13	9	15	8	1	25	1	7	2	5	10
4637	27	9	59	1580	172	1	12	0	18	12	13	9	1	29	2	9	3	7	11
4638	9	4	30	490	91	0	0	0	7	10	8	5	0	28	1	5	2	7	7
4639	10	4	30	541	103	0	0	0	3	5	7	4	0	23	0	5	2	6	7
4640	14	5	32	744	151	0	1	0	16	7	10	10	0	13	0	6	2	3	9
4641	9	4	30	490	91	0	0	0	7	10	8	5	0	28	1	5	2	7	7
4642	7	2	26	776	216	0	1	0	13	9	8	7	0	15	4	9	3	4	9
4643	8	3	16	275	45	0	0	0	1	2	3	2	0	7	0	2	0	2	4
4644	8	3	17	270	44	0	0	0	1	2	3	1	0	6	1	2	0	2	4
4645	7	3	20	247	79	0	0	0	1	3	4	3	0	12	0	4	1	3	9
4646	9	4	19	326	53	0	0	0	1	2	4	2	0	8	1	3	0	3	5
4647	10	4	20	338	57	0	0	0	2	2	6	3	0	11	0	3	1	3	5
4648	25	11	54	900	139	2	1	0	3	7	9	6	1	20	7	13	2	7	13
4649	11	4	38	218	12	0	0	0	2	2	2	1	0	5	0	1	1	11	3
4650	14	4	40	581	79	2	1	0	2	4	12	5	1	4	1	6	2	3	7
4651	17	6	53	627	207	0	1	2	28	9	14	11	1	15	2	12	3	6	11

Meat, Poultry, Fish

Food No.	Food Description & Amount	wt gm	wt oz	cal	% cal fat	prot gm	carbo gm	fiber gm
4652	Sausage, pickled (Include Penrose hot or firecracker sausage) [2 sausages]	28	1.0	81	72%	4	1	0.0
4653	Sausage, Polish [1 sausage (10" x 1¼")]	227	8.0	704	79%	30	5	0.0
4654	Sausage, pork and beef [1 patty, cooked]	27	1.0	107	82%	4	1	0.0
4655	Sausage, pork and beef, brown and serve, cooked [1 patty]	27	1.0	107	82%	4	1	0.0
4656	Sausage, pork, brown and serve, cooked [1 patty]	27	1.0	100	76%	5	0	0.0
4657	Sausage, pork, country style, fresh, cooked [1 patty (raw dimensions: 3-7/8" dia x ¼")]	27	1.0	100	76%	5	0	0.0
4658	Sausage, pork, fresh, bulk, patty or link, cooked (Include breakfast sausage) [1 patty (raw dimensions: 3-7/8" dia x ¼")]	27	1.0	100	76%	5	0	0.0
4659	Sausage, pork rice links, brown and serve, cooked [2 links, cooked]	50	1.8	120	71%	7	1	0.0
4660	Sausage, smoked link, pork and beef [1 link (4" long x 1-1/8" dia)]	68	2.4	228	81%	9	1	0.0
4661	Sausage, smoked link, pork [1 link (4" x 1-1/8")]	68	2.4	265	73%	15	1	0.0
4662	Sausage, smoked, pork [1 link, (4" long)]	68	2.4	265	73%	15	1	0.0
4663	Sausage, turkey breakfast, bulk [1 patty]	42	1.5	86	42%	12	0	0.0
4664	Sausage, turkey, smoked (Include chicken sausage) [2 slices]	56	2.0	111	69%	8	1	0.0
4665	Sausage, turkey and pork, fresh, bulk, patty or link, cooked [2 oz, cooked]	56	2.0	172	67%	13	0	0.0
4666	Sausage, turkey, pork, and beef, reduced fat, smoked [1 sausage (2" x 1-5/8")]	39	1.4	94	63%	7	1	0.0
4667	Sausage, Vienna, canned [2 sausages (2" x 7/8")]	32	1.1	89	81%	3	1	0.0
4668	Sausage, Vienna, chicken, canned [2 sausages]	32	1.1	82	68%	4	2	0.0
4669	Scrapple, cooked [2 slices (2¾" x 2-1/8" x ¼")]	50	1.8	114	57%	5	8	0.4
4670	Souse [2 slices (3-7/8" sq x 1/8")]	56	2.0	97	67%	7	0	0.0
4671	Sweetbreads, cooked [2 oz, cooked]	56	2.0	97	22%	18	0	0.0
4672	Thuringer (Include summer sausage) [2 slices (4-1/8" dia x 1/8") (10 per 8 oz pkg)]	46	1.6	154	79%	7	0	0.0
4673	Tongue, braised (Include beef, pork, lamb, veal) [2 oz, cooked]	56	2.0	158	66%	12	0	0.0
4674	Tongue, deviled (Include beef, pork, lamb, veal) [½ cup]	113	4.0	326	71%	21	1	0.0
4675	Tongue, pot roast, Puerto Rican style (Lengua al caldero) [1 slice (5" x 2" x 1")]	110	3.9	352	66%	27	1	0.1
4676	Tongue, smoked, cured, or pickled, cooked (Include beef, pork, lamb, veal) [2 slices (3" x 2" x 1/8")]	40	1.4	110	66%	9	0	0.0
4677	Tripe, battered, fried [4 pieces (1 cubic inch, raw)]	44	1.6	71	49%	6	3	0.1
4678	Tripe, cooked [2 oz, cooked]	56	2.0	58	36%	9	0	0.0
	Fish and Shellfish (weight column is for cooked, edible portion)							
4750	Anchovy, canned [1 can (2 oz) drained]	45	1.6	95	42%	13	0	0.0
4751	Barracuda, baked or broiled (Include sauteed; fried with no coating) [2 oz, boneless, cooked]	56	2.0	119	52%	13	0	0.0
4752	Barracuda, floured or breaded, fried [2 oz, boneless, cooked]	56	2.0	139	53%	13	2	0.1
4753	Barracuda, steamed or poached [2 oz, boneless, cooked]	56	2.0	112	45%	14	0	0.0
4754	Carp, baked or broiled (Include sauteed; fried with no coating; bream, buffalofish, chub, sucker) [2 oz, boneless, cooked]	56	2.0	115	52%	13	0	0.0
4755	Carp, floured or breaded, fried (Include bream, buffalofish, chub, sucker) [2 oz, boneless, cooked]	56	2.0	157	51%	12	7	0.2
4756	Carp, smoked (Include bream, buffalofish, sucker) [1 oz]	56	2.0	111	40%	16	0	0.0
4757	Carp, steamed or poached (Include bream, buffalofish, chub, sucker) [1 oz, boneless, cooked]	56	2.0	90	40%	13	0	0.0
4758	Catfish, baked or broiled (Include sauteed; fried with no coating; bullhead) [1 medium catfish]	272	9.6	591	60%	55	2	0.1
4759	Catfish, battered, fried (Include bullhead) [1 filet]	81	2.9	236	66%	12	8	0.3
4760	Catfish, breaded or battered, baked [2 oz, boneless, cooked]	56	2.0	171	58%	10	7	0.2
4761	Catfish, floured or breaded, fried (Include bullhead) [1 medium]	332	11.7	968	56%	62	42	1.4
4762	Catfish, steamed or poached [2 oz, boneless, cooked]	56	2.0	95	51%	11	0	0.0
4763	Cod, baked or broiled (Include sauteed; fried with no coating) [2 oz, boneless, cooked]	56	2.0	69	27%	12	0	0.0
4764	Cod, battered, fried [2 oz, boneless, cooked]	56	2.0	97	41%	10	4	0.1
4765	Cod, breaded or battered, baked [1 filet]	56	2.0	112	41%	11	5	0.2

Food No.	fat gm	sat fat gm	choles mg	sodium mg	potas mg	% of Daily Value													
						vit A	vit E	vit C	thia	ribo	niac	vit B-6	fola	vit B-12	calc	phos	mag	iron	zinc
4652	6	3	21	444	64	0	0	0	5	7	6	3	0	20	0	4	1	5	5
4653	62	22	152	2443	615	0	2	0	35	29	33	20	3	61	10	34	9	18	31
4654	10	3	19	217	51	0	0	0	6	2	5	1	0	2	0	3	1	2	3
4655	10	3	19	217	51	0	0	0	6	2	5	1	0	2	0	3	1	2	3
4656	8	3	22	349	97	0	0	1	13	4	6	4	0	8	1	5	1	2	5
4657	8	3	22	349	97	0	0	1	13	4	6	4	0	8	1	5	1	2	5
4658	8	3	22	349	97	0	0	1	13	4	6	4	0	8	1	5	1	2	5
4659	9	3	35	325	105	0	1	1	21	5	7	5	1	11	1	5	2	3	6
4660	21	7	48	643	129	0	1	0	12	7	11	6	0	17	1	7	2	5	10
4661	22	8	46	1020	228	0	1	2	32	10	15	12	1	18	2	11	3	4	13
4662	22	8	46	1020	228	0	1	2	32	10	15	12	1	18	2	11	3	4	13
4663	4	1	34	289	116	0	1	0	2	4	11	8	1	2	1	8	3	4	8
4664	9	3	55	492	111	0	1	0	2	5	10	6	1	3	5	7	2	5	6
4665	13	4	47	492	189	0	1	1	19	8	12	10	1	12	2	11	3	5	12
4666	7	2	25	373	80	0	0	0	5	3	6	5	0	3	1	6	2	2	6
4667	8	3	17	305	32	0	0	0	2	2	3	2	0	5	0	2	1	2	3
4668	6	2	32	438	27	1	0	0	1	2	5	5	0	1	3	3	1	4	2
4669	7	3	23	382	122	0	0	0	4	2	4	2	0	2	0	3	1	2	5
4670	7	2	37	578	14	0	1	0	1	5	3	4	0	8	1	3	1	3	4
4671	2	1	263	37	192	0	2	69	2	5	6	3	0	20	0	38	2	6	12
4672	14	6	35	571	125	0	0	0	5	9	10	6	0	42	1	5	2	6	8
4673	12	5	60	34	101	0	1	0	1	12	6	4	1	55	0	8	2	11	18
4674	26	11	124	1609	185	0	1	0	3	7	7	8	1	94	2	13	4	17	28
4675	26	11	130	77	226	0	2	1	2	25	12	6	1	89	2	17	6	24	39
4676	8	3	42	416	70	0	1	0	1	8	4	3	0	38	0	6	2	7	12
4677	4	1	36	48	91	0	2	2	2	5	1	1	0	8	1	5	1	5	6
4678	2	1	56	27	159	0	0	3	0	6	0	1	0	11	1	5	1	6	10
4750	4	1	38	1651	245	1	10	0	2	10	45	5	1	7	10	11	8	12	7
4751	7	2	31	76	271	2	4	3	5	16	27	10	0	41	2	8	5	4	3
4752	8	2	29	213	256	1	5	2	6	16	27	9	0	39	1	8	5	5	3
4753	6	2	33	55	245	1	3	2	4	16	25	9	0	44	2	8	4	5	3
4754	7	1	47	66	244	3	4	4	5	2	6	6	3	16	3	30	5	5	7
4755	9	2	55	115	212	1	5	1	7	5	7	5	3	13	5	25	5	7	7
4756	5	1	58	382	291	1	3	2	6	3	7	7	3	19	4	36	6	6	9
4757	4	1	47	31	201	1	2	1	4	2	5	5	2	15	3	26	5	5	7
4758	39	9	164	336	1072	17	28	15	80	16	40	30	8	122	4	71	20	10	17
4759	17	4	49	66	224	1	12	1	17	7	10	6	2	21	3	16	5	5	4
4760	11	2	44	186	193	8	8	0	15	6	9	5	2	17	3	13	4	5	4
4761	60	13	267	705	1150	10	38	3	90	36	55	32	12	105	18	80	26	31	23
4762	5	1	33	33	178	1	4	1	13	3	7	5	1	24	1	13	4	2	3
4763	2	0	24	66	269	2	2	4	1	2	6	12	1	9	1	12	4	1	2
4764	4	1	28	51	215	0	3	2	3	3	6	9	1	7	2	10	3	2	2
4765	5	1	33	147	241	5	4	2	4	4	7	10	1	8	2	11	4	3	2

Meat, Poultry, Fish

Food No.	Food Description & Amount	wt gm	wt oz	cal	% cal fat	prot gm	carbo gm	fiber gm
4766	Cod, dried, salted [1 piece (5½" x 1½" x ½")]	80	2.8	232	7%	50	0	0.0
4767	Cod, dried, salted, salt removed in water [2 oz, dried, soaked in water]	68	2.4	56	7%	12	0	0.0
4768	Cod, floured or breaded, fried [1 filet]	87	3.1	185	46%	17	7	0.2
4769	Cod, smoked [2 oz, boneless]	56	2.0	46	7%	10	0	0.0
4770	Cod, steamed or poached [2 oz, boneless, cooked]	56	2.0	57	7%	13	0	0.0
4771	Croaker, baked or broiled (Incl. sauteed; fried with no coating; angelfish, butterflyfish, drumfish, goatfish, kingfish, sea trout, freshwater sheepshead, spadefish, spot, surgeonfish, weakfish, weke) [1 filet]	62	2.2	120	47%	15	0	0.0
4772	Croaker, breaded or battered, baked (Include angelfish, butterflyfish, drumfish, goatfish, kingfish, sea trout, freshwater sheepshead, spadefish, spot, surgeonfish, weakfish, weke) [1 filet]	81	2.9	179	47%	16	7	0.2
4773	Croaker, floured or breaded, fried (Include angelfish, butterflyfish, drumfish, goatfish, kingfish, sea trout, freshwater sheepshead, spadefish, spot, surgeonfish, weakfish, weke) [2 oz, boneless, cooked]	56	2.0	160	48%	12	8	0.3
4774	Croaker, steamed or poached (Include angelfish, butterflyfish, drumfish, goatfish, kingfish, sea trout, freshwater sheepshead, spadefish, spot, surgeonfish, weakfish, weke) [2 oz, boneless, cooked]	56	2.0	74	27%	13	0	0.0
4775	Eel, smoked [2 oz, boneless]	56	2.0	162	57%	16	0	0.0
4776	Eel, steamed or poached [2 oz, boneless, cooked]	56	2.0	130	57%	13	0	0.0
4777	Fish sticks, baked or broiled [2 sticks]	48	1.7	131	40%	8	11	0.0
4778	Fish sticks, battered, fried [2 sticks]	48	1.7	99	50%	9	3	0.1
4779	Fish sticks, breaded or battered, baked [2 sticks]	48	1.7	131	40%	8	11	0.0
4780	Fish sticks, cooked [2 sticks]	48	1.7	131	40%	8	11	0.0
4781	Fish sticks, floured or breaded, fried [2 sticks]	48	1.7	106	45%	10	4	0.1
4782	Flounder, baked or broiled (Include sauteed; fried with no coating; dab, fluke, halibut, sole, turbot) [1 filet (6" x 2½" x ¼")]	57	2.0	76	29%	13	0	0.0
4783	Flounder, battered, fried (Include dab, fluke, halibut, sole, turbot) [2 oz, boneless, cooked]	56	2.0	115	51%	10	4	0.1
4784	Flounder, breaded or battered, baked (Include dab, fluke, halibut, sole, turbot [1 filet]	56	2.0	117	42%	12	5	0.2
4785	Flounder, floured or breaded, fried (Include fried dab, fluke, halibut, sole, turbot) [1 filet]	81	2.9	179	46%	16	7	0.2
4786	Flounder, raw (Include dab, fluke, halibut, sole, turbot) [2 oz, boneless, raw]	56	2.0	51	12%	11	0	0.0
4787	Flounder, smoked (Include dab, fluke, halibut, sole, turbot) [2 oz, boneless]	56	2.0	123	12%	25	0	0.0
4788	Flounder, steamed or poached (Include dab, fluke, halibut, sole, turbot) [2 oz, boneless, cooked]	56	2.0	64	12%	13	0	0.0
4789	Haddock, baked or broiled (Include sauteed; fried with no coating; burbot, cusk, hake, ling, monkfish, pollock, scrod) [2 oz, boneless, cooked]	56	2.0	73	26%	12	0	0.0
4790	Haddock, battered, fried (Include burbot, cusk, hake, ling, monkfish, pollock, scrod) [1 filet]	178	6.3	316	41%	33	12	0.4
4791	Haddock, breaded or battered, broiled (Include burbot, cusk, hake, ling, monkfish, pollock, scrod) [2 oz, boneless, cooked]	56	2.0	115	41%	12	5	0.2
4792	Haddock, floured or breaded, fried (Include burbot, cusk, hake, ling, monkfish, pollock, scrod) [1 filet]	81	2.9	176	45%	16	7	0.2
4793	Haddock, smoked (Include burbot, cusk, hake, ling, monkfish, pollock, scrod white fish) [2 oz, boneless]	56	2.0	65	7%	14	0	0.0
4794	Haddock, steamed or poached (Include burbot, cusk, hake, ling, monkfish, pollock, scrod) [2 oz, boneless, cooked]	56	2.0	62	7%	13	0	0.0
4795	Herring, baked or broiled (Include sauteed; fried with no coating; alewife, milkfish, shad) [2 oz, boneless, cooked]	56	2.0	137	59%	13	0	0.0
4796	Herring, dried, salted (Include alewife, milkfish, shad) [2 oz, boneless]	56	2.0	225	51%	25	0	0.0
4797	Herring, floured or breaded, fried (Include alewife, milkfish, shad) [2 oz, boneless, cooked]	56	2.0	176	56%	12	7	0.2
4798	Herring, pickled (Include in wine sauce) [2 oz, boneless]	56	2.0	147	62%	8	5	0.0

Food No.	fat gm	sat fat gm	choles mg	sodium mg	potas mg	vit A	vit E	vit C	thia	ribo	niac	vit B-6	fola	vit B-12	calc	phos	mag	iron	zinc
						% of Daily Value													
4766	2	0	122	5622	1166	3	2	5	14	11	30	35	5	133	13	76	27	11	8
4767	0	0	29	1227	240	1	1	1	3	2	6	7	1	27	3	17	6	3	2
4768	9	2	50	151	364	2	6	3	5	6	12	16	2	12	3	17	6	5	3
4769	0	0	24	30	231	1	1	1	3	2	5	6	1	8	1	11	4	1	2
4770	0	0	26	45	240	0	1	3	1	2	6	11	1	9	0	11	4	1	2
4771	6	2	51	89	295	5	6	4	4	5	17	11	3	31	1	18	8	2	2
4772	9	2	67	201	303	8	8	0	8	8	19	11	3	30	4	19	9	5	3
4773	9	2	56	135	223	2	7	0	7	7	15	8	3	21	4	14	7	5	3
4774	2	1	43	36	208	1	3	0	3	4	13	9	2	25	1	13	6	1	2
4775	10	2	111	45	239	83	16	2	9	2	15	3	3	35	2	19	4	2	9
4776	8	2	89	33	164	63	13	2	6	2	11	2	2	30	1	14	3	2	8
4777	6	2	54	279	125	1	3	0	4	5	5	1	2	14	1	9	3	2	2
4778	5	1	37	48	158	1	4	0	3	6	8	6	1	20	4	10	7	2	2
4779	6	2	54	279	125	1	3	0	4	5	5	1	2	14	1	9	3	2	2
4780	6	2	54	279	125	1	3	0	4	5	5	1	2	14	1	9	3	2	2
4781	5	1	43	90	179	1	3	0	3	7	9	6	1	22	4	11	8	3	2
4782	2	1	32	74	245	2	7	3	4	3	9	6	1	15	1	12	5	1	2
4783	6	1	32	54	187	1	8	1	4	4	8	5	1	12	2	10	4	2	2
4784	5	1	39	152	218	5	8	1	6	5	10	6	2	14	3	12	5	4	2
4785	9	2	55	148	307	2	12	2	8	7	14	8	2	18	4	16	7	5	3
4786	1	0	27	45	202	1	5	2	3	3	8	6	1	14	1	10	4	1	2
4787	2	0	65	110	488	1	12	3	7	6	19	13	2	31	2	25	10	3	4
4788	1	0	34	51	215	1	6	1	3	3	9	6	1	15	1	12	5	1	2
4789	2	0	37	64	210	3	2	2	1	1	12	9	2	12	2	12	6	4	2
4790	14	3	120	158	537	3	12	0	10	10	34	22	6	30	9	35	17	14	6
4791	5	1	44	145	191	6	4	0	4	4	12	8	2	10	4	12	6	6	2
4792	9	2	62	138	268	2	6	0	5	5	18	11	3	15	5	17	9	8	3
4793	1	0	43	427	232	1	1	0	2	2	14	11	2	15	3	14	8	4	2
4794	1	0	40	43	187	1	1	0	1	1	11	9	2	12	2	12	6	4	2
4795	9	2	44	93	243	4	5	3	4	10	12	10	2	124	4	17	6	4	5
4796	13	3	85	952	464	3	5	1	7	19	23	19	3	242	9	34	12	9	9
4797	11	2	52	140	209	2	6	1	7	11	12	8	2	114	6	15	6	7	5
4798	10	1	7	487	39	14	3	0	1	5	9	5	0	40	4	5	1	4	2

Meat, Poultry, Fish

Food No.	Food Description & Amount	wt gm	wt oz	cal	% cal fat	prot gm	carbo gm	fiber gm
4799	Herring, pickled, in cream sauce [2 oz, boneless]	56	2.0	141	66%	7	5	0.0
4800	Herring, raw (Include alewife, milkfish, shad) [2 oz, boneless, raw]	56	2.0	88	51%	10	0	0.0
4801	Herring, smoked, kippered [2 oz, boneless]	56	2.0	122	51%	14	0	0.0
4802	Jellyfish, pickled [1 cup]	58	2.0	21	35%	3	0	0.0
4803	Mackerel, baked or broiled (Include sauteed; fried with no coating; enenui, garfish, ono, needlefish, wahoo) [2 oz, boneless, cooked]	56	2.0	125	56%	13	0	0.0
4804	Mackerel, canned [2 oz, boneless]	56	2.0	87	36%	13	0	0.0
4805	Mackerel, dried (Include enenui, garfish, ono, needlefish, wahoo) [2 oz, boneless]	56	2.0	171	74%	10	0	0.0
4806	Mackerel, floured or breaded, fried (Include fried enenui, garfish, ono, needlefish, wahoo) [2 oz, boneless, cooked]	56	2.0	164	59%	12	5	0.2
4807	Mackerel, pickled (Include enenui, garfish, ono, needlefish, wahoo) [2 oz, boneless]	56	2.0	144	61%	13	0	0.0
4808	Mackerel, raw (Include enenui, garfish, ono, needlefish, wahoo) [2 oz, boneless, raw]	56	2.0	94	50%	11	0	0.0
4809	Mackerel, salted [2 oz, dried, soaked, drained, and cooked]	44	1.6	134	74%	8	0	0.0
4810	Mackerel, smoked (Include enenui, garfish, ono, needlefish, wahoo) [2 oz, boneless]	56	2.0	112	45%	14	0	0.0
4811	Mullet, baked or broiled (Include sauteed; fried with no coating) [1 filet (6" x 2½" x ¼")]	57	2.0	111	45%	14	0	0.0
4812	Mullet, floured or breaded, fried (Include fried) [2 oz, boneless, cooked]	56	2.0	154	47%	12	7	0.2
4813	Mullet, raw [2 oz, raw]	56	2.0	66	29%	11	0	0.0
4814	Mullet, steamed or poached [2 oz, boneless, cooked]	56	2.0	83	29%	14	0	0.0
4815	Ocean perch, baked or broiled (Include sauteed; fried with no coating; bocaccio, menpachi, orange roughy, redfish, rockfish) [2 oz, boneless, cooked]	56	2.0	77	32%	12	0	0.0
4816	Ocean perch, battered, fried (Include bocaccio, menpachi, orange roughy, redfish, rockfish) [2 oz, boneless, cooked]	56	2.0	116	52%	10	4	0.1
4817	Ocean perch, breaded or battered, baked (Include bocaccio, menpachi, orange roughy, redfish, rockfish) [2 oz, boneless, cooked]	56	2.0	104	32%	12	5	0.2
4818	Ocean perch, floured or breaded, fried (Include bocaccio, menpachi, orange roughy, redfish, rockfish) [2 oz, boneless, cooked]	56	2.0	125	48%	11	5	0.2
4819	Ocean perch, raw (Include bocaccio, menpachi, orange roughy, redfish, rockfish) [2 oz, boneless, raw]	56	2.0	53	16%	10	0	0.0
4820	Ocean perch, steamed or poached (Include bocaccio, orange roughy, menpachi, redfish, rockfish) [2 oz, boneless, cooked]	56	2.0	66	16%	13	0	0.0
4821	Octopus, cooked [2 oz, cooked]	56	2.0	106	39%	9	6	0.2
4822	Octopus, dried [2 oz]	56	2.0	175	11%	32	5	0.0
4823	Octopus, dried, boiled [1 cup, cooked]	106	3.7	174	11%	32	5	0.0
4824	Octopus, smoked [2 oz, boneless, cooked]	56	2.0	78	11%	14	2	0.0
4825	Octopus, steamed [2 oz, cooked]	56	2.0	92	11%	17	2	0.0
4826	Perch, baked or broiled (Include sauteed; fried with no coating; freshwater bass, bluegill, crappie, sunfish, walleye) [2 oz, boneless, cooked]	56	2.0	75	27%	13	0	0.0
4827	Perch, battered, fried (Include freshwater bass, bluegill, crappie, sunfish, walleye) [2 oz, boneless, cooked]	56	2.0	102	41%	11	4	0.1
4828	Perch, breaded or battered, baked (Include freshwater bass, bluegill, crappie, sunfish, walleye) [2 oz, boneless, cooked]	56	2.0	102	29%	12	5	0.2
4829	Perch, floured or breaded, fried (Include fried freshwater bass, bluegill, crappie, sunfish, walleye) [2 oz, boneless, cooked]	56	2.0	148	43%	13	8	0.3
4830	Perch, steamed or poached [2 oz, boneless, cooked]	56	2.0	64	9%	14	0	0.0
4831	Pike, baked or broiled (Include sauteed; fried with no coating; muskellunge, pickerel) [2 oz, boneless, cooked]	56	2.0	73	26%	13	0	0.0
4832	Pike, battered, fried (Include muskellunge, pickerel) [2 oz, boneless, cooked]	56	2.0	114	50%	10	4	0.1
4833	Pike, floured or breaded, fried (Include muskellunge, pickerel) [2 oz, boneless, cooked]	56	2.0	122	45%	11	5	0.2

Food No.	fat gm	sat fat gm	choles mg	sodium mg	potas mg	% of Daily Value													
						vit A	vit E	vit C	thia	ribo	niac	vit B-6	fola	vit B-12	calc	phos	mag	iron	zinc
4799	10	3	11	395	47	14	2	0	1	5	7	4	1	32	5	5	1	3	2
4800	5	1	34	50	183	2	3	1	3	8	9	8	1	128	3	13	4	3	4
4801	7	2	46	514	250	2	3	1	5	11	12	12	2	175	5	18	6	5	5
4802	1	0	3	5620	2	0	0	0	0	0	1	0	0	0	0	1	0	7	2
4803	8	2	42	71	259	3	4	3	6	12	22	11	0	43	1	12	8	4	3
4804	4	1	44	212	109	7	4	1	1	7	17	6	1	65	13	17	5	6	4
4805	14	4	53	2492	291	3	7	0	1	6	9	11	2	112	4	14	8	4	4
4806	11	3	47	101	227	2	6	1	7	12	20	10	1	35	3	11	7	6	3
4807	10	2	49	63	220	4	5	0	8	13	32	14	0	102	1	15	13	6	3
4808	5	1	36	44	218	2	3	1	5	10	18	11	0	48	1	10	6	3	2
4809	11	3	42	1958	229	2	5	0	1	5	7	9	2	88	3	11	7	3	3
4810	6	2	33	223	290	1	3	2	5	18	30	11	0	39	2	9	5	5	3
4811	6	1	36	80	267	5	5	4	4	3	18	14	1	2	3	16	5	4	3
4812	8	2	46	126	226	3	6	1	7	6	17	11	2	3	5	15	5	7	3
4813	2	1	27	36	200	2	3	1	3	3	15	12	1	2	2	12	4	3	2
4814	3	1	35	41	215	2	3	1	3	3	16	12	1	2	3	14	5	4	2
4815	3	0	28	69	183	2	5	2	4	4	6	7	1	10	7	14	5	3	2
4816	7	1	29	51	145	1	7	1	5	5	6	5	1	8	6	12	4	4	2
4817	4	1	37	130	176	3	5	1	7	6	8	7	2	9	8	14	5	5	3
4818	7	1	35	99	165	1	6	1	6	6	7	6	2	8	7	13	5	5	2
4819	1	0	24	42	153	1	3	1	4	4	6	6	1	9	6	12	4	3	2
4820	1	0	29	47	162	1	4	1	4	4	6	6	1	10	7	14	5	4	2
4821	5	1	40	188	213	3	5	4	4	4	8	9	3	166	5	12	5	19	7
4822	2	0	102	490	745	8	12	17	4	4	21	36	8	674	11	40	16	63	24
4823	2	0	102	488	668	9	6	14	4	5	20	34	6	636	11	30	16	56	24
4824	1	0	46	219	334	4	5	8	2	2	10	16	4	302	5	18	7	28	11
4825	1	0	54	258	353	5	6	7	2	3	11	18	3	336	6	16	8	30	13
4826	2	0	59	60	180	2	2	3	3	4	5	4	1	19	5	13	5	3	5
4827	5	1	54	47	148	1	3	1	4	5	5	3	1	15	5	11	4	4	4
4828	3	1	64	122	173	3	2	1	5	6	6	4	1	18	6	13	5	5	5
4829	7	1	71	133	180	1	4	1	6	7	7	4	2	16	7	14	6	7	5
4830	1	0	63	39	160	1	1	1	3	4	5	3	1	19	6	13	5	4	5
4831	2	0	26	45	174	3	2	5	2	2	7	4	2	20	4	15	5	2	3
4832	6	1	28	34	138	1	4	2	4	4	7	3	2	15	4	12	4	3	3
4833	6	1	33	80	157	2	4	3	4	4	8	3	2	17	5	13	5	4	3

Meat, Poultry, Fish

Food No.	Food Description & Amount	wt gm	wt oz	cal	% cal fat	prot gm	carbo gm	fiber gm
4834	Pike, steamed or poached (Include muskellunge, pickerel) [2 oz, boneless, cooked]	56	2.0	62	7%	14	0	0.0
4835	Pompano, baked or broiled (Include sauteed; fried with no coating; akule, blackfish, bluefish, butterfish, dolphinfish, jack, mahimahi, paplo, parrot fish, sablefish, scad, tilefish, ulva, yellowtail) [2 oz, boneless, cooked]	56	2.0	143	60%	13	0	0.0
4836	Pompano, battered, fried (Include akule, blackfish, bluefish, butterfish, dolphinfish, jack, mahimahi, paplo, parrot fish, sablefish, scad, tilefish, ulva, yellowtail) [2 oz, boneless, cooked]	56	2.0	150	63%	10	4	0.1
4837	Pompano, floured or breaded, fried (Include akule, blackfish, bluefish, butterfish, dolphinfish, jack, mahimahi, paplo, parrot fish, sablefish, scad, tilefish, ulva, yellowtail) [2 oz, boneless, cooked]	56	2.0	179	56%	12	7	0.2
4838	Pompano, raw (Include akule, blackfish, bluefish, butterfish, dolphinfish, jack, mahimahi, paplo, parrot fish, sablefish, scad, tilefish, ulva, yellowtail) [2 oz, boneless, raw]	56	2.0	92	52%	10	0	0.0
4839	Pompano, smoked (Incl. akule, blackfish, bluefish, butterfish, dolphinfish, jack, mahimahi, paplo, parrot fish, sablefish, scad, tilefish, ulva, yellowtail) [2 oz, boneless]	56	2.0	108	52%	12	0	0.0
4840	Pompano, steamed or poached (Include akule, blackfish, bluefish, butterfish, dolphinfish, jack, mahimahi, paplo, parrot fish, sablefish, scad, tilefish, ulva, yellowtail) [2 oz, boneless, cooked]	56	2.0	115	52%	13	0	0.0
4841	Porgy, baked or broiled (Include sauteed; fried with no coating; scup, sea bream, marine sheepshead, snapper) [2 oz, boneless, cooked]	56	2.0	109	44%	14	0	0.0
4842	Porgy, battered, fried (Include scup, sea bream, marine sheepshead, snapper) [2 oz, boneless, cooked]	56	2.0	164	61%	10	6	0.2
4843	Porgy, breaded or battered, baked (Include scup, sea bream, marine sheepshead, snapper) [2 oz, boneless, cooked]	56	2.0	149	50%	11	7	0.2
4844	Porgy, floured or breaded, fried (Include scup, sea bream, marine sheepshead, snapper) [2 oz, boneless, cooked]	56	2.0	161	47%	12	8	0.3
4845	Porgy, raw (Include scup, sea bream, marine sheepshead, snapper) [2 oz, boneless, raw]	56	2.0	59	23%	11	0	0.0
4846	Porgy, steamed or poached (Include scup, sea bream, marine sheepshead, snapper) [2 oz, boneless, cooked]	56	2.0	74	23%	13	0	0.0
4847	Ray, baked or broiled (Include sauteed; fried with no coating; skate) [2 oz, boneless, cooked]	56	2.0	114	41%	16	0	0.0
4848	Ray, floured or breaded, fried (Include fried; skate) [2 oz, boneless, cooked]	56	2.0	161	47%	13	7	0.2
4849	Ray, steamed or poached (Include skate) [2 oz, boneless, cooked]	56	2.0	92	31%	15	0	0.0
4850	Roe, cod and shad, cooked [2 oz]	56	2.0	110	51%	14	1	0.0
4851	Roe, herring [2 Tbs]	28	1.0	39	41%	6	0	0.0
4852	Roe, sturgeon (Include caviar) [2 Tbs]	32	1.1	81	64%	8	1	0.0
4853	Salmon, baked or broiled (Include sauteed; fried with no coating; saltwater trout) [2 oz, boneless, cooked]	56	2.0	97	40%	14	0	0.0
4854	Salmon, battered, fried (Include saltwater trout) [2 oz, boneless, cooked]	56	2.0	127	54%	10	4	0.1
4855	Salmon, canned [2 oz]	56	2.0	79	40%	11	0	0.0
4856	Salmon, dried [2 oz, boneless]	56	2.0	81	27%	14	0	0.0
4857	Salmon, floured or breaded, fried (Include fried saltwater trout) [2 oz, boneless, cooked]	56	2.0	134	44%	12	6	0.2
4858	Salmon, raw (Include saltwater trout) [2 oz, boneless, raw]	56	2.0	82	37%	12	0	0.0
4859	Salmon, smoked (Include lox) [2 oz, boneless]	56	2.0	66	33%	10	0	0.0
4860	Salmon, steamed or poached (Include saltwater trout) [2 oz, boneless, cooked]	56	2.0	81	27%	14	0	0.0
4861	Sardines, canned in oil [1 can (3.75 oz), drained]	92	3.2	191	50%	23	0	0.0
4862	Sardines, cooked [2 oz, cooked]	56	2.0	116	50%	14	0	0.0
4863	Sardines, dried [4 sardines (5" long)]	28	1.0	57	51%	6	0	0.0
4864	Sardines, skinless, boneless, packed in water [1 can (4.375 oz, 4 sardines), drained]	84	3.0	182	51%	21	0	0.0

Food No.	fat gm	sat fat gm	choles mg	sodium mg	potas mg	% of Daily Value													
						vit A	vit E	vit C	thia	ribo	niac	vit B-6	fola	vit B-12	calc	phos	mag	iron	zinc
4834	0	0	28	25	156	1	1	3	2	2	7	3	2	20	4	14	5	2	3
4835	10	3	36	79	281	5	2	3	26	5	11	7	3	12	2	14	5	2	3
4836	10	3	33	46	197	1	4	0	17	5	8	5	2	10	2	11	4	3	3
4837	11	3	47	126	239	2	4	0	21	8	11	6	3	10	4	13	5	6	4
4838	5	2	28	36	213	2	0	0	21	4	8	6	2	12	1	11	4	2	3
4839	6	2	33	43	251	2	1	0	23	5	10	6	2	12	1	13	4	2	3
4840	7	2	35	41	227	2	1	0	21	4	9	6	2	13	2	12	4	2	3
4841	5	1	39	70	223	5	4	3	5	4	15	10	3	16	3	14	4	2	2
4842	11	2	37	43	149	1	7	0	6	6	11	6	2	10	4	11	3	4	2
4843	8	2	44	180	167	8	6	0	7	6	12	7	2	11	5	11	4	5	3
4844	8	2	51	127	191	2	5	0	8	7	15	8	3	12	5	13	5	6	3
4845	2	0	29	24	161	2	1	0	4	3	11	8	2	13	2	10	3	2	2
4846	2	0	36	26	171	2	2	0	4	4	12	8	2	14	3	12	4	2	2
4847	5	1	38	81	123	7	5	2	2	3	10	13	1	17	3	16	9	3	2
4848	8	2	47	134	117	4	6	0	5	6	11	11	1	13	4	14	8	6	3
4849	3	1	36	50	96	4	3	0	2	2	9	11	0	15	2	13	8	3	2
4850	6	1	241	84	147	7	22	16	9	28	6	5	11	102	2	25	3	2	4
4851	2	0	105	25	62	2	9	6	4	12	3	2	5	37	1	11	1	1	2
4852	6	1	188	480	58	18	10	0	4	12	0	5	4	107	9	11	24	21	2
4853	4	1	35	68	223	4	4	2	7	2	24	6	1	25	1	16	4	3	2
4854	8	1	34	47	169	2	6	0	7	4	18	5	1	19	2	13	4	4	2
4855	4	1	29	307	188	1	4	0	1	6	18	9	2	33	12	18	5	3	4
4856	2	0	36	47	226	2	3	0	8	2	25	6	1	26	1	16	5	3	3
4857	7	1	44	108	201	2	5	0	8	5	22	6	1	21	3	15	5	5	3
4858	3	1	25	26	237	2	2	1	4	5	20	15	1	39	2	15	4	2	2
4859	2	1	13	439	98	1	3	0	1	3	13	8	0	30	1	9	3	3	1
4860	2	0	36	42	192	2	3	0	6	2	21	6	1	30	1	14	4	3	3
4861	11	1	131	465	365	6	1	0	5	12	24	8	3	137	35	45	9	15	8
4862	6	1	80	283	222	4	1	0	3	7	15	5	2	83	21	27	5	9	5
4863	3	1	22	32	117	1	2	0	2	5	6	5	1	61	2	8	3	2	2
4864	10	2	69	771	375	3	4	1	7	16	18	17	3	262	7	27	10	7	8

Meat, Poultry, Fish

Food No.	Food Description & Amount	wt gm	wt oz	cal	% cal fat	prot gm	carbo gm	fiber gm
4865	Sea bass, baked or broiled (Include sauteed; fried with no coating; grouper, striped bass, wreakfish) [2 oz, boneless, cooked]	56	2.0	84	36%	13	0	0.0
4866	Sea bass, breaded or battered, baked (Include grouper, striped bass, wreakfish) [2 oz, boneless, cooked]	56	2.0	106	34%	12	5	0.2
4867	Sea bass, floured or breaded, fried (Include fried grouper, striped bass, wreakfish) [2 oz, boneless, cooked]	56	2.0	124	42%	12	6	0.2
4868	Sea bass, pickled (Mero en escabeche) [2 oz, boneless]	56	2.0	154	80%	7	1	0.1
4869	Sea bass, steamed or poached (Include grouper, striped bass, wreakfish) [2 oz, boneless, cooked]	56	2.0	68	19%	13	0	0.0
4870	Shark, baked or broiled (Include sauteed; fried with no coating; dogfish, grayfish) [2 oz, boneless, cooked]	56	2.0	101	41%	14	0	0.0
4871	Shark, steamed or poached (Include dogfish, grayfish) [2 oz, boneless, cooked]	56	2.0	92	31%	15	0	0.0
4872	Smelt, baked or broiled (Include sauteed; capelin) [2 oz, boneless, cooked]	56	2.0	95	42%	13	0	0.0
4873	Smelt, battered, fried [2 oz, boneless, cooked]	56	2.0	146	59%	9	5	0.2
4874	Smelt, floured or breaded, fried (Include capelin) [2 oz, boneless, cooked]	56	2.0	143	46%	12	7	0.2
4875	Smelt, steamed or poached (Include capelin) [2 oz, boneless, cooked]	56	2.0	69	22%	12	0	0.0
4876	Squid, baked, broiled (Include sauteed; cuttlefish, calamari) [1 squid]	272	9.6	377	31%	51	10	0.0
4877	Squid, breaded, fried [2 oz, cooked]	56	2.0	111	38%	10	7	0.2
4878	Squid, canned (Include calameres en su tinta, squid in its own ink) [1 cup]	187	6.6	199	13%	34	7	0.0
4879	Squid, dried (Include cuttlefish, calamari) [2 oz, boneless]	56	2.0	196	13%	33	7	0.0
4880	Squid, pickled [2 oz, boneless]	56	2.0	53	13%	9	2	0.0
4881	Squid, raw (Include cuttlefish) [2 oz, boneless, raw]	56	2.0	52	14%	9	2	0.0
4882	Squid, steamed or boiled [2 oz, boneless, cooked]	56	2.0	60	13%	10	2	0.0
4883	Sturgeon, baked or broiled (Include sauteed; fried with no coating) [2 oz, boneless, cooked]	56	2.0	76	35%	12	0	0.0
4884	Sturgeon, floured or breaded, fried (Include fried) [2 oz, boneless, cooked]	56	2.0	131	54%	10	5	0.2
4885	Sturgeon, smoked [2 oz, boneless]	56	2.0	97	23%	17	0	0.0
4886	Sturgeon, steamed [2 oz, boneless, cooked]	56	2.0	74	35%	11	0	0.0
4887	Swordfish, baked or broiled (Include sauteed; fried with no coating; marlin) [2 oz, boneless, cooked]	56	2.0	100	42%	13	0	0.0
4888	Swordfish, floured or breaded, fried (Include marlin) [2 oz, boneless, cooked]	56	2.0	140	51%	12	5	0.2
4889	Swordfish, steamed or poached (Include marlin) [2 oz, boneless, cooked]	56	2.0	86	30%	14	0	0.0
4890	Trout, baked or broiled (Include sauteed; fried with no coating; cisco, lake herring, steelhead, whitefish) [2 oz, boneless, cooked]	56	2.0	106	44%	14	0	0.0
4891	Trout, battered, fried (Include cisco, lake herring, steelhead, whitefish) [2 oz, boneless, cooked]	56	2.0	130	52%	11	4	0.1
4892	Trout, breaded or battered, baked (Include cisco, lake herring, steelhead, whitefish) [2 oz, boneless, cooked]	56	2.0	120	35%	14	5	0.2
4893	Trout, floured or breaded, fried (Include cisco, lake herring, steelhead, whitefish) [2 oz, boneless, cooked]	56	2.0	152	49%	13	6	0.2
4894	Trout, smoked (Include chub, cisco, lake herring, steelhead, whitefish) [2 oz, boneless]	56	2.0	149	40%	21	0	0.0
4895	Trout, steamed or poached (Include cisco, lake herring, steelhead, whitefish) [2 oz, boneless, cooked]	56	2.0	98	35%	15	0	0.0
4896	Tuna, canned, oil pack (Include low sodium) [2 oz]	56	2.0	111	37%	16	0	0.0
4897	Tuna, canned, water pack (Include low sodium) [2 oz]	56	2.0	65	6%	14	0	0.0
4898	Tuna, fresh, baked or broiled (Include sauteed; fried with no coating; ahi, aku, bonito) [2 oz, boneless, cooked]	56	2.0	86	24%	15	0	0.0
4899	Tuna, fresh, dried (Include ahi, aku, bonito) [1 cup]	42	1.5	76	31%	12	0	0.0
4900	Tuna, fresh, floured or breaded, fried (Include ahi, aku, bonito) [2 oz, boneless, cooked]	56	2.0	133	42%	14	5	0.2
4901	Tuna, fresh, raw (Include ahi, aku, bonito) [2 oz, boneless, raw]	56	2.0	60	8%	13	0	0.0
4902	Tuna, fresh, smoked (Include ahi, aku, bonito) [2 oz, boneless]	56	2.0	113	45%	14	0	0.0

Food No.	fat gm	sat fat gm	choles mg	sodium mg	potas mg	vit A	vit E	vit C	thia	ribo	niac	vit B-6	fola	vit B-12	calc	phos	mag	iron	zinc
						% of Daily Value													
4865	3	1	28	69	178	5	3	2	5	5	5	12	1	3	1	13	7	1	2
4866	4	1	37	126	166	6	3	0	7	6	6	11	1	3	2	13	7	3	2
4867	6	1	38	108	164	3	4	0	6	7	7	11	1	3	3	13	7	4	2
4868	14	2	16	44	111	2	8	0	3	3	3	7	1	2	1	8	4	1	1
4869	1	0	29	43	152	3	2	0	4	4	5	11	1	3	1	12	6	1	2
4870	5	1	34	71	109	6	4	2	2	2	10	12	1	12	2	14	8	3	2
4871	3	1	36	50	96	4	3	0	2	2	9	11	0	15	2	13	8	3	2
4872	4	1	51	75	215	4	3	3	1	5	5	5	1	37	4	17	5	4	8
4873	10	2	44	49	151	1	7	0	3	6	5	3	1	24	4	12	4	4	6
4874	7	2	58	124	189	2	5	0	4	7	7	4	1	29	6	15	5	6	7
4875	2	0	50	38	175	1	2	0	0	5	4	4	1	35	4	15	5	4	8
4876	13	3	768	242	815	11	24	25	4	64	34	9	4	68	11	73	27	12	34
4877	5	1	142	85	156	1	5	3	3	15	8	2	1	11	4	14	5	5	6
4878	3	1	504	86	425	2	12	12	2	42	19	5	2	35	7	38	16	8	22
4879	3	1	496	94	524	2	12	16	3	41	22	6	2	44	7	47	18	8	22
4880	1	0	129	25	138	0	3	3	1	13	6	1	1	11	2	12	5	2	6
4881	1	0	130	25	138	1	3	4	1	14	6	2	1	12	2	12	5	2	6
4882	1	0	151	26	127	1	4	4	1	13	6	1	1	11	2	11	5	2	7
4883	3	1	43	39	204	14	2	0	3	3	28	6	2	23	1	15	6	3	2
4884	8	2	45	88	171	10	5	0	5	4	24	5	2	18	2	13	6	4	2
4885	2	1	45	414	212	16	1	0	3	3	31	8	3	27	1	16	7	3	2
4886	3	1	42	30	159	13	2	0	3	3	28	6	2	24	1	12	5	2	2
4887	5	1	26	84	199	4	3	3	2	4	31	10	0	18	0	18	5	3	5
4888	8	2	33	107	173	2	5	1	4	5	28	8	1	15	2	16	4	5	5
4889	3	1	28	57	174	2	2	1	1	4	29	9	0	18	0	17	4	3	5
4890	5	1	39	42	300	6	1	4	9	3	27	18	2	35	4	19	5	1	2
4891	7	1	38	42	194	1	3	0	12	11	12	5	2	59	3	14	3	6	3
4892	5	1	48	95	233	2	1	0	14	13	15	6	2	69	4	16	4	8	3
4893	8	2	47	100	222	2	3	0	14	13	15	6	2	65	4	15	4	7	3
4894	7	1	58	52	362	2	1	1	21	19	21	9	3	117	4	25	6	8	4
4895	4	1	42	22	272	5	0	3	8	3	25	18	2	38	5	18	5	1	2
4896	5	1	10	198	116	1	3	0	1	4	35	3	1	21	1	17	4	4	3
4897	0	0	17	189	133	1	1	0	1	2	37	10	1	28	1	9	4	5	3
4898	2	0	30	44	296	3	3	3	17	2	31	27	0	5	1	13	8	3	2
4899	3	1	20	20	132	31	2	0	8	7	22	11	0	74	0	13	7	3	2
4900	6	1	37	79	256	1	5	1	16	4	28	22	1	5	3	12	8	5	3
4901	1	0	25	21	249	1	1	1	16	2	27	25	0	5	1	11	7	2	2
4902	6	2	34	62	292	1	3	2	5	18	30	11	0	39	2	9	5	5	3

Meat, Poultry, Fish

Food No.	Food Description & Amount	wt gm	wt oz	cal	% cal fat	prot gm	carbo gm	fiber gm
4903	Tuna, fresh, steamed or poached (Include ahi, aku, bonito) [2 oz, boneless, cooked]	56	2.0	77	8%	17	0	0.0
4904	Whiting, baked or broiled (Include sauteed; fried with no coating) [2 oz, boneless, cooked]	56	2.0	74	30%	12	0	0.0
4905	Whiting, battered, fried [2 oz, boneless, cooked]	56	2.0	101	43%	10	4	0.1
4906	Whiting, breaded or battered, baked [2 oz, boneless, cooked]	56	2.0	116	42%	11	5	0.2
4907	Whiting, floured or breaded, fried (Include fried) [2 oz, boneless, cooked]	56	2.0	123	47%	11	5	0.2
4908	Whiting, steamed or poached [2 oz, boneless, cooked]	56	2.0	64	13%	13	0	0.0
4909	Abalone, floured or breaded, fried [2 oz, cooked]	56	2.0	107	32%	11	6	0.1
4910	Abalone, steamed or poached [2 oz, cooked]	56	2.0	118	7%	19	7	0.0
4911	Clams, baked or broiled (Include sauteed) [1 cup (8 large clams, 12 medium clams, 15 small clams)]	150	5.3	210	45%	23	5	0.0
4912	Clams, canned [2 oz]	56	2.0	52	12%	9	2	0.0
4913	Clams, floured or breaded, fried (Include baked) [1 cup (8 large clams, 12 medium clams, 15 small clams)]	150	5.3	271	40%	22	17	0.4
4914	Clams, raw [4 clams]	64	2.3	47	12%	8	2	0.0
4915	Clams, smoked, in oil [2 oz]	56	2.0	98	59%	8	2	0.0
4916	Clams, steamed or boiled [1 cup (8 large clams, 12 medium clams, 15 small clams)]	150	5.3	139	12%	24	5	0.0
4917	Conch, battered, fried [2 oz, raw]	50	1.8	104	44%	10	4	0.1
4918	Conch, baked or broiled [2 oz, raw]	34	1.2	44	8%	9	1	0.0
4919	Crab, baked or broiled (Include sauteed) [1 cup, flaked and pieces]	118	4.2	163	42%	23	0	0.0
4920	Crab, canned (Include white or king meat) [2 oz]	56	2.0	55	11%	11	0	0.0
4921	Crab, hard shell, steamed (Include boiled) [1 cup, flaked and pieces]	118	4.2	120	16%	24	0	0.0
4922	Crab, soft shell, floured or breaded, fried [2 oz, cooked]	56	2.0	187	54%	11	10	0.3
4923	Crayfish, boiled or steamed [2 oz, without shell, cooked]	56	2.0	49	12%	9	0	0.0
4924	Crayfish, floured or breaded, fried [2 oz, without shell, cooked]	56	2.0	124	47%	10	6	0.2
4925	Lobster, baked or broiled (Include sauteed) [1 cup, cooked, diced]	145	5.1	169	23%	29	2	0.0
4926	Lobster, battered, fried [1 cup]	145	5.1	306	47%	28	11	0.3
4927	Lobster, canned [2 oz]	56	2.0	55	5%	11	1	0.0
4928	Lobster, floured or breaded, fried [2 oz, without shell, cooked]	56	2.0	123	46%	11	5	0.2
4929	Lobster, steamed or boiled [1 cup, cooked, diced]	145	5.1	142	5%	30	2	0.0
4930	Mussels, raw [4 mussels]	64	2.3	55	23%	8	2	0.0
4931	Mussels, steamed or poached [4 mussels]	32	1.1	55	23%	8	2	0.0
4932	Oysters, baked or broiled (Include sauteed) [4 eastern oysters]	48	1.7	51	60%	3	2	0.0
4933	Oysters, battered, fried [4 eastern oysters]	32	1.1	68	54%	3	5	0.1
4934	Oysters, canned [1 cup, drained]	162	5.7	122	32%	12	7	0.0
4935	Oysters, floured or breaded, fried [4 eastern oysters]	32	1.1	64	57%	3	4	0.1
4936	Oysters, raw [4 eastern oysters]	60	2.1	41	33%	4	2	0.0
4937	Oysters, smoked [6 oysters]	30	1.1	33	33%	3	2	0.0
4938	Oysters, steamed [4 eastern oyster]	48	1.7	41	33%	4	2	0.0
4939	Scallops, baked or broiled (Include sauteed) [4 scallops]	100	3.5	134	27%	20	3	0.0
4940	Scallops, battered, fried [4 scallops]	32	1.1	74	45%	6	4	0.1
4941	Scallops, floured or breaded, fried [4 scallops]	100	3.5	218	45%	18	11	0.3
4942	Scallops, steamed or boiled [4 scallops]	100	3.5	107	27%	16	2	0.0
4943	Sea urchin (roe) [2 Tbs]	24	0.8	35	52%	4	0	0.0
4944	Shrimp, baked or broiled (Include sauteed; prawn) [1 cup, cooked]	145	5.1	226	30%	36	2	0.0
4945	Shrimp, canned [1 cup]	128	4.5	154	15%	30	1	0.0
4946	Shrimp, dried [20 shrimp]	10	0.4	30	15%	6	0	0.0
4947	Shrimp, floured or breaded, fried (Include prawn) [1 cup, cooked]	129	4.6	318	45%	27	15	0.5
4948	Shrimp, steamed or boiled (Include prawn) [1 cup, cooked]	145	5.1	202	15%	39	2	0.0
	Your Additions							

Food No.	fat gm	sat fat gm	choles mg	sodium mg	potas mg	vit A	vit E	vit C	thia	ribo	niac	vit B-6	fola	vit B-12	calc	phos	mag	iron	zinc
						% of Daily Value													
4903	1	0	32	24	268	1	2	1	16	2	30	26	0	5	1	12	8	3	2
4904	3	0	44	67	167	3	2	2	2	2	4	5	2	23	3	15	4	1	4
4905	5	1	43	52	138	1	3	0	4	3	5	4	2	18	4	13	3	2	3
4906	5	1	49	147	157	6	4	0	4	4	5	4	2	19	5	14	4	3	4
4907	6	1	48	97	152	2	4	0	4	4	5	4	2	19	4	13	4	3	4
4908	1	0	47	46	150	2	1	0	2	2	4	4	2	23	3	14	3	1	4
4909	4	1	53	189	160	0	13	2	8	4	5	4	1	6	2	12	8	12	4
4910	1	0	95	287	196	0	20	3	13	5	6	7	1	8	3	15	11	18	6
4911	11	2	60	202	559	22	14	36	9	18	15	5	7	1382	8	30	4	137	16
4912	1	0	24	39	198	6	3	12	4	8	6	2	2	519	3	9	2	49	6
4913	12	2	85	246	518	14	13	26	14	24	18	5	6	1039	12	29	6	122	16
4914	1	0	22	36	201	6	3	14	3	8	6	2	3	527	3	11	1	50	6
4915	6	1	21	35	197	6	6	13	3	8	6	2	3	516	3	11	1	49	6
4916	2	0	64	105	530	15	9	33	10	22	15	5	6	1391	9	24	4	131	17
4917	5	1	31	69	72	0	14	0	3	3	3	1	17	33	5	9	23	4	5
4918	0	0	22	52	55	0	10	0	1	2	2	1	15	30	3	7	20	3	4
4919	8	1	111	375	363	6	9	6	7	3	18	10	14	135	12	23	9	6	31
4920	1	0	50	186	209	0	3	3	3	3	4	4	6	4	6	15	5	3	15
4921	2	0	118	329	382	0	5	6	8	3	19	11	15	144	12	24	10	6	33
4922	11	2	69	187	180	1	8	2	9	6	11	5	6	48	7	12	5	6	14
4923	1	0	74	53	166	1	4	1	2	3	6	2	6	20	3	15	5	3	7
4924	7	1	85	70	168	2	10	1	6	5	8	3	5	15	3	15	4	5	5
4925	4	2	111	571	496	7	7	0	1	6	8	5	4	73	9	26	12	3	27
4926	16	3	113	511	474	3	16	0	6	10	10	5	4	56	11	27	12	6	25
4927	0	0	40	213	197	1	3	0	0	2	3	2	2	29	3	10	5	1	11
4928	6	1	63	217	166	2	7	0	3	4	6	2	2	7	4	9	4	3	12
4929	1	0	104	551	510	4	7	0	1	6	8	6	4	75	9	27	13	3	28
4930	1	0	18	183	205	3	2	9	7	8	5	2	7	128	2	13	5	14	7
4931	1	0	18	156	143	3	2	6	6	6	4	1	5	77	2	9	5	13	7
4932	3	1	24	122	72	3	3	3	3	2	3	1	1	139	2	6	5	17	274
4933	4	1	32	82	55	2	3	1	4	4	3	1	1	77	2	5	4	12	168
4934	4	1	97	197	403	16	7	15	18	17	11	8	4	562	8	24	24	66	1068
4935	4	1	23	98	58	1	3	2	3	3	3	1	1	84	2	5	4	13	185
4936	1	0	32	127	94	2	2	4	4	3	4	2	2	195	3	8	7	22	363
4937	1	0	26	103	76	1	2	3	3	3	3	2	1	158	2	7	6	18	295
4938	1	0	32	127	84	2	2	3	4	3	4	2	1	175	3	6	7	20	363
4939	4	1	40	231	392	5	8	6	1	4	7	9	5	29	3	27	17	2	8
4940	4	1	26	68	101	1	3	1	2	3	3	2	1	7	1	7	4	2	2
4941	11	2	54	259	341	2	10	4	5	8	9	7	4	22	5	24	15	6	7
4942	3	1	32	185	282	4	6	4	1	4	5	7	3	22	2	16	14	1	6
4943	2	0	74	18	32	1	8	6	2	11	2	2	5	40	1	10	1	1	2
4944	7	1	267	312	327	12	10	6	3	3	21	9	1	32	9	36	16	24	13
4945	3	0	221	216	269	2	5	5	2	3	18	7	1	24	8	30	13	19	11
4946	0	0	44	43	53	0	1	1	0	1	3	1	0	5	1	6	3	4	2
4947	16	3	238	261	256	9	12	3	10	11	19	7	3	21	9	28	12	22	11
4948	3	1	290	240	247	9	7	5	3	3	18	9	1	22	10	27	15	23	14

Meat, Poultry, Fish

Food No.	Food Description & Amount	wt gm	wt oz	cal	% cal fat	prot gm	carbo gm	fiber gm
Your Additions								

						% of Daily Value													
Food No.	fat gm	sat fat gm	choles mg	sodium mg	potas mg	vit A	vit E	vit C	thia	ribo	niac	vit B-6	fola	vit B-12	calc	phos	mag	iron	zinc

Soups, Sauces, Fats, Miscellaneous

Soups, Sauces, Fats, Misc.

Food No.	Food Description & Amount	wt gm	wt oz	cal	% cal fat	prot gm	carbo gm	fiber gm
	Soups							
5000	Asparagus soup, cream of, made with milk [1 cup]	248	8.7	149	40%	6	17	0.5
5001	Asparagus soup, cream of, made with water [1 cup]	244	8.6	87	43%	2	11	0.5
5002	Bacon soup, cream of, made with water (Include Albertson brand) [1 cup]	244	8.6	521	71%	22	15	0.5
5003	Barley soup (Include beef barley, chicken barley, mushroom barley soup) [1 cup]	244	8.6	96	7%	5	18	3.6
5004	Barley soup, sweet, with or without nuts, Oriental Style [1 cup]	244	8.6	217	13%	2	47	3.0
5005	Bean soup (Include Navy bean soup) [1 cup]	253	8.9	137	26%	7	19	8.6
5006	Bean soup, home recipe [1 cup]	247	8.7	141	3%	9	27	6.7
5007	Bean soup, mixed beans [1 cup]	238	8.4	129	10%	8	22	6.2
5008	Bean with bacon or pork soup [1 cup]	253	8.9	173	31%	8	23	7.9
5009	Bean soup with ham, chunky style [1 cup]	243	8.6	224	29%	11	29	4.9
5010	Bean and ham soup, canned, reduced sodium, prepared with water or ready-to-serve [1 cup]	249	8.8	184	13%	10	34	10.0
5011	Bean soup with macaroni (Include Pasta e Fagiole without meat; Pasta e Fagioli) [1 cup]	253	8.9	156	22%	8	22	3.7
5012	Bean soup with macaroni and meat (Include Pasta Fagiole) [1 cup]	253	8.9	205	50%	6	20	3.1
5013	Bean and rice soup [1 cup]	253	8.9	155	22%	8	23	3.5
5014	Bean soup with vegetables, rice, and pork [1 cup]	243	8.6	193	30%	9	25	3.4
5015	Bean soup with vegetables and rice, canned, reduced sodium, prepared with water or ready-to-serve [1 cup]	241	8.5	140	6%	5	27	5.5
5016	Beef, broth, bouillon, or consomme [1 cup]	240	8.5	17	28%	3	0	0.0
5017	Beef, broth, bouillon, or consomme, canned, low sodium [1 cup]	240	8.5	38	34%	5	1	0.0
5018	Beef, broth, bouillon, or consomme, dry, not reconstituted [1 cube]	4	0.1	7	28%	1	1	0.0
5019	Beef, broth, bouillon, or consomme, low sodium, dry, not reconstituted [1 cube]	4	0.1	10	47%	1	1	0.0
5020	Beef broth, without tomato, home recipe [1 cup]	240	8.5	31	6%	5	3	0.0
5021	Beef dumpling soup [1 cup]	241	8.5	314	40%	24	21	0.7
5022	Beef and mushroom soup [1 cup]	256	9.0	553	61%	43	8	0.3
5023	Beef and mushroom soup, canned, low sodium, chunky style (Include beef soup, canned, low sodium or no salt added) [1 cup]	251	8.9	173	30%	11	19	0.5
5024	Beef noodle soup [1 cup]	244	8.6	84	33%	5	9	0.8
5025	Beef noodle soup, canned, undiluted [1 cup]	251	8.9	168	33%	10	18	1.5
5026	Beef noodle soup, chunky style [1 cup]	240	8.5	152	24%	15	13	1.1
5027	Beef noodle soup, home recipe [1 cup]	244	8.6	167	33%	19	8	1.2
5028	Beef noodle soup, Puerto Rican style (Sopa de carne y fideos) [1 cup]	250	8.8	140	22%	15	12	1.6
5029	Beef rice soup [1 cup]	241	8.5	111	25%	8	12	0.5
5030	Beef and rice soup, Puerto Rican style [1 cup]	250	8.8	140	22%	15	12	1.5
5031	Beef and rice noodle soup, Oriental style (Vietnamese Pho Bo) [1 cup]	244	8.6	174	20%	17	17	1.0
5032	Beef stroganoff soup, chunky style (Include creamed beef soup) [1 cup]	240	8.5	235	42%	12	22	1.4
5033	Beef vegetable soup with potato, stew type (Include chunky style) [1 cup]	240	8.5	170	27%	12	20	1.4
5034	Beef vegetable soup with noodles, stew type, chunky style [1 cup]	240	8.5	182	25%	12	23	1.5
5035	Beef vegetable soup with rice, stew type, chunky style [1 cup]	240	8.5	181	24%	11	23	1.4
5036	Beef vegetable soup, Mexican style (Sopa caldo de Res) [1 cup]	239	8.4	141	37%	12	11	1.6
5037	Beer soup, made with milk [1 cup]	245	8.6	109	30%	5	11	0.6
5038	Beet soup (borscht) [1 cup]	245	8.6	78	46%	3	8	2.1
5039	Bird's nest soup (chicken, ham, and noodles) [1 cup]	244	8.6	112	22%	14	6	0.0
5040	Black bean soup [1 cup]	247	8.7	116	12%	6	20	4.4
5041	Bouillabaisse [1 cup]	227	8.0	241	33%	34	5	0.6
5042	Broccoli cheese soup, made with milk [1 cup]	239	8.4	177	50%	7	16	1.7
5043	Broccoli soup (Include cream of broccoli soup) [1 cup]	237	8.4	207	54%	9	17	2.0
5044	Cabbage soup [1 cup]	245	8.6	67	45%	4	6	1.7
5045	Cabbage with meat soup [1 cup]	245	8.6	121	35%	14	5	1.4
5046	Carrot soup with rice and milk [1 cup]	245	8.6	89	16%	5	13	1.3
5047	Cauliflower soup, cream of, made with milk [1 cup]	248	8.7	199	55%	8	15	1.5
5048	Carrot soup with milk [1 cup]	237	8.4	60	24%	5	6	1.3

Food no.	fat gm	sat fat gm	choles mg	sodium mg	potas mg	% of Daily Value													
						vit A	vit E	vit C	thia	ribo	niac	vit B-6	fola	vit B-12	calc	phos	mag	iron	zinc
5000	7	3	16	1044	363	10	3	6	6	16	4	3	7	7	18	16	5	5	9
5001	4	1	5	985	173	5	3	4	4	5	4	1	6	1	3	4	1	5	6
5002	41	13	55	1155	564	17	11	3	31	25	29	13	8	20	14	31	8	8	15
5003	1	0	0	723	184	0	0	0	3	4	14	4	2	3	2	8	6	5	3
5004	3	0	0	8	104	0	1	0	3	3	5	4	2	0	1	6	6	3	5
5005	4	1	3	918	357	5	1	2	5	8	2	2	5	1	7	11	9	9	6
5006	0	0	0	39	602	66	2	8	9	4	2	9	18	0	10	11	15	19	9
5007	1	0	5	76	421	2	2	10	13	5	5	8	23	1	4	13	11	12	7
5008	6	2	3	956	403	9	2	3	6	2	3	2	8	1	8	13	11	11	7
5009	7	1	12	339	595	51	6	4	19	8	10	8	13	2	7	15	13	23	10
5010	3	1	5	466	393	24	2	5	9	4	4	6	8	1	9	3	12	14	9
5011	4	1	0	445	490	3	3	18	9	7	14	8	10	2	6	12	9	13	6
5012	11	4	12	201	256	0	1	1	10	3	4	3	9	1	4	7	9	11	6
5013	4	1	0	440	487	3	3	18	9	5	14	8	10	2	6	12	9	13	6
5014	6	2	16	711	554	2	1	15	19	7	14	9	12	6	4	13	9	21	8
5015	1	0	2	472	352	3	2	4	9	3	4	4	9	0	7	9	8	9	4
5016	1	0	0	782	130	0	0	0	0	3	9	1	1	3	1	3	1	2	0
5017	1	0	0	72	206	0	0	0	0	4	16	1	1	4	1	7	1	3	2
5018	0	0	0	738	15	0	0	0	0	1	1	0	0	1	0	1	0	0	0
5019	1	0	0	38	11	1	0	0	0	1	0	0	0	0	1	1	1	0	0
5020	0	0	0	475	444	0	1	0	5	13	10	7	19	0	2	7	4	4	3
5021	14	5	117	1324	350	5	3	0	15	20	22	14	4	35	13	28	8	19	23
5022	38	14	156	854	570	0	6	2	6	23	53	23	5	85	5	33	9	26	63
5023	6	4	15	63	351	49	1	13	7	16	14	8	4	11	3	13	1	14	18
5024	3	1	5	956	99	6	0	1	4	3	5	2	1	3	2	5	2	6	11
5025	6	2	10	1905	198	13	0	1	9	7	11	4	2	7	3	9	3	12	21
5026	4	1	48	495	239	28	1	2	8	10	15	9	3	21	2	14	6	13	21
5027	6	2	66	92	419	56	1	4	10	13	13	12	3	44	3	20	7	15	38
5028	3	1	40	55	584	3	2	35	8	11	15	15	5	27	2	17	8	13	23
5029	3	1	15	573	210	17	0	1	6	5	13	8	2	12	2	9	4	7	7
5030	3	1	38	55	582	3	2	35	8	10	15	15	5	27	2	16	8	13	22
5031	4	1	42	522	334	2	1	7	6	10	15	14	4	31	2	17	10	12	25
5032	11	6	50	1044	336	20	7	0	6	13	1	7	4	10	5	12	1	12	18
5033	5	3	14	866	336	26	1	12	4	9	14	7	3	10	3	12	1	13	18
5034	5	2	19	801	315	24	1	11	6	9	14	6	3	10	3	12	2	14	17
5035	5	2	13	801	317	24	1	11	5	8	14	7	3	10	3	12	2	13	17
5036	6	2	24	462	676	30	2	17	10	15	16	15	19	11	4	15	8	9	14
5037	4	1	101	63	144	6	1	1	4	15	3	5	5	7	9	11	4	2	3
5038	4	2	7	496	288	4	1	15	3	5	7	5	12	2	5	6	5	4	2
5039	3	1	27	747	246	0	1	0	7	7	26	9	1	5	1	13	3	5	6
5040	2	0	0	1198	274	5	0	1	5	3	3	5	6	0	4	11	10	12	9
5041	9	2	90	416	733	9	9	20	16	11	25	19	7	173	8	34	18	22	12
5042	10	4	17	955	299	16	9	54	8	15	4	6	7	5	17	15	7	5	5
5043	12	4	16	204	480	26	11	80	8	23	4	8	10	6	26	22	10	5	7
5044	3	1	0	310	307	4	5	21	7	9	6	8	13	26	3	6	3	3	2
5045	5	1	31	282	430	3	4	18	30	17	14	15	11	26	3	16	6	6	9
5046	2	1	2	622	268	83	1	2	5	6	13	7	3	4	5	9	3	5	3
5047	12	4	16	193	364	17	6	39	7	20	3	7	8	6	23	20	8	3	6
5048	2	1	2	566	279	89	1	2	2	7	12	6	3	4	5	9	3	3	3

Soups, Sauces, Fats, Misc.

Food No.	Food Description & Amount	wt gm	wt oz	cal	% cal fat	prot gm	carbo gm	fiber gm
5049	Celery soup, canned, undiluted [1 cup]	251	8.9	181	56%	3	18	1.5
5050	Celery soup, cream of, made with milk [1 cup]	248	8.7	153	48%	6	15	0.8
5051	Celery soup, cream of, made with water [1 cup]	244	8.6	90	56%	2	9	0.8
5052	Cheddar cheese soup [1 cup]	251	8.9	218	54%	9	16	1.0
5053	Cheddar cheese soup, canned, undiluted [1 cup]	257	9.1	311	61%	11	21	2.1
5054	Chicken corn soup, home recipe [1 cup]	251	8.9	203	30%	14	25	1.5
5055	Chicken and mushroom soup, cream of, made with milk (Include turkey and mushroom soup) [1 cup]	248	8.7	200	53%	8	15	0.3
5056	Chicken, broth, bouillon, or consomme (Include chicken broth powder, reconstituted; Lipton's Trim Chicken Cup-a-Soup) [1 cup]	244	8.6	39	32%	5	1	0.0
5057	Chicken broth, bouillion, or consomme, dry, not reconstituted [1 cube]	4	0.1	11	47%	1	1	0.0
5058	Chicken broth, without tomato, home recipe [1 cup]	240	8.5	86	30%	6	8	0.0
5059	Chicken broth soup stock, Mexican style[1 cup]	242	8.5	130	16%	6	22	2.4
5060	Chicken broth, canned, reduced sodium [1 cup]	240	8.5	17	0%	3	1	0.0
5061	Chicken broth, canned, low sodium [1 cup]	240	8.5	17	13%	2	1	1.0
5062	Chicken gumbo soup [1 cup]	244	8.6	56	23%	3	8	2.0
5063	Chicken noodle soup (Include chicken and stars soup) [1 cup]	241	8.5	75	27%	4	9	0.7
5064	Chicken noodle soup, canned, low sodium, ready-to-serve [1 cup]	246	8.7	76	29%	4	10	0.7
5065	Chicken noodle soup, canned, reduced sodium, ready-to-serve (Include Campbell's, Healthy Choice) [1 cup]	238	8.4	84	24%	8	7	1.0
5066	Chicken noodle soup, canned, undiluted [1 cup]	246	8.7	150	27%	8	19	1.5
5067	Chicken noodle soup, chunky style [1 cup]	240	8.5	175	31%	13	17	3.8
5068	Chicken noodle soup, with carrots [1 cup]	241	8.5	128	19%	18	7	1.0
5069	Chicken noodle soup, cream of [1 cup]	245	8.6	137	32%	8	15	0.7
5070	Chicken or turkey soup, cream of, canned, undiluted [1 cup]	251	8.9	233	57%	7	19	0.5
5071	Chicken or turkey soup, cream of, made with milk [1 cup]	248	8.7	179	50%	7	15	0.3
5072	Chicken or turkey soup, cream of, made with water (Include instant) [1 cup]	244	8.6	117	57%	3	9	0.3
5073	Chicken or turkey soup, cream of, canned, made with water, reduced sodium [1 cup]	244	8.6	73	20%	2	12	0.5
5074	Chicken or turkey vegetable soup, stew type (Include chunky style; chicken or turkey vegetable soup with noodles) [1 cup]	240	8.5	170	33%	12	17	1.4
5075	Chicken soup with vegetables (broccoli, carrots, celery, potatoes and onions), Oriental style [1 cup]	228	8.0	54	25%	6	4	0.8
5076	Chicken or turkey rice soup, home recipe [1 cup]	231	8.1	161	25%	15	14	0.7
5077	Chicken vegetable soup with noodles, stew type, chunky style [1 cup]	240	8.5	167	29%	11	20	2.8
5078	Chicken vegetable soup with rice, Mexican style (Sopa / Caldo de Pollo) [1 cup]	242	8.5	177	20%	13	22	2.1
5079	Chicken vegetable soup with rice, stew type, chunky style, made with milk [1 cup]	242	8.5	131	27%	9	15	0.8
5080	Chicken or turkey vegetable soup, home recipe [1 cup]	239	8.4	133	26%	14	11	1.4
5081	Chicken rice soup [1 cup]	241	8.5	60	29%	4	7	0.6
5082	Chicken rice soup, canned, reduced sodium, ready-to-serve (Include Campbell's) [1 cup]	241	8.5	116	24%	7	14	0.7
5083	Chicken rice soup, canned, undiluted [1 cup]	246	8.7	121	29%	7	14	1.2
5084	Chicken rice soup, chunky style (Include turkey rice soup) [1 cup]	240	8.5	127	23%	12	13	1.0
5085	Chicken rice soup, Puerto Rican style (Sopa de pollo con arroz) [1 cup]	220	7.8	200	39%	16	14	1.0
5086	Chicken soup with dumplings and potatoes [1 cup]	251	8.9	113	41%	6	11	0.9
5087	Chicken soup with dumplings [1 cup]	241	8.5	97	51%	6	6	0.5
5088	Chicken soup with noodles and potatoes, Puerto Rican style [1 cup]	220	7.8	165	29%	14	14	1.1
5089	Chicken soup [1 cup]	241	8.5	75	30%	4	9	0.7
5090	Chicken soup, canned, undiluted [1 cup]	246	8.7	150	27%	8	19	1.5
5091	Chicken soup with vegetables and fruit, Oriental Style [1 cup]	234	8.3	136	25%	16	9	1.2
5092	Chili beef soup [1 cup]	250	8.8	170	35%	7	21	9.5
5093	Chili beef soup, chunky style [1 cup]	240	8.5	192	34%	16	16	4.5
5094	Chunky pea and ham soup [1 cup]	240	8.5	185	19%	11	27	4.1

Food no.	fat gm	sat fat gm	choles mg	sodium mg	potas mg	vit A	vit E	vit C	thia	ribo	niac	vit B-6	fola	vit B-12	calc	phos	mag	iron	zinc
						% of Daily Value													
5049	11	3	28	1900	246	6	2	1	4	6	3	1	1	2	8	8	3	7	2
5050	8	3	24	1012	313	9	1	2	5	14	2	3	2	7	19	15	6	4	4
5051	6	1	14	954	123	3	1	0	2	3	2	1	1	1	4	4	2	4	1
5052	13	8	40	1022	344	17	1	2	4	19	3	4	2	7	29	25	5	4	7
5053	21	13	59	1920	308	22	2	0	2	16	4	3	2	0	29	27	2	8	9
5054	7	2	32	460	365	6	3	9	6	14	23	13	15	4	7	18	9	5	10
5055	12	4	21	1033	348	17	0	2	4	18	9	5	2	7	18	14	6	5	10
5056	1	0	0	776	210	0	0	0	1	4	17	1	1	4	1	7	1	3	2
5057	1	0	1	743	12	1	0	0	0	1	0	0	0	0	1	1	1	0	0
5058	3	1	7	343	252	0	1	1	6	12	19	7	13	0	1	6	2	3	2
5059	2	1	5	261	692	81	2	29	10	12	20	16	13	0	2	10	7	7	4
5060	0	0	0	554	204	0	0	2	0	2	8	1	1	2	2	4	1	3	1
5061	0	0	0	379	192	0	0	28	0	1	6	1	1	2	1	3	1	3	1
5062	1	0	5	954	76	1	0	8	2	3	3	3	1	0	2	2	1	5	3
5063	2	1	6	931	55	6	0	0	4	4	8	1	1	3	2	4	2	4	2
5064	2	1	7	74	57	7	0	0	3	4	7	1	1	2	2	4	1	4	3
5065	2	1	13	459	303	24	1	4	2	6	20	8	3	4	4	10	3	10	4
5066	5	1	12	1862	111	13	1	0	9	8	15	3	1	5	3	7	2	8	4
5067	6	1	19	850	108	12	4	0	5	10	22	2	1	5	2	7	2	8	6
5068	3	1	61	79	290	49	2	6	8	9	34	13	3	4	2	16	7	6	9
5069	5	2	17	990	245	12	1	2	7	15	8	4	2	9	16	15	5	5	5
5070	15	4	20	1973	176	11	1	0	4	7	8	2	1	3	7	8	1	7	8
5071	10	4	21	1049	278	12	1	2	5	15	5	3	2	7	18	15	5	4	7
5072	7	2	10	990	88	6	1	0	2	4	4	1	0	1	4	4	1	3	4
5073	2	1	8	452	341	15	0	0	0	2	4	1	0	1	2	3	1	1	1
5074	6	2	29	850	168	12	1	2	5	10	21	2	1	4	2	11	2	9	6
5075	1	0	16	567	142	18	1	11	2	4	7	6	3	1	2	5	4	3	4
5076	4	1	38	323	284	31	1	3	8	11	25	11	8	1	2	12	5	7	8
5077	5	1	22	834	460	70	2	11	9	7	20	13	7	2	3	13	8	8	6
5078	4	1	27	246	655	70	2	25	11	13	27	18	12	1	3	13	8	8	8
5079	4	1	11	885	259	47	1	5	4	10	12	4	2	6	10	11	4	8	6
5080	4	1	34	511	459	23	5	31	8	11	28	18	12	2	3	13	7	8	8
5081	2	0	6	819	100	7	0	0	1	1	6	1	0	3	2	2	0	4	2
5082	3	1	14	482	422	20	1	4	4	7	25	7	3	6	2	14	3	5	4
5083	4	1	12	1636	202	13	0	0	2	3	11	2	1	5	3	4	0	8	4
5084	3	1	12	888	108	59	0	6	2	6	21	2	1	5	3	7	2	10	6
5085	9	2	52	206	440	2	1	15	7	7	27	16	3	3	2	15	7	7	9
5086	5	1	31	800	210	5	1	6	3	4	10	6	1	3	1	7	3	4	3
5087	6	1	33	865	116	5	1	0	1	4	9	2	1	3	2	6	1	4	3
5088	5	1	48	211	441	1	1	16	9	9	21	14	3	3	2	14	7	7	11
5089	2	1	7	1106	55	7	0	0	4	4	7	1	1	2	2	4	1	4	3
5090	5	1	12	1862	111	13	1	0	9	8	15	3	1	5	3	7	2	8	4
5091	4	1	46	172	261	2	1	11	6	7	19	12	3	2	2	10	6	6	8
5092	7	3	13	1035	525	15	1	7	4	4	5	8	4	5	4	15	8	12	9
5093	7	3	31	407	487	2	1	12	9	10	16	10	21	15	3	16	10	16	18
5094	4	2	7	965	305	49	1	12	8	6	13	11	1	4	3	18	10	12	21

Soups, Sauces, Fats, Misc.

Food No.	Food Description & Amount	wt gm	wt oz	cal	% cal fat	prot gm	carbo gm	fiber gm
5095	Clam chowder, Manhattan (Include chunky style) [1 cup]	240	8.5	106	24%	5	15	2.2
5096	Clam chowder, New England, canned, reduced sodium, ready-to-serve [1 cup]	251	8.9	123	17%	6	20	1.1
5097	Clam chowder, New England, made with milk [1 cup]	248	8.7	151	30%	10	17	0.8
5098	Clam chowder, New England, made with water [1 cup]	244	8.6	95	27%	5	12	1.5
5099	Codfish soup with noodles, Puerto Rican style [1 cup]	245	8.6	174	24%	14	18	1.4
5100	Codfish, rice, and vegetable soup, Puerto Rican style [1 cup]	245	8.6	166	22%	13	19	1.0
5101	Corn soup, cream of, made with milk [1 cup]	248	8.7	226	47%	8	24	1.4
5102	Corn soup, cream of, made with water [1 cup]	244	8.6	168	50%	6	16	0.8
5103	Crab soup, made with milk (Include crab bisque, seafood bisque) [1 cup]	248	8.7	236	45%	20	12	0.3
5104	Crab soup, tomato-base [1 cup]	244	8.6	169	38%	14	12	1.1
5105	Cucumber soup, cream of, made with milk [1 cup]	248	8.7	199	56%	7	15	0.5
5106	Duck soup [1 cup]	244	8.6	410	81%	16	2	0.3
5107	Egg drop soup [1 cup]	244	8.6	73	47%	8	1	0.0
5108	Escarole soup [1 cup]	245	8.6	252	57%	9	18	1.0
5109	Fish and vegetable soup, Puerto Rican style (Sopa de pescado) [1 cup]	250	8.8	101	21%	16	3	0.6
5110	Fish broth [1 cup]	244	8.6	41	43%	6	0	0.0
5111	Fish chowder (Include fisherman's soup, seafood chowder) [1 cup]	244	8.6	194	25%	24	12	0.7
5112	Fish soup, with potatoes (Sopa de Pescado) [1 cup]	241	8.5	113	18%	16	6	0.6
5113	Fruit soup[1 cup]	242	8.5	176	1%	1	46	3.9
5114	Garbanzo or chickpea soup [1 cup]	253	8.9	208	14%	10	36	9.3
5115	Garlic egg soup, Puerto Rican style (Sopa de ajo) [1 cup]	202	7.1	180	53%	10	11	0.4
5116	Gazpacho [1 cup]	244	8.6	56	4%	7	1	0.5
5117	Gazpacho, canned, undiluted [1 can (10.5 oz), undiluted]	298	10.5	69	4%	9	1	0.6
5118	Ham, noodle, and vegetable soup, Puerto Rican style [1 cup]	250	8.8	154	24%	17	12	1.5
5119	Ham, pasta, and vegetable soup [1 cup]	244	8.6	62	14%	5	8	1.6
5120	Ham, rice, and potato soup, Puerto Rican style [1 cup]	240	8.5	157	33%	9	17	1.2
5121	Hot and sour soup (Include hot and spicy Chinese soup) [1 cup]	244	8.6	162	45%	15	5	0.5
5122	Instant soup [1 cup]	240	8.5	50	20%	3	7	0.7
5123	Instant soup, cream of [1 cup]	254	9.0	104	46%	2	12	0.4
5124	Instant soup, cream of, low sodium [1 cup]	254	9.0	104	48%	2	12	0.3
5125	Instant soup, noodle (Include meat and/or vegetable flavors) [1 cup]	240	8.5	44	19%	2	6	0.4
5126	Instant soup, noodle with egg, shrimp or chicken [1 cup]	240	8.5	184	23%	12	23	1.0
5127	Instant soup, rice (Include meat or chicken flavor) [1 cup]	240	8.5	58	21%	2	9	0.7
5128	Lamb, pasta, and vegetable soup, Puerto Rican style [1 cup]	250	8.8	168	39%	13	13	1.9
5129	Leek soup, cream of, made with milk [1 cup]	248	8.7	173	41%	7	19	0.5
5130	Leek soup, made from dry mix [1 cup]	254	9.0	71	26%	2	11	3.0
5131	Lentil soup [1 cup]	248	8.7	219	34%	12	26	13.1
5132	Lima bean soup [1 cup]	253	8.9	111	24%	5	17	5.1
5133	Liquid from stewed kidney beans, Puerto Rican style [1 cup]	228	8.0	75	87%	4	6	0.2
5134	Lobster bisque [1 cup]	248	8.7	253	47%	20	13	0.2
5135	Lobster gumbo [1 cup]	244	8.6	178	35%	10	20	3.0
5136	Macaroni and potato soup [1 cup]	244	8.6	212	14%	7	40	3.1
5137	Matzo ball soup [1 cup]	241	8.5	119	42%	7	10	0.4
5138	Meatball soup, Mexican style (Sopa de Albondigas) [1 cup]	237	8.4	195	61%	10	9	1.5
5139	Meat broth, Puerto Rican style (Caldo) [1 cup]	240	8.5	17	28%	3	0	0.0
5140	Minestrone soup, canned, reduced sodium, ready-to-serve (Include Campbell's, Healthy Choice, Progresso) [1 cup]	239	8.4	120	14%	5	22	5.7
5141	Minestrone soup, home recipe [1 cup]	235	8.3	234	49%	9	22	3.8
5142	Meat and hominy soup, Mexican style (Pozole) [1 cup]	238	8.4	188	31%	16	15	1.5
5143	Mushroom soup, canned, undiluted (Include cream of mushroom soup, undiluted) [1 cup]	251	8.9	259	66%	4	19	0.8
5144	Mushroom soup, cream of, made with milk [1 cup]	248	8.7	192	57%	6	15	0.4
5145	Mushroom soup, cream of, made with water [1 cup]	244	8.6	129	66%	2	9	0.4
5146	Mushroom soup, cream of, low sodium, made with water [1 cup]	244	8.6	129	63%	2	9	0.5

Food no.	fat gm	sat fat gm	choles mg	sodium mg	potas mg	% of Daily Value vit A	vit E	vit C	thia	ribo	niac	vit B-6	fola	vit B-12	calc	phos	mag	iron	zinc
5095	3	1	8	785	284	21	2	13	3	3	7	9	2	99	5	6	4	12	9
5096	2	1	14	558	289	4	3	11	4	6	5	5	2	315	4	9	3	31	5
5097	5	2	16	995	304	6	1	6	4	14	5	6	2	170	19	16	6	8	8
5098	3	0	5	915	146	0	0	3	1	3	5	4	1	133	4	5	2	8	5
5099	5	1	46	199	365	3	4	22	12	6	12	11	4	9	3	18	10	8	5
5100	4	1	27	200	376	3	4	23	10	4	11	13	3	8	3	16	9	7	4
5101	12	4	15	340	396	16	6	10	7	21	6	4	9	6	21	21	9	5	6
5102	9	3	12	649	237	11	4	5	4	12	5	3	5	4	12	12	5	4	5
5103	12	3	86	584	489	14	9	8	11	17	15	10	12	96	25	30	12	6	25
5104	7	1	60	475	527	10	10	33	9	5	15	13	12	73	8	16	9	8	19
5105	12	4	16	192	359	18	6	5	7	20	3	4	3	6	24	20	8	3	6
5106	37	13	89	93	351	6	2	6	15	19	28	10	4	4	2	20	6	19	14
5107	4	1	103	729	220	4	1	0	2	11	15	3	4	8	2	11	1	4	3
5108	16	5	19	780	459	14	8	5	10	27	4	5	9	12	31	25	10	4	8
5109	2	0	29	605	473	3	2	13	5	7	19	10	4	12	7	17	6	4	3
5110	2	0	2	381	351	0	14	0	5	11	14	5	12	28	1	14	4	0	1
5111	5	2	56	180	711	6	2	12	11	16	14	18	4	21	15	30	12	4	7
5112	2	0	29	622	523	1	1	4	5	6	20	12	4	13	7	21	7	4	4
5113	0	0	0	9	392	8	1	3	2	3	3	7	0	0	2	4	5	7	2
5114	3	0	0	18	345	0	2	4	9	6	3	8	26	0	6	17	12	16	11
5115	11	2	160	724	223	7	5	0	7	17	16	4	5	8	5	14	3	8	5
5116	0	0	0	739	224	26	2	12	3	1	5	7	2	0	2	4	2	5	2
5117	0	0	0	903	274	32	3	14	4	2	6	9	3	0	3	4	2	7	2
5118	4	1	38	1052	606	4	2	35	28	11	22	20	5	8	3	20	8	7	12
5119	1	0	8	267	223	21	1	17	10	5	8	6	4	1	3	6	5	5	5
5120	6	2	21	484	294	0	1	6	12	5	12	13	2	3	2	11	6	4	7
5121	8	3	34	1011	384	0	1	1	18	15	25	10	3	7	3	19	7	11	10
5122	1	0	2	1222	29	0	0	0	4	3	4	0	0	0	3	3	2	3	1
5123	5	2	1	1148	151	6	3	4	43	9	8	2	2	3	5	7	2	2	6
5124	6	1	0	61	94	0	6	6	80	6	3	1	2	2	3	5	3	3	2
5125	1	0	2	1101	53	0	0	1	6	3	4	3	0	0	2	3	2	2	1
5126	5	1	110	562	218	4	1	1	12	13	20	5	5	9	3	16	6	12	7
5127	1	0	2	931	10	0	0	0	0	0	2	1	0	1	1	1	0	0	1
5128	7	3	42	53	525	5	2	66	8	10	23	13	7	21	3	15	8	10	20
5129	8	3	26	1016	313	9	4	4	6	16	3	4	3	7	18	15	6	4	4
5130	2	1	3	965	89	0	1	4	3	1	1	1	2	0	3	3	3	3	2
5131	8	3	5	48	330	20	3	6	7	5	4	8	17	0	3	17	10	17	10
5132	3	1	3	89	418	42	2	6	7	3	3	7	13	0	4	9	11	9	5
5133	7	3	9	5	930	0	0	0	15	12	4	3	19	1	3	20	21	25	7
5134	13	4	64	450	547	20	10	3	6	21	5	7	4	43	27	31	12	3	18
5135	7	1	23	441	607	18	10	45	14	7	11	10	17	17	11	13	14	9	10
5136	3	1	7	65	715	5	2	34	15	11	12	25	6	4	12	16	12	4	6
5137	5	1	63	757	190	2	3	0	5	10	15	2	3	5	3	9	2	7	3
5138	13	5	54	145	441	54	3	18	6	10	15	10	8	14	3	11	6	8	12
5139	1	0	0	782	130	0	0	0	0	3	9	1	1	3	1	3	1	2	0
5140	2	0	0	514	445	20	2	23	10	6	8	7	8	0	5	8	8	10	5
5141	13	4	9	494	584	19	5	14	16	14	14	12	29	0	4	15	11	13	7
5142	6	2	42	408	318	1	1	2	11	15	25	12	11	2	2	14	6	8	14
5143	19	5	3	1737	168	0	12	4	4	10	8	1	2	4	7	9	3	6	8
5144	12	4	12	930	274	6	6	3	5	16	5	3	2	8	18	16	5	3	7
5145	10	3	1	872	84	0	6	2	2	5	4	1	1	2	3	4	2	3	4
5146	9	2	2	49	100	0	6	2	3	6	4	1	1	1	5	5	1	3	4

Soups, Sauces, Fats, Misc.

Food No.	Food Description & Amount	wt gm	wt oz	cal	% cal fat	prot gm	carbo gm	fiber gm
5147	Mushroom soup, cream of, canned, made with milk, reduced sodium [1 cup]	248	8.7	128	33%	6	16	0.8
5148	Mushroom soup, cream of, canned, made with water, reduced sodium [1 cup]	244	8.6	65	29%	2	10	0.8
5149	Mushroom soup, cream of, canned, undiluted, reduced sodium [1 cup]	251	8.9	131	29%	3	20	1.5
5150	Mushroom soup, made from dry mix [1 cup]	253	8.9	96	45%	2	11	0.8
5151	Mushroom soup, with meat broth, made with water (Include Campbell's Beefy Mushroom) [1 cup]	244	8.6	85	42%	3	9	0.1
5152	Mushroom with chicken soup, cream of, made with milk [1 cup]	248	8.7	200	53%	8	15	0.3
5153	Noodle (mostly) soup (Include spaghetti soup, Top Ramen, Oriental Noodle Soup, meat flavors, saimin soup) [1 cup]	244	8.6	165	38%	4	22	1.2
5154	Noodle and potato soup, Puerto Rican style [1 cup]	245	8.6	72	5%	2	16	2.0
5155	Noodle soup, made with milk [1 cup]	248	8.7	177	31%	9	21	0.9
5156	Noodle soup with vegetables, Oriental style [1 cup]	228	8.0	112	25%	6	14	0.7
5157	Noodle soup with fish ball, shrimp, and dark green leafy vegetable [1 cup]	234	8.3	164	32%	11	16	1.2
5158	Onion soup, cream of, canned, undiluted [1 cup]	251	8.9	221	43%	6	26	1.0
5159	Onion soup, cream of, made with milk [1 cup]	248	8.7	173	41%	7	19	0.5
5160	Onion soup, dry mix, not reconstituted [1 pkg (1.5 oz)]	39	1.4	115	18%	5	21	4.1
5161	Onion soup, French [1 cup]	241	8.5	58	27%	4	8	1.0
5162	Onion soup, made from dry mix [1 cup]	246	8.7	27	19%	1	5	1.0
5163	Oxtail soup [1 cup]	244	8.6	68	32%	3	9	0.5
5164	Oyster stew [1 cup]	245	8.6	212	57%	12	11	0.0
5165	Pea soup, canned, low sodium, made with water [1 cup]	250	8.8	165	16%	9	27	0.8
5166	Pea soup, instant type [1 cup]	271	9.6	133	11%	8	23	3.0
5167	Pea soup, made with milk [1 cup]	254	9.0	227	22%	13	32	2.9
5168	Pea soup, made with lowfat milk [1 cup]	254	9.0	219	19%	13	32	2.9
5169	Pea soup, made with water [1 cup]	250	8.8	165	16%	9	27	2.8
5170	Pepperpot (tripe) soup (Include Menudo; Mondongo soup; pork, potatoes, yuca) [1 cup]	241	8.5	104	40%	6	9	0.5
5171	Pigeon pea asopao [1 cup]	250	8.8	245	26%	10	38	6.2
5172	Pinto bean soup [1 cup]	253	8.9	191	3%	11	36	12.6
5173	Plantain soup, Puerto Rican style (Sopa de platano) [1 cup]	245	8.6	97	11%	6	18	1.3
5174	Pork, rice, and vegetable soup [1 cup]	244	8.6	124	32%	12	8	0.7
5175	Pork, vegetable soup with potatoes, stew type [1 cup]	240	8.5	136	16%	13	17	4.2
5176	Pork with vegetable (no carrots, broccoli, or dark-green leafy) soup, Oriental Style [1 cup]	228	8.0	77	35%	11	1	0.5
5177	Portuguese bean soup [1 cup]	253	8.9	145	10%	9	25	5.8
5178	Potato soup, instant, made from dry mix (Include Lipton's) [1 cup]	249	8.8	68	8%	2	15	1.5
5179	Potato soup, made with milk [1 cup]	248	8.7	137	33%	6	17	0.5
5180	Potato soup, made with water [1 cup]	244	8.6	74	29%	2	11	0.5
5181	Potato and cheese soup [1 cup]	248	8.7	188	40%	10	19	1.1
5182	Potato chowder (Include corn chowder) [1 cup]	248	8.7	221	55%	7	19	1.3
5183	Rice and potato soup, Puerto Rican style [1 cup]	245	8.6	185	23%	4	31	1.1
5184	Rice soup, made with tea [1 cup]	241	8.5	75	17%	2	14	0.7
5185	Salmon soup, cream style [1 cup]	248	8.7	261	44%	28	7	0.2
5186	Scotch broth (lamb, vegetables, and barley) [1 cup]	241	8.5	80	30%	5	9	1.2
5187	Seafood soup with potatoes and vegetables (including carrots, broccoli, and/or dark-green leafy) [1 cup]	244	8.6	151	14%	21	11	1.3
5188	Seafood soup with potatoes and vegetables (no carrots, broccoli, or dark-green leafy) [1 cup]	244	8.6	160	14%	20	13	1.2
5189	Seafood soup with vegetables (including carrots, broccoli, and/or dark-green leafy (no potatoes)) [1 cup]	244	8.6	143	15%	20	9	1.6
5190	Seafood soup with vegetables (no carrots, broccoli, dark-green leafy, or potatoes) [1 cup]	244	8.6	154	15%	21	12	1.3
5191	Seaweed soup [1 cup]	230	8.1	83	40%	8	6	0.6
5192	Shav soup [1 cup]	240	8.5	58	59%	2	4	0.9

Food no.	fat gm	sat fat gm	choles mg	sodium mg	potas mg	% of Daily Value: vit A	vit E	vit C	thia	ribo	niac	vit B-6	fola	vit B-12	calc	phos	mag	iron	zinc
5147	5	2	14	542	660	6	1	2	6	26	2	5	4	6	16	18	6	4	6
5148	2	1	4	484	469	0	1	0	3	14	1	3	2	0	2	6	2	3	3
5149	4	1	8	961	939	0	1	0	7	28	2	5	5	1	3	13	3	7	6
5150	5	1	0	1020	200	0	3	2	19	7	3	1	1	4	7	8	1	3	1
5151	4	2	8	974	158	13	0	2	2	6	6	2	2	0	1	4	2	5	9
5152	12	4	21	1032	348	17	0	2	4	18	9	5	2	7	18	14	6	5	10
5153	7	2	0	862	53	0	11	0	2	1	1	1	1	0	1	3	3	2	1
5154	0	0	3	14	364	6	2	31	7	4	6	9	5	0	3	5	6	4	3
5155	6	3	29	121	353	31	2	3	10	21	4	7	4	10	25	23	9	5	7
5156	3	1	17	833	177	2	2	3	7	6	16	3	3	3	2	9	4	7	4
5157	6	1	46	638	327	3	3	7	9	8	18	7	5	7	3	15	6	9	5
5158	11	3	30	1908	246	6	8	4	7	9	5	3	4	2	7	8	3	7	2
5159	8	3	26	1016	313	9	4	4	6	16	3	4	3	7	18	15	6	4	4
5160	2	1	2	3493	260	0	2	1	7	14	10	2	2	0	5	13	6	3	2
5161	2	0	0	1053	67	0	1	2	2	1	3	2	4	0	3	1	1	4	4
5162	1	0	0	849	64	0	0	0	2	3	2	0	0	0	1	3	1	1	0
5163	2	1	2	1166	81	0	0	0	2	1	4	1	1	4	1	6	2	1	0
5164	13	8	80	341	393	18	5	6	9	20	6	6	3	255	24	26	16	32	516
5165	3	1	0	25	190	2	0	3	7	4	6	3	1	0	3	13	10	11	11
5166	2	0	3	1220	238	1	1	0	15	9	7	2	11	5	2	13	12	6	4
5167	6	3	11	979	381	8	1	4	10	15	6	5	2	6	18	24	14	11	15
5168	5	2	7	977	383	9	1	4	10	15	6	5	2	6	18	24	14	11	15
5169	3	1	0	918	190	2	0	3	7	4	6	3	0	0	3	13	10	11	11
5170	5	2	10	971	152	9	0	2	4	3	6	3	2	3	2	4	1	5	8
5171	7	2	8	226	855	9	4	68	27	13	14	11	36	1	5	17	22	12	9
5172	1	0	0	11	528	0	1	6	14	6	4	9	32	0	7	20	17	16	8
5173	1	1	0	1429	508	6	1	16	2	7	19	10	5	5	3	8	7	6	1
5174	4	2	41	55	206	30	1	2	17	8	13	10	2	4	2	10	4	6	13
5175	2	1	20	668	681	54	3	50	20	10	18	18	10	3	6	16	11	11	10
5176	3	1	30	34	318	0	2	2	20	8	12	11	1	4	1	12	3	3	9
5177	2	1	5	25	586	56	4	18	11	6	7	10	16	0	4	14	13	14	8
5178	1	0	2	129	249	0	0	5	1	3	4	2	2	0	4	6	4	3	2
5179	5	3	17	1062	327	9	1	2	5	14	3	4	2	7	17	16	4	3	7
5180	2	1	6	1004	137	3	0	0	2	2	3	2	1	1	2	5	1	3	4
5181	8	5	26	169	553	12	2	16	7	20	5	10	4	9	29	24	9	4	8
5182	14	5	21	232	483	8	2	15	7	15	6	10	4	7	16	17	8	3	6
5183	5	2	7	188	176	1	1	10	13	2	9	7	1	1	2	6	5	8	4
5184	1	0	0	14	147	21	2	1	5	2	3	4	5	0	1	3	4	4	2
5185	13	3	75	1541	526	6	8	1	3	17	48	20	6	93	29	46	11	9	11
5186	3	1	5	1012	159	22	0	2	1	3	6	4	2	4	1	6	1	5	11
5187	2	1	42	257	707	15	3	16	10	13	22	20	18	13	5	21	13	8	5
5188	3	1	42	248	645	1	2	11	11	12	23	18	12	13	3	21	10	5	5
5189	2	1	42	264	658	71	4	13	10	14	22	18	18	13	5	21	13	7	5
5190	3	1	43	255	575	2	2	7	11	12	22	16	12	13	3	21	10	5	5
5191	4	1	14	1149	223	2	4	4	3	12	14	4	21	12	10	11	16	12	10
5192	4	1	157	18	61	21	4	11	2	6	1	4	11	5	5	7	2	4	3

Soups, Sauces, Fats, Misc.

Food No.	Food Description & Amount	wt gm	wt oz	cal	% cal fat	prot gm	carbo gm	fiber gm
5193	Shrimp gumbo [1 cup]	244	8.6	170	36%	10	19	2.7
5194	Shrimp soup, cream of, made with milk (Include shrimp bisque) [1 cup]	248	8.7	267	48%	22	13	0.2
5195	Shrimp soup, cream of, made with water [1 cup]	244	8.6	90	52%	3	8	0.2
5196	Sopa seca (dry soup) [1 cup]	218	7.7	340	42%	7	43	2.2
5197	Sopa seca de arroz (dry rice soup) [1 cup]	218	7.7	351	39%	6	47	2.0
5198	Sopa Seca de Fideo (dry pasta soup) [1 cup]	218	7.7	328	45%	8	38	2.4
5199	Sopa de Fideo Aguada, Mexican style noodle soup [1 cup]	242	8.5	194	39%	8	22	0.9
5200	Sopa de tortilla, Mexican style tortilla soup [1 cup]	240	8.5	238	52%	10	19	1.4
5201	Sour cherry soup [1 cup]	242	8.5	208	31%	3	35	1.3
5202	Soybean soup, made with milk [1 cup]	253	8.9	214	53%	14	13	3.7
5203	Soybean soup, miso broth [1 cup]	240	8.5	85	36%	6	8	2.0
5204	Spanish vegetable soup, Puerto Rican style (Caldo gallego) [1 cup]	250	8.8	289	57%	18	13	2.6
5205	Spinach soup [1 cup]	245	8.6	204	54%	9	16	1.7
5206	Split pea soup [1 cup]	250	8.8	165	16%	9	27	2.8
5207	Split pea soup, canned, reduced sodium, prepared with water or ready-to-serve [1 cup]	250	8.8	178	12%	10	30	4.8
5208	Split pea and ham soup [1 cup]	253	8.9	195	19%	12	28	4.3
5209	Split pea and ham soup, canned, reduced sodium, prepared with water or ready-to serve [1 cup]	253	8.9	172	9%	10	29	4.8
5210	Sweet and sour soup [1 cup]	244	8.6	72	10%	3	14	1.6
5211	Tomato beef noodle soup, made with water [1 cup]	244	8.6	139	28%	4	21	1.5
5212	Tomato beef rice soup, made with water [1 cup]	244	8.6	126	21%	3	22	1.6
5213	Tomato beef soup, made with water [1 cup]	244	8.6	139	28%	4	21	1.5
5214	Tomato noodle soup, cream of (Include tomato macaroni made with milk) [1 cup]	248	8.7	185	28%	7	28	2.7
5215	Tomato noodle soup, made with water (Include tomato macaroni soup) [1 cup]	244	8.6	144	15%	4	27	1.0
5216	Tomato rice soup, canned, undiluted [1 can undiluted]	312	11.0	290	21%	5	53	4.1
5217	Tomato rice soup, made with water (Include Spanish rice soup) [1 cup]	247	8.7	119	21%	2	22	1.5
5218	Tomato soup, canned, low sodium, ready-to-serve (Include condensed made with water) [1 can ready-to-serve]	298	10.5	104	21%	2	20	0.6
5219	Tomato soup, canned, undiluted [1 cup]	251	8.9	171	20%	4	33	1.0
5220	Tomato soup, cream of (Include tomato bisque, canned tomato soup prepared with milk) [1 cup]	248	8.7	148	27%	6	22	0.5
5221	Tomato soup, instant type, made with water [1 cup]	265	9.3	103	21%	2	19	0.5
5222	Tomato soup, made with water [1 cup]	244	8.6	85	20%	2	17	0.5
5223	Tomato vegetable soup with noodles, made with water [1 cup]	241	8.5	72	24%	2	12	0.5
5224	Tomato vegetable soup, made with water [1 cup]	241	8.5	53	14%	2	10	0.5
5225	Turkey noodle soup [1 cup]	244	8.6	69	26%	4	9	0.8
5226	Turkey noodle soup, home recipe [1 cup]	244	8.6	149	18%	21	8	1.2
5227	Turkey noodle soup, chunky style [1 cup]	236	8.3	177	28%	15	16	1.3
5228	Turtle and vegetable soup (Include snapper soup) [1 cup]	244	8.6	118	32%	13	4	0.7
5229	Vegetable bean soup, made with water (Include minestrone) [1 cup]	241	8.5	83	27%	4	11	1.0
5230	Vegetable beef noodle soup, made with water [1 cup]	244	8.6	81	28%	5	10	0.6
5231	Vegetable beef soup, home recipe [1 cup]	241	8.5	231	47%	16	15	2.5
5232	Vegetable beef soup, made with lowfat milk [1 cup]	248	8.7	134	24%	10	16	2.0
5233	Vegetable beef soup with noodles or pasta, home recipe [1 cup]	241	8.5	245	42%	16	20	2.6
5234	Vegetable beef soup with rice, home recipe [1 cup]	244	8.6	242	43%	16	19	2.5
5235	Vegetable beef soup, chunky style [1 cup]	240	8.5	157	26%	11	18	2.8
5236	Vegetable beef soup, canned, undiluted [1 can]	305	10.8	192	22%	14	25	4.9
5237	Vegetable beef soup, made with water (Include vegetable with meat soups) [1 cup]	244	8.6	79	22%	6	10	2.0
5238	Vegetable beef soup with rice, made with water or ready-to-serve [1 cup]	244	8.6	96	17%	6	15	0.5
5239	Vegetable broth, bouillon (Include onion broth, pot liquor) [1 cup]	240	8.5	17	1%	2	2	0.0
5240	Vegetable chicken or turkey soup, canned, undiluted [1 cup]	246	8.7	149	36%	7	17	1.5

Food no.	fat gm	sat fat gm	choles mg	sodium mg	potas mg	vit A	vit E	vit C	thia	ribo	niac	vit B-6	fola	vit B-12	calc	phos	mag	iron	zinc
						% of Daily Value													
5193	7	1	51	343	516	16	9	42	13	6	13	10	15	5	10	13	13	13	6
5194	14	4	130	311	454	19	9	6	7	20	11	8	3	22	27	34	13	11	11
5195	5	3	17	976	59	1	4	0	1	2	2	2	1	10	2	3	2	3	5
5196	16	4	7	631	417	8	12	21	22	9	21	10	4	1	3	11	8	15	6
5197	15	4	7	614	402	8	12	20	19	5	19	11	4	1	3	10	7	16	6
5198	16	4	7	649	433	8	12	21	25	13	23	9	4	1	3	11	9	14	5
5199	8	1	7	322	365	3	7	15	15	16	24	10	14	0	1	9	5	7	4
5200	14	4	19	346	349	5	6	11	7	15	17	10	13	2	13	18	7	5	6
5201	7	4	80	20	125	13	2	2	4	7	1	4	3	4	5	6	3	4	2
5202	13	3	8	352	554	6	10	9	9	20	8	10	10	6	18	26	15	18	8
5203	3	1	0	988	361	45	3	7	4	9	13	8	14	3	6	10	9	10	6
5204	18	6	63	561	603	2	2	35	10	10	24	16	8	11	5	18	10	11	16
5205	12	4	14	636	596	60	9	13	11	29	4	12	26	9	32	22	21	15	8
5206	3	1	0	918	190	2	0	3	7	4	6	3	0	0	3	13	10	11	11
5207	2	1	5	415	458	18	1	0	12	4	6	9	13	0	4	14	9	11	7
5208	4	2	8	1017	321	51	1	12	8	6	13	11	1	4	4	19	10	13	22
5209	2	1	8	496	516	22	1	4	14	6	9	6	12	1	4	14	9	10	8
5210	1	0	5	1292	227	3	2	28	6	4	5	6	4	0	3	4	4	3	2
5211	4	2	5	917	220	5	4	0	6	5	9	4	2	3	2	6	2	6	5
5212	3	1	1	1185	388	7	3	24	4	4	10	4	4	1	3	5	2	5	3
5213	4	2	5	917	220	5	4	0	6	5	9	4	2	3	2	6	2	6	5
5214	6	3	26	642	396	10	10	97	12	14	9	8	5	7	14	15	6	12	3
5215	2	0	20	528	215	6	9	83	12	5	10	5	4	1	2	7	4	13	4
5216	7	1	3	1981	802	18	9	60	10	7	13	9	9	0	6	8	3	11	8
5217	3	1	2	815	331	8	4	25	4	3	5	4	3	0	2	3	1	4	3
5218	2	0	0	60	322	8	14	135	8	4	9	7	4	0	1	4	2	12	2
5219	4	1	0	1391	527	14	23	222	12	6	14	11	7	0	3	7	4	20	3
5220	5	2	11	757	454	13	12	113	9	14	8	8	5	6	16	15	6	10	5
5221	2	1	0	943	294	8	4	8	4	3	4	5	2	1	5	7	3	2	1
5222	2	0	0	699	264	7	12	111	6	3	7	6	3	0	2	3	2	10	2
5223	2	0	0	822	210	30	4	2	4	3	5	3	3	0	2	3	2	6	3
5224	1	0	0	1092	99	2	4	10	4	3	4	2	2	0	1	3	5	3	1
5225	2	1	5	819	75	3	0	0	5	4	7	2	1	3	1	5	2	5	4
5226	3	1	66	86	398	56	2	4	9	12	23	18	3	5	3	21	8	10	16
5227	5	1	59	531	229	30	1	2	8	9	18	11	3	4	3	14	6	10	10
5228	4	1	59	472	281	4	4	12	6	9	8	5	4	9	7	12	5	6	4
5229	3	1	1	915	313	23	3	2	3	3	5	5	4	0	4	6	2	5	5
5230	2	1	5	871	137	13	1	2	4	3	5	3	2	4	2	4	1	6	10
5231	12	5	47	255	621	20	2	21	10	16	15	16	14	16	3	17	9	14	29
5232	4	2	12	852	366	26	0	5	5	14	6	6	4	11	17	16	6	7	13
5233	11	4	52	234	573	18	2	19	13	15	16	15	13	15	3	18	10	15	27
5234	12	5	45	244	600	19	2	20	12	15	16	16	14	16	3	17	9	14	28
5235	4	2	22	892	397	53	2	17	10	10	14	12	7	9	3	13	7	13	18
5236	5	2	12	1925	421	46	0	10	6	7	13	9	6	13	4	10	4	15	25
5237	2	1	5	795	173	19	0	4	2	3	5	4	3	5	2	4	2	6	11
5238	2	1	5	801	167	18	1	4	2	3	5	4	3	5	2	5	2	6	10
5239	0	0	0	3180	55	0	0	0	0	1	3	1	1	2	1	4	2	1	0
5240	6	2	10	1857	331	51	1	2	5	6	11	5	2	5	3	8	2	9	7

Soups, Sauces, Fats, Misc.

Food No.	Food Description & Amount	wt gm	wt oz	cal	% cal fat	prot gm	carbo gm	fiber gm
5241	Vegetable chicken or turkey soup, made with water or ready-to-serve [1 can ready to-serve]	298	10.5	92	36%	4	11	0.9
5242	Vegetable chicken soup, canned, made with water, low sodium [1 cup]	241	8.5	166	26%	12	19	1.0
5243	Vegetable noodle soup, home recipe [1 cup]	241	8.5	121	37%	5	15	1.9
5244	Vegetable noodle soup, canned, reduced sodium, prepared with water or ready-to-serve [1 cup]	244	8.6	99	10%	4	18	3.4
5245	Vegetable chicken rice soup, made with water or ready-to-serve [1 cup]	241	8.5	67	32%	4	8	0.8
5246	Vegetable chicken noodle soup, made with water or ready-to-serve [1 cup]	241	8.5	75	31%	4	9	0.8
5247	Vegetable noodle soup, made with water (Include vegetable with dumplings, alphabet vegetable soup) [1 cup]	241	8.5	72	24%	2	12	0.6
5248	Vegetable rice soup, made with water [1 cup]	241	8.5	106	15%	3	20	0.7
5249	Vegetable soup, home recipe [1 cup]	234	8.3	100	40%	4	12	2.1
5250	Vegetable soup, canned, low sodium, made with water or ready-to-serve [1 cup]	241	8.5	82	26%	2	13	0.8
5251	Vegetable soup, canned, undiluted [1 cup]	246	8.7	162	21%	6	26	3.2
5252	Vegetable soup, chunky style [1 cup]	240	8.5	122	27%	4	19	1.2
5253	Vegetable soup, cream of, made with milk [1 cup]	248	8.7	213	42%	9	22	0.7
5254	Vegetable soup, dark leafy-greens, with meat, Oriental style [1 cup]	228	8.0	52	30%	7	2	1.0
5255	Vegetable soup, cream of, made from dry mix, low sodium, made with water [1 cup]	260	9.2	167	3%	19	22	1.4
5256	Vegetable soup, dark leafy-greens, meatless, Oriental style [1 cup]	226	8.0	38	93%	0	1	0.5
5257	Vegetable soup, dry mix, not reconstituted [1 Tbs]	1	0.0	4	14%	0	1	0.0
5258	Vegetable soup, made from dry mix [1 cup]	253	8.9	53	19%	3	8	0.5
5259	Vegetable soup, made from dry mix, low sodium (Include Hain brand) [1 cup]	253	8.9	56	12%	2	10	0.5
5260	Vegetable soup, made with water [1 cup]	241	8.5	81	21%	3	13	1.6
5261	Vegetable soup, Spanish style, stew type [1 cup]	227	8.0	192	33%	14	18	4.4
5262	Vegetable soup with chicken broth, Mexican style (Sopa Ranchera) [1 cup]	232	8.2	140	42%	6	16	1.7
5263	Vegetable soup with pasta, chunky style (Include Campbell's Chunky Mediterranean Vegetable) [1 cup]	240	8.5	127	20%	5	21	5.8
5264	Vegetarian bouillon, dry [1 cube]	4	0.1	13	14%	0	2	0.1
5265	Vegetarian vegetable soup, made with water [1 cup]	241	8.5	72	24%	2	12	0.6
5266	Vegetarian vegetable soup, undiluted [1 cup]	246	8.7	145	24%	4	24	1.2
5267	Vichyssoise soup [1 cup]	248	8.7	137	33%	6	17	0.5
5268	Watercress soup [1 cup]	245	8.6	26	14%	5	0	0.1
5269	White bean soup, Puerto Rican style (Sopon de habichuelas blancas) [1 cup]	275	9.7	242	26%	9	36	3.9
5270	Won-Ton soup [1 cup]	241	8.5	182	35%	14	14	0.9
5271	Zucchini soup, cream of [1 cup]	248	8.7	171	53%	6	14	1.3
	Sauces, Gravies, and Dips							
5300	Barbecue sauce (Include Szechuan sauce) [½ cup]	125	4.4	94	22%	2	16	1.5
5301	Barbecue sauce, low sodium [½ cup]	125	4.4	94	22%	2	16	3.8
5302	Black bean sauce [½ cup]	138	4.9	129	43%	3	14	2.0
5303	Cheese sauce made with lowfat cheese [½ cup]	122	4.3	162	52%	11	8	0.1
5304	Cheese sauce [½ cup]	122	4.3	134	50%	7	10	0.4
5305	Clam sauce, white [½ cup]	120	4.2	301	64%	21	5	0.2
5306	Cranberry-raspberry sauce [½ cup]	140	4.9	219	1%	0	57	2.7
5307	Cocktail sauce [½ cup]	137	4.8	119	7%	2	30	3.8
5308	Duck sauce (Include hoisin sauce) [2 Tbs]	30	1.1	70	52%	0	7	0.0
5309	Enchilada sauce, green [½ cup]	125	4.4	93	69%	2	7	1.9
5310	Enchilada sauce, red [½ cup]	125	4.4	161	88%	1	5	1.0
5311	Fish sauce (bagoong) [½ cup]	136	4.8	48	0%	7	5	0.0
5312	Green tomato-chile sauce, cooked (Salsa verde) [½ cup]	123	4.3	91	69%	1	7	2.4
5313	Green tomato-chile sauce, raw (Salsa de tomate verde cruda) [½ cup]	120	4.2	31	24%	1	6	1.9
5314	Hoisin sauce [2 Tbs]	36	1.3	79	14%	1	16	1.0
5315	Lobster sauce [½ cup]	117	4.1	193	57%	12	7	0.7
5316	Miso [2 Tbs]	34	1.2	70	27%	4	10	1.8

Food no.	fat gm	sat fat gm	choles mg	sodium mg	potas mg	% of Daily Value: vit A	vit E	vit C	thia	ribo	niac	vit B-6	fola	vit B-12	calc	phos	mag	iron	zinc
5241	4	1	6	1149	204	32	1	1	3	4	7	3	1	3	2	5	2	6	4
5242	5	1	17	84	369	60	1	9	3	10	17	5	3	4	3	11	2	8	14
5243	5	1	8	413	470	26	5	16	9	11	11	10	15	0	4	9	7	7	4
5244	1	0	3	465	301	22	2	4	14	7	9	5	7	0	5	8	8	7	3
5245	2	1	8	880	128	17	0	1	2	2	6	2	1	2	2	3	1	4	2
5246	3	1	7	940	105	17	0	1	3	4	7	2	1	2	2	4	2	5	2
5247	2	0	0	827	210	30	1	2	4	3	5	3	3	0	2	3	2	6	3
5248	2	0	0	840	192	26	1	2	4	3	5	4	2	0	2	4	3	6	4
5249	5	1	0	395	534	26	5	19	7	10	10	11	15	0	4	8	7	6	4
5250	2	0	0	43	267	40	2	7	3	3	4	7	3	0	4	2	1	6	14
5251	4	1	2	1626	386	42	0	8	7	5	10	6	5	0	3	8	3	11	11
5252	4	1	0	1010	396	59	3	10	5	4	6	10	4	0	6	7	2	9	21
5253	10	4	20	1197	440	11	6	8	80	27	3	5	4	9	30	27	10	4	8
5254	2	1	17	476	234	15	3	34	12	6	9	9	15	3	4	7	7	4	4
5255	1	0	2	600	583	10	1	27	9	32	3	7	9	10	33	29	12	13	10
5256	4	1	0	20	96	11	5	6	1	2	1	2	6	0	2	1	4	3	1
5257	0	0	0	81	7	0	0	1	0	0	0	0	0	0	0	0	0	0	0
5258	1	1	0	1002	76	2	0	2	2	2	2	3	2	4	1	4	6	5	2
5259	1	1	0	51	104	2	4	10	3	3	4	3	3	0	1	3	5	4	1
5260	2	0	1	814	192	21	0	3	3	3	5	3	2	0	2	4	2	5	6
5261	7	2	28	346	588	28	2	37	12	9	15	16	12	15	4	17	10	12	15
5262	7	2	10	235	430	7	6	33	9	11	17	11	13	0	2	9	7	5	3
5263	3	1	5	864	612	43	3	8	4	7	6	12	8	0	6	11	4	10	10
5264	0	0	0	269	24	0	1	2	1	1	1	1	1	0	0	1	1	1	0
5265	2	0	0	827	210	30	1	2	4	3	5	3	3	0	2	3	2	6	3
5266	4	1	0	1653	421	60	3	5	7	5	9	6	5	0	4	7	4	12	6
5267	5	3	17	1062	327	9	1	2	5	14	3	4	2	8	17	16	4	3	7
5268	0	0	35	92	63	3	1	4	1	1	3	2	0	4	2	5	3	3	2
5269	7	2	9	184	504	1	2	19	15	4	10	10	11	1	6	11	11	17	9
5270	7	2	53	543	316	10	2	6	27	15	23	10	5	7	3	15	5	10	7
5271	10	3	13	159	452	16	6	8	7	18	4	6	5	5	20	19	10	3	5
5300	2	0	0	1019	218	11	6	15	3	1	6	5	1	0	2	3	6	6	2
5301	2	0	0	166	761	11	6	15	3	1	6	5	4	0	2	3	6	6	2
5302	6	1	0	861	187	1	3	4	5	3	2	3	9	0	3	5	5	5	3
5303	9	4	19	612	200	11	5	2	5	16	2	3	2	9	33	36	5	3	10
5304	7	4	23	682	241	5	1	2	4	14	1	3	1	8	25	19	5	1	3
5305	21	3	56	94	534	14	15	32	9	21	14	5	6	1372	8	28	4	131	15
5306	0	0	0	25	60	0	1	11	1	3	2	1	1	0	1	1	2	2	1
5307	1	0	0	1254	551	10	7	32	6	5	7	10	8	0	3	5	7	5	3
5308	4	1	4	1	36	0	1	11	1	0	0	0	1	0	0	0	0	0	0
5309	7	4	22	15	270	8	2	19	3	5	7	5	2	1	4	6	5	3	2
5310	16	8	46	18	168	17	4	17	3	4	2	4	2	1	3	4	2	2	1
5311	0	0	0	10499	392	0	0	1	1	5	16	27	17	11	6	1	60	6	2
5312	7	2	3	2	313	2	5	24	3	3	10	6	2	0	1	5	6	4	2
5313	1	0	0	3	249	2	2	22	3	2	8	5	2	0	1	4	5	3	2
5314	1	0	1	581	43	0	0	0	0	5	2	1	2	0	1	1	2	2	1
5315	12	2	85	347	230	3	8	2	14	11	12	9	7	7	2	14	4	5	8
5316	2	0	0	1240	56	0	0	0	2	5	1	4	3	0	2	5	4	5	8

Soups, Sauces, Fats, Misc.

Food No.	Food Description & Amount	wt gm	wt oz	cal	% cal fat	prot gm	carbo gm	fiber gm
5317	Miso sauce [½ cup]	120	4.2	188	16%	6	35	2.9
5318	Mole poblano (sauce) [½ cup]	133	4.7	157	66%	5	11	2.4
5319	Mole verde (sauce) [½ cup]	133	4.7	119	56%	7	8	1.9
5320	Natto [½ cup]	88	3.1	186	47%	16	13	4.7
5321	Oyster sauce (Include scalloped oysters) [½ cup]	128	4.5	163	58%	7	10	0.2
5322	Oyster-flavored sauce [½ cup]	117	4.1	62	0%	0	16	0.1
5323	Peanut sauce [2 Tbs]	28	1.0	87	76%	4	3	0.9
5324	Plum sauce, Oriental-style [2 Tbs]	39	1.4	78	2%	0	20	0.4
5325	Puerto Rican ground seasoning [½ cup]	120	4.2	94	71%	1	7	1.7
5326	Salsa, cruda (uncooked salsa, tomato, pepper, onion, coriander) [½ cup]	120	4.2	22	11%	1	5	1.3
5327	Salsa, cooked (Include taco sauce; creole sauce; picante sauce; salsa de chile rojo) [½ cup]	137	4.8	30	9%	2	7	2.6
5328	Salsa, red, cooked, homemade [½ cup]	117	4.1	105	80%	1	5	1.2
5329	Sofrito, Puerto Rican seasoning [½ cup]	120	4.2	307	78%	10	7	1.6
5330	Soy sauce (Include shoyu) [2 Tbs]	36	1.3	19	1%	2	3	0.3
5331	Soy sauce, low sodium [2 Tbs]	36	1.3	19	1%	2	3	0.3
5332	Spaghetti sauce (Include marinara sauce, cacciatore sauce, pizza sauce, spaghetti sauce with mushrooms) [1 cup]	250	8.8	143	33%	4	21	4.0
5333	Spaghetti sauce, fat free [1 cup]	250	8.8	103	16%	2	22	3.5
5334	Spaghetti sauce with meat, canned, no extra meat added [1 cup]	250	8.8	178	39%	7	19	3.8
5335	Spaghetti sauce, low sodium (Include marinara sauce, cacciatore sauce, pizza sauce, spaghetti sauce with mushrooms) [1 cup]	250	8.8	273	40%	5	40	7.5
5336	Steak sauce, tomato-base (Include A1) [2 Tbs]	31	1.1	19	3%	0	5	0.5
5337	Sweet and sour sauce (Include Vietnamese sauce) [2 Tbs]	30	1.1	28	0%	0	7	0.0
5338	Teriyaki sauce (Include Oriental barbecue sauce) [½ cup]	144	5.1	121	0%	9	23	0.1
5339	Teriyaki sauce, reduced sodium [1 cup]	255	9.0	214	0%	15	41	0.3
5340	Tomato and sofrito stewing sauce, Puerto Rican style [½ cup]	120	4.2	223	79%	6	7	1.5
5341	Tomato sauce [½ cup]	122	4.3	37	5%	2	9	1.7
5342	Tomato sauce, low sodium [½ cup]	122	4.3	37	6%	2	9	1.8
5343	White sauce, milk sauce [½ cup]	125	4.4	185	66%	5	11	0.2
5344	Worcestershire sauce [2 Tbs]	34	1.2	23	0%	0	6	0.0
5345	Gravy, brown nut meatless [2 Tbs]	30	1.1	37	77%	1	2	0.3
5346	Gravy, Chinese, or sauce,(soy sauce, stock or bouillon, cornstarch) [½ cup]	117	4.1	48	5%	1	11	0.1
5347	Gravy, flour and water [½ cup]	120	4.2	96	2%	3	20	0.7
5348	Gravy, giblet (Include any poultry gravy with pieces of meat) [½ cup]	119	4.2	89	48%	6	6	0.4
5349	Gravy, meat or poultry, made with water [½ cup]	118	4.2	93	65%	2	6	0.5
5350	Gravy, meat or poultry, made with water, low sodium [½ cup]	118	4.2	63	41%	4	6	0.4
5351	Gravy, beef or meat, low sodium [½ cup]	118	4.2	63	41%	4	6	0.4
5352	Gravy, meat, with fruit (Include French sauce) [½ cup]	119	4.2	74	44%	3	8	0.5
5353	Gravy, meat, with wine [1 cup]	118	4.2	76	40%	2	5	0.3
5354	Gravy, meat-based, from Puerto-Rican style beef stew [½ cup]	104	3.7	86	92%	0	2	0.3
5355	Gravy, meat-based, from Puerto-Rican style stuffed pot roast [½ cup]	136	4.8	334	100%	0	0	0.0
5356	Gravy, milk quick gravy [½ cup]	125	4.4	178	65%	5	11	0.2
5357	Gravy, mushroom [½ cup]	119	4.2	32	11%	1	6	0.5
5358	Gravy, poultry-based from Puerto Rican-style chicken fricasse [½ cup]	120	4.2	254	91%	1	6	1.2
5359	Gravy, swiss steak [½ cup]	117	4.1	62	40%	4	6	0.5
5360	Chili con queso (tomato, pepper, and cheese dip) [½ cup]	120	4.2	251	64%	14	9	0.4
5361	Dip, bean, made with refried beans (Include garbanzo bean dip; jalapeno pepper bean dip; bean dip) [½ cup]	131	4.6	188	34%	8	24	9.0
5362	Dip, cheese base other than cream cheese [½ cup]	128	4.5	372	66%	21	11	0.0
5363	Dip, cream cheese base [½ cup]	120	4.2	391	87%	8	6	0.0
5364	Dip, eggplant (Include Baba Ghanoush) [½ cup]	117	4.1	190	72%	5	12	3.1
5365	Dip, shrimp, cream cheese base (Include clam dip) [½ cup]	118	4.2	290	77%	12	5	0.5
5366	Dip, sour cream base (Include buttermilk type; onion dip) [½ cup]	122	4.3	268	81%	5	10	1.0

Food no.	fat gm	sat fat gm	choles mg	sodium mg	potas mg	vit A	vit E	vit C	thia	ribo	niac	vit B-6	fola	vit B-12	calc	phos	mag	iron	zinc
						% of Daily Value													
5317	3	0	0	1965	100	0	0	0	4	8	2	6	4	0	4	8	6	9	12
5318	12	3	1	223	284	2	8	7	5	5	9	5	3	1	4	14	15	9	7
5319	7	1	1	387	419	4	2	78	5	6	13	7	6	2	2	23	22	17	9
5320	10	1	0	6	638	0	0	19	9	10	0	6	2	0	19	15	25	42	18
5321	10	3	39	309	245	10	8	7	10	13	6	4	2	184	10	14	11	26	385
5322	0	0	0	2530	1	0	0	0	0	0	0	0	0	0	0	0	0	0	0
5323	7	1	0	68	105	0	7	5	1	1	10	3	3	0	1	5	6	1	3
5324	0	0	0	233	45	3	1	1	0	1	1	1	0	0	1	1	1	1	0
5325	7	1	0	7	241	6	9	79	4	3	3	8	5	0	2	3	3	3	1
5326	0	0	0	8	184	5	1	26	3	2	3	5	3	0	1	2	3	2	1
5327	0	0	0	354	253	9	4	46	4	3	5	8	5	0	6	3	4	5	3
5328	9	2	2	7	185	4	8	21	3	2	2	4	3	0	1	2	2	2	1
5329	27	9	41	1083	353	4	4	45	11	6	9	12	4	4	2	13	5	5	8
5330	0	0	0	2057	65	0	0	0	1	3	6	3	1	0	1	4	3	4	1
5331	0	0	0	1200	65	0	0	0	1	3	6	3	1	0	1	4	3	4	1
5332	5	1	0	1030	738	10	14	33	9	6	13	14	6	0	6	8	11	10	3
5333	2	0	0	1365	995	20	17	55	11	18	14	24	9	0	3	10	13	11	5
5334	8	2	15	982	742	9	14	31	9	7	17	16	6	8	5	10	11	12	8
5335	12	2	0	75	960	31	17	47	10	9	19	44	13	0	7	9	15	9	4
5336	0	0	0	454	126	3	2	8	1	1	2	2	0	0	1	1	2	2	1
5337	0	0	0	96	9	0	0	0	0	0	0	0	0	0	0	0	1	0	0
5338	0	0	0	5520	324	0	0	0	3	6	9	7	7	0	4	22	22	14	1
5339	0	0	0	4534	574	0	0	0	5	11	16	13	13	0	6	39	39	24	2
5340	20	7	26	524	256	5	4	66	10	5	8	11	4	2	1	7	4	4	5
5341	0	0	0	738	453	12	8	27	5	4	7	9	3	0	2	4	6	5	2
5342	0	0	0	13	453	12	8	27	6	4	7	10	3	0	2	4	6	5	2
5343	14	4	10	187	196	17	8	2	6	13	3	2	2	6	15	12	4	2	3
5344	0	0	0	333	272	0	0	7	2	3	1	0	0	0	4	2	1	10	0
5345	3	0	0	57	24	0	4	0	1	1	1	0	0	0	1	2	2	1	1
5346	0	0	0	767	22	0	0	0	0	1	1	1	0	1	0	2	1	1	0
5347	0	0	0	4	28	0	0	0	11	7	7	1	1	0	1	3	2	7	1
5348	5	1	50	625	138	30	1	1	2	10	7	3	11	36	1	6	1	8	9
5349	7	2	2	681	129	13	1	0	1	3	3	1	1	2	2	3	1	3	6
5350	3	1	4	21	96	0	0	0	2	3	4	1	1	2	1	4	1	5	8
5351	3	1	4	21	96	0	0	0	2	3	4	1	1	2	1	4	1	5	8
5352	4	1	2	502	129	5	1	10	3	2	3	1	1	1	1	3	1	3	5
5353	3	1	2	472	110	5	0	0	1	2	2	1	1	1	1	3	1	3	5
5354	9	4	9	100	65	2	2	9	1	1	1	2	1	0	1	1	1	1	0
5355	37	15	30	3	0	0	9	0	0	0	0	0	0	0	0	0	0	0	0
5356	13	6	20	61	196	6	2	2	5	13	2	2	2	6	15	12	4	2	3
5357	0	0	0	646	26	0	0	1	2	2	2	1	0	1	2	2	1	1	1
5358	26	5	6	537	201	5	15	49	3	2	3	7	3	0	2	2	4	4	1
5359	3	1	3	652	94	0	0	0	2	2	4	1	1	2	1	3	1	5	8
5360	18	11	46	1178	292	18	3	11	4	22	2	6	2	5	48	60	7	3	15
5361	7	1	0	6	396	4	7	31	9	4	2	7	24	0	4	14	13	11	6
5362	27	17	71	1722	310	24	4	0	4	32	1	7	2	9	72	91	9	2	22
5363	38	22	110	400	153	43	6	1	2	12	1	3	3	8	9	11	2	7	4
5364	15	2	0	12	325	1	4	17	29	3	9	6	9	0	4	21	9	8	8
5365	25	14	123	300	169	28	5	3	2	8	5	4	3	10	7	14	5	9	5
5366	24	15	50	910	225	22	3	2	4	13	3	1	3	6	14	13	5	1	2

Soups, Sauces, Fats, Misc.

Food No.	Food Description & Amount	wt gm	wt oz	cal	% cal fat	prot gm	carbo gm	fiber gm
5367	Dip, sour cream base, reduced calorie [½ cup]	120	4.2	176	71%	4	10	0.9
5368	Dip, spinach, sour cream base [½ cup]	120	4.2	215	73%	3	14	1.7
5369	Hummus [½ cup]	120	4.2	205	44%	6	24	6.1
	Fats and Oils							
5400	Almond oil (Include apricot oil) [1 Tbs]	14	0.5	120	100%	0	0	0.0
5401	Bacon grease or meat drippings (Include ham, sausage, lamb, chicken) [1 Tbs]	13	0.5	114	100%	0	0	0.0
5402	Butter replacement, fat-free powder (Include Butter Buds) [1 Tbs]	5	0.2	19	2%	0	4	0.0
5403	**Butter, regular,** salted (Include seasoned butter, garlic butter) [1 Tbs]	14	0.5	102	100%	0	0	0.0
5404	Butter, regular, unsalted [1 Tbs]	14	0.5	102	100%	0	0	0.0
5405	Butter, whipped, salted [1 Tbs]	9	0.3	67	100%	0	0	0.0
5406	Butter, whipped, unsalted [1 Tbs]	9	0.3	67	100%	0	0	0.0
5407	Butter, whipped, stick, salted [1 Tbs]	9	0.3	67	100%	0	0	0.0
5408	Butter, whipped, stick, unsalted [1 Tbs]	9	0.3	67	100%	0	0	0.0
5409	Butter, light, stick, salted [1 Tbs]	14	0.5	71	99%	0	0	0.0
5410	Butter, light, stick, unsalted [1 Tbs]	14	0.5	71	99%	0	0	0.0
5411	Butter, light, whipped, tub, salted [1 Tbs]	10	0.3	47	99%	0	0	0.0
5412	Butter-margarine blend, stick, unsalted [1 Tbs]	14	0.5	102	100%	0	0	0.0
5413	Butter-margarine or vegetable oil blend (Include Blue Bonnet Butter Spread) [1 Tbs]	14	0.5	102	100%	0	0	0.0
5414	Margarine, imitation (Include Shedd's Spread) [1 Tbs]	15	0.5	50	100%	0	0	0.0
5415	Margarine, liquid, salted [1 Tbs]	14	0.5	102	100%	0	0	0.0
5416	**Margarine, regular**, stick, salted [1 Tbs]	14	0.5	102	100%	0	0	0.0
5417	Margarine, regular, tub, salted [1 Tbs]	14	0.5	102	100%	0	0	0.0
5418	Margarine, tub, unsalted [1 Tbs]	14	0.5	102	100%	0	0	0.0
5419	Margarine, whipped, stick, salted [1 Tbs]	9	0.3	68	100%	0	0	0.0
5420	Margarine, whipped, tub, unsalted [1 Tbs]	9	0.3	67	100%	0	0	0.0
5421	Margarine-like spread, liquid, salted [1 Tbs]	14	0.5	88	100%	0	0	0.0
5422	Margarine-like spread, liquid, salted, fat free [1 Tbs]	14	0.5	6	63%	0	0	0.0
5423	Margarine-like spread, reduced calorie, about 40% fat, stick, salted [1 Tbs]	15	0.5	53	100%	0	0	0.0
5424	Margarine-like spread, stick, unsalted [1 Tbs]	14	0.5	77	100%	0	0	0.0
5425	Margarine-like spread, tub, fat free, salted [1 Tbs]	15	0.5	5	39%	0	0	0.0
5426	Margarine-like spread, tub, reduced calorie, about 20% fat, salted [1 Tbs]	15	0.5	26	100%	0	0	0.0
5427	Margarine-like spread, tub, reduced calorie, about 20% fat, unsalted [1 Tbs]	15	0.5	27	100%	0	0	0.0
5428	Margarine-like spread, tub, salted [1 Tbs]	14	0.5	77	100%	0	0	0.0
5429	Margarine-like spread, tub, sweetened [1 Tbs]	14	0.5	76	88%	0	2	0.0
5430	Margarine-like spread, tub, unsalted [1 Tbs]	14	0.5	76	100%	0	0	0.0
5431	Margarine-like spread, tub, whipped, salted [1 Tbs]	10	0.4	54	101%	0	0	0.0
5432	Corn oil [1 Tbs]	14	0.5	120	100%	0	0	0.0
5433	Corn and canola oil [1 Tbs]	14	0.5	124	100%	0	0	0.0
5434	Cottonseed oil [1 Tbs]	14	0.5	120	100%	0	0	0.0
5435	Ghee, clarified butter (Include butter oil) [1 Tbs]	13	0.5	112	100%	0	0	0.0
5436	Flaxseed oil [1 Tbs]	14	0.5	120	100%	0	0	0.0
5437	Honey butter [1 Tbs]	18	0.6	85	62%	0	9	0.0
5438	Lard with annatto, Puerto Rican (Manteca con achiote) [1 Tbs]	15	0.5	135	100%	0	0	0.0
5439	Lard [1 Tbs]	13	0.5	115	100%	0	0	0.0
5440	Olive oil [1 Tbs]	14	0.5	119	100%	0	0	0.0
5441	Peanut oil [1 Tbs]	14	0.5	119	100%	0	0	0.0
5442	Rapeseed oil (Include canola oil; Puritan) [1 Tbs]	14	0.5	120	100%	0	0	0.0
5443	Safflower oil [1 Tbs]	14	0.5	120	100%	0	0	0.0
5444	Sesame oil [1 Tbs]	14	0.5	120	100%	0	0	0.0
5445	Shortening, animal (Include Spry) [1 Tbs]	13	0.5	115	100%	0	0	0.0
5446	Shortening, vegetable (Include Crisco, Fluffo, Frymax) [1 Tbs]	13	0.5	113	100%	0	0	0.0
5447	Soybean and sunflower oil [1 Tbs]	14	0.5	120	100%	0	0	0.0
5448	Soybean oil (Include Crisco, Wesson) [1 Tbs]	14	0.5	120	100%	0	0	0.0

Food no.	fat gm	sat fat gm	choles mg	sodium mg	potas mg	% of Daily Value: vit A	vit E	vit C	thia	ribo	niac	vit B-6	fola	vit B-12	calc	phos	mag	iron	zinc
5367	14	8	43	846	203	12	2	2	4	13	3	1	3	6	13	13	4	1	4
5368	17	6	22	383	199	38	9	17	11	7	2	5	13	3	9	6	7	6	3
5369	10	2	0	293	209	0	5	16	7	4	2	24	18	0	6	13	9	10	9
5400	14	1	0	0	0	0	24	0	0	0	0	0	0	0	0	0	0	0	0
5401	13	6	13	70	0	0	1	0	0	0	0	0	0	0	0	0	0	0	0
5402	0	0	0	60	0	0	0	0	0	0	0	0	0	0	0	0	0	1	0
5403	12	7	31	117	4	11	1	0	0	0	0	0	0	0	0	0	0	0	0
5404	12	7	31	2	4	11	1	0	0	0	0	0	0	0	0	0	0	0	0
5405	8	5	21	78	2	7	1	0	0	0	0	0	0	0	0	0	0	0	0
5406	8	5	21	1	2	7	1	0	0	0	0	0	0	0	0	0	0	0	0
5407	8	5	21	78	2	7	1	0	0	0	0	0	0	0	0	0	0	0	0
5408	8	5	21	1	2	7	1	0	0	0	0	0	0	0	0	0	0	0	0
5409	8	5	15	64	10	10	1	0	0	1	0	0	0	0	1	0	0	1	0
5410	8	5	15	5	10	10	1	0	0	1	0	0	0	0	1	0	0	1	0
5411	5	3	10	43	7	6	0	0	0	0	0	0	0	0	0	0	0	1	0
5412	11	4	10	4	5	14	6	0	0	0	0	0	0	0	0	0	0	0	0
5413	11	4	12	127	5	11	5	0	0	0	0	0	0	0	0	0	0	0	0
5414	6	1	0	139	4	12	2	0	0	0	0	0	0	0	0	0	0	0	0
5415	11	2	0	111	13	11	3	0	0	1	0	0	0	1	1	1	0	0	0
5416	11	2	0	134	6	11	8	0	0	0	0	0	0	0	0	0	0	0	0
5417	11	2	0	153	5	11	8	0	0	0	0	0	0	0	0	0	0	0	0
5418	11	2	0	4	5	11	8	0	0	0	0	0	0	0	0	0	0	0	0
5419	8	1	0	89	4	8	5	0	0	0	0	0	0	0	0	0	0	0	0
5420	8	1	0	3	4	8	5	0	0	0	0	0	0	0	0	0	0	0	0
5421	10	2	0	141	4	15	5	0	0	0	0	0	0	0	0	0	0	0	0
5422	0	0	0	118	7	11	0	0	0	0	0	0	0	0	1	0	0	0	0
5423	6	1	0	149	5	16	3	0	0	0	0	0	0	0	0	0	0	0	0
5424	9	2	0	0	4	11	6	0	0	0	0	0	0	0	0	0	0	0	0
5425	0	0	0	94	0	14	0	0	0	0	0	0	0	0	0	0	0	0	0
5426	3	0	0	110	4	14	3	0	0	0	0	0	0	0	0	0	0	0	0
5427	3	0	0	4	5	16	2	0	0	0	0	0	0	0	0	0	0	0	0
5428	9	1	0	142	4	11	6	0	0	0	0	0	0	0	0	0	0	0	0
5429	7	1	0	77	4	15	9	0	0	0	0	0	0	0	0	0	0	0	0
5430	9	1	0	4	4	11	6	0	0	0	0	0	0	0	0	0	0	0	0
5431	6	1	0	99	3	8	4	0	0	0	0	0	0	0	0	0	0	0	0
5432	14	2	0	0	0	0	13	0	0	0	0	0	0	0	0	0	0	0	0
5433	14	1	0	0	0	0	13	0	0	0	0	0	0	0	0	0	0	0	0
5434	14	4	0	0	0	0	24	0	0	0	0	0	0	0	0	0	0	0	0
5435	13	8	33	0	1	12	2	0	0	0	0	0	0	0	0	0	0	0	0
5436	14	1	0	0	0	0	11	0	0	0	0	0	0	0	0	0	0	0	0
5437	6	4	16	60	7	5	1	0	0	0	0	0	0	0	0	0	0	0	0
5438	15	6	14	0	0	0	1	0	0	0	0	0	0	0	0	0	0	0	0
5439	13	5	12	0	0	0	1	0	0	0	0	0	0	0	0	0	0	0	0
5440	14	2	0	0	0	0	8	0	0	0	0	0	0	0	0	0	0	0	0
5441	14	2	0	0	0	0	8	0	0	0	0	0	0	0	0	0	0	0	0
5442	14	1	0	0	0	0	13	0	0	0	0	0	0	0	0	0	0	0	0
5443	14	1	0	0	0	0	27	0	0	0	0	0	0	0	0	0	0	0	0
5444	14	2	0	0	0	0	3	0	0	0	0	0	0	0	0	0	0	0	0
5445	13	5	12	0	0	0	1	0	0	0	0	0	0	0	0	0	0	0	0
5446	13	3	0	0	0	0	7	0	0	0	0	0	0	0	0	0	0	0	0
5447	14	2	0	0	0	0	26	0	0	0	0	0	0	0	0	0	0	0	0
5448	14	2	0	0	0	0	11	0	0	0	0	0	0	0	0	0	0	0	0

Food No.	Food Description & Amount	wt gm	wt oz	cal	% cal fat	prot gm	carbo gm	fiber gm
5449	Sunflower oil (Include Wesson Sunlite) [1 Tbs]	14	0.5	120	100%	0	0	0.0
5450	Vegetable oil-butter spread, tub, salted [1 Tbs]	14	0.5	51	99%	0	0	0.0
5451	Vegetable oil-butter spread, tub, salted, reduced calorie, [1 Tbs]	13	0.5	59	100%	0	0	0.0
5452	Vegetable oil-butter spread, stick, salted, reduced calorie, [1 Tbs]	13	0.5	60	100%	0	0	0.0
5453	Walnut oil [1 Tbs]	14	0.5	120	100%	0	0	0.0
5454	Wheat germ oil [1 Tbs]	14	0.5	120	100%	0	0	0.0
	Dressings							
5500	Bacon and tomato dressing [2 Tbs]	30	1.1	98	97%	1	1	0.1
5501	Bacon and tomato dressing, low calorie [2 Tbs]	32	1.1	65	95%	1	1	0.1
5502	Bacon dressing (hot) [2 Tbs]	29	1.0	103	96%	1	1	0.0
5503	Blue or roquefort cheese dressing [2 Tbs]	31	1.1	154	93%	1	2	0.0
5504	Blue or roquefort cheese dressing, low-calorie [2 Tbs]	31	1.1	30	65%	2	1	0.0
5505	Blue or roquefort cheese dressing, reduced calorie [2 Tbs]	31	1.1	27	28%	1	4	0.0
5506	Blue or roquefort cheese dressing, reduced calorie, fat-free, cholesterol-free [2 Tbs]	33	1.2	38	6%	1	8	1.1
5507	Caesar dressing [2 Tbs]	29	1.0	155	98%	0	1	0.0
5508	Caesar dressing, low-calorie [2 Tbs]	30	1.1	33	36%	0	6	0.0
5509	Celery seed dressing (Include celery seed and onion dressing) [2 Tbs]	31	1.1	196	88%	0	7	0.3
5510	Coleslaw dressing [2 Tbs]	31	1.1	122	77%	0	7	0.0
5511	Coleslaw dressing, reduced calorie [2 Tbs]	34	1.2	69	88%	0	13	0.1
5512	Cream cheese dressing (Include Philadelphia brand) [2 Tbs]	31	1.1	130	95%	1	2	0.0
5513	Creamy dressing, made with sour cream and oil (Include French made with sour cream, Creamy Cucumber, Seven Seas Southern with Bacon, Wishbone Creamy Bacon, Creamy Italian) [2 Tbs]	29	1.0	147	97%	0	2	0.0
5514	Creamy dressing, made with sour cream and/or buttermilk and oil, reduced calorie (Include Kraft Reduced Calorie Creamy Cucumber Dressing) [2 Tbs]	30	1.1	48	79%	0	2	0.0
5515	Creamy dressing, made with sour cream and/or buttermilk and oil, reduced calorie, cholesterol-free [2 Tbs]	30	1.1	42	51%	0	5	0.0
5516	Creamy dressing, made with sour cream and/or buttermilk and oil, reduced calorie, fat-free, cholesterol-free [2 Tbs]	33	1.2	35	23%	0	7	0.0
5517	Feta cheese dressing (Include Marzetties') [2 Tbs]	29	1.0	160	97%	1	1	0.0
5518	French dressing (Include Catalina, Ranch Style other than Hidden Valley, Sweet 'n Saucy, Holsum's 1867, Richelieu's Western dressing) [2 Tbs]	31	1.1	134	86%	0	5	0.0
5519	French dressing, low-calorie [2 Tbs]	32	1.1	43	39%	0	7	0.0
5520	French dressing, reduced calorie [2 Tbs]	32	1.1	65	59%	0	9	0.0
5521	French dressing, reduced calorie, fat-free, cholesterol-free [2 Tbs]	32	1.1	43	21%	0	7	0.1
5522	Fruit dressing, made with cream [2 Tbs]	30	1.1	62	56%	1	6	0.0
5523	Fruit dressing, made with honey, oil, and water (Include with herbs, lemon juice) [2 Tbs]	29	1.0	149	85%	0	7	0.0
5524	Green Goddess dressing (Include Marie's Avocado Goddess Dressing) [2 Tbs]	31	1.1	155	88%	1	5	0.0
5525	Honey mustard dressing (Include Naturally Fresh Honey Mustard dressing) [2 Tbs]	31	1.1	102	49%	0	14	0.2
5526	Italian dressing, low-calorie (Include Wishbone Lite Dijon Vinegarette, McDonald's Lite Vinaigrette) [2 Tbs]	30	1.1	32	84%	0	1	0.0
5527	Italian dressing, made with vinegar, oil, and garlic (Include Christie's Greek dressing, California Onion dressing, Green Onion dressing, Kraft Presto dressing, vinegarette dressing, Seven Seas Viva Italian dressing) [2 Tbs]	29	1.0	137	93%	0	3	0.0
5528	Italian dressing, reduced calorie [2 Tbs]	28	1.0	56	90%	0	2	0.1
5529	Italian dressing, reduced calorie, fat-free [2 Tbs]	28	1.0	13	40%	0	2	0.1
5530	Korean dressing, or marinade, made with ginseng, garlic, onion, chili pepper, salt [2 Tbs]	30	1.1	10	3%	0	2	0.2
5531	Mayonnaise, imitation [2 Tbs]	30	1.1	69	75%	0	5	0.0
5532	Mayonnaise, imitation, no cholesterol [2 Tbs]	30	1.1	145	89%	0	5	0.0
5533	Mayonnaise, low-calorie or diet [2 Tbs]	31	1.1	72	75%	0	5	0.0

Food no.	fat gm	sat fat gm	choles mg	sodium mg	potas mg	% of Daily Value vit A	vit E	vit C	thia	ribo	niac	vit B-6	fola	vit B-12	calc	phos	mag	iron	zinc
5449	14	1	0	0	0	0	31	0	0	0	0	0	0	0	0	0	0	0	0
5450	6	1	0	112	5	11	3	0	0	0	0	0	0	0	0	0	0	0	0
5451	7	2	9	79	5	11	3	0	0	0	0	0	0	0	0	0	0	0	0
5452	7	2	7	76	1	12	5	0	0	0	0	0	0	0	0	0	0	0	0
5453	14	1	0	0	0	0	2	0	0	0	0	0	0	0	0	0	0	0	0
5454	14	3	0	0	0	0	119	0	0	0	0	0	0	0	0	0	0	0	0
5500	10	2	1	325	32	1	5	4	1	0	1	1	0	0	0	1	0	0	0
5501	7	1	1	351	35	1	6	5	1	0	1	1	0	0	0	1	0	0	0
5502	11	2	2	46	30	0	8	0	1	0	1	0	0	1	0	1	1	1	1
5503	16	3	5	335	11	2	13	1	0	2	0	1	1	1	2	2	0	0	1
5504	2	1	0	367	2	0	1	0	0	2	0	0	0	1	3	3	1	1	1
5505	1	0	3	502	16	0	1	0	0	1	0	0	0	1	2	1	0	0	1
5506	0	0	1	265	64	0	1	0	1	2	0	0	0	1	2	4	1	0	0
5507	17	3	1	317	9	0	7	0	0	0	0	0	0	0	1	1	0	0	0
5508	1	0	1	323	9	0	1	0	0	0	0	0	0	0	1	1	0	0	0
5509	19	2	0	1	47	2	17	3	1	1	0	2	1	0	1	1	1	2	0
5510	10	2	8	222	3	2	9	0	0	0	0	0	0	1	0	1	0	0	0
5511	7	1	8	538	17	0	7	0	0	0	0	0	0	1	1	1	0	0	0
5512	14	3	8	22	11	3	9	0	0	1	0	0	0	1	1	1	0	1	0
5513	16	2	1	2	8	1	14	0	0	0	0	0	0	0	0	0	0	0	0
5514	4	1	0	307	11	0	3	0	0	0	0	0	1	0	0	0	0	0	0
5515	2	0	0	280	15	0	7	0	0	1	0	0	0	1	1	3	0	0	0
5516	1	0	0	330	44	0	1	0	0	1	0	0	0	0	1	3	0	0	0
5517	17	3	7	91	13	1	9	0	1	4	0	2	1	2	4	3	1	1	2
5518	13	3	0	427	25	4	12	0	0	0	0	0	0	1	0	0	0	1	0
5519	2	0	0	255	26	4	2	0	0	0	0	0	0	0	0	0	0	1	0
5520	4	1	0	324	26	4	2	0	0	0	0	0	0	0	0	0	0	1	0
5521	1	0	0	252	25	4	2	0	0	0	0	0	0	0	0	0	0	1	0
5522	4	2	36	11	33	5	1	7	1	2	0	1	2	1	1	2	1	1	1
5523	14	2	0	1	4	0	12	0	0	0	0	0	0	0	0	0	0	0	0
5524	15	2	12	331	18	0	11	0	0	1	0	0	0	1	1	1	1	1	1
5525	6	1	0	74	20	0	5	0	0	0	0	0	0	0	1	1	1	1	1
5526	3	0	2	236	5	0	2	0	0	0	0	0	0	0	0	0	0	0	0
5527	14	2	0	231	4	1	14	0	0	0	0	0	0	1	0	0	0	0	0
5528	6	1	0	398	9	0	1	0	0	0	0	0	1	0	0	0	0	0	0
5529	1	0	0	258	37	0	1	0	0	0	0	0	1	0	0	0	0	0	0
5530	0	0	0	83	32	0	0	17	0	0	1	1	1	0	1	1	1	1	0
5531	6	1	7	149	3	0	9	0	0	0	0	0	0	0	0	0	0	0	0
5532	14	2	0	106	3	0	13	0	0	0	0	0	0	0	0	0	0	0	0
5533	6	1	7	155	3	0	9	0	0	0	0	0	0	0	0	0	0	0	0

Soups, Sauces, Fats, Misc.

Food No.	Food Description & Amount	wt gm	wt oz	cal	% cal fat	prot gm	carbo gm	fiber gm
5534	Mayonnaise, low-calorie or diet, low sodium [2 Tbs]	28	1.0	65	75%	0	4	0.0
5535	Mayonnaise, made with tofu [2 Tbs]	30	1.1	94	75%	3	3	0.2
5536	Mayonnaise, made with yogurt (Include Yogannaise) [2 Tbs]	28	1.0	27	47%	1	3	0.0
5537	Mayonnaise, reduced calorie or diet, cholesterol-free [2 Tbs]	29	1.0	97	90%	0	2	0.0
5538	Mayonnaise, regular (Include McDonald's House dressing) [2 Tbs]	28	1.0	198	100%	0	1	0.0
5539	Mayonnaise-type dressing (Include Miracle Whip) [2 Tbs]	29	1.0	115	77%	0	7	0.0
5540	Mayonnaise-type dressing, cholesterol free (Include Miracle Whip (cholesterol-free)) [2 Tbs]	30	1.1	206	100%	0	0	0.0
5541	Mayonnaise-type dressing, fat-free [2 Tbs]	32	1.1	24	31%	0	4	1.2
5542	Mayonnaise-type dressing, low-calorie or diet (Include Miracle Whip Light) [2 Tbs]	28	1.0	73	66%	0	7	0.0
5543	Mayonnaise-type dressing, low-calorie or diet cholesterol-free (Include Miracle Whip Light (cholesterol-free)) [2 Tbs]	30	1.1	96	80%	0	4	0.0
5544	Milk, vinegar, and artificial sweetener dressing [2 Tbs]	31	1.1	24	44%	1	3	0.0
5545	Milk, vinegar, and sugar dressing [2 Tbs]	33	1.2	42	23%	1	8	0.0
5546	Peppercorn dressing [2 Tbs]	27	0.9	151	98%	0	1	0.0
5547	Poppy seed dressing (Include Naturally Fresh brand) [2 Tbs]	29	1.0	130	83%	0	6	0.0
5548	Russian dressing [2 Tbs]	31	1.1	151	93%	0	3	0.0
5549	Russian dressing, low-calorie [2 Tbs]	32	1.1	46	25%	0	9	0.1
5550	Salad dressing, low-calorie (Include Nutri-System salad dressing) [2 Tbs]	32	1.1	41	65%	0	4	0.1
5551	Sandwich spread [2 Tbs]	31	1.1	119	79%	0	7	0.1
5552	Sesame dressing [2 Tbs]	29	1.0	156	95%	0	3	0.2
5553	Sour cream dressing, filled, sour, non-dairy (Include King Sour, Zest) [2 Tbs]	29	1.0	52	84%	1	1	0.0
5554	Sweet and sour dressing [2 Tbs]	31	1.1	5	0%	0	1	0.0
5555	Thousand Island dressing (Include McDonald's Big Mac sauce) [2 Tbs]	31	1.1	118	85%	0	5	0.0
5556	Thousand Island dressing, low-calorie [2 Tbs]	31	1.1	49	61%	0	5	0.4
5557	Thousand Island dressing, reduced calorie, fat-free, cholesterol-free [2 Tbs]	32	1.1	36	16%	0	10	0.1
5558	Vinegar, sugar, and water dressing [2 Tbs]	32	1.1	17	0%	0	5	0.0
5559	Yogurt dressing [2 Tbs]	31	1.1	23	46%	1	2	0.0
	Condiments							
5600	Beans, string, green, pickled [½ cup]	68	2.4	19	3%	1	4	2.0
5601	Beets, pickled (Include pickled beets with onions, beet salad) [½ cup, sliced]	84	3.0	53	2%	1	13	2.0
5602	Cabbage, fresh, pickled, Japanese style [½ cup]	75	2.6	16	4%	1	3	2.3
5603	Cabbage, Kim Chee style [½ cup]	75	2.6	16	9%	1	3	0.9
5604	Cabbage, mustard, salted [½ cup]	64	2.3	13	5%	1	3	2.0
5605	Cabbage, red, pickled (Include sweet and sour red cabbage) [½ cup]	75	2.6	110	1%	0	29	0.6
5606	Catsup, tomato [2 Tbs]	34	1.2	35	3%	1	9	0.4
5607	Catsup, tomato, low sodium [2 Tbs]	34	1.2	35	3%	1	9	0.4
5608	Cauliflower, pickled [½ cup]	63	2.2	27	6%	1	6	1.2
5609	Celery, pickled [½ cup]	75	2.6	11	7%	0	3	1.1
5610	Chinese preserved sweet zucchini (Include other vegetables) [5 slices]	60	2.1	222	0%	0	57	0.2
5611	Chutney [2 Tbs]	34	1.2	52	3%	0	13	0.8
5612	Corn relish [2 Tbs]	31	1.1	26	6%	1	6	0.5
5613	Cucumber pickles, dill or sour [1 small]	37	1.3	7	10%	0	2	0.4
5614	Cucumber pickles, dill, reduced salt (Include Vlasic Half the Salt Kosher Crunchy Dill Spears; Vlasic Half the Salt Hamburger Dill Chips) [1 pickle (3¾" long)]	65	2.3	7	16%	0	1	0.8
5615	Cucumber pickles, fresh (Include bread and butter) [½ cup]	85	3.0	62	2%	1	15	1.3
5616	Cucumber pickles, relish (Include Indian sweet relish) [½ cup]	123	4.3	159	3%	0	43	1.3
5617	Cucumber pickles, sweet (Include candied dill spears, semi-sweet) [1 Gherkin (2-1/8" long)]	6	0.2	7	2%	0	2	0.1
5618	Cucumber pickles, sweet, reduced salt (Include Vlasic Half the Salt Sweet Butter Chips) [5 slices]	30	1.1	35	2%	0	10	0.5
5619	Cucumber, Kim Chee style [½ cup]	75	2.6	16	4%	1	4	1.1
5620	Eggplant, pickled [½ cup]	68	2.4	23	19%	1	5	1.7

Food no.	fat gm	sat fat gm	choles mg	sodium mg	potas mg	vit A	vit E	vit C	thia	ribo	niac	vit B-6	fola	vit B-12	calc	phos	mag	iron	zinc
						% of Daily Value													
5534	5	1	7	31	3	0	5	0	0	0	0	0	0	0	0	0	0	0	0
5535	8	1	0	200	20	0	6	0	1	1	0	0	1	0	2	1	4	0	1
5536	1	1	12	139	27	0	1	0	0	2	0	0	0	1	2	2	0	1	0
5537	10	1	0	214	20	0	9	0	0	0	0	0	0	0	0	0	0	0	0
5538	22	3	16	157	9	2	15	0	0	0	0	8	1	1	0	1	0	1	0
5539	10	1	8	209	3	2	5	0	0	0	0	0	0	1	0	1	0	0	0
5540	23	3	0	146	4	0	16	0	0	1	0	0	0	0	0	1	0	0	0
5541	1	0	0	380	30	0	2	0	0	0	0	0	0	0	0	0	0	0	0
5542	5	1	7	199	3	2	5	0	0	0	0	0	0	1	0	1	0	0	0
5543	9	1	0	204	0	0	6	0	0	0	0	0	0	0	0	0	0	0	0
5544	1	1	5	17	62	1	0	0	0	3	0	0	0	0	4	3	2	1	1
5545	1	1	4	15	56	1	0	0	0	3	0	0	0	0	4	3	2	1	1
5546	16	3	13	285	47	0	4	0	0	0	0	1	2	1	1	1	0	1	0
5547	12	2	0	127	5	0	10	0	0	0	0	0	0	0	0	0	1	0	0
5548	16	2	6	266	48	6	14	3	1	1	1	0	1	2	1	1	0	1	1
5549	1	0	2	281	51	1	1	3	0	0	0	0	0	1	1	1	0	1	0
5550	3	0	2	270	17	2	2	0	0	0	0	0	0	0	0	1	0	1	0
5551	10	2	23	306	11	3	10	0	0	0	0	0	0	1	0	1	0	0	2
5552	16	2	0	285	14	0	3	0	0	0	0	1	0	0	0	0	0	0	0
5553	5	4	2	14	47	0	0	0	1	3	0	0	1	2	3	3	1	0	1
5554	0	0	0	65	10	0	0	4	0	0	0	0	0	0	0	0	0	0	0
5555	11	2	8	218	35	3	2	0	0	0	0	0	0	1	0	1	0	1	0
5556	3	0	5	306	35	3	2	0	0	0	0	0	0	1	0	1	0	1	0
5557	1	0	1	273	52	0	1	0	1	1	0	1	0	1	1	1	1	1	0
5558	0	0	0	1	10	0	0	0	0	0	0	0	0	0	0	0	1	0	0
5559	1	1	3	12	45	1	0	1	1	2	0	0	1	2	3	2	1	0	1
5600	0	0	0	4	128	4	1	14	3	3	2	2	5	0	2	2	4	4	1
5601	0	0	0	53	205	0	1	3	1	2	1	2	10	0	1	3	4	3	2
5602	0	0	0	208	640	1	0	1	0	2	1	4	8	0	4	3	2	2	1
5603	0	0	0	498	188	21	1	66	2	3	2	8	11	0	7	3	3	4	1
5604	0	0	0	459	157	6	0	0	2	3	2	10	12	0	4	2	2	2	1
5605	0	0	0	14	159	0	0	26	1	1	1	3	2	0	4	2	5	4	1
5606	0	0	0	405	164	3	2	9	2	1	2	3	1	0	1	1	2	1	1
5607	0	0	0	7	164	3	2	9	2	1	2	3	1	0	1	1	2	1	1
5608	0	0	0	11	129	2	0	34	2	2	1	5	4	0	1	2	2	2	1
5609	0	0	0	196	177	1	1	6	2	2	1	2	3	0	3	2	2	2	1
5610	0	0	0	1	49	1	0	2	1	1	0	1	1	0	0	1	1	1	0
5611	0	0	0	7	139	2	1	13	2	1	1	2	1	0	1	1	2	2	0
5612	0	0	0	4	60	2	0	13	1	1	1	2	2	0	0	1	1	1	1
5613	0	0	0	474	43	1	0	1	0	1	0	0	0	0	0	1	1	1	0
5614	0	0	0	12	15	1	0	1	0	0	0	0	0	0	0	1	1	1	0
5615	0	0	0	572	170	1	1	13	0	2	0	0	1	0	3	2	0	2	0
5616	1	0	0	993	31	2	0	2	0	2	1	1	0	0	0	2	2	6	1
5617	0	0	0	56	2	0	0	0	0	0	0	0	0	0	0	0	0	0	0
5618	0	0	0	5	10	0	0	1	0	1	0	0	0	0	0	0	0	1	0
5619	0	0	0	766	88	2	1	4	2	1	2	4	4	0	1	1	2	20	3
5620	0	0	0	1138	8	0	0	0	2	3	2	5	3	0	2	1	1	3	1

Soups, Sauces, Fats, Misc.

Food No.	Food Description & Amount	wt gm	wt oz	cal	% cal fat	prot gm	carbo gm	fiber gm
5621	Horseradish [2 Tbs]	30	1.1	16	33%	0	3	3.0
5622	Hotdog relish (Include chow chow, Mustard pickles) [2 Tbs]	31	1.1	36	7%	0	8	0.5
5623	Mushrooms, pickled [½ cup]	78	2.8	18	14%	1	4	0.8
5624	Mustard (Include horseradish mustard, Chinese mustard) [1 Tbs]	15	0.5	11	53%	1	1	0.4
5625	Mustard sauce [2 Tbs]	20	0.7	50	84%	0	2	0.2
5626	Okra, pickled [5 pods]	55	1.9	19	2%	1	4	1.5
5627	Olives, green [½ cup]	67	2.3	77	99%	1	1	0.7
5628	Olives, green, stuffed [½ cup]	73	2.6	76	96%	1	1	0.8
5629	Olives, ripe [10 small]	34	1.2	36	82%	0	2	1.0
5630	Pepper, hot, pickled (Include pickled jalapeno pepper; hot pepper) [½ cup]	56	2.0	27	3%	1	7	0.7
5631	Peppers, hot, sauce (Include Tabasco sauce) [1 Tbs]	15	0.5	3	5%	0	1	0.3
5632	Peppers, pickled [½ cup]	68	2.4	27	4%	1	7	1.1
5633	Pickled green bananas, Puerto Rican style (Guineos verdes en escabeche) [½ cup]	75	2.6	242	83%	1	12	1.3
5634	Pickles, mixed [½ cup]	78	2.7	106	3%	0	29	0.9
5635	Radishes, pickled, Hawaiian style [½ cup]	75	2.6	17	12%	1	3	1.7
5636	Recaito (Puerto Rican little coriander) (Include Recaito congelado) [½ cup]	120	4.2	24	26%	3	3	2.8
5637	Seaweed, pickled [2 Tbs]	19	0.7	28	1%	0	7	0.1
5638	Tomato chili sauce (catsup-type) [2 Tbs]	34	1.2	35	3%	1	8	2.0
5639	Tomato relish (Include tomato preserves) [2 Tbs]	40	1.4	58	2%	1	15	0.7
5640	Tsukemono, Japanese pickles (Include nara zuke, takuan zuke, wasabi zuke) [½ cup]	68	2.4	15	8%	1	3	1.8
5641	Turnip, pickled [½ cup]	78	2.7	32	3%	1	8	1.2
5642	Vegetable relish [½ cup]	70	2.5	25	5%	1	6	0.6
5643	Vegetables, pickled (Include giardiniera) [½ cup]	82	2.9	22	5%	1	5	1.7
5644	Vegetables, pickled, Hawaiian style [½ cup]	75	2.6	19	13%	1	4	2.0
5645	Zucchini, pickled [½ cup]	85	3.0	30	6%	1	7	1.0
	Miscellaneous Foods							
5700	Adobo fresco (Include adobo criollo, creole seasoning) [2 Tbs]	36	1.3	81	83%	1	7	0.5
5701	Ensure Plus liquid nutrition [1 cup]	252	8.9	365	33%	14	50	0.0
5702	Ensure with fiber, liquid [1 cup]	248	8.7	253	30%	9	37	3.2
5703	Formulated diet meal, powdered, soy protein isolate, with herbs (Include Optimum Plus) [1 oz]	28	1.0	39	32%	1	5	0.3
5704	Gelatin, plain, drink [1 cup]	244	8.6	19	0%	5	0	0.0
5705	Gelatin, plain, powder, dry [1 envelope (1 Tbs)]	7	0.2	23	0%	6	0	0.0
5706	Gelatin, plain, prepared [1 package, prepared]	480	16.9	283	0%	6	67	0.0
5707	Hi-protein wafers (Include hi-protein oatmeal wafer) [25 wafers]	60	2.1	200	11%	25	23	1.6
5708	Lecithin [1 Tbs]	8	0.3	61	100%	0	0	0.0
5709	Meal replacement or supplement, liquid, predigested protein (Include Pro-Linn, E.M.F.) [1 fl oz]	37	1.3	70	0%	17	0	0.0
5710	Meal replacement or supplement, liquid, soy-base, high protein (Include Ensure liquid nutrition) [1 cup]	252	8.9	350	32%	13	47	2.5
5711	Meal replacement or supplement, liquid, soy-based (Include Isocal liquid nutrition) [1 cup]	247	8.7	262	35%	8	31	0.5
5712	Meal replacement, soy-milk base, powder, reconstituted [1 cup]	218	7.7	267	33%	9	34	1.3
5713	Meal supplement or replacement, gelatin-based, powder, not reconstituted (Include Physicians Weight Loss Chicken Nutrient) [1 packet]	15	0.5	51	0%	11	1	0.1
5714	Meal supplement or replacement, gelatin-based, powder, reconstituted (Include Physicians Weight Loss Chicken Nutrient) [1 cup]	252	8.9	69	0%	15	2	0.1
5715	Protein diet powder with soy and casein (Include Nature Slim, Herbalife) [1 serving]	20	0.7	78	8%	11	6	0.2
5716	Protein powder [1 Tbs]	28	1.0	112	20%	9	14	1.4
5717	Protein supplement, powdered (Include Shaklee Instant Protein, Trim n' Easy, Slender Now, Slender, MLV Protein Additive) [3 Tbs]	28	1.0	109	8%	16	8	1.4
5718	Protein supplement, tablets (Include milk tablets) [10 tablets]	10	0.4	40	8%	6	3	0.5

Food no.	fat gm	sat fat gm	choles mg	sodium mg	potas mg	% of Daily Value													
						vit A	vit E	vit C	thia	ribo	niac	vit B-6	fola	vit B-12	calc	phos	mag	iron	zinc
5621	1	0	0	94	74	0	0	2	0	0	1	1	4	0	2	1	2	1	2
5622	0	0	0	161	61	0	0	3	0	0	0	0	0	0	1	1	2	2	0
5623	0	0	0	3	232	0	0	3	4	16	12	3	2	0	0	6	2	5	3
5624	1	0	0	188	20	0	1	0	1	0	0	1	0	0	1	1	1	2	1
5625	5	1	0	61	17	0	4	0	0	0	0	0	0	0	0	0	1	1	0
5626	0	0	0	4	135	3	1	13	5	2	2	4	7	0	4	3	7	2	2
5627	8	1	0	1596	37	2	9	0	0	0	0	0	0	0	4	1	4	6	1
5628	8	1	0	1518	51	5	9	15	0	0	0	1	1	0	4	1	4	7	1
5629	3	0	0	299	3	1	5	1	0	0	0	0	0	0	3	0	0	6	0
5630	0	0	0	469	150	23	1	163	3	2	2	6	3	0	1	2	3	3	1
5631	0	0	0	4	85	1	0	17	0	0	1	1	0	0	0	0	0	0	0
5632	0	0	0	1	105	16	2	117	2	1	1	7	3	0	1	1	2	1	1
5633	22	3	0	1	184	0	13	6	2	2	1	12	2	0	1	2	4	2	1
5634	0	0	0	662	20	1	0	1	0	2	1	1	0	0	0	1	1	4	1
5635	0	0	0	592	250	0	0	0	1	1	1	4	2	0	2	2	2	1	1
5636	1	0	0	32	553	32	14	12	5	8	4	5	2	0	11	4	7	12	3
5637	0	0	0	27	36	1	0	1	0	1	0	0	2	0	1	1	2	2	0
5638	0	0	0	457	126	2	5	9	2	1	3	3	4	0	1	2	1	2	0
5639	0	0	0	947	157	6	1	39	2	1	1	3	1	0	2	2	3	3	0
5640	0	0	0	360	400	1	0	0	0	1	1	3	4	0	3	2	2	1	1
5641	0	0	0	33	115	3	0	24	2	1	1	3	2	0	2	2	2	1	1
5642	0	0	0	6	124	2	0	9	2	1	1	2	2	0	1	2	2	2	1
5643	0	0	0	166	174	56	1	47	3	2	2	6	3	0	2	2	2	2	1
5644	0	0	0	795	148	3	0	0	2	3	2	7	6	0	3	2	2	2	1
5645	0	0	0	3	170	5	1	22	3	1	1	4	3	0	1	3	4	2	1
5700	8	1	0	6175	67	1	4	3	1	1	1	0	0	0	4	1	2	6	1
5701	13	2	0	287	532	9	24	89	35	36	36	35	36	36	18	18	18	18	27
5702	8	1	0	193	389	25	30	83	25	25	25	25	25	26	17	17	17	17	25
5703	1	0	0	27	49	2	0	7	5	4	4	4	1	4	2	2	2	2	4
5704	0	0	0	18	1	0	0	0	0	1	0	0	0	0	1	0	1	0	1
5705	0	0	0	14	1	0	0	0	0	1	0	0	1	0	0	0	0	0	0
5706	0	0	0	202	5	0	0	0	0	1	0	0	0	0	1	11	1	1	1
5707	3	0	0	406	235	0	0	0	7	4	4	1	26	0	12	47	6	48	16
5708	8	1	0	0	0	0	2	0	0	0	0	0	0	0	0	0	0	0	0
5709	0	0	0	281	73	12	0	12	11	1	6	0	8	0	16	14	5	7	5
5710	12	2	0	247	444	18	1	61	42	37	37	37	12	37	15	15	18	18	37
5711	10	3	0	131	326	6	9	65	33	33	32	32	13	33	16	13	13	13	17
5712	10	2	0	165	336	11	4	55	33	31	30	30	11	30	13	12	14	14	24
5713	0	0	0	262	46	0	0	1	1	1	1	1	1	1	7	2	2	1	0
5714	0	0	0	359	62	0	0	1	1	1	1	1	2	1	10	3	3	1	1
5715	1	0	0	131	76	0	0	0	92	85	35	18	9	1	35	18	2	49	5
5716	3	0	0	431	112	19	1	19	17	2	10	0	12	0	25	22	8	11	8
5717	1	0	0	183	106	0	0	0	128	119	49	25	12	0	12	25	3	69	7
5718	0	0	0	68	39	0	0	0	48	44	18	9	4	0	18	9	1	26	3

Soups, Sauces, Fats, Misc.

Food No.	Food Description & Amount	wt gm	wt oz	cal	% cal fat	prot gm	carbo gm	fiber gm
5719	Textured vegetable protein, dry [2 Tbs]	8	0.3	28	3%	4	3	1.5
5720	Vinegar [2 Tbs]	30	1.1	4	0%	0	2	0.0
5721	Yeast (Include brewers yeast) [1 Tbs, dry]	8	0.3	24	14%	3	3	1.7
5722	Yeast extract spread (Include Vegemite, Marmite, Promite) [1 tsp]	6	0.2	10	0%	2	1	0.2
	Your Additions							

						% of Daily Value													
Food no.	fat gm	sat fat gm	choles mg	sodium mg	potas mg	vit A	vit E	vit C	thia	ribo	niac	vit B-6	fola	vit B-12	calc	phos	mag	iron	zinc
5719	0	0	0	2	203	0	0	0	4	1	1	2	6	0	2	6	6	4	1
5720	0	0	0	0	30	0	0	0	0	0	0	0	0	0	0	0	2	1	0
5721	0	0	0	4	160	0	0	0	13	26	16	6	47	0	1	10	2	7	3
5722	0	0	0	216	156	0	0	0	39	50	29	4	15	1	1	1	3	1	1

Mixed Dishes and Fast Foods

Mixed Dishes & Fast Foods

Food No.	Food Description & Amount	wt gm	wt oz	cal	% cal fat	prot gm	carbo gm	fiber gm
	Beef and Veal Dishes							
6000	Beef and barbecue sauce [1 cup]	263	9.3	457	41%	56	8	0.7
6001	Beef and cream or white sauce [1 cup]	256	9.0	368	55%	25	15	0.3
6002	Beef and macaroni with cheese sauce (mixture) [1 cup]	246	8.7	348	42%	21	27	0.8
6003	Beef and noodles with sauce made from cream of mushroom soup [1 cup]	249	8.8	373	36%	33	25	1.0
6004	Beef and noodles with cream or white sauce [1 cup]	249	8.8	390	45%	27	25	0.8
6005	Beef and noodles with gravy [1 cup]	249	8.8	302	28%	31	21	1.1
6006	Beef and noodles with tomato-based sauce (Include beef casserole; Hamburger Helper; Hamburger Helper Chili Tomato; Hamburger Helper Lasagna) [1 cup]	249	8.8	275	23%	29	24	2.1
6007	Beef and noodles, seasoned, no sauce (Include Hamburger Helper Beef Noodle) [1 cup]	156	5.5	262	29%	24	21	0.9
6008	Beef and potatoes with sauce made from cream of mushroom soup [1 cup]	252	8.9	325	35%	27	24	1.8
6009	Beef and potatoes with cheese sauce [1 cup]	249	8.8	510	55%	34	23	2.4
6010	Beef and potatoes with cream or white sauce (Include Hamburger Helper Potato Stroganoff) [1 cup]	252	8.9	304	35%	25	23	1.4
6011	Beef and potatoes with gravy in pie crust [1/6 of 8" square]	216	7.6	321	37%	18	32	2.5
6012	Beef and potatoes, seasoned, but no sauce [1 cup]	190	6.7	284	26%	30	21	1.9
6013	Beef and rice with sauce made from cream of mushroom soup [1 cup]	248	8.7	412	45%	21	34	0.7
6014	Beef and rice with cream sauce [1 cup]	248	8.7	417	44%	20	37	0.6
6015	Beef and rice with gravy [1 cup]	222	7.8	292	34%	18	30	0.7
6016	Beef and rice with tomato-based sauce, onions [1 cup]	244	8.6	307	29%	20	35	3.0
6017	Beef, sweet and sour (beef, pineapple, sweet and sour sauce) [1 cup]	252	8.9	336	49%	16	28	1.7
6018	Beef and vegetables (no carrots, broccoli, dark-green leafy, or potatoes), sauce made from cream of mushroom soup [1 cup]	252	8.9	360	57%	26	12	2.4
6019	Beef and vegetables (no carrots, broccoli, dark-green leafy, or potatoes), gravy [1 cup]	252	8.9	223	22%	27	15	3.9
6020	Beef and vegetables (no carrots, broccoli, dark-green leafy, or potatoes), seasoned, but no sauce [1 cup]	162	5.7	238	47%	15	17	1.7
6021	Beef and vegetables (no carrots, broccoli, dark-green leafy, or potatoes), soy-based sauce [1 cup]	217	7.7	247	42%	16	21	4.0
6022	Beef and vegetables (no carrots, broccoli, dark-green leafy, or potatoes), tomato-based sauce [1 cup]	249	8.8	288	54%	22	12	2.2
6023	Beef and vegetables (Including carrots, broccoli, and/or dark-green leafy, no potatoes), sauce made from cream of mushroom soup [1 cup]	252	8.9	369	54%	25	16	3.3
6024	Beef and vegetables (Including carrots, broccoli, and/or dark-green leafy, no potatoes), gravy [1 cup]	252	8.9	216	25%	28	11	2.1
6025	Beef and vegetables (Including carrots, broccoli, and/or dark-green leafy, no potatoes), seasoned, but no sauce [1 cup]	162	5.7	244	48%	16	17	1.8
6026	Beef and vegetables (Including carrots, broccoli, and/or dark-green leafy, no potatoes), soy-based sauce [1 cup]	217	7.7	196	47%	16	11	3.9
6027	Beef and vegetables (Including carrots, broccoli, and/or dark-green leafy, no potatoes), tomato-based sauce [1 cup]	249	8.8	183	25%	24	9	2.3
6028	Beef and vegetables, Hawaiian style (Includes seaweed, bamboo shoots, taro, carrots, burdock root, soy sauce) [1 cup]	252	8.9	212	16%	10	37	4.9
6029	Beef in barbeque sauce on bun (Include Sloppy Joe) [1 beef with sauce on bun]	186	6.6	358	37%	18	36	2.4
6030	Beef bourguignonne [1 cup]	244	8.6	200	38%	21	9	1.6
6031	Beef burgundy [1 cup]	244	8.6	291	36%	35	9	1.4
6032	Beef chow mein or chop suey with noodles [1 cup]	220	7.8	421	51%	22	31	3.7
6033	Beef chow mein or chop suey, no noodles [1 cup]	220	7.8	271	50%	22	12	2.7
6034	Beef curry [1 cup]	236	8.3	436	65%	27	13	2.7
6035	Beef goulash with noodles [1 cup]	249	8.8	361	35%	30	27	1.7
6036	Beef goulash with potatoes [1 cup]	244	8.6	299	37%	27	19	1.9
6037	Beef goulash [1 cup]	249	8.8	270	39%	33	7	1.0
6038	Beef hash, made from roast beef [1 cup]	190	6.7	312	46%	21	21	2.3
6039	Meat loaf, beef (Include meatball or patty, with breading, no sauce) [1 slice]	108	3.8	231	54%	18	7	0.4

Food No.	fat gm	sat fat gm	choles mg	sodium mg	potas mg	% of Daily Value: vit A	vit E	vit C	thia	ribo	niac	vit B-6	fola	vit B-12	calc	phos	mag	iron	zinc
6000	21	8	160	632	913	5	4	7	11	23	41	31	4	113	4	46	15	36	85
6001	22	6	68	300	585	22	11	2	12	30	18	13	3	43	20	35	11	17	29
6002	16	7	61	704	265	4	1	1	19	23	20	6	3	19	10	19	9	15	27
6003	15	5	100	651	518	2	5	1	15	21	27	20	4	51	7	35	12	22	35
6004	20	6	80	240	500	17	9	2	17	25	21	17	4	42	16	34	12	17	26
6005	9	3	91	606	453	0	1	0	16	16	26	19	4	47	2	29	10	22	35
6006	7	2	86	667	740	10	7	21	18	17	28	25	5	45	3	29	14	22	30
6007	8	2	82	74	320	2	2	0	15	13	21	16	3	38	1	24	9	18	25
6008	13	4	76	561	579	1	4	12	11	18	22	25	5	44	5	27	10	19	47
6009	31	14	115	885	761	12	4	12	10	26	33	28	6	51	31	43	14	16	43
6010	12	4	65	164	690	10	4	11	14	23	19	26	4	39	15	31	12	14	37
6011	13	3	38	462	563	3	7	12	17	15	22	23	5	23	3	19	9	14	25
6012	8	3	88	62	589	0	1	13	11	16	23	28	5	49	2	27	10	20	52
6013	21	7	61	803	345	3	7	2	12	16	28	13	3	34	10	22	8	17	29
6014	20	7	55	409	351	6	7	1	17	18	25	14	3	31	14	23	9	16	24
6015	11	4	47	878	247	0	1	0	13	8	24	11	2	25	2	15	6	16	26
6016	10	4	47	83	825	15	15	21	17	12	28	22	4	26	3	23	14	22	20
6017	18	6	54	930	336	3	5	36	8	11	13	16	3	27	3	15	8	15	26
6018	23	8	88	801	506	2	5	10	5	16	31	16	9	46	6	22	9	19	38
6019	5	2	71	853	416	4	2	18	16	17	20	17	11	38	4	26	10	22	45
6020	12	4	49	271	380	6	4	33	6	10	21	13	8	25	2	14	7	12	22
6021	11	2	39	464	458	7	9	27	10	15	14	13	10	27	5	17	11	17	20
6022	17	7	75	732	742	14	10	94	9	14	32	26	6	38	3	19	11	17	31
6023	22	8	86	638	653	190	6	14	9	16	33	20	7	45	6	23	9	17	36
6024	6	2	81	91	462	66	2	9	10	17	18	18	6	43	4	25	8	20	48
6025	13	4	51	283	403	35	4	34	7	11	22	13	8	26	3	15	8	12	22
6026	10	3	44	339	457	161	11	79	6	14	11	18	11	18	6	16	8	14	31
6027	5	2	70	116	473	93	2	16	8	14	16	18	5	37	4	22	8	17	42
6028	4	1	13	1747	811	79	10	11	11	13	17	20	21	10	11	20	22	15	13
6029	15	5	46	1008	368	7	6	10	19	16	29	11	5	25	9	15	9	20	21
6030	8	2	56	112	549	3	3	7	7	13	16	16	5	41	3	23	10	16	32
6031	12	3	94	114	844	1	5	7	13	29	34	22	6	68	3	38	13	27	53
6032	24	5	43	950	519	10	8	33	24	21	29	20	11	28	4	26	14	23	23
6033	15	4	50	924	556	12	9	39	12	15	21	21	11	33	4	24	10	16	23
6034	31	7	69	802	978	37	27	41	12	20	27	24	5	51	4	29	15	24	40
6035	14	3	95	130	549	2	11	7	19	19	29	19	5	45	2	32	13	23	31
6036	12	3	65	179	912	2	11	29	11	16	27	26	6	42	2	29	13	19	29
6037	12	3	84	225	698	3	8	15	10	18	29	23	5	54	2	34	11	20	35
6038	16	5	57	470	587	0	6	12	11	12	19	25	4	30	2	20	9	14	33
6039	14	5	90	133	295	2	1	1	5	16	20	7	3	28	4	16	6	11	24

Mixed Dishes & Fast Foods

Food No.	Food Description & Amount	wt gm	wt oz	cal	% cal fat	prot gm	carbo gm	fiber gm
6040	Beef roll, stuffed with vegetables or meat mixture (Include roulades, paupiettes, bracciola) [1 beef roll]	134	4.7	279	46%	27	9	1.0
6041	Beef salad [1 cup]	182	6.4	495	70%	33	2	0.8
6042	Beef shishkabob [1 shishkabob]	202	7.1	178	27%	24	9	2.1
6043	Sloppy Joe (not including bun) [1 cup]	251	8.9	402	51%	28	23	2.4
6044	Beef steak with onions, Puerto Rican style (Biftec encebollado) (Include Puerto Rican style stewed steak) [1 cup]	179	6.3	589	69%	38	7	1.4
6045	Beef stew, from dried beef, Puerto Rican style (Tasajo guisado, carne cecina guisada) [1 cup]	200	7.1	491	67%	34	6	1.0
6046	Beef stew, seasoned ground beef with potatoes, Mexican style (Picadillo de carne de rez con papas) [1 cup]	222	7.8	385	63%	24	10	1.4
6047	Beef stew, Mexican style, no potatoes, tomato-based sauce (Carne guisada sin papas) [1 cup]	244	8.6	455	35%	57	14	2.0
6048	Beef stew, Mexican style, no potatoes, tomato-based sauce with chili peppers (Carne guisada con chile) [1 cup]	244	8.6	386	31%	45	21	3.2
6049	Beef stew, Puerto Rican style, meat with gravy [1 cup]	235	8.3	437	68%	30	3	0.6
6050	Beef stew, Puerto-Rican style (Carne a la Judia) [1 cup]	195	6.9	422	59%	29	13	1.6
6051	Beef stew with potatoes and vegetables (no carrots, broccoli, dark-green leafy), gravy [1 cup]	252	8.9	298	40%	25	18	2.4
6052	Beef stew with potatoes and vegetables (no carrots, broccoli, dark-green leafy), tomato-based sauce [1 cup]	252	8.9	292	40%	25	19	2.5
6053	Beef stew with potatoes and vegetables (including carrots, broccoli, and/or dark-green leafy), gravy [1 cup]	252	8.9	176	18%	17	19	2.9
6054	Beef stew with potatoes and vegetables (including carrots, broccoli, and/or dark-green leafy), tomato-based sauce (Include meatball stew) [1 cup]	252	8.9	176	18%	17	20	3.1
6055	Beef stew with potatoes, gravy [1 cup]	252	8.9	221	21%	23	20	1.8
6056	Beef stew with potatoes, tomato-based sauce [1 cup]	252	8.9	230	20%	23	22	2.1
6057	Beef stroganoff with noodles (Include Hamburger Helper Beef Stroganoff) [1 cup]	256	9.0	344	50%	20	23	1.5
6058	Beef stroganoff [1 cup]	256	9.0	408	60%	26	16	1.4
6059	Beef wellington [1 slice]	116	4.1	355	57%	25	12	0.5
6060	Beef with tomato-based sauce (Include beef with tomatoes, meatballs with tomato sauce) [1 cup]	249	8.8	449	62%	32	10	2.1
6061	Beef and dumplings and vegetables (no carrots, broccoli, dark-green leafy), gravy [1 cup]	249	8.8	269	41%	19	21	2.6
6062	Beef and dumplings and vegetables (including carrots, broccoli, and/or dark-green leafy), gravy [1 cup]	249	8.8	230	43%	16	17	2.1
6063	Ground beef patty (Includes egg and onion) [1 patty]	85	3.0	218	59%	20	1	0.1
6064	Beef and noodles and vegetables (no carrots, broccoli, dark-green leafy), sauce of cream of mushroom soup [1 cup]	249	8.8	342	52%	18	23	2.0
6065	Beef and noodles and vegetables (no carrots, broccoli, dark-green leafy), gravy [1 cup]	249	8.8	276	36%	19	25	2.8
6066	Beef and noodles and vegetables (no carrots, broccoli, dark-green leafy), seasoned, but no sauce [1 cup]	162	5.7	206	23%	19	20	2.3
6067	Beef and noodles and vegetables (no carrots, broccoli, dark-green leafy), soy-based sauce [1 cup]	217	7.7	226	28%	12	28	2.0
6068	Beef and noodles and vegetables (no carrots, broccoli, dark-green leafy), tomato-based sauce [1 cup]	249	8.8	231	18%	20	27	2.6
6069	Beef and noodles and vegetables (including carrots, broccoli, and/or dark-green leafy), sauce made with cream of mushroom soup [1 cup]	249	8.8	342	52%	18	23	2.1
6070	Beef and noodles and vegetables (including carrots, broccoli, and/or dark-green leafy), gravy [1 cup]	249	8.8	269	38%	18	24	2.4
6071	Beef and noodles and vegetables (including carrots, broccoli, and/or dark-green leafy), seasoned, but no sauce [1 cup]	162	5.7	205	23%	19	20	2.4
6072	Beef and noodles and vegetables (including carrots, broccoli, and/or dark-green leafy), soy-based sauce [1 cup]	217	7.7	222	28%	13	27	2.4
6073	Beef and noodles and vegetables (including carrots, broccoli, and/or dark-green leafy), tomato-based sauce [1 cup]	249	8.8	215	17%	18	26	2.9

Food No.	fat gm	sat fat gm	choles mg	sodium mg	potas mg	% of Daily Value													
						vit A	vit E	vit C	thia	ribo	niac	vit B-6	fola	vit B-12	calc	phos	mag	iron	zinc
6040	14	5	76	218	492	36	2	5	14	16	23	22	4	46	2	25	8	16	28
6041	39	9	130	291	418	3	18	5	7	19	15	26	5	45	4	27	7	23	73
6042	5	2	58	59	626	6	3	55	10	13	20	23	6	40	2	23	9	15	25
6043	23	9	97	1100	935	11	9	30	9	17	38	25	7	53	5	24	13	22	40
6044	45	12	114	84	643	0	23	7	10	17	27	30	6	68	3	35	11	21	40
6045	37	7	56	4465	673	4	29	18	7	15	30	14	4	37	2	23	12	31	40
6046	27	11	97	95	625	3	2	47	7	18	30	17	5	38	2	21	9	16	35
6047	18	6	157	591	1301	6	8	18	20	36	49	36	7	113	4	57	21	41	86
6048	13	4	118	450	1363	13	10	409	21	33	42	41	11	84	5	48	23	38	67
6049	33	12	109	226	370	2	5	14	7	16	19	18	3	54	2	25	7	20	50
6050	28	9	86	291	868	3	11	24	10	15	28	25	4	45	2	30	12	19	30
6051	13	6	67	110	591	2	1	19	9	12	16	14	6	31	2	22	9	19	41
6052	13	5	65	138	620	3	1	24	9	12	17	14	6	30	3	22	9	19	40
6053	4	1	39	114	654	71	2	20	11	12	17	17	6	28	3	19	9	14	24
6054	4	1	38	140	686	71	2	24	12	12	18	17	7	28	3	19	10	15	24
6055	5	2	58	73	869	0	1	25	11	15	23	23	5	42	2	25	11	18	34
6056	5	2	58	188	794	2	2	26	12	14	24	26	5	42	2	25	12	17	34
6057	19	7	74	468	394	7	7	2	14	18	19	10	4	30	7	24	9	18	24
6058	27	11	85	677	556	10	11	3	12	23	23	14	5	43	9	31	10	20	33
6059	22	7	94	80	361	2	6	1	12	25	21	17	6	44	1	23	7	24	30
6060	31	12	114	403	808	10	8	36	8	19	44	24	5	55	5	26	12	23	46
6061	12	5	44	908	353	2	2	8	13	13	22	10	6	23	8	18	6	17	26
6062	11	4	41	820	350	62	2	4	8	11	19	11	4	21	6	15	5	14	24
6063	14	6	102	74	250	1	1	1	2	11	23	11	3	39	1	15	4	11	28
6064	20	8	69	769	279	6	5	5	8	15	18	9	5	21	17	23	8	14	23
6065	11	5	58	795	331	2	1	8	13	11	22	10	6	22	3	18	7	18	27
6066	5	2	64	82	258	3	1	10	14	12	15	12	6	26	3	19	8	17	30
6067	7	1	45	592	275	2	5	32	13	10	15	12	5	15	2	15	8	13	12
6068	5	1	62	315	503	6	3	24	18	15	21	14	8	31	3	22	11	20	27
6069	20	8	68	775	286	43	6	5	8	14	18	10	4	21	17	23	8	13	22
6070	11	5	59	788	336	40	2	4	10	11	21	11	4	22	3	16	7	17	26
6071	5	2	64	80	264	41	1	8	14	12	15	13	6	26	3	19	8	17	30
6072	7	1	43	584	286	28	6	28	13	10	14	12	8	15	4	15	9	13	12
6073	4	1	55	288	516	60	3	24	17	14	19	14	7	27	4	21	11	18	24

Mixed Dishes & Fast Foods

Food No.	Food Description & Amount	wt gm	wt oz	cal	% cal fat	prot gm	carbo gm	fiber gm
6074	Beef and potatoes and vegetables (no carrots, broccoli, dark-green leafy), sauce made with cream of mushroom soup [1 cup]	252	8.9	402	52%	27	21	2.2
6075	Beef and potatoes and vegetables (no carrots, broccoli, dark-green leafy), seasoned, but no sauce [1 cup]	162	5.7	183	23%	19	16	2.6
6076	Beef and potatoes and vegetables (including carrots, broccoli, and/or dark-green leafy), sauce made with cream of mushroom soup [1 cup]	252	8.9	403	51%	27	22	2.4
6077	Beef and potatoes and vegetables (including carrots, broccoli, and/or dark-green leafy), no sauce [1 cup]	162	5.7	182	24%	18	16	2.7
6078	Beef and rice and vegetables (no carrots, broccoli, dark-green leafy), sauce made with cream of mushroom soup [1 cup]	249	8.8	363	43%	21	30	2.0
6079	Beef and rice and vegetables (no carrots, broccoli, dark-green leafy), gravy [1 cup]	249	8.8	313	44%	21	22	2.1
6080	Beef and rice and vegetables (no carrots, broccoli, dark-green leafy), seasoned, but no sauce [1 cup]	162	5.7	204	20%	18	22	1.9
6081	Beef and rice and vegetables (no carrots, broccoli, dark-green leafy), soy-based sauce [1 cup]	217	7.7	209	35%	13	21	1.4
6082	Beef and rice and vegetables (no carrots, broccoli, dark-green leafy), tomato-based sauce [1 cup]	249	8.8	210	14%	16	28	2.9
6083	Beef and rice and vegetables (including carrots, broccoli, and/or dark-green leafy), sauce made with mushroom soup [1 cup]	249	8.8	367	42%	21	31	2.3
6084	Beef and rice and vegetables (including carrots, broccoli, and/or dark-green leafy), gravy [1 cup]	249	8.8	334	44%	22	23	2.2
6085	Beef and rice and vegetables (including carrots, broccoli, and/or dark-green leafy), seasoned, but no sauce [1 cup]	162	5.7	203	20%	18	22	2.0
6086	Beef and rice and vegetables (including carrots, broccoli, and/or dark-green leafy), soy-based sauce [1 cup]	217	7.7	200	34%	12	21	2.0
6087	Beef and rice and vegetables (including carrots, broccoli, and/or dark-green leafy), tomato-based sauce [1 cup]	249	8.8	213	15%	17	28	2.5
6088	Beef and tofu and vegetables (no carrots, broccoli, dark-green leafy, or potatoes), soy-based sauce [1 cup]	217	7.7	277	46%	23	17	3.1
6089	Beef and tofu and vegetables (including carrots, broccoli, and/or dark-green leafy (no potatoes)), soy-based sauce [1 cup]	217	7.7	272	47%	22	16	2.6
6090	Brunswick stew [1 cup]	243	8.6	321	39%	29	19	2.8
6091	Chili con carne without beans [1 cup]	254	9.0	351	48%	25	21	3.7
6092	Chili con carne with beans [1 cup]	254	9.0	322	40%	22	27	7.5
6093	Chili con carne with beans and cheese [1 cup]	254	9.0	378	47%	26	25	6.9
6094	Chili con carne (pork) with beans [1 cup]	254	9.0	275	27%	24	27	7.5
6095	Corned beef hash [1 cup]	190	6.7	344	56%	17	20	1.0
6096	Corned beef with tomato sauce and onion, Puerto Rican style [1 cup]	235	8.3	472	55%	45	5	1.0
6097	Corned beef and potatoes and vegetables (no carrots, broccoli, and dark-green leafy), seasoned, but no sauce [1 cup]	162	5.7	180	42%	10	17	2.3
6098	Corned beef and potatoes and vegetables (including carrots, broccoli, and/or dark-green leafy), seasoned, but no sauce [1 cup]	162	5.7	169	40%	9	17	2.6
6099	Creamed chipped or dried beef [1 cup]	246	8.7	328	56%	18	18	0.3
6100	Ground beef patty (Includes onion) with gravy [1 patty with gravy]	115	4.1	138	30%	20	3	0.3
6101	Ground beef with tomato sauce and taco seasonings on a cornbread crust (Include Hamburger Helper Taco Bake) [1 cup]	179	6.3	364	39%	18	37	4.1
6102	Ground beef, stewed seasoned Mexican style (Picadillo de carne de rez) [1 cup]	222	7.8	462	69%	31	3	0.5
6103	Ground beef, stewed seasoned, Puerto Rican style (Picadillo guisado, picadillo de carne) [1 cup]	200	7.1	577	73%	32	5	1.1
6104	Ground beef, stewed seasoned, Puerto Rican style (Picadillo para relleno) [1 cup]	150	5.3	481	70%	30	5	1.1
6105	Liver (beef or calf) and onions, fried, seasoned [1 slice with onions]	143	5.0	215	30%	24	12	0.8
6106	Mexican style beef stew with potatoes, tomato-based sauce (Carne guisada con papas) [1 cup]	244	8.6	274	32%	32	13	1.6
6107	Pepper steak [1 cup]	217	7.7	320	58%	28	6	1.3
6108	Salisbury steak with gravy [1 steak with gravy]	129	4.6	218	56%	16	7	0.4

Food No.	fat gm	sat fat gm	choles mg	sodium mg	potas mg	% of Daily Value													
						vit A	vit E	vit C	thia	ribo	niac	vit B-6	fola	vit B-12	calc	phos	mag	iron	zinc
6074	23	8	89	642	781	0	5	22	8	16	36	23	6	47	5	24	10	19	39
6075	5	2	50	88	418	3	1	16	11	11	15	18	7	28	2	18	8	14	31
6076	23	8	88	628	788	49	5	22	8	16	36	24	6	46	5	24	10	19	38
6077	5	2	50	85	424	44	1	14	10	11	15	19	6	28	3	18	8	14	31
6078	17	6	65	573	417	0	4	5	13	12	30	15	5	34	5	20	8	19	30
6079	15	6	65	359	448	3	4	61	10	11	29	20	6	36	3	18	8	17	27
6080	4	2	46	79	262	3	1	10	14	10	15	13	6	26	3	18	7	16	30
6081	8	2	32	437	307	0	3	11	10	12	16	12	6	13	3	15	7	13	15
6082	3	1	34	306	485	6	3	25	16	12	18	15	9	24	3	19	9	17	23
6083	17	6	65	558	428	61	4	6	14	12	31	15	5	34	5	20	8	19	30
6084	16	6	69	393	488	74	3	8	11	12	31	17	5	38	4	20	8	17	29
6085	4	2	46	77	269	40	1	8	13	10	15	14	5	26	3	17	7	16	30
6086	7	2	29	410	334	45	4	25	10	9	14	13	7	12	3	14	7	12	14
6087	3	1	36	285	521	60	3	24	16	12	19	16	7	26	3	19	10	17	24
6088	14	3	36	1225	433	2	7	13	14	13	12	14	10	28	15	26	37	47	31
6089	14	3	36	1243	442	39	7	6	12	12	11	14	8	29	15	25	36	46	30
6090	14	4	77	393	634	9	5	16	33	18	32	22	7	8	5	26	14	12	20
6091	19	7	81	911	830	16	11	47	13	18	35	23	7	44	6	23	13	22	34
6092	14	5	60	912	765	12	8	35	13	16	27	18	11	32	6	23	14	21	27
6093	20	9	76	965	724	17	8	33	13	19	25	17	11	33	20	32	14	20	29
6094	8	3	51	892	793	12	8	36	45	21	24	22	11	7	7	26	14	16	16
6095	21	7	63	1026	380	0	2	0	1	10	20	8	4	20	2	13	7	21	29
6096	29	11	142	1837	387	3	7	13	4	16	22	14	5	42	3	20	8	21	40
6097	8	3	42	493	344	0	1	22	7	6	12	17	5	12	2	9	6	6	15
6098	8	2	37	452	347	43	1	20	7	6	11	17	5	10	3	9	6	6	13
6099	20	6	33	1469	499	24	11	3	11	27	13	10	4	25	27	28	10	12	18
6100	5	2	54	62	364	0	1	1	6	12	16	11	2	39	1	19	6	13	30
6101	16	5	76	975	414	9	6	16	14	18	24	14	4	25	9	36	9	16	21
6102	35	14	127	121	515	1	2	15	5	22	35	13	3	50	2	24	9	19	44
6103	47	16	126	1219	693	5	14	22	11	22	36	18	4	43	3	29	11	18	41
6104	38	12	105	1185	644	4	12	19	31	21	31	21	3	25	3	29	10	13	29
6105	7	2	424	415	410	943	3	38	14	215	64	66	50	1638	2	42	7	31	33
6106	10	3	87	329	862	4	5	16	12	21	29	24	4	62	2	33	13	24	48
6107	20	4	70	563	550	2	15	45	9	14	22	24	7	48	3	26	9	17	29
6108	14	6	60	438	292	0	1	1	5	14	17	6	2	20	3	14	5	12	24

Mixed Dishes & Fast Foods

Food No.	Food Description & Amount	wt gm	wt oz	cal	% cal fat	prot gm	carbo gm	fiber gm
6109	Soup meat, seasoned, shredded , Puerto Rican style (Ropa vieja, sopa de carne ripiada) [1 cup]	133	4.7	275	56%	24	5	1.2
6110	Steak tartare (raw ground beef seasoned with onion, egg yolk, anchovy) [1 cup]	224	7.9	511	65%	40	1	0.2
6111	Tripe, stewed Puerto Rican style, with potatoes (Mondongo) [1 cup]	280	9.9	318	33%	27	27	5.2
6112	Stuffed cabbage rolls with rice [1 roll]	103	3.6	126	45%	8	9	1.3
6113	Stuffed grape leaves with beef and rice [1 roll]	21	0.7	50	69%	2	2	0.7
6114	Stuffed green pepper, Puerto Rican style (Pimiento relleno) [1 pepper (3½" x 3½" x 2")]	250	8.8	433	40%	22	43	4.6
6115	Stuffed pot roast, Puerto Rican style, with gravy and stuffing [1 slice with gravy and stuffing]	134	4.7	379	70%	26	1	0.2
6116	Swedish meatballs with cream or white sauce [1 cup]	246	8.7	405	51%	31	17	0.6
6117	Swiss steak (floured, braised; cooked with tomato-vegetable sauce) [1 piece with sauce]	170	6.0	177	39%	20	7	1.1
6118	Swiss steak, with gravy [1 steak with gravy]	92	3.2	182	46%	15	8	3.4
6119	Variety meats, stewed Puerto Rican style (mostly liver) (Gandinga) [1 cup]	165	5.8	166	24%	23	8	1.4
6120	Veal and noodles with cream or white sauce [1 cup]	224	7.9	378	47%	27	22	0.7
6121	Veal cordon bleu [1 roll (with ham and sauce)]	229	8.1	476	67%	33	4	0.7
6122	Veal fricassee, Puerto Rican style (ternera en fricase) [1 cup]	230	8.1	391	42%	38	18	2.3
6123	Veal goulash with vegetables (no carrots, broccoli, dark-green leafy, or potatoes), tomato-base sauce (Include veal marengo, veal stew) [1 cup]	252	8.9	243	34%	32	7	1.0
6124	Veal goulash with vegetables (including carrots, broccoli, and/or dark-green leafy (no potatoes)), tomato-base sauce (Include veal marengo, veal stew) [1 cup]	252	8.9	248	34%	33	7	1.1
6125	Veal Marsala [1 slice with sauce]	96	3.4	267	66%	12	6	0.2
6126	Veal parmigiana [1 piece with sauce and cheese]	182	6.4	359	53%	26	16	1.1
6127	Veal scallopini [1 slice with sauce]	96	3.4	238	64%	18	1	0.4
6128	Veal stew with potatoes and vegetables (no carrots, broccoli, or dark-green leafy), tomato-based sauce) [1 cup]	252	8.9	198	30%	16	18	2.5
6129	Veal stew with potatoes and vegetables (including carrots, broccoli, and/or dark-green leafy), tomato-based sauce [1 cup]	252	8.9	190	31%	16	16	2.8
6130	Veal with butter sauce [1 piece with sauce]	99	3.5	156	54%	16	2	0.1
6131	Veal with cream sauce (Include veal paprikash) [1 cup]	246	8.7	281	39%	36	5	0.6
6132	Veal with gravy [1 slice with gravy]	65	2.3	100	44%	12	1	0.1
6133	Veal with vegetables (no carrots, broccoli, dark-green leafy, or potatoes), cream or white sauce [1 cup]	241	8.5	292	46%	30	9	1.2
6134	Veal with vegetables (including carrots, broccoli, and/or dark-green leafy (no potatoes)), cream or white sauce [1 cup]	241	8.5	251	44%	26	9	1.8
	Pork Dishes							
6200	Chitterlings, stewed Puerto Rican style (cuajo guisado) [1 cup]	240	8.5	618	83%	17	11	2.3
6201	Cabbage with ham hocks [1 cup]	200	7.1	191	55%	16	6	3.1
6202	Greens with ham or pork [1 cup]	144	5.1	81	38%	6	7	3.1
6203	Ham and noodles with cream or white sauce [1 cup]	244	8.6	381	39%	27	30	1.0
6204	Ham and noodles, no sauce [1 cup]	157	5.5	239	26%	19	24	1.1
6205	Ham and rice mixed with cream of mushroom soup [1 cup]	248	8.7	332	35%	17	35	0.7
6206	Ham and vegetables (no carrots, broccoli, dark-green leafy, or potatoes), seasoned, but no sauce [1 cup]	162	5.7	220	57%	19	5	2.2
6207	Ham and vegetables (including carrots, broccoli, and/or dark-green leafy (no potatoes)), seasoned, but no sauce [1 cup]	162	5.7	228	55%	19	7	2.1
6208	Ham croquette [1 croquette (1½" x 2")]	62	2.2	151	53%	9	8	0.2
6209	Ham loaf (not luncheon meat) (Include pork meatball, with breading, no sauce) [1 slice]	108	3.8	207	38%	25	6	0.3
6210	Ham or pork and potatoes with cheese sauce [1 cup]	249	8.8	385	52%	26	20	2.0
6211	Ham or pork and potatoes with gravy [1 cup]	252	8.9	255	34%	21	21	1.8
6212	Ham or pork and rice, no sauce [1 cup]	196	6.9	295	22%	21	34	0.5
6213	Ham or pork salad [1 cup]	182	6.4	396	69%	27	2	0.8
6214	Ham or pork with sauce made from cream of mushroom soup [1 slice with sauce]	65	2.3	97	48%	10	2	0.1

Food No.	fat gm	sat fat gm	choles mg	sodium mg	potas mg	vit A	vit E	vit C	thia	ribo	niac	vit B-6	fola	vit B-12	calc	phos	mag	iron	zinc
						% of Daily Value													
6109	17	5	60	64	442	3	8	43	7	11	19	14	4	36	2	25	7	18	35
6110	37	15	240	268	617	5	4	1	9	33	49	29	7	74	4	33	11	24	58
6111	12	3	118	571	1070	14	9	94	15	19	11	21	21	23	5	26	14	24	28
6112	6	2	42	206	293	4	2	23	4	6	10	6	5	11	3	8	5	7	11
6113	4	1	5	15	47	13	2	3	1	2	2	2	1	2	2	2	2	2	2
6114	19	7	61	921	859	16	12	182	26	24	37	29	10	24	12	22	16	29	27
6115	29	10	93	381	260	0	5	1	7	13	16	14	2	42	1	21	5	16	41
6116	23	10	163	407	573	9	1	4	20	31	33	16	5	40	12	33	11	18	37
6117	8	2	49	142	496	21	5	14	8	12	19	14	3	32	3	20	8	13	21
6118	9	1	0	620	136	0	8	0	45	26	37	43	14	29	2	25	4	9	9
6119	4	1	281	92	465	429	4	80	24	165	66	25	34	278	2	30	7	115	37
6120	20	6	105	235	390	15	9	1	14	27	26	11	5	24	16	30	11	11	33
6121	35	19	172	599	503	20	4	8	14	24	49	23	6	27	18	37	11	8	28
6122	18	4	129	760	963	4	16	43	12	23	57	31	8	19	3	31	14	13	29
6123	9	3	115	237	695	3	9	15	8	24	68	26	7	18	2	35	12	9	24
6124	9	3	119	251	736	50	9	15	9	25	71	27	6	18	2	36	12	10	24
6125	19	9	70	144	212	8	4	3	4	9	25	10	2	8	2	13	4	4	9
6126	21	8	145	648	538	13	11	12	11	25	43	21	5	15	20	34	11	12	20
6127	17	5	65	278	253	10	8	1	3	14	26	10	3	15	5	17	5	5	19
6128	7	3	55	160	614	3	2	24	9	13	34	21	7	9	3	19	9	8	14
6129	7	3	55	167	548	60	2	20	9	13	34	20	7	9	4	19	9	8	14
6130	9	5	73	218	197	8	1	0	3	10	24	8	2	9	1	12	3	4	11
6131	12	5	139	158	696	12	4	3	8	29	77	27	6	21	4	40	13	10	27
6132	5	2	43	190	142	0	1	0	2	7	16	6	2	10	1	10	3	3	14
6133	15	6	115	333	545	9	6	4	8	28	50	17	7	22	11	31	11	8	22
6134	12	5	95	309	689	58	7	42	10	29	42	22	25	18	15	28	20	16	21
6200	57	17	214	189	358	8	13	121	6	11	5	13	6	26	6	11	9	35	52
6201	12	4	41	802	320	2	1	45	32	13	17	20	7	7	5	16	6	4	11
6202	3	1	11	528	265	58	5	50	10	7	6	9	3	2	6	6	4	4	4
6203	17	5	70	1466	468	8	7	1	30	28	25	14	3	11	19	34	12	13	19
6204	7	2	63	788	208	3	2	0	38	13	22	15	2	8	2	20	8	12	14
6205	13	4	30	1405	317	3	7	2	31	16	22	15	2	8	10	22	8	12	15
6206	14	5	50	966	392	3	1	20	36	14	20	19	6	9	4	20	7	7	14
6207	14	5	50	998	416	129	3	29	35	14	20	23	3	9	5	20	7	7	14
6208	9	2	18	494	153	5	5	1	17	9	10	8	1	5	5	10	3	4	6
6209	9	3	104	986	355	3	4	6	29	18	24	16	2	10	3	25	6	8	17
6210	22	10	80	1266	688	10	4	11	35	25	26	25	4	13	26	42	12	8	22
6211	10	3	57	651	821	0	2	25	37	16	30	25	4	9	2	26	10	10	16
6212	7	2	39	984	270	3	3	0	46	12	27	22	2	8	2	22	8	12	16
6213	31	6	76	1618	474	3	19	5	49	17	27	36	5	14	3	26	7	7	19
6214	5	2	26	208	162	0	2	1	22	8	10	9	1	5	2	9	3	3	6

Mixed Dishes & Fast Foods

Food No.	Food Description & Amount	wt gm	wt oz	cal	% cal fat	prot gm	carbo gm	fiber gm
6215	Ham or pork with barbecue sauce [1 slice with sauce]	58	2.0	104	46%	12	2	0.1
6216	Ham or pork with gravy [1 slice with gravy]	65	2.3	77	38%	10	2	0.1
6217	Ham or pork with stuffing [1 stuffed pork chop]	155	5.5	287	28%	26	24	1.0
6218	Ham or pork with tomato-based sauce [1 slice with sauce]	65	2.3	85	49%	8	3	0.6
6219	Ham or pork, noodles and vegetables (no carrots, broccoli, or dark-green leafy), cheese sauce [1 cup]	241	8.5	444	44%	33	28	2.5
6220	Ham or pork, noodles, and vegetables (including carrots, broccoli, and/or dark-green leafy), tomato-based sauce [1 cup]	249	8.8	418	43%	31	29	2.9
6221	Ham pot pie [1 piece (1/6 of pie)]	105	3.7	251	54%	9	19	1.3
6222	Ham stroganoff (Include ham with cream or white sauce) [1 cup]	244	8.6	356	63%	21	11	1.4
6223	Ham, potatoes, and vegetables (no carrots, broccoli, or dark-green leafy), no sauce [1 cup]	162	5.7	176	48%	13	10	2.3
6224	Ham, potatoes, and vegetables (including carrots, broccoli, and/or dark-green leafy), no sauce [1 cup]	162	5.7	229	49%	17	11	1.9
6225	Pork and onions with soy-based sauce (mixture) [1 cup]	256	9.0	531	49%	34	35	2.0
6226	Pork and rice with tomato-based sauce [1 cup]	244	8.6	349	29%	25	35	1.2
6227	Pork and vegetables (no carrots, broccoli, dark-green leafy, or potatoes), tomato-based sauce [1 cup]	249	8.8	286	42%	33	7	1.7
6228	Pork and vegetables (no carrots, broccoli, or dark-green leafy), soy-based sauce [1 cup]	217	7.7	259	45%	16	21	4.0
6229	Pork and vegetables (no carrots, broccoli, dark-green leafy, or potatoes), no sauce [1 cup]	162	5.7	211	42%	22	8	2.0
6230	Pork and vegetables (including carrots, broccoli, and/or dark-green leafy (no potatoes)), no sauce (Include chow yuk) [1 cup]	162	5.7	223	40%	22	12	4.1
6231	Pork and vegetables (including carrots, broccoli, and/or dark-green leafy (no potatoes)), tomato-based sauce [1 cup]	249	8.8	288	40%	33	9	2.3
6232	Pork and vegetables (including carrots, broccoli, and/or dark-green leafy), soy-based sauce [1 cup]	217	7.7	247	42%	14	22	3.2
6233	Pork and vegetables, Hawaiian style [1 cup]	252	8.9	223	43%	14	20	4.9
6234	Pork and watercress with soy-based sauce [1 cup]	162	5.7	248	55%	20	8	0.7
6235	Pork chop stewed with vegetables, Puerto Rican style (Chuletas a la jardinera) [1 cup]	235	8.3	224	28%	26	15	2.4
6236	Pork chow mein or chop suey with noodles [1 cup]	220	7.8	448	54%	22	31	3.7
6237	Pork chow mein or chop suey, no noodles [1 cup]	220	7.8	286	53%	22	12	2.7
6238	Pork hash, Hawaiian style ground pork, vegetables (no carrots, broccoli, dark-green leafy, or potatoes), soy-based sauce [1 cup]	190	6.7	349	62%	26	6	1.0
6239	Pork or ham with soy-based sauce [1 cup]	244	8.6	337	50%	34	5	0.1
6240	Pork roast, stuffed, Puerto Rican style [1 slice (3" x ¾") with stuffing]	120	4.2	237	48%	27	3	0.5
6241	Pork with chili and tomatoes (Puerco con chile) [1 cup]	236	8.3	226	38%	28	6	1.5
6242	Pork, potatoes, and vegetables (no carrots, broccoli, or dark-green leafy), gravy [1 cup]	252	8.9	227	28%	16	25	3.5
6243	Pork, potatoes, and vegetables (no carrots, broccoli, or dark-green leafy), no sauce [1 cup]	162	5.7	197	34%	14	18	2.3
6244	Pork, potatoes, and vegetables (no carrots, broccoli, or dark-green leafy), tomato-based sauce [1 cup]	252	8.9	230	26%	17	26	4.4
6245	Pork, potatoes, and vegetables (including carrots, broccoli, and/or dark-green leafy), gravy [1 cup]	252	8.9	218	29%	15	24	3.0
6246	Pork, potatoes, and vegetables (including carrots, broccoli, and/or dark-green leafy), no sauce [1 cup]	162	5.7	204	33%	14	20	3.3
6247	Pork, potatoes, and vegetables (including carrots, broccoli, and/or dark-green leafy), tomato-based sauce [1 cup]	252	8.9	220	27%	16	26	4.0
6248	Pork, rice, and vegetables (no carrots, broccoli, or dark-green leafy), soy-based sauce (Include pork chow mein or chop suey with rice) [1 cup]	217	7.7	241	29%	19	23	1.5
6249	Pork, rice, and vegetables (no carrots, broccoli, or dark-green leafy), tomato-based sauce [1 cup]	249	8.8	254	26%	17	30	2.9

Food No.	fat gm	sat fat gm	choles mg	sodium mg	potas mg	% of Daily Value													
						vit A	vit E	vit C	thia	ribo	niac	vit B-6	fola	vit B-12	calc	phos	mag	iron	zinc
6215	5	2	33	430	187	1	1	2	24	8	12	9	1	5	1	11	3	4	8
6216	3	1	30	180	125	0	0	1	15	7	8	7	1	4	1	9	2	2	7
6217	9	3	62	1261	432	0	2	0	64	24	34	22	8	11	4	27	8	13	18
6218	5	1	22	465	273	3	3	8	14	6	11	8	1	3	1	9	4	4	6
6219	21	9	90	1143	539	19	7	8	49	33	27	21	8	14	29	45	13	15	25
6220	20	7	86	1114	622	124	8	17	51	28	30	28	5	12	21	38	13	17	24
6221	15	3	13	450	207	16	8	7	17	10	14	6	3	3	1	10	4	8	6
6222	25	11	65	1620	429	11	9	3	35	19	23	18	4	12	10	26	8	7	17
6223	9	3	34	652	334	1	1	29	27	10	15	19	5	6	3	14	6	4	9
6224	13	4	46	894	467	64	3	34	34	12	20	24	3	8	4	19	8	7	13
6225	29	5	87	758	797	3	18	18	56	25	38	28	10	12	8	35	13	15	20
6226	11	4	63	803	562	6	5	13	58	16	31	27	3	8	3	24	11	14	17
6227	13	4	96	196	837	7	6	63	61	24	39	33	5	12	4	35	12	11	21
6228	13	2	39	465	468	7	10	28	35	18	17	15	10	7	6	17	11	10	11
6229	10	4	56	78	405	3	1	11	50	17	22	20	5	8	3	20	8	8	13
6230	10	4	56	76	451	40	2	6	45	20	22	20	5	8	4	22	10	8	14
6231	13	4	94	205	885	102	6	26	60	24	39	31	5	12	5	35	13	11	21
6232	12	2	35	456	538	147	9	15	31	13	15	17	6	6	5	16	8	6	10
6233	11	3	35	45	807	69	8	18	32	15	16	25	10	4	6	19	11	9	14
6234	15	4	53	315	584	61	4	32	42	20	21	24	8	8	7	21	10	8	12
6235	7	2	65	348	727	6	3	27	44	20	31	25	9	9	6	28	12	10	16
6236	27	5	48	848	489	2	12	34	52	25	31	21	10	7	4	25	13	18	17
6237	17	4	56	926	527	12	9	39	43	20	24	22	10	8	5	23	10	10	16
6238	24	8	112	284	598	1	3	9	40	25	29	19	4	14	4	29	9	11	26
6239	19	6	100	2223	653	0	2	1	56	25	46	25	2	16	3	41	10	11	23
6240	13	4	93	289	422	2	4	15	35	18	26	20	2	10	1	20	6	10	27
6241	10	3	75	383	736	7	4	54	48	21	32	27	4	10	3	29	11	9	16
6242	7	2	36	583	501	5	2	17	29	11	18	20	7	5	3	16	9	7	11
6243	7	3	36	57	462	3	2	14	34	10	18	21	4	5	2	14	8	6	9
6244	7	2	36	682	814	13	8	34	31	13	21	26	8	4	4	17	12	10	12
6245	7	2	37	505	524	103	2	12	26	10	17	24	4	5	4	14	8	6	10
6246	7	3	35	58	485	21	2	12	31	12	18	21	4	5	3	15	9	6	10
6247	7	2	37	604	843	113	8	30	29	12	21	30	5	4	4	15	12	9	11
6248	8	3	48	495	533	5	3	37	37	14	27	20	3	6	5	21	9	12	12
6249	7	2	37	654	652	13	9	28	34	13	23	23	6	4	4	17	11	13	13

Mixed Dishes & Fast Foods

Food No.	Food Description & Amount	wt gm	wt oz	cal	% cal fat	prot gm	carbo gm	fiber gm
6250	Pork, rice, and vegetables (including carrots, broccoli, and/or dark-green leafy), soy-based sauce [1 cup]	217	7.7	247	29%	20	23	1.6
6251	Pork, rice, and vegetables (including carrots, broccoli, and/or dark-green leafy), tomato-based sauce [1 cup]	249	8.8	230	27%	16	27	2.7
6252	Pork stew, Mexican style, no potatoes, tomato-based sauce (mixture) (cerdo guisado sin papas) [1 cup]	244	8.6	290	37%	35	9	1.2
6253	Mexican style pork stew, with potatoes, tomato-based sauce (mixture) (cerdo guisado con papas) [1 cup]	244	8.6	283	35%	32	13	1.6
6254	Pork, tofu, and vegetables (no carrots, broccoli, dark-green leafy, or potatoes), soy-based sauce [1 cup]	217	7.7	309	51%	23	17	3.1
6255	Pork, tofu, and vegetables (including carrots, broccoli, and/or dark-green leafy (no potatoes)), soy-base sauce [1 cup]	217	7.7	303	52%	22	16	2.7
6256	Sausage and noodles with cream or white sauce [1 cup]	244	8.6	397	48%	17	34	2.7
6257	Sausage and peppers, no sauce [1 cup]	154	5.4	387	70%	24	4	0.4
6258	Sausage and rice mixed with cream of mushroom soup [1 cup]	244	8.6	439	55%	16	32	0.6
6259	Sausage and rice with cheese sauce [1 cup]	244	8.6	461	51%	21	34	0.7
6260	Sausage and rice with tomato-based sauce [1 cup]	244	8.6	502	47%	20	45	3.3
6261	Sausage and vegetables (no carrots, broccoli, dark-green leafy, or potatoes), tomato-based sauce [1 cup]	249	8.8	443	71%	23	9	1.9
6262	Sausage and vegetables (including carrots, broccoli, and/or dark-green leafy (no potatoes)), tomato-based sauce [1 cup]	249	8.8	408	69%	21	11	2.6
6263	Sausage gravy [1 cup]	240	8.5	393	65%	17	17	0.3
6264	Sausage with tomato-based sauce [1 link with sauce]	42	1.5	55	65%	3	2	0.4
6265	Sausage, noodles, and vegetables (no carrots, broccoli, or dark-green leafy), tomato-based sauce [1 cup]	249	8.8	379	50%	20	27	2.4
6266	Sausage, noodles, and vegetables (including carrots, broccoli, and/or dark-green leafy), tomato-based sauce [1 cup]	249	8.8	375	50%	20	27	2.5
6267	Sausage, potatoes, and vegetables (no carrots, broccoli, or dark-green leafy), gravy [1 cup]	252	8.9	409	55%	18	28	3.4
6268	Sausage, potatoes, and vegetables (including carrots, broccoli, and/or dark-green leafy), gravy [1 cup]	252	8.9	403	57%	17	27	2.8
6269	Stewed pig's feet, Puerto Rican style (Patitas de cerdo guisadas) [1 cup with bones]	184	6.5	220	55%	16	8	0.8
6270	Stewed pork, Puerto Rican style [1 cup]	200	7.1	385	56%	37	5	1.0
6271	Stewed beans with pork, tomatoes, and chili peppers, Mexican style (Frijoles a la charra) [1 cup]	242	8.5	350	59%	13	24	4.7
6272	Sweet and sour pork with rice [1 cup]	244	8.6	270	21%	13	40	1.5
6273	Sweet and sour pork [1 cup]	226	8.0	231	32%	15	25	1.6
	Lamb Dishes and Other Meat Dishes							
6400	Lamb curry [1 cup]	236	8.3	256	49%	28	3	1.0
6401	Lamb or mutton and noodles with gravy [1 cup]	249	8.8	367	43%	21	30	1.3
6402	Lamb or mutton and potatoes with gravy [1 cup]	252	8.9	256	36%	20	20	1.8
6403	Lamb or mutton and potatoes with tomato-based sauce [1 cup]	252	8.9	265	35%	21	22	2.3
6404	Lamb or mutton goulash [1 cup]	249	8.8	310	46%	33	8	1.1
6405	Lamb or mutton loaf [1 medium slice]	108	3.8	196	51%	15	9	0.4
6406	Lamb or mutton stew with potatoes and vegetables (no carrots, broccoli, or dark-green leafy), gravy [1 cup]	252	8.9	253	22%	24	25	3.1
6407	Lamb or mutton stew with potatoes and vegetables (no carrots, broccoli, or dark-green leafy), tomato-based sauce [1 cup]	252	8.9	241	19%	22	26	3.7
6408	Lamb or mutton stew with potatoes and vegetables (including carrots, broccoli, and/or dark-green leafy), gravy [1 cup]	252	8.9	261	21%	24	28	4.6
6409	Lamb or mutton stew with potatoes and vegetables (including carrots, broccoli, and/or dark-green leafy), tomato-based sauce [1 cup]	252	8.9	249	19%	22	29	5.1
6410	Lamb or mutton stew with vegetables (no carrots, broccoli, or dark-green leafy (no potatoes)), gravy [1 cup]	252	8.9	285	34%	34	12	2.4

Food No.	fat gm	sat fat gm	choles mg	sodium mg	potas mg	% of Daily Value													
						vit A	vit E	vit C	thia	ribo	niac	vit B-6	fola	vit B-12	calc	phos	mag	iron	zinc
6250	8	3	49	509	554	39	2	17	38	14	28	20	3	6	5	22	9	12	12
6251	7	2	34	628	720	39	9	28	31	15	21	23	15	4	8	16	16	18	13
6252	12	4	99	349	816	4	6	13	61	26	40	31	3	13	4	37	12	11	24
6253	11	4	89	315	873	4	6	17	56	24	38	31	4	12	4	34	12	11	22
6254	18	4	35	1214	450	3	8	14	34	15	17	16	10	4	15	26	37	42	15
6255	18	4	35	1220	464	46	8	7	32	15	16	16	8	4	15	25	37	41	14
6256	21	10	74	1116	332	14	2	18	32	21	16	11	7	13	21	27	10	15	15
6257	30	11	91	1021	399	2	2	43	47	17	23	21	2	24	3	19	6	11	19
6258	27	9	51	1499	341	1	6	4	40	15	23	14	2	20	8	20	7	12	16
6259	26	11	73	1465	489	5	1	4	42	24	20	16	2	25	28	34	10	10	15
6260	26	9	69	1081	518	3	8	16	56	15	31	23	7	24	5	23	8	15	18
6261	35	12	92	1925	671	7	3	72	56	19	29	26	5	30	7	23	9	11	20
6262	31	11	82	1754	729	105	3	27	52	18	27	23	4	27	8	23	9	11	18
6263	28	9	56	817	493	19	7	4	32	29	14	12	3	23	26	29	9	6	13
6264	4	1	10	340	155	3	2	7	7	3	4	4	1	4	1	3	2	2	3
6265	21	7	84	1063	545	7	6	34	42	17	25	21	5	16	5	21	11	17	17
6266	21	7	82	1044	550	20	6	38	42	17	25	20	5	16	4	21	11	17	16
6267	25	9	44	1215	797	9	6	42	30	17	21	22	8	14	15	24	11	11	17
6268	25	9	45	1205	846	75	6	39	28	17	20	23	5	14	16	23	11	10	16
6269	13	4	73	281	424	5	5	19	7	7	7	10	2	4	4	9	5	6	9
6270	24	6	108	453	822	5	11	17	61	26	41	32	3	14	4	38	12	12	25
6271	23	8	23	274	566	3	2	15	21	7	10	11	20	5	5	20	15	14	10
6272	6	2	28	618	311	2	4	24	36	10	19	19	2	4	3	14	9	11	10
6273	8	2	39	839	386	3	5	33	37	12	18	21	3	6	3	15	9	8	10
6400	14	4	89	323	496	0	5	2	6	17	40	10	7	48	4	28	10	17	44
6401	17	4	81	654	240	12	9	0	19	16	27	7	5	25	2	20	9	17	22
6402	10	4	65	73	761	0	1	24	9	13	32	17	7	33	3	22	11	13	32
6403	10	4	65	147	872	3	2	36	11	14	34	19	8	33	4	23	12	15	32
6404	16	5	107	272	613	3	10	16	17	23	47	18	13	75	4	32	12	18	53
6405	11	5	92	200	237	3	1	1	4	14	20	5	4	24	5	16	5	8	21
6406	6	2	62	334	545	2	1	18	15	12	27	18	8	26	3	18	11	15	30
6407	5	2	60	575	687	7	4	28	16	13	28	21	9	25	3	18	13	15	28
6408	6	2	62	541	576	26	2	14	12	14	27	18	8	26	3	19	12	15	31
6409	5	2	60	572	716	30	5	24	13	15	27	21	8	25	4	19	14	15	29
6410	11	4	98	466	408	7	2	11	15	18	33	10	10	42	4	24	10	21	45

Mixed Dishes & Fast Foods

Food No.	Food Description & Amount	wt gm	wt oz	cal	% cal fat	prot gm	carbo gm	fiber gm
6411	Lamb or mutton stew with vegetables (including carrots, broccoli, and/or dark-green leafy (no potatoes)), gravy [1 cup]	252	8.9	299	32%	35	16	4.6
6412	Lamb or mutton with gravy [1 slice with gravy]	43	1.5	56	37%	8	1	0.1
6413	Lamb or mutton, rice, and vegetables (no carrots, broccoli, or dark-green leafy), gravy [1 cup]	252	8.9	270	21%	18	35	4.4
6414	Lamb or mutton, rice, and vegetables (including carrots, broccoli, and/or dark-green leafy), gravy [1 cup]	252	8.9	255	35%	19	21	1.5
6415	Lamb or mutton, rice, and vegetables (including carrots, broccoli, and/or dark-green leafy), tomato-based sauce [1 cup]	252	8.9	251	21%	16	34	3.8
6416	Lamb shishkabob [1 shishkabob]	202	7.1	245	41%	27	9	2.1
6417	Rabbit, stewed Puerto Rican style (Fricase de conejo) [1 cup, boneless]	219	7.7	470	53%	38	16	1.7
6418	Deer loaf (Include deer meatball, with breading, no sauce) [1 medium slice]	108	3.8	148	20%	22	6	0.4
6419	Venison and noodles with cream or white sauce [1 cup]	249	8.8	344	41%	27	23	0.7
6420	Venison stew with potatoes and vegetables (no carrots, broccoli, or dark-green leafy), tomato-based sauce [1 cup]	252	8.9	163	10%	19	18	3.2
6421	Venison stew with potatoes and vegetables (including carrots, broccoli, and/or dark-green leafy), tomato-based sauce [1 cup]	252	8.9	161	10%	18	18	3.3
6422	Venison with gravy [1 slice with gravy]	65	2.3	78	23%	13	1	0.1
6423	Venison with tomato-based sauce [1 cup]	249	8.8	227	17%	40	6	1.1
6424	Venison, noodles, and vegetables (no carrots, broccoli, or dark-green leafy), tomato-based sauce [1 cup]	249	8.8	191	11%	16	26	2.9
6425	Venison, noodles, and vegetables (including carrots, broccoli, and/or dark-green leafy), tomato-based sauce [1 cup]	249	8.8	203	10%	16	29	3.2
6426	Venison, potatoes, and vegetables (no carrots, broccoli, or dark-green leafy), gravy [1 cup]	252	8.9	170	10%	19	18	2.8
6427	Venison, potatoes, and vegetables (including carrots, broccoli, and/or dark-green leafy), gravy [1 cup]	252	8.9	162	10%	18	19	3.2
6428	Stewed goat, Puerto Rican style (Cabrito en fricase, chilindron de chivo) (Include Puerto Rican stewed kid) [1 piece with gravy]	88	3.1	230	61%	20	2	0.4
	Chicken and Turkey Dishes							
6500	Almond chicken [1 cup]	242	8.5	280	47%	22	16	3.4
6501	Chicken cornbread [1 piece (2½" x 2½" x 1½")]	67	2.4	117	43%	10	6	0.5
6502	Chicken curry [1 cup]	236	8.3	294	49%	27	10	2.2
6503	Chicken fricassee, Puerto Rican style (Fricase de pollo) (Include stewed chicken (Pollo guisado)) [1 cup, boneless]	223	7.9	430	64%	24	15	2.0
6504	Chicken kiev [1 serving (1 whole breast)]	258	9.1	643	46%	73	10	0.3
6505	Chicken livers, chopped, with eggs and onion [1 cup]	208	7.3	472	70%	27	6	1.0
6506	Chicken or turkey a la king with vegetables (no carrots, broccoli, dark-green leafy, or potatoes), cream, white, or soup-based sauce [1 cup]	241	8.5	469	66%	25	15	1.2
6507	Chicken or turkey a la king with vegetables (including carrots, broccoli, and/or dark-green leafy (no potatoes)), cream, white, or soup-based sauce [1 cup]	241	8.5	476	65%	25	17	1.5
6508	Chicken or turkey and noodles with soup-based (cream of mushroom) sauce [1 cup]	224	7.9	312	32%	22	30	1.2
6509	Chicken or turkey and noodles with cheese sauce [1 cup]	224	7.9	330	30%	25	32	1.4
6510	Chicken or turkey and noodles with cream or white sauce [1 cup]	224	7.9	320	31%	22	32	1.2
6511	Chicken or turkey and noodles with gravy [1 cup]	224	7.9	304	36%	20	27	1.2
6512	Chicken or turkey and noodles, no sauce [1 cup]	157	5.5	254	28%	20	24	1.1
6513	Chicken or turkey and noodles, tomato-based sauce [1 cup]	224	7.9	291	29%	20	31	2.4
6514	Chicken or turkey and potatoes with gravy (Include Chicken Helper Chicken, Potatoes, and Gravy) [1 cup]	242	8.5	277	40%	19	22	1.7
6515	Chicken or turkey and rice, no sauce [1 cup]	196	6.9	314	24%	23	34	0.5
6516	Chicken or turkey and rice with soup-based (cream of mushroom) sauce [1 cup]	248	8.7	455	43%	28	35	0.9
6517	Chicken with rice, Puerto Rican style (Arroz con Pollo) [1 cup]	163	5.7	462	38%	18	51	1.1
6518	Chicken or turkey and rice with cream sauce (Include Chicken Helper Mushroom Chicken with Long Grain and Wild Rice) [1 cup]	248	8.7	358	38%	22	32	1.4

Food No.	fat gm	sat fat gm	choles mg	sodium mg	potas mg	% of Daily Value													
						vit A	vit E	vit C	thia	ribo	niac	vit B-6	fola	vit B-12	calc	phos	mag	iron	zinc
6411	11	4	98	464	459	46	3	5	10	21	32	9	10	42	5	25	12	20	46
6412	2	1	22	121	97	0	0	0	2	5	8	2	1	11	0	6	2	4	9
6413	6	2	38	548	464	4	3	54	19	11	23	20	14	16	3	18	11	15	23
6414	10	3	57	239	330	40	3	5	13	13	25	10	7	29	4	17	8	13	29
6415	6	2	37	476	500	80	5	49	15	9	21	21	10	16	4	15	10	13	20
6416	11	4	88	79	572	6	3	55	11	19	33	15	11	45	3	24	10	15	42
6417	27	5	102	308	857	2	16	24	8	14	47	24	5	84	4	32	12	21	21
6418	3	1	100	111	328	2	1	1	11	29	26	9	2	68	4	21	6	18	13
6419	16	4	99	218	420	16	8	2	19	38	27	11	3	70	15	30	11	23	17
6420	2	1	56	249	743	6	4	49	15	23	28	20	9	52	3	21	12	19	14
6421	2	1	55	245	771	74	4	44	15	23	27	20	8	51	3	20	11	19	13
6422	2	1	45	181	156	0	1	0	5	15	13	5	1	39	0	10	3	11	9
6423	4	2	144	529	592	7	7	17	14	43	34	17	2	107	2	25	10	35	25
6424	2	1	62	351	493	6	4	17	17	19	20	13	5	36	3	18	12	20	12
6425	2	1	61	342	484	45	4	16	18	20	21	14	5	35	3	18	12	21	12
6426	2	1	59	74	606	2	1	23	15	23	27	16	6	54	2	20	10	19	13
6427	2	1	54	77	610	70	2	23	15	22	26	16	6	50	3	19	10	18	12
6428	16	3	56	324	343	1	7	7	6	25	15	2	2	14	2	16	1	15	25
6500	15	2	40	526	549	4	17	11	6	12	47	22	7	5	7	25	15	11	11
6501	6	1	70	64	77	5	3	0	4	7	10	5	2	3	1	7	3	4	5
6502	16	3	84	629	626	20	14	31	9	13	51	25	5	5	4	25	13	12	14
6503	31	6	81	770	704	15	17	74	11	11	39	25	5	5	3	23	11	11	13
6504	33	16	283	454	623	22	7	0	17	21	160	69	4	15	6	56	18	18	17
6505	37	11	753	92	256	458	11	30	12	106	21	32	184	304	4	36	7	46	30
6506	34	12	195	493	400	35	13	9	12	23	36	20	6	10	15	30	9	11	15
6507	34	12	195	367	434	120	14	10	11	24	34	23	6	10	16	29	9	11	14
6508	11	3	81	550	220	3	4	1	15	15	27	10	3	5	7	20	9	14	14
6509	11	4	95	581	321	5	1	2	16	21	24	11	4	9	21	30	12	12	13
6510	11	3	81	139	276	10	4	1	17	20	25	10	4	6	13	24	11	13	13
6511	12	3	78	590	145	3	2	0	15	12	25	8	3	3	3	16	8	13	11
6512	8	2	82	47	130	1	1	0	14	10	25	9	3	4	2	15	8	12	12
6513	9	2	74	658	478	14	10	20	18	13	29	15	4	3	3	18	12	16	13
6514	12	4	54	1117	625	3	2	24	9	10	27	19	4	2	2	15	9	10	11
6515	8	2	62	513	171	1	2	0	16	8	31	15	2	3	2	16	7	13	13
6516	22	5	66	1170	395	16	13	2	14	10	63	21	2	5	6	27	10	15	11
6517	20	5	54	340	264	3	7	8	23	7	35	14	2	3	3	18	8	19	12
6518	15	4	56	415	326	14	8	6	17	15	37	16	4	7	12	23	9	13	13

Mixed Dishes & Fast Foods

Food No.	Food Description & Amount	wt gm	wt oz	cal	% cal fat	prot gm	carbo gm	fiber gm
6519	Chicken or turkey and rice with soy-based sauce (Include Chicken Helper Chicken Teriyaki) [1 cup]	244	8.6	323	18%	42	22	0.2
6520	Chicken or turkey and rice with tomato-based sauce [1 cup]	244	8.6	229	10%	19	33	2.8
6521	Chicken or turkey and vegetables (no carrots, broccoli, dark-green leafy, or potatoes), cheese sauce [1 cup]	249	8.8	309	37%	29	20	2.9
6522	Chicken or turkey and vegetables (no carrots, broccoli, dark-green leafy, or potatoes), gravy [1 cup]	252	8.9	289	43%	23	18	3.0
6523	Chicken or turkey and vegetables (no carrots, broccoli, dark-green leafy, or potatoes), no sauce [1 cup]	162	5.7	153	23%	17	13	2.7
6524	Chicken or turkey and vegetables (no carrots, broccoli, dark-green leafy, or potatoes), soy-based sauce [1 cup]	162	5.7	292	58%	22	8	0.9
6525	Chicken or turkey and vegetables (including carrots, broccoli, and/or dark-green leafy (no potatoes)), cheese sauce [1 cup]	249	8.8	321	42%	34	12	2.1
6526	Chicken or turkey and vegetables (including carrots, broccoli, and/or dark-green leafy (no potatoes)), gravy [1 cup]	252	8.9	281	45%	23	15	2.9
6527	Chicken or turkey and vegetables (including carrots, broccoli, and/or dark-green leafy (no potatoes)), no sauce [1 cup]	162	5.7	148	24%	17	12	2.5
6528	Chicken or turkey and vegetables (including carrots, broccoli, and/or dark-green leafy (no potatoes)), soy-based sauce [1 cup]	162	5.7	289	60%	22	6	0.8
6529	Chicken or turkey cacciatore (Include chicken or turkey with tomato-based sauce, chicken or turkey with tomatoes) [½ chicken breast with sauce]	128	4.5	241	50%	22	7	1.0
6530	Chicken or turkey cake, patty, or croquette [1 cake or patty]	85	3.0	219	53%	14	11	0.3
6531	Chicken or turkey chow mein or chop suey with noodles [1 cup]	220	7.8	275	45%	19	20	2.3
6532	Chicken or turkey chow mein or chop suey, no noodles [1 cup]	220	7.8	193	39%	20	10	2.1
6533	Chicken or turkey cordon bleu [1 roll (½ breast with ham and sauce)]	229	8.1	494	53%	44	11	0.5
6534	Chicken or turkey creole, without rice [1 cup]	246	8.7	192	19%	29	9	2.1
6535	Chicken or turkey divan [1 cup]	236	8.3	324	39%	41	8	3.0
6536	Chicken or turkey fricassee [1 cup]	244	8.6	323	51%	29	8	0.3
6537	Chicken or turkey fricassee, no potatoes, Puerto Rican style (with sauce) [1 cup]	223	7.9	457	68%	30	6	1.2
6538	Chicken or turkey fricassee, no sauce, no potatoes, Puerto Rican style [1 cup]	223	7.9	561	60%	52	0	0.0
6539	Chicken or turkey fricassee, with sauce, no potatoes, Puerto Rican style (potatoes reported separately) (Include pollo en salsa, Puerto Rican style chicken or turkey in sauce) [1 cup]	223	7.9	470	61%	40	4	0.7
6540	Chicken or turkey garden salad (chicken and/or turkey, other vegetables but no tomato or carrots), no dressing [1 cup]	90	3.2	64	19%	11	2	0.8
6541	Chicken or turkey garden salad (chicken and/or turkey, tomato and/or carrots, other vegetables), no dressing (Include McDonald's Chicken Salad Oriental) [1 fast food order]	252	8.9	161	18%	27	6	2.5
6542	Chicken or turkey hash [1 cup]	190	6.7	212	36%	18	16	2.3
6543	Chicken or turkey loaf (Include with breading, no sauce; chicken or turkey meatball, with breading, no sauce) [1 slice]	108	3.8	184	32%	22	8	0.6
6544	Chicken or turkey parmigiana [1 piece with sauce and cheese]	182	6.4	320	44%	28	16	1.1
6545	Chicken or turkey pate with vegetables, diet (Include Nu System Cuisine Chicken Pate with Vegetables) [1 container (3 oz)]	85	3.0	127	18%	24	0	0.0
6546	Chicken or turkey pot pie [1 pie (8 oz, frozen)]	227	8.0	490	52%	20	38	3.1
6547	Chicken or turkey salad with egg [1 cup]	182	6.4	385	68%	28	3	0.7
6548	Chicken or turkey salad [1 cup]	182	6.4	417	69%	30	2	0.8
6549	Chicken or turkey souffle [1 cup]	159	5.6	283	58%	20	9	0.2
6550	Chicken or turkey teriyaki (chicken or turkey with soy-based sauce) [½ chicken breast with sauce]	128	4.5	178	19%	27	7	0.4
6551	Chicken or turkey tetrazzini [1 cup]	246	8.7	366	48%	19	28	1.7
6552	Chicken or turkey with soup-based (cream of mushroom) sauce [½ chicken breast with sauce]	129	4.6	188	44%	21	4	0.1
6553	Chicken or turkey with barbecue sauce [½ chicken breast with sauce]	123	4.3	234	43%	28	3	0.3
6554	Chicken or turkey with cheese sauce [1 cup]	241	8.5	368	40%	44	9	0.3
6555	Chicken or turkey with cream sauce [½ chicken breast with sauce]	129	4.6	210	53%	16	8	0.1

Food No.	fat gm	sat fat gm	choles mg	sodium mg	potas mg	% of Daily Value													
						vit A	vit E	vit C	thia	ribo	niac	vit B-6	fola	vit B-12	calc	phos	mag	iron	zinc
6519	7	2	126	719	533	2	3	6	15	19	78	28	3	7	6	37	17	15	21
6520	3	1	49	94	698	15	14	22	16	10	42	22	4	3	4	20	14	16	11
6521	13	4	83	499	641	9	4	17	13	20	41	25	8	9	17	33	15	11	15
6522	14	4	76	94	449	5	3	30	10	12	40	19	7	3	3	21	11	10	11
6523	4	1	45	125	359	5	2	18	6	8	21	13	5	2	3	12	8	7	9
6524	19	5	83	627	379	4	4	5	6	10	39	17	3	4	2	19	7	7	11
6525	15	5	101	604	558	76	6	36	9	23	46	31	7	11	21	35	12	9	17
6526	14	4	79	104	467	57	3	31	10	11	39	18	5	4	3	20	10	11	11
6527	4	1	45	130	353	32	2	17	6	8	21	14	5	2	3	12	7	7	9
6528	19	5	85	642	346	5	4	13	5	10	40	16	3	4	2	20	7	8	11
6529	13	3	67	130	362	7	7	13	7	10	37	19	2	4	3	16	7	9	11
6530	13	3	39	176	180	7	6	2	7	11	22	10	2	4	7	13	5	7	7
6531	14	2	43	793	371	1	4	15	14	16	37	17	9	3	4	18	10	13	12
6532	8	2	50	651	415	1	5	17	8	13	35	19	13	4	4	19	9	10	11
6533	29	15	188	665	487	21	4	3	20	24	81	36	4	13	23	45	13	14	18
6534	4	1	70	436	710	10	9	55	10	10	70	31	5	5	5	27	14	10	8
6535	14	6	134	445	433	29	9	66	8	20	46	24	9	8	31	39	14	10	14
6536	18	5	86	504	295	1	3	0	8	14	40	13	3	6	2	19	6	10	14
6537	35	7	86	642	411	9	18	39	15	13	35	22	4	6	3	20	9	11	16
6538	38	9	165	142	352	9	9	0	7	18	59	23	3	7	3	29	10	14	25
6539	32	7	122	441	394	9	12	23	12	16	46	23	3	6	3	25	10	13	20
6540	1	0	29	37	187	2	1	11	3	3	24	12	7	2	2	9	4	3	3
6541	3	1	69	91	536	23	4	37	10	9	58	30	18	5	4	22	10	9	7
6542	8	2	43	245	585	1	9	19	8	8	21	25	6	3	4	16	9	8	14
6543	7	2	93	139	240	4	2	6	7	13	33	17	3	5	5	18	6	8	11
6544	16	5	137	641	471	15	11	14	12	20	42	18	4	7	20	32	11	13	16
6545	3	1	64	70	157	3	1	0	2	6	35	14	1	3	1	14	5	4	5
6546	28	9	62	246	355	74	11	16	24	21	33	11	7	3	6	20	9	17	12
6547	29	6	214	448	311	9	17	6	5	18	27	22	8	10	5	20	6	9	14
6548	32	6	106	290	331	5	19	5	5	11	33	25	5	5	4	18	7	9	15
6549	18	5	221	234	266	22	9	1	7	25	20	13	5	10	11	23	6	8	11
6550	4	1	82	1683	309	2	2	5	5	11	44	23	3	5	3	20	9	10	13
6551	19	7	49	705	200	11	7	10	13	15	25	10	3	5	14	22	8	12	13
6552	9	3	63	411	217	2	3	1	4	10	33	17	1	5	4	16	5	6	11
6553	11	3	89	262	275	5	2	2	5	10	47	23	2	5	2	20	7	8	13
6554	16	6	136	739	535	7	2	1	10	27	60	33	3	15	25	43	13	9	21
6555	12	3	47	164	242	12	6	1	6	14	22	12	2	6	11	17	6	5	9

Mixed Dishes & Fast Foods

Food No.	Food Description & Amount	wt gm	wt oz	cal	% cal fat	prot gm	carbo gm	fiber gm
6556	Chicken or turkey with dumplings (Include Chicken Helper Chicken and Dumplings) [1 cup]	244	8.6	373	46%	26	22	0.7
6557	Chicken or turkey with stuffing (Include Chicken Helper Chicken and Stuffing) [1 cup]	200	7.1	273	18%	35	19	0.8
6558	Chicken or turkey, dumplings, and vegetables (no carrots, broccoli, or dark-green leafy), gravy [1 cup]	249	8.8	273	34%	22	22	2.5
6559	Chicken or turkey, dumplings, and vegetables (including carrots, broccoli, and/or dark-green leafy), gravy [1 cup]	249	8.8	264	30%	23	23	3.2
6560	Chicken or turkey, noodles, and vegetables (no carrots, broccoli, or dark-green leafy), cheese sauce [1 cup]	244	8.6	389	38%	32	28	2.6
6561	Chicken or turkey, noodles, and vegetables (no carrots, broccoli, or dark-green leafy), cream or white sauce [1 cup]	244	8.6	340	34%	27	28	2.1
6562	Chicken or turkey, noodles, and vegetables (no carrots, broccoli, or dark-green leafy), gravy [1 cup]	224	7.9	257	35%	17	25	2.4
6563	Chicken or turkey, noodles, and vegetables (no carrots, broccoli, or dark-green leafy), no sauce [1 cup]	162	5.7	184	18%	15	22	2.7
6564	Chicken or turkey, noodles, and vegetables (no carrots, broccoli, or dark-green leafy), tomato-based sauce [1 cup]	224	7.9	285	35%	18	28	2.7
6565	Chicken or turkey, noodles, and vegetables (no carrots, broccoli, or dark-green leafy), cream, white, or cream of mushroom soup-based sauce [1 cup]	224	7.9	294	37%	19	28	2.4
6566	Chicken or turkey, noodles, and vegetables (including carrots, broccoli, and/or dark-green leafy), cheese sauce [1 cup]	244	8.6	356	39%	30	24	2.1
6567	Chicken or turkey, noodles, and vegetables (including carrots, broccoli, and/or dark-green leafy), cream or white sauce [1 cup]	224	7.9	306	35%	18	31	2.9
6568	Chicken or turkey, noodles, and vegetables (including carrots, broccoli, and/or dark-green leafy), gravy [1 cup]	224	7.9	267	35%	16	27	2.7
6569	Chicken or turkey, noodles, and vegetables (including carrots, broccoli, and/or dark-green leafy), no sauce [1 cup]	162	5.7	178	19%	15	21	2.4
6570	Chicken or turkey, noodles, and vegetables (including carrots, broccoli, and/or dark-green leafy), tomato-based sauce [1 cup]	224	7.9	293	34%	18	30	3.0
6571	Chicken or turkey, potatoes, and vegetables (no carrots, broccoli, or dark-green leafy), no sauce [1 cup]	162	5.7	201	25%	24	12	2.0
6572	Chicken or turkey, potatoes, and vegetables (including carrots, broccoli, and/or dark-green leafy), no sauce [1 cup]	162	5.7	195	26%	23	12	1.8
6573	Chicken or turkey, rice, and vegetables (no carrots, broccoli, or dark-green leafy), cream of mushroom soup-based sauce [1 cup]	252	8.9	372	38%	22	35	4.0
6574	Chicken or turkey, rice, and vegetables (no carrots, broccoli, or dark-green leafy), cheese sauce [1 cup]	249	8.8	347	30%	30	29	1.4
6575	Chicken or turkey, rice, and vegetables (no carrots, broccoli, or dark-green leafy), gravy [1 cup]	252	8.9	381	39%	23	34	2.7
6576	Chicken or turkey, rice, and vegetables (no carrots, broccoli, or dark-green leafy), no sauce [1 cup]	162	5.7	190	16%	16	23	2.2
6577	Chicken or turkey, rice, and vegetables (no carrots, broccoli, or dark-green leafy), soy-based sauce [1 cup]	217	7.7	228	40%	15	19	1.7
6578	Chicken or turkey, rice, and vegetables (no carrots, broccoli, or dark-green leafy), tomato-based sauce [1 cup]	249	8.8	354	36%	22	34	3.4
6579	Chicken or turkey, rice, and vegetables (including carrots, broccoli, and/or dark-green leafy), cream of mushroom soup-based sauce [1 cup]	252	8.9	338	42%	20	29	2.9
6580	Chicken or turkey, rice, and vegetables (including carrots, broccoli, and/or dark-green leafy), cheese sauce [1 cup]	249	8.8	277	29%	24	25	3.2
6581	Chicken or turkey, rice, and vegetables (including carrots, broccoli, and/or dark-green leafy), gravy [1 cup]	252	8.9	345	40%	21	30	2.6
6582	Chicken or turkey, rice, and vegetables (including carrots, broccoli, and/or dark-green leafy), no sauce [1 cup]	162	5.7	191	18%	17	21	1.7
6583	Chicken or turkey, rice, and vegetables (including carrots, broccoli, and/or dark-green leafy), soy-based sauce [1 cup]	217	7.7	241	38%	15	22	2.3

Food No.	fat gm	sat fat gm	choles mg	sodium mg	potas mg	% of Daily Value: vit A	vit E	vit C	thia	ribo	niac	vit B-6	fola	vit B-12	calc	phos	mag	iron	zinc
6556	19	5	89	244	297	5	4	3	15	18	47	15	3	5	13	26	9	14	13
6557	5	1	105	511	403	2	3	5	15	18	66	23	7	6	4	29	12	13	17
6558	10	3	56	735	394	10	3	8	15	15	35	18	7	5	13	22	8	13	15
6559	9	2	57	421	417	59	3	9	15	16	36	21	8	5	13	23	9	13	14
6560	16	6	102	378	456	15	5	9	17	26	39	17	8	8	24	39	15	15	21
6561	13	3	89	283	327	6	6	6	16	19	30	14	6	6	10	24	11	14	16
6562	10	3	40	712	190	2	2	0	13	10	23	6	3	1	2	15	8	12	11
6563	4	1	53	209	178	4	1	6	13	9	19	8	6	2	2	14	7	11	10
6564	11	3	66	437	332	7	7	7	14	11	26	9	3	2	3	17	10	15	12
6565	12	3	63	545	291	5	6	1	17	16	24	10	5	6	11	22	10	13	13
6566	16	6	97	370	428	21	8	26	12	24	35	16	8	8	24	36	13	13	18
6567	12	3	64	337	348	147	6	3	15	18	21	15	5	6	12	20	10	12	12
6568	10	3	61	494	238	131	3	2	13	11	21	13	4	3	4	14	8	12	10
6569	4	1	54	145	194	80	1	2	12	8	19	11	4	2	3	13	7	10	10
6570	11	3	66	307	367	92	7	8	13	12	24	12	4	2	4	16	10	15	11
6571	6	2	67	132	368	3	2	11	8	10	29	18	6	3	2	16	8	8	13
6572	6	2	67	86	381	62	2	8	6	9	29	20	4	3	3	15	8	7	12
6573	16	4	63	709	348	7	4	18	23	12	40	16	9	3	5	23	11	18	15
6574	12	4	84	596	400	6	3	3	14	18	34	17	4	8	18	30	11	12	17
6575	17	5	72	545	352	8	3	8	17	11	40	15	6	4	4	22	9	16	14
6576	3	1	39	35	234	2	1	9	13	8	21	14	7	2	3	14	8	9	11
6577	10	3	41	919	195	2	2	0	9	7	23	8	3	1	2	14	7	10	11
6578	14	4	68	241	491	11	7	15	18	11	41	18	7	3	4	22	11	17	13
6579	16	4	63	374	391	16	8	57	14	12	36	16	12	3	7	21	10	15	13
6580	9	3	63	461	448	19	7	62	13	17	27	17	14	6	17	26	12	12	15
6581	15	4	68	421	365	16	6	43	15	11	37	17	11	3	6	21	10	14	13
6582	4	1	44	57	213	54	2	17	10	7	22	14	4	2	3	13	7	9	10
6583	10	3	41	707	252	125	3	2	7	8	20	13	3	1	4	12	7	9	9

Mixed Dishes & Fast Foods

Food No.	Food Description & Amount	wt gm	wt oz	cal	% cal fat	prot gm	carbo gm	fiber gm
6584	Chicken or turkey, rice, and vegetables (including carrots, broccoli, and/or dark-green leafy), tomato-based sauce [1 cup]	249	8.8	352	37%	21	33	2.7
6585	Chicken or turkey, stuffing, and vegetables (no carrots, broccoli, or dark-green leafy), gravy [1 cup]	244	8.6	324	44%	21	24	2.6
6586	Chicken or turkey, stuffing, and vegetables (no carrots, broccoli, or dark-green leafy), no sauce [1 cup]	162	5.7	207	18%	21	20	1.7
6587	Chicken or turkey, stuffing, and vegetables (including carrots, broccoli, and/or dark-green leafy), gravy [1 cup]	244	8.6	359	36%	25	32	4.4
6588	Chicken or turkey, stuffing, and vegetables (including carrots, broccoli, and/or dark-green leafy), no sauce [1 cup]	162	5.7	232	35%	15	22	3.3
6589	Chicken or turkey, sweet and sour [½ chicken breast with sauce]	131	4.6	118	25%	8	15	0.9
6590	Chicken wing with hot pepper sauce (Include Buffalo chicken wing) [2 wings]	32	1.1	98	64%	8	0	0.0
6591	Chicken with gravy [2 slices with gravy]	44	1.6	59	44%	7	1	0.1
6592	Gizzards, stewed, Puerto Rican style (Mollejitas guisadas) [1 cup]	260	9.2	501	50%	45	13	1.9
6593	General Tso chicken [1 cup]	146	5.1	293	52%	19	16	0.8
6594	Kung pao chicken (Include cashew chicken) [1 cup]	162	5.7	431	64%	29	11	2.2
6595	Moo Goo Gai Pan [1 cup]	216	7.6	272	62%	15	12	2.7
6596	Soupy rice with chicken, Puerto Rican style (Asopao de pollo) [1 cup, boneless]	263	9.3	346	39%	19	33	1.7
6597	Spaghetti sauce with poultry, home-made style [1 cup]	249	8.8	261	48%	16	21	4.2
6598	Stew, chicken or turkey, with potatoes and vegetables (no carrots, broccoli, or dark-green leafy), gravy [1 cup]	252	8.9	217	16%	28	16	2.5
6599	Stew, chicken or turkey, with potatoes and vegetables (no carrots, broccoli, or dark-green leafy), tomato-based sauce [1 cup]	247	8.7	227	16%	29	19	3.0
6600	Stew, chicken or turkey, with potatoes and vegetables (including carrots, broccoli, and/or dark-green leafy), gravy [1 cup]	252	8.9	291	44%	24	15	2.0
6601	Stew, chicken or turkey, with potatoes and vegetables (including carrots, broccoli, and/or dark-green leafy), tomato-based sauce [1 cup]	247	8.7	218	16%	27	18	2.7
6602	Stewed chicken with tomato-based sauce, Mexican style (Pollo guisado con tomate) [½ chicken breast with sauce]	128	4.5	135	46%	15	3	0.5
6603	Stuffed chicken, drumstick or breast, Puerto Rican style (Muslo de pollo o pechuga rellena) [1 breast (4" x 3" x ¾")]	210	7.4	470	30%	62	16	0.7
6604	Turkey with gravy [1 cup]	244	8.6	266	29%	38	6	0.5
	Fish Dishes							
6700	Biscayne codfish, Puerto Rican style (Bacalao a la Vizcaina) [1 cup]	175	6.2	341	54%	16	24	2.7
6701	Chow mein or chop suey, no noodles [1 cup]	220	7.8	284	51%	23	12	2.7
6702	Clam cake or patty (Include deviled) [1 cake or patty]	120	4.2	423	40%	24	38	1.2
6703	Clams Casino [2 clams]	60	2.1	70	40%	5	6	0.7
6704	Clams, stuffed [1 large (6 in 11 oz package)]	52	1.8	101	52%	5	7	0.4
6705	Codfish ball or cake [1 ball]	63	2.2	125	48%	9	8	0.7
6706	Codfish salad, Puerto Rican style (Ensalada de bacalao) [1 cup]	150	5.3	220	63%	12	9	1.7
6707	Codfish salad, Puerto Rican style (Gazpacho de bacalao) [1 cup salad and 1 slice toast]	170	6.0	270	53%	14	18	2.0
6708	Codfish salad, Puerto Rican style (Serenata) (Include oil, vinegar, onion, olives, tomatoes) [1 cup]	145	5.1	257	79%	10	5	0.9
6709	Codfish with starchy vegetables, Puerto Rican style (Serenata de bacalao) [1 cup]	173	6.1	237	35%	6	34	4.7
6710	Crab cake [1 cake]	120	4.2	203	43%	27	1	0.1
6711	Crab imperial (Include stuffed crab) [1 stuffed crab]	194	6.8	292	48%	30	6	0.3
6712	Crab salad made with imitation crab [1 cup]	208	7.3	299	37%	18	28	0.8
6713	Crab salad [1 cup]	208	7.3	282	44%	27	11	0.7
6714	Crab, deviled [1 cup]	175	6.2	346	46%	23	23	1.0
6715	Crabs in tomato-based sauce, Puerto Rican style (Salmorejo de jueyes) [1 cup]	170	6.0	289	57%	27	4	0.5
6716	Fish a la creole, Puerto Rican style (Pescado frito con mojo) [1 slice (4" x 3½" x ½") with sauce]	213	7.5	324	59%	26	8	1.7
6717	Fish and noodles with cream of mushroom soup-based sauce [1 cup]	224	7.9	260	33%	18	25	1.0
6718	Fish and rice with cream of mushroom soup-based sauce [1 cup]	248	8.7	318	31%	19	34	0.7
6719	Fish and rice with cream sauce [1 cup]	248	8.7	367	36%	21	36	0.6

Food No.	fat gm	sat fat gm	choles mg	sodium mg	potas mg	% of Daily Value													
						vit A	vit E	vit C	thia	ribo	niac	vit B-6	fola	vit B-12	calc	phos	mag	iron	zinc
6584	15	4	70	147	542	95	7	14	17	10	43	19	4	3	4	21	11	16	12
6585	16	4	51	836	360	16	7	6	14	14	34	18	9	4	6	18	8	12	14
6586	4	1	59	420	340	2	3	7	13	13	40	15	8	3	4	19	9	10	11
6587	14	3	58	582	482	66	8	11	18	16	40	24	11	4	6	23	14	16	14
6588	9	2	29	388	351	54	6	8	13	10	17	15	8	3	5	15	10	12	12
6589	3	1	23	506	185	2	3	20	4	5	15	9	1	1	2	8	5	5	4
6590	7	2	26	25	59	2	1	0	1	2	10	7	0	1	0	5	2	2	4
6591	3	1	20	148	77	3	0	0	1	3	10	5	0	2	1	5	1	2	4
6592	28	6	305	537	911	36	26	38	10	30	55	16	25	63	7	37	15	52	49
6593	17	4	65	906	250	5	9	21	7	11	31	14	4	4	3	15	6	8	9
6594	31	5	64	907	428	6	18	13	10	9	66	29	11	4	5	26	16	11	10
6595	19	4	35	304	488	14	17	57	11	20	22	16	11	5	13	20	8	9	11
6596	15	4	59	326	319	6	4	27	17	9	34	15	5	3	3	19	9	14	12
6597	14	3	46	881	1078	25	24	63	13	14	26	29	7	2	6	18	16	18	14
6598	4	1	83	142	621	4	2	27	14	14	53	25	8	5	3	26	13	12	15
6599	4	1	83	246	780	8	3	42	15	15	55	28	8	5	5	27	14	14	16
6600	14	4	87	113	632	73	2	20	10	12	45	22	5	4	3	22	11	10	13
6601	4	1	82	226	822	72	4	38	12	14	54	28	6	5	5	26	14	12	15
6602	7	1	46	174	244	3	6	11	4	7	27	11	2	3	1	12	5	5	7
6603	15	6	323	713	687	14	7	12	21	35	117	44	8	21	24	64	19	19	22
6604	9	3	93	805	491	0	2	0	7	19	41	28	3	9	3	29	8	17	31
6700	21	3	33	509	867	4	15	36	9	6	14	23	5	10	4	19	12	9	5
6701	16	4	60	941	524	12	9	39	19	16	27	22	10	18	4	22	10	14	21
6702	19	4	121	380	505	17	13	20	24	33	23	5	7	974	22	37	6	122	16
6703	3	1	10	118	163	5	3	21	5	5	5	4	2	192	3	5	2	20	3
6704	6	1	12	117	169	8	5	7	5	8	6	2	2	258	3	7	2	30	4
6705	7	1	35	175	275	1	4	4	5	4	7	8	2	6	2	11	5	2	2
6706	15	2	71	319	419	5	10	26	8	7	8	13	6	9	3	15	8	5	4
6707	16	2	72	427	468	6	10	33	12	11	12	14	7	9	4	18	10	8	5
6708	23	3	22	175	360	3	14	18	5	3	7	9	4	7	2	12	7	4	2
6709	9	1	10	87	716	63	10	30	7	6	6	19	6	3	4	11	9	5	3
6710	10	2	181	434	428	9	10	6	8	8	19	11	13	130	14	28	11	7	36
6711	16	4	244	504	517	15	14	17	12	17	21	14	18	157	19	34	13	9	38
6712	12	2	74	748	430	4	8	4	4	12	16	14	4	47	7	22	17	4	4
6713	14	2	142	700	536	4	13	12	10	5	23	14	20	163	16	29	12	8	38
6714	18	4	168	946	515	20	17	19	17	15	22	12	15	110	15	26	12	13	28
6715	18	2	132	375	539	3	17	21	10	5	24	15	18	161	15	28	13	9	38
6716	21	4	83	479	698	8	19	22	9	9	31	25	7	51	4	32	17	7	5
6717	10	3	38	769	240	4	6	1	10	12	40	10	2	27	8	18	8	13	9
6718	11	3	21	945	293	5	8	2	14	12	46	14	2	30	10	20	9	14	10
6719	15	4	26	411	363	18	10	1	16	17	46	15	3	31	17	25	11	14	9

Mixed Dishes & Fast Foods

Food No.	Food Description & Amount	wt gm	wt oz	cal	% cal fat	prot gm	carbo gm	fiber gm
6720	Fish and rice with tomato-based sauce [1 cup]	248	8.7	283	16%	19	40	0.8
6721	Fish and vegetables (no carrots, broccoli, dark-green leafy, or potatoes), tomato-based sauce [1 cup]	224	7.9	187	26%	28	7	1.7
6722	Fish and vegetables (no carrots, broccoli, dark-green leafy, or potatoes), soy-based sauce [1 cup]	162	5.7	146	26%	21	5	1.1
6723	Fish and vegetables (including carrots, broccoli, and/or dark-green leafy (no potatoes)), soy-based sauce 1 cup]	162	5.7	159	26%	23	5	1.0
6724	Fish and vegetables (including carrots, broccoli, and/or dark-green leafy (no potatoes)), tomato-based sauce [1 cup]	224	7.9	195	25%	28	8	2.0
6725	Fish cake (Kamaboko) tempura [2 oz, cooked]	56	2.0	94	33%	7	8	0.1
6726	Fish cake or patty [1 cake or patty]	120	4.2	237	48%	16	15	1.4
6727	Fish moochim (Korean style), dried fish with soy sauce [½ cup]	20	0.7	68	41%	7	2	0.2
6728	Fish timbale or mousse [1 cup]	175	6.2	331	69%	22	3	0.0
6729	Fish with cream or white sauce, not tuna or lobster [1 cup]	249	8.8	332	49%	28	13	0.3
6730	Fish with tomato-based sauce (Include fish with tomatoes) [1 cup]	222	7.8	223	28%	35	4	0.9
6731	Fish, noodles, and vegetables (no carrots, broccoli, or dark-green leafy), cheese sauce [1 cup]	244	8.6	291	22%	27	29	3.0
6732	Fish, noodles, and vegetables (including carrots, broccoli, and/or dark-green leafy), cheese sauce [1 cup]	224	7.9	245	23%	24	22	2.0
6733	Fish, tofu, and vegetables, tempura, Hawaiian style [1 cup]	63	2.2	146	68%	6	7	1.0
6734	Flounder, stuffed [1 piece]	210	7.4	334	29%	43	13	0.7
6735	Gefilte fish [5 balls]	41	1.4	47	30%	7	0	0.0
6736	Haddock cake or patty [1 cake or patty]	120	4.2	237	48%	16	15	1.4
6737	Kamaboko (Japanese fish cake) [2 slices]	32	1.1	37	5%	4	4	0.0
6738	Lau lau (pork and fish wrapped in taro or spinach leaves) [1 lau lau]	214	7.5	318	59%	30	2	1.4
6739	Lobster creole, Puerto Rican style (Langosta a la criolla) [1 cup]	242	8.5	395	57%	30	12	2.3
6740	Lobster newburg (Include lobster thermidor, lobster with cream or white sauce) [1 cup]	244	8.6	611	73%	30	11	0.1
6741	Lobster salad [1 cup]	182	6.4	150	46%	11	10	1.3
6742	Lobster with butter sauce (Include Lobster Norfolk) [1 cup]	188	6.6	448	71%	30	2	0.0
6743	Lobster, stuffed, baked [1 lobster]	400	14.1	730	40%	63	43	2.0
6744	Lomi salmon [1 cup]	234	8.3	151	32%	18	8	2.1
6745	Mackerel cake or patty [1 cake or patty]	120	4.2	297	54%	19	15	1.5
6746	Marinated fish, Puerto Rican style (Ceviche) [1 cup]	250	8.8	172	10%	29	10	1.3
6747	Mussels with tomato-based sauce [1 cup]	240	8.5	269	19%	30	24	3.5
6748	Octopus salad, Puerto Rican style (Ensalada de pulpo) [1 cup]	180	6.3	297	63%	17	10	1.7
6749	Oyster fritter [2 fritters]	80	2.8	243	47%	8	24	0.8
6750	Oyster pie (Include pot pie) [1/6 of pie]	109	3.8	274	58%	6	22	0.9
6751	Oysters Rockefeller [4 oysters]	96	3.4	129	51%	7	9	1.4
6752	Paella, with meat, Valenciana style (Paella Valenciana) [1 cup, boneless]	183	6.5	530	50%	35	28	0.9
6753	Paella, seafood Puerto Rican style (Paella a la marinera) [1 cup]	230	8.1	333	28%	37	22	1.7
6754	Salmon cake or patty (Include salmon croquette) [1 cake or patty]	120	4.2	261	54%	16	14	1.3
6755	Salmon loaf [1 slice]	105	3.7	208	49%	17	9	0.4
6756	Salmon salad [1 cup]	208	7.3	405	66%	27	6	1.3
6757	Sardines with mustard sauce [4 sardines (3" x 1" x ½") with sauce]	48	1.7	85	61%	8	0	0.0
6758	Sardines with tomato-based sauce [4 sardines (3" x 1" x ½") with sauce]	48	1.7	85	61%	8	0	0.0
6759	Scallops and noodles with cheese sauce [1 cup]	224	7.9	361	37%	31	27	0.8
6760	Scallops with cheese sauce [1 cup]	244	8.6	271	31%	35	14	0.4
6761	Seafood garden salad with seafood, eggs, tomato and/or carrots, other vegetables, no dressing (Include Hardee's Seafod Salad) [1 cup]	95	3.4	52	25%	7	2	0.9
6762	Seafood garden salad with seafood, eggs, vegetables (no tomato or carrots), no dressing [1 cup]	95	3.4	54	26%	8	2	0.8
6763	Seafood garden salad with seafood, tomato and/or carrots, other vegetables, no dressing [1 cup]	95	3.4	43	13%	7	3	1.0

						% of Daily Value													
Food No.	fat gm	sat fat gm	choles mg	sodium mg	potas mg	vit A	vit E	vit C	thia	ribo	niac	vit B-6	fola	vit B-12	calc	phos	mag	iron	zinc
6720	5	1	20	809	434	10	12	88	16	10	49	18	4	28	8	19	9	19	8
6721	5	1	67	443	712	11	19	40	11	9	23	20	6	34	4	24	12	6	5
6722	4	1	49	539	605	2	5	30	7	6	14	17	5	13	3	26	11	5	4
6723	5	1	54	572	616	21	6	31	8	6	15	18	4	14	3	28	12	5	4
6724	5	1	68	432	721	76	19	40	12	9	24	21	5	34	4	24	13	6	5
6725	3	1	29	33	132	0	2	0	2	4	6	5	0	17	2	8	6	2	1
6726	13	3	67	334	523	3	7	8	9	8	12	16	3	11	3	21	9	4	4
6727	3	0	17	1001	177	0	1	1	3	2	5	6	1	19	3	12	5	3	2
6728	25	15	212	163	423	29	11	3	7	15	14	11	4	27	8	25	9	4	5
6729	18	5	172	701	705	13	10	3	12	27	14	17	6	26	19	41	14	7	9
6730	7	1	87	334	857	12	20	26	13	10	30	22	5	37	6	35	17	6	6
6731	7	3	58	750	458	8	3	9	18	20	53	19	8	40	21	34	15	15	11
6732	6	3	52	684	393	12	4	23	12	17	47	16	5	37	20	29	12	12	8
6733	11	2	101	40	116	25	12	4	2	8	2	3	3	4	4	8	6	8	3
6734	11	2	160	470	803	10	21	10	18	16	34	21	11	90	12	44	19	11	19
6735	2	0	28	21	97	1	1	1	2	2	4	3	1	8	2	9	3	1	2
6736	13	3	67	334	523	3	7	8	9	8	12	16	3	11	3	21	9	4	4
6737	0	0	16	20	79	0	0	0	1	2	4	3	0	11	1	5	4	1	1
6738	21	6	90	212	762	40	17	19	29	19	29	22	21	25	8	29	19	13	15
6739	25	3	140	916	859	12	29	44	6	8	16	15	6	21	10	24	16	9	32
6740	50	30	369	647	607	52	9	1	7	24	8	8	8	67	24	40	14	6	27
6741	8	1	112	314	403	11	7	32	5	10	5	7	8	23	4	13	7	5	9
6742	35	22	198	905	523	36	10	0	1	7	8	6	4	76	10	28	13	4	28
6743	32	18	275	1751	1091	33	16	1	21	26	28	13	12	144	26	59	29	20	57
6744	5	1	45	467	603	9	7	44	7	13	31	18	12	60	20	31	12	9	6
6745	18	4	91	479	350	10	12	8	8	14	27	15	3	63	19	27	10	11	7
6746	2	0	50	90	734	20	4	121	7	1	3	34	6	68	6	29	14	3	4
6747	6	1	67	1489	913	14	17	42	28	31	22	10	26	432	7	39	22	50	26
6748	21	3	52	234	534	8	18	32	6	5	11	21	8	292	7	20	11	34	13
6749	13	3	73	294	117	5	8	2	14	13	11	3	3	128	12	15	7	26	279
6750	18	5	30	132	178	8	10	3	13	13	9	3	3	95	8	11	7	19	197
6751	7	3	37	303	250	34	4	19	11	9	8	5	13	150	8	11	12	25	280
6752	30	7	138	207	561	10	12	26	26	19	50	21	6	309	5	33	11	50	23
6753	10	2	168	423	554	18	13	62	12	8	17	22	6	147	12	29	15	33	20
6754	16	4	57	506	387	3	12	7	6	11	27	19	5	37	18	28	8	5	6
6755	11	3	122	506	292	11	8	4	6	17	23	11	6	39	19	28	8	7	7
6756	30	6	216	837	501	11	22	6	7	24	38	29	12	87	27	45	12	10	11
6757	6	1	29	199	164	3	8	1	1	7	10	3	3	72	12	18	4	6	4
6758	6	1	29	199	164	3	8	1	1	7	10	3	3	72	12	18	4	6	4
6759	15	5	84	537	613	17	12	1	17	18	13	7	5	24	32	50	20	24	26
6760	9	4	88	1010	820	9	9	2	12	19	9	9	5	34	39	60	22	21	27
6761	1	0	71	82	199	16	2	13	3	5	4	4	8	5	4	9	4	5	6
6762	2	0	78	88	194	5	2	18	3	5	4	5	10	6	4	10	4	5	6
6763	1	0	37	79	207	16	2	14	3	2	4	4	8	4	4	9	5	5	6

Mixed Dishes & Fast Foods

Food No.	Food Description & Amount	wt gm	wt oz	cal	% cal fat	prot gm	carbo gm	fiber gm
6764	Seafood garden salad with seafood, vegetables (no tomato or carrots), no dressing [1 cup]	95	3.4	41	13%	7	2	1.0
6765	Seafood newburg (Include shrimp newburg, crabmeat thermidor) [1 cup]	244	8.6	613	74%	30	10	0.1
6766	Seafood restructured (Include Delicaseas, Sea Tails, Sea Stix, imitation crabmeat) [1 cup, chunks or flakes]	126	4.4	146	5%	17	16	0.2
6767	Seafood salad [1 cup]	208	7.3	328	63%	26	5	0.7
6768	Seafood souffle [1 cup]	159	5.6	253	57%	17	9	0.2
6769	Seafood stew with potatoes and vegetables (no carrots, broccoli, or dark-green leafy), tomato-base sauce [1 cup]	252	8.9	174	19%	20	15	2.0
6770	Seafood stew with potatoes and vegetables (including carrots, broccoli, and/or dark-green leafy), tomato-base sauce [1 cup]	252	8.9	177	19%	21	15	2.1
6771	Shellfish mixture and noodles, tomato-based sauce [1 cup]	224	7.9	251	21%	15	34	1.9
6772	Shellfish mixture and vegetables (no carrots, broccoli, dark-green leafy, or potatoes), cream of mushroom soup-based sauce [1 cup]	244	8.6	244	41%	21	15	2.2
6773	Shellfish mixture and vegetables (no carrots, broccoli, dark-green leafy, or potatoes), soy-base sauce [1 cup]	162	5.7	163	49%	10	12	2.7
6774	Shellfish mixture and vegetables (including carrots, broccoli, and/or dark-green leafy (no potatoes)), cream of mushroom soup-based sauce [1 cup]	224	7.9	216	48%	14	15	2.5
6775	Shellfish mixture and vegetables (including carrots, broccoli, and/or dark-green leafy (no potatoes)), soy-base sauce [1 cup]	162	5.7	164	50%	10	11	2.7
6776	Shrimp and noodles with cheese sauce [1 cup]	224	7.9	349	38%	29	24	0.8
6777	Shrimp and pasta garden salad (shrimp, pasta salad, tomato and/or carrots, other vegetables), no dressing (Include Burger King Shrimp and Pasta Salad) [1 fast food order]	261	9.2	165	34%	13	15	2.8
6778	Shrimp and vegetables (no carrots, broccoli, dark-green leafy, or potatoes), soy-based sauce [1 cup]	162	5.7	174	56%	8	12	3.0
6779	Shrimp and vegetables (including carrots, broccoli, and/or dark-green leafy (no potatoes)), soy-based sauce [1 cup]	162	5.7	175	54%	8	13	3.3
6780	Shrimp cake or patty (Include shrimp burger; shrimp stick, battered) [1 cake or patty]	120	4.2	247	48%	17	15	1.3
6781	Shrimp chow mein or chop suey with noodles [1 cup]	220	7.8	272	42%	17	24	2.8
6782	Shrimp chow mein or chop suey, no noodles [1 cup]	220	7.8	154	32%	16	11	2.0
6783	Shrimp cocktail (shrimp with cocktail sauce) [1 cup]	230	8.1	218	11%	28	21	4.9
6784	Shrimp creole, no rice [1 cup]	246	8.7	309	38%	36	11	1.5
6785	Shrimp creole, with rice (Include shrimp jambalaya) [1 cup]	243	8.6	310	27%	27	28	1.4
6786	Shrimp garden salad (shrimp, eggs, tomato and/or carrots, other vegetables), no dressing (Include McDonald's Shrimp Salad) [1 cup]	95	3.4	60	24%	9	2	0.7
6787	Shrimp garden salad (shrimp, eggs, vegetables but not tomato or carrots), no dressing [1 cup]	95	3.4	69	25%	11	2	0.6
6788	Shrimp in garlic sauce, Puerto Rican style (Camarones al ajillo) [1 cup]	212	7.5	653	74%	37	6	0.5
6789	Shrimp salad [1 cup]	182	6.4	282	54%	27	6	0.8
6790	Shrimp scampi (Include shrimp in butter sauce) [1 cup]	136	4.8	311	64%	26	1	0.0
6791	Shrimp teriyaki (shrimp with soy-based sauce) [1 cup]	201	7.1	248	11%	39	12	0.7
6792	Shrimp with lobster sauce [1 cup]	185	6.5	292	38%	35	7	0.6
6793	Shrimp, curried [1 cup]	236	8.3	298	43%	28	14	0.4
6794	Shrimp, stuffed [4 stuffed shrimp]	64	2.3	127	44%	13	4	0.1
6795	Stewed codfish, Puerto Rican style (Bacalao guisado) [1 cup]	200	7.1	240	35%	18	21	3.1
6796	Stewed codfish, Puerto Rican style [1 cup]	227	8.0	322	27%	44	14	3.6
6797	Stewed salmon, Puerto Rican style (Salmon guisado) [1 cup]	212	7.5	318	45%	26	18	2.2
6798	Stuffed rice with chicken, Dominican style (Arroz relleno Dominicano) [1 cup]	200	7.1	573	37%	43	43	1.7
6799	Sushi, with egg, no vegetables, no fish, rolled in seaweed [2 pieces]	52	1.8	63	36%	3	7	0.1
6800	Sushi, with vegetables and fish [1 cup]	166	5.9	232	3%	9	47	1.9
6801	Sushi, with vegetables, no fish [1 cup]	166	5.9	240	2%	5	53	2.2
6802	Sushi, with vegetables, rolled in seaweed [1 cup]	166	5.9	194	2%	4	43	0.9
6803	Sweet and sour shrimp [1 cup]	176	6.2	481	56%	12	46	1.1
6804	Tuna and rice with cream of mushroom soup-based sauce [1 cup]	248	8.7	352	37%	20	34	0.8

Food No.	fat gm	sat fat gm	choles mg	sodium mg	potas mg	% of Daily Value													
						vit A	vit E	vit C	thia	ribo	niac	vit B-6	fola	vit B-12	calc	phos	mag	iron	zinc
6764	1	0	37	77	210	6	2	21	4	3	4	4	12	4	4	9	4	5	6
6765	50	30	426	551	533	53	8	5	9	23	15	11	11	83	25	39	14	13	27
6766	1	0	62	77	310	1	1	0	3	9	14	12	1	44	5	19	15	3	3
6767	23	3	132	352	503	5	18	21	5	6	12	9	8	31	9	28	14	11	22
6768	16	4	223	302	270	21	10	2	7	22	14	8	6	18	13	23	7	9	10
6769	4	1	96	509	795	12	8	70	13	12	17	18	9	399	8	22	11	51	12
6770	4	1	97	521	817	43	8	50	13	13	18	17	9	404	8	23	11	52	13
6771	6	1	81	348	284	8	6	15	18	10	15	7	5	150	5	20	12	28	10
6772	11	3	77	754	565	13	10	25	11	19	17	8	8	620	10	28	9	77	15
6773	9	2	41	174	339	4	8	55	7	7	8	10	7	160	6	13	7	29	6
6774	11	3	64	756	458	77	13	106	7	11	12	10	8	244	8	20	8	36	10
6775	9	2	43	185	388	61	9	59	9	7	9	9	8	165	6	14	8	29	6
6776	15	5	216	499	339	21	8	4	15	17	20	9	3	27	24	31	15	25	17
6777	6	1	73	384	411	20	9	36	10	6	11	8	18	8	6	15	10	13	7
6778	11	2	37	197	313	2	9	65	8	5	7	10	8	4	6	11	8	13	4
6779	10	2	36	182	331	69	9	63	9	5	8	11	8	4	5	11	8	13	4
6780	13	3	144	300	329	3	10	9	6	6	13	11	2	13	6	20	10	12	7
6781	13	2	82	710	391	2	6	16	15	14	22	9	11	10	6	22	13	19	9
6782	5	1	93	674	407	1	7	18	6	9	17	9	11	11	6	20	11	14	7
6783	3	0	196	1129	576	7	16	43	7	6	22	13	12	21	9	31	15	21	11
6784	13	2	256	521	580	19	15	40	9	7	26	14	3	28	13	38	19	27	14
6785	9	2	181	370	439	13	11	28	20	6	24	11	3	20	10	30	16	24	12
6786	2	0	88	72	184	8	2	11	3	4	5	4	6	7	3	10	5	7	4
6787	2	0	111	87	175	3	3	7	2	5	6	4	6	9	4	12	5	8	5
6788	54	9	269	536	417	39	39	60	5	4	22	14	3	33	12	38	18	26	14
6789	17	3	206	392	367	4	15	10	3	4	16	14	4	22	9	28	13	19	10
6790	22	13	247	392	240	21	6	4	2	3	15	6	1	21	7	27	12	17	9
6791	3	1	269	3104	486	9	7	8	6	8	30	14	4	31	11	39	22	31	15
6792	12	2	261	474	422	4	11	5	13	12	25	14	6	26	8	37	15	21	16
6793	14	4	177	342	443	18	11	6	8	17	16	8	3	23	23	37	15	17	12
6794	6	1	102	168	165	4	6	3	5	5	10	5	5	42	5	14	6	7	11
6795	9	1	39	209	737	6	10	101	12	6	16	26	6	12	4	20	13	8	5
6796	10	1	102	4186	1063	9	12	122	16	12	28	39	11	106	11	55	22	12	7
6797	16	3	65	918	925	4	17	25	7	15	44	28	8	83	27	44	16	11	10
6798	24	7	156	487	490	8	9	18	23	21	69	32	5	9	10	36	14	23	23
6799	3	1	70	176	43	5	1	1	3	6	2	2	2	2	1	4	2	3	2
6800	1	0	11	93	218	14	3	7	19	4	15	8	4	6	3	11	7	13	6
6801	0	0	0	88	169	15	1	7	20	4	13	7	4	0	2	8	6	14	6
6802	0	0	0	5	106	7	1	4	14	3	10	7	3	0	2	6	5	9	5
6803	30	4	71	2019	362	5	31	15	4	7	14	11	2	8	5	15	11	14	6
6804	15	4	13	928	277	7	9	11	12	13	42	8	2	22	10	27	9	13	10

Mixed Dishes & Fast Foods

Food No.	Food Description & Amount	wt gm	wt oz	cal	% cal fat	prot gm	carbo gm	fiber gm
6805	Tuna cake or patty [1 cake or patty]	120	4.2	300	52%	22	14	1.3
6806	Tuna casserole with vegetables and cream of mushroom soup-based sauce, no noodles [1 cup]	224	7.9	398	47%	29	23	2.0
6807	Tuna loaf [1 slice]	105	3.7	245	46%	22	10	0.5
6808	Tuna noodle casserole with cream of mushroom soup-based sauce [1 cup]	224	7.9	401	40%	27	32	1.2
6809	Tuna noodle casserole with cream or white sauce [1 cup]	224	7.9	426	40%	28	34	1.2
6810	Tuna noodle casserole with vegetables and cream of mushroom soup-based sauce [1 cup]	224	7.9	381	38%	25	33	2.2
6811	Tuna noodle casserole with vegetables, cream or white sauce [1 cup]	224	7.9	349	35%	21	35	2.7
6812	Tuna pot pie [1 cup]	252	8.9	563	53%	23	42	3.4
6813	Tuna salad with cheese [1 cup]	208	7.3	358	44%	30	20	0.8
6814	Tuna salad with egg [1 cup]	208	7.3	314	40%	28	19	0.8
6815	Tuna salad [1 cup]	208	7.3	296	33%	29	20	1.0
6816	Tuna with cream or white sauce [1 cup]	237	8.4	392	53%	32	12	0.3
	Other Mixed Dishes							
6900	Antipasto with ham, fish, cheese, vegetables [1 cup]	115	4.1	151	58%	11	4	1.1
6901	Bacon strips, meatless (Include Morning Star Breakfast Strips, Stripple) [4 strips]	20	0.7	62	86%	2	1	0.5
6902	Baked beans [1 cup]	253	8.9	390	30%	16	55	10.1
6903	Baked beans, low sodium [1 cup]	253	8.9	235	4%	12	52	13.9
6904	Baked beans, with pork and sweet sauce [1 cup]	253	8.9	281	12%	13	53	13.2
6905	Baked beans, with tomato sauce (Include vegetarian baked beans) [1 cup]	255	9.0	237	4%	12	52	12.8
6906	Beans and franks [1 cup]	259	9.1	368	42%	17	40	17.9
6907	Beans, cooked with ground beef [1 cup]	266	9.4	416	25%	28	52	8.9
6908	Beans, cooked with pork [1 cup]	178	6.3	252	15%	12	43	6.8
6909	Bierock (turnover filled with ground beef and cabbage mixture) [1 bierock]	215	7.6	517	33%	21	64	3.7
6910	Biscuit with gravy (Include Hardee's) [1 biscuit with gravy]	221	7.8	429	49%	13	44	1.1
6911	Black beans, Cuban style (Habichuelas negras guisadas a la Cubana) [1 cup]	270	9.5	302	14%	16	50	11.8
6912	Boston baked beans [1 cup]	253	8.9	390	30%	16	55	10.1
6913	Bread stuffing made with egg [1 cup]	170	6.0	300	44%	6	35	4.6
6914	Breaded brains, Puerto Rican style (Sesos rebosados) [2 fritters (3½"x2½"x½")]	120	4.2	307	56%	13	20	0.6
6915	Breakfast links, patties, or slices, meatless (Include Prosage, Morningstar) [2 links]	50	1.8	128	64%	9	5	1.4
6916	Calzone, with cheese, meatless (Include stromboli, Pizza Hut Calizza) [1 calzone or stromboli]	424	15.0	1641	51%	81	117	5.0
6917	Calzone, with meat and cheese (Include stromboli, Pizza Hut Calizza) [1 calzone or stromboli]	424	15.0	1474	46%	64	131	5.7
6918	Cannelloni, cheese and spinach-filled, no sauce [1 cannelloni]	74	2.6	119	39%	5	13	0.9
6919	Cassava pie stuffed with crabmeat, Puerto Rican style (Empanada de jueyes) [1 empanada (5"x 2½"x½")]	126	4.4	311	46%	14	29	1.9
6920	Chalupas with beans and cheese [1 chalupa]	164	5.8	285	48%	10	28	7.0
6921	Chalupas with chicken and cheese [1 chalupa]	150	5.3	296	47%	17	23	5.4
6922	Chayote relleno (stuffed christophine, Puerto Rican style) [¼ chayote (4½" x 2" x 1")]	123	4.3	256	66%	16	6	2.6
6923	Cheese fondue [1 cup]	215	7.6	446	59%	31	8	0.1
6924	Cheese souffle [1 cup]	95	3.4	196	69%	9	6	0.1
6925	Cheese turnovers, Puerto Rican style (Pastelillos de queso; Empandillas) [2 turnovers]	42	1.5	172	52%	4	16	0.5
6926	Chickpeas stewed with pig's feet, Puerto Rican style (Garbanzos guisados con patitos de cerdo) [1 cup, with bones]	202	7.1	268	51%	17	16	3.8
6927	Chiles rellenos [1 chili]	143	5.0	365	74%	17	8	1.3
6928	Chiles rellenos, filled with meat and cheese [1 chili]	143	5.0	222	65%	10	10	1.8
6929	Chili beans, barbecue beans, ranch style beans or Mexican-style beans (Include beans in chili sauce) [1 cup]	253	8.9	223	10%	13	43	10.6
6930	Chili con carne with beans and macaroni [1 cup]	253	8.9	336	31%	21	38	6.7
6931	Chili con carne with beans and rice [1 cup]	250	8.8	297	27%	11	45	7.2

						% of Daily Value													
Food No.	fat gm	sat fat gm	choles mg	sodium mg	potas mg	vit A	vit E	vit C	thia	ribo	niac	vit B-6	fola	vit B-12	calc	phos	mag	iron	zinc
6805	17	4	43	422	326	3	11	6	7	9	46	11	3	23	3	25	8	8	6
6806	21	5	18	1054	320	11	13	8	16	18	57	7	6	31	11	31	11	15	10
6807	13	3	99	346	193	11	8	4	7	15	38	5	4	24	7	22	6	8	6
6808	18	4	38	830	248	8	11	1	15	16	51	6	3	27	9	29	11	16	10
6809	19	4	42	460	296	16	11	1	17	20	51	6	3	28	14	32	12	16	10
6810	16	4	35	784	255	9	10	6	18	16	47	6	5	24	9	27	11	16	10
6811	14	3	33	663	318	10	9	16	18	19	36	7	5	17	14	27	11	16	10
6812	33	9	31	536	378	89	18	10	26	22	51	8	7	21	6	29	10	19	8
6813	18	6	54	1070	364	10	9	4	4	12	65	20	4	53	17	30	10	11	11
6814	14	3	130	810	332	9	10	4	4	12	65	20	6	54	4	22	8	12	7
6815	11	2	41	853	352	5	8	4	4	7	75	22	4	57	3	21	9	12	7
6816	23	6	134	779	403	13	14	2	9	28	53	9	6	41	18	42	11	10	10
6900	10	4	112	724	241	60	4	7	8	15	12	9	5	13	14	17	5	7	9
6901	6	1	0	293	34	0	6	0	59	6	8	5	2	0	0	1	1	3	1
6902	13	5	13	236	1082	0	2	4	14	5	3	13	31	1	18	20	33	35	16
6903	1	0	0	3	749	4	6	13	25	9	5	16	15	0	13	26	20	4	24
6904	4	1	18	850	673	3	6	13	8	9	4	11	24	0	15	27	22	23	25
6905	1	0	0	1012	755	4	6	13	25	9	5	16	14	0	13	27	20	4	24
6906	17	6	16	1114	609	4	6	10	10	9	12	6	19	0	12	27	18	25	32
6907	12	4	51	1146	987	4	5	11	12	14	20	16	19	23	13	26	23	32	32
6908	4	2	7	312	725	1	2	4	12	5	4	8	21	1	11	15	19	24	12
6909	19	6	44	48	319	1	6	15	38	32	38	12	13	23	4	20	8	29	22
6910	23	7	40	1373	405	5	10	3	24	27	16	5	3	15	24	44	36	15	7
6911	5	1	2	31	891	2	3	26	30	7	6	11	41	0	11	25	27	23	17
6912	13	5	13	236	1082	0	2	4	14	5	3	13	31	1	18	20	33	35	16
6913	15	3	43	881	131	15	11	0	15	13	12	4	8	2	6	9	5	10	4
6914	19	4	1499	102	340	1	14	20	17	24	23	8	2	132	7	28	5	16	10
6915	9	1	0	444	116	3	5	0	78	12	28	21	3	0	3	11	5	10	5
6916	93	44	253	2051	558	73	34	0	70	106	49	14	39	21	190	152	28	51	54
6917	76	26	190	1073	678	46	35	0	88	98	74	18	52	32	77	91	22	59	51
6918	5	2	34	60	129	16	2	3	7	10	4	4	8	2	9	8	5	8	4
6919	16	4	49	373	983	5	10	69	18	15	13	20	10	43	22	23	21	21	14
6920	15	6	23	165	476	9	8	12	12	8	4	11	29	2	18	23	15	13	10
6921	15	6	45	181	417	9	7	10	10	10	13	13	20	3	17	24	14	12	12
6922	19	6	133	270	386	5	3	18	22	17	15	15	6	9	4	19	7	8	16
6923	29	19	97	286	225	27	2	0	3	25	2	5	2	17	103	66	13	5	28
6924	15	6	136	225	125	18	6	0	4	17	1	3	4	6	18	18	4	4	7
6925	10	4	15	137	31	3	2	0	8	7	5	1	1	1	11	9	2	6	3
6926	15	4	68	255	418	7	6	14	6	7	5	8	11	2	6	13	7	10	11
6927	30	12	168	522	386	25	21	188	6	23	5	13	7	8	40	31	9	9	14
6928	16	5	110	130	342	16	14	58	6	13	10	12	5	10	11	14	6	9	10
6929	3	0	0	1834	1139	0	2	7	7	22	5	34	16	0	8	39	28	26	34
6930	12	4	47	722	623	9	7	28	17	16	25	12	10	19	5	22	13	21	24
6931	9	4	26	1171	598	5	6	4	15	10	10	15	9	0	8	28	20	36	24

Mixed Dishes & Fast Foods

Food No.	Food Description & Amount	wt gm	wt oz	cal	% cal fat	prot gm	carbo gm	fiber gm
6932	Chili con carne with chicken or turkey and beans [1 cup]	254	9.0	217	22%	17	27	7.4
6933	Chili con carne with venison and beans [1 cup]	254	9.0	251	17%	26	27	7.5
6934	Chilaquiles, with egg [1 cup]	232	8.2	441	64%	14	28	4.3
6935	Chilaquiles, without egg [1 cup]	232	8.2	445	65%	10	32	5.1
6936	Chimichanga with beans and cheese, meatless [1 chimichanga]	118	4.2	256	56%	8	21	3.2
6937	Chimichanga with beef [1 chimichanga]	118	4.2	388	60%	13	25	1.7
6938	Chimichanga with beef and beans [1 chimichanga]	118	4.2	241	52%	8	21	3.2
6939	Chimichanga with beef and cheese [1 chimichanga]	118	4.2	341	63%	13	19	1.5
6940	Chimichanga with beef and rice [1 chimichanga]	288	10.2	643	52%	19	59	4.4
6941	Chimichanga with chicken and cheese [1 chimichanga]	183	6.5	560	61%	24	31	2.3
6942	Chimichanga with chicken and sour cream, no cheese [1 chimichanga]	118	4.2	278	64%	9	17	1.2
6943	Chow fun noodles with meat and vegetables [1 cup]	152	5.4	192	34%	10	22	1.7
6944	Chow fun noodles with vegetables, meatless [1 cup]	152	5.4	160	12%	4	32	1.2
6945	Chow mein or chop suey, with noodles [1 cup]	220	7.8	412	51%	21	31	3.7
6946	Chop suey, meatless [1 cup]	220	7.8	248	26%	5	40	2.1
6947	Chow mein or chop suey, various types of meat, with noodles [1 cup]	220	7.8	420	52%	21	31	3.7
6948	Codfish fritters, Puerto Rican style (Bacalaitos) [2 fritters (3½" x 3½")]	68	2.4	372	69%	12	17	0.6
6949	Corned beef patty [1 patty]	100	3.5	181	56%	9	11	0.5
6950	Cornmeal dressing with chicken or turkey and vegetables [1 cup]	161	5.7	383	55%	12	31	2.5
6951	Cornmeal fritters, Puerto Rican style (Arepa; arepitas) [2 fritters (2½"x2½"x¼")]	80	2.8	219	60%	6	16	1.5
6952	Cornmeal sticks, Puerto Rican style (Surullos) [4 sticks (3" x ¾")]	80	2.8	327	45%	6	38	3.6
6953	Cowpeas, cooked with pork (Include blackeye peas with pork, field peas with pork) [1 cup]	179	6.3	239	18%	24	25	7.9
6954	Creamed dried beef on toast [1 slice toast with sauce]	145	5.1	230	43%	11	21	0.7
6955	Crepe, with creamy chicken-mushroom filling, no sauce on top [1 crepe]	123	4.3	239	48%	18	13	0.6
6956	Crepe, with creamy beef-mushroom filling, creamy mushroom sauce on top [1 crepe]	154	5.4	292	52%	22	12	0.8
6957	Croissant, filled with broccoli and cheese (Include Sara Lee Le Sanwich with broccoli and cheese) [1 croissant]	113	4.0	303	51%	8	29	1.4
6958	Dim sum, egg roll type, meat filled (Include shrimp, pork, ham) [1 dim sum]	28	1.0	50	42%	3	4	0.2
6959	Dirty rice [1 cup]	198	7.0	281	31%	11	36	0.6
6960	Dressing with chicken and vegetables [1 cup]	161	5.7	351	47%	12	34	2.3
6961	Dressing with meat and vegetables (Include with sausage, ground beef, pepperoni, ham, bacon, salami) [1 cup]	161	5.7	421	58%	11	33	2.1
6962	Dressing with oysters [1 cup]	161	5.7	309	54%	8	28	2.0
6963	Dumplings, fried, pork [1 dumpling]	100	3.5	341	55%	13	25	0.8
6964	Dumplings, fried, Puerto Rican style [2 dumplings]	64	2.3	236	57%	4	22	0.7
6965	Dumplings, meat-filled (Include pierogi, piroshki, kreplach) [1 dumpling]	97	3.4	362	59%	11	25	0.9
6966	Dumplings, plain [2 dumplings]	64	2.3	80	24%	2	13	0.4
6967	Dumplings, potato or cheese-filled (Include pierogi) [1 dumpling]	57	2.0	104	22%	4	17	0.8
6968	Dumplings, steamed, filled with meat, poultry, or seafood (Include shui-mai, steamed dim sum) [2 dumplings]	74	2.6	81	20%	8	7	0.4
6969	Egg foo yung, beef [1 patty]	86	3.0	119	60%	8	3	0.5
6970	Egg foo yung, chicken [1 patty]	86	3.0	121	59%	8	4	0.5
6971	Egg foo yung, pork [1 patty]	86	3.0	125	60%	8	4	0.5
6972	Egg foo yung, shrimp (Include Tortas de Carmaron) [1 cup]	175	6.2	317	70%	17	7	1.5
6973	Egg roll, meatless [1 egg roll]	64	2.3	101	52%	3	10	0.8
6974	Egg roll, with chicken or turkey [1 egg roll]	64	2.3	103	48%	4	9	0.6
6975	Egg roll, with meat (Include Chinese rolls, spring rolls, lumpia) [1 egg roll]	64	2.3	113	49%	5	9	0.7
6976	Egg roll, with shrimp [1 egg roll]	64	2.3	105	49%	4	10	0.7
6977	Eggplant parmesan casserole, low-calorie [1 cup]	198	7.0	181	44%	14	13	3.6
6978	Eggplant parmesan casserole, regular [1 cup]	198	7.0	319	62%	14	17	3.2
6979	Enchilada with beans, meatless [1 enchilada]	118	4.2	207	36%	6	29	6.4
6980	Enchilada with beans and cheese, meatless [1 enchilada]	131	4.6	252	46%	9	26	5.4
6981	Enchilada with beef, no beans [1 enchilada]	114	4.0	207	40%	11	21	3.0

Food No.	fat gm	sat fat gm	choles mg	sodium mg	potas mg	% of Daily Value													
						vit A	vit E	vit C	thia	ribo	niac	vit B-6	fola	vit B-12	calc	phos	mag	iron	zinc
6932	5	1	33	874	682	12	8	36	15	13	26	18	14	2	6	20	13	15	10
6933	5	1	72	893	785	12	8	35	16	31	26	13	10	46	6	26	15	28	16
6934	32	9	198	217	416	26	17	24	9	23	6	13	10	8	20	25	13	12	11
6935	32	9	23	193	429	21	17	28	8	12	6	12	6	1	21	21	14	10	9
6936	16	5	17	305	291	9	12	18	9	9	7	6	4	2	15	14	7	10	7
6937	26	6	35	233	216	1	17	5	13	11	18	7	2	19	6	13	5	13	16
6938	14	3	17	230	323	4	12	18	9	8	11	8	4	8	5	10	7	11	10
6939	24	7	39	282	199	8	13	10	10	12	12	6	4	13	18	18	5	10	13
6940	37	7	39	573	668	12	32	41	30	20	33	18	9	21	11	22	14	26	22
6941	38	11	67	487	248	11	21	9	16	20	21	9	7	6	31	30	9	14	15
6942	20	6	30	155	179	8	11	9	9	9	11	4	4	2	7	9	4	7	5
6943	7	2	20	206	269	3	4	11	20	8	14	16	5	3	3	11	5	4	7
6944	2	0	0	80	94	1	1	8	5	1	6	9	4	0	2	6	6	3	3
6945	23	4	58	965	449	11	8	34	30	20	29	17	10	12	5	24	14	21	16
6946	7	1	0	466	272	1	7	32	17	9	15	12	7	0	3	11	8	12	6
6947	24	5	42	1150	477	11	8	33	36	23	32	19	10	11	4	25	13	20	17
6948	29	4	24	51	253	1	24	1	11	8	11	7	2	8	2	14	6	7	3
6949	11	4	33	540	200	0	1	0	1	5	11	4	2	11	1	7	4	11	15
6950	23	5	140	357	228	77	15	7	13	27	13	9	29	47	16	18	7	21	12
6951	15	5	16	106	54	5	8	0	7	8	5	3	2	1	12	9	3	5	5
6952	17	4	8	57	90	4	13	0	17	12	11	6	4	1	6	8	6	12	4
6953	5	2	28	719	506	0	2	1	44	12	17	17	63	11	4	33	18	20	22
6954	11	3	17	865	277	12	6	1	12	18	11	6	3	13	16	16	7	10	10
6955	13	6	119	168	247	10	3	2	9	16	36	15	4	6	6	18	6	8	6
6956	17	6	109	515	282	13	7	2	8	20	26	11	4	20	17	26	9	11	19
6957	17	11	48	539	131	20	3	12	14	15	9	3	6	2	16	15	4	9	6
6958	2	1	18	34	44	0	1	1	5	3	3	2	1	2	1	3	1	2	3
6959	10	5	104	461	221	75	3	7	15	22	27	8	21	48	2	15	5	22	11
6960	18	4	104	494	200	68	10	7	19	27	17	8	28	41	10	13	7	22	11
6961	27	8	31	1105	215	8	7	3	27	16	19	5	6	3	9	11	6	18	8
6962	18	4	23	560	232	17	13	8	16	13	13	5	7	121	10	12	10	26	254
6963	21	5	27	86	198	1	11	1	35	16	18	10	2	5	3	13	5	10	7
6964	15	3	0	119	70	2	9	0	11	9	7	1	1	1	9	7	2	8	2
6965	24	6	28	119	115	0	10	0	15	12	13	5	2	14	1	10	3	13	15
6966	2	1	1	131	41	1	1	0	7	6	4	1	1	1	9	6	2	5	1
6967	2	1	33	101	84	3	1	2	9	8	6	3	2	2	3	6	2	6	2
6968	2	0	39	325	132	1	1	2	8	6	11	5	1	4	2	8	3	5	4
6969	8	2	166	131	139	9	5	5	3	13	3	6	6	11	3	10	3	6	7
6970	8	2	167	132	136	9	5	5	3	14	4	6	6	6	3	10	3	5	5
6971	8	2	167	131	157	9	5	5	9	15	4	7	6	7	3	11	3	5	6
6972	25	5	379	522	329	49	15	6	6	28	8	12	10	16	7	24	7	13	10
6973	6	1	30	274	97	2	4	5	5	6	4	2	3	1	1	4	2	4	2
6974	6	1	38	164	73	2	3	4	5	6	5	2	3	1	2	4	2	5	2
6975	6	1	37	274	124	2	4	4	11	7	6	5	2	2	2	6	3	5	3
6976	6	1	40	293	100	2	4	4	5	6	5	3	2	2	2	5	2	5	2
6977	9	5	25	671	513	13	4	14	9	12	7	11	6	7	38	29	9	5	11
6978	22	9	55	684	447	17	12	13	9	15	8	10	6	7	37	28	9	7	10
6979	8	2	5	128	456	13	6	21	8	5	5	10	20	0	8	18	13	10	6
6980	13	6	21	262	464	23	6	26	7	8	5	11	15	2	20	25	13	9	9
6981	9	3	28	183	395	17	5	23	5	9	13	12	3	11	8	19	10	9	15

Mixed Dishes & Fast Foods

Food No.	Food Description & Amount	wt gm	wt oz	cal	% cal fat	prot gm	carbo gm	fiber gm
6982	Enchilada with beef and beans [1 enchilada]	116	4.1	207	37%	8	25	4.9
6983	Enchilada with beef and cheese, no beans [1 enchilada]	105	3.7	209	50%	10	17	2.6
6984	Enchilada with beef, beans, and cheese (Include Taco Bell enchirito) [1 enchilada or enchirito]	129	4.6	242	45%	10	24	4.7
6985	Enchilada with cheese, meatless, no beans [1 enchilada]	102	3.6	225	55%	10	17	2.5
6986	Enchilada with chicken [1 enchilada]	126	4.4	202	30%	14	22	3.2
6987	Enchilada with chicken and beans [1 enchilada]	113	4.0	185	35%	9	22	4.6
6988	Enchilada with chicken and cheese, no beans [1 enchilada]	126	4.4	235	45%	14	20	3.0
6989	Enchilada with chicken, beans, and cheese [1 enchilada]	126	4.4	227	43%	11	23	4.5
6990	Enchilada with ham and cheese, no beans [1 enchilada]	105	3.7	201	45%	9	20	2.7
6991	Enchilada with seafood [1 enchilada]	126	4.4	179	24%	12	23	3.3
6992	Fajita with beef [fajita with 1 tortilla]	223	7.9	399	41%	23	36	3.2
6993	Fajita with chicken [fajita with 1 tortilla]	223	7.9	363	30%	20	44	5.1
6994	Falafel [4 patties (2¼" dia)]	68	2.4	227	48%	9	22	8.9
6995	Flauta with beef [1 flauta]	113	4.0	354	70%	14	13	1.9
6996	Flauta with chicken [1 flauta]	113	4.0	330	70%	13	12	1.7
6997	Flavored pasta (Include Lipton Beef Flavor, Lipton Chicken Flavor) [1 cup]	185	6.5	210	36%	7	27	1.0
6998	Flavored rice mixture (Include Ricearoni, all flavors; Liptons rice and sauce; Uncle Ben's Rice Oriental) [1 cup]	218	7.7	277	29%	4	44	0.9
6999	Flavored rice mixture with cheese (Include rice au gratin) [1 cup]	230	8.1	198	34%	5	29	1.8
7000	Flavored rice, brown and wild [1 cup]	217	7.7	236	24%	6	40	2.8
7001	Flavored rice, white and wild [1 cup]	182	6.4	172	17%	5	31	1.3
7002	Flavored rice and pasta mixture, beef flavor [1 cup]	184	6.5	207	27%	5	33	1.2
7003	Flavored rice and pasta mixture, chicken flavor [1 cup]	208	7.3	234	27%	5	37	1.3
7004	Fried chickpeas, Puerto Rican style (Garbanzos fritos) [1 cup]	120	4.2	377	58%	13	28	8.0
7005	Fried rice, Puerto Rican style (arroz frito) [1 cup]	173	6.1	222	25%	25	15	1.0
7006	Gnocchi, cheese [1 cup]	70	2.5	128	60%	7	6	0.2
7007	Gnocchi, potato [1 cup]	188	6.6	268	44%	5	33	1.8
7008	Grape leaves stuffed with rice [1 roll]	56	2.0	91	64%	1	8	1.7
7009	Gumbo with rice (New Orleans type with shellfish, pork, and/or poultry, tomatoes, okra, rice) [1 cup]	244	8.6	193	35%	14	17	1.9
7010	Gumbo, no rice (New Orleans type with shellfish, pork, and/or poultry, tomatoes, okra) [1 cup]	244	8.6	179	43%	15	11	2.0
7011	Hallacas, Puerto Rican style (hominy, pork or ham, vegetables) [1 hallaca (5¾" x 2½" x ½")]	95	3.4	148	62%	6	9	1.0
7012	Hash [1 cup]	190	6.7	344	56%	17	20	1.0
7013	Italian pie with meat (Include Priazzo; Pizza Hut Priazzo Roma, Priazzo Milano, Priazzo Portofino, Priazzo Verona) [1/8 of 12" dia]	191	6.7	569	36%	21	69	3.5
7014	Italian pie, meatless (Include Pizza Hut Priazzo Florentine) [1/8 of 12" dia]	163	5.7	444	30%	18	59	3.0
7015	Jambalaya with meat and rice [1 cup]	244	8.6	398	49%	26	23	1.2
7016	Julienne salad (meat, cheese, eggs, vegetables), no dressing (Include Burger King Chef's Salad; Hardee's Chef's Salad; McDonald's Chef's Salad) [1 cup]	76	2.7	72	52%	7	2	0.6
7017	Kibby, Puerto Rican style (beef and bulgar) (Plato Arabe) [2 fritters (3" x 3" x ½")]	110	3.9	190	39%	10	20	4.8
7018	Kidney bean salad [1 cup]	231	8.1	349	37%	13	45	11.3
7019	Kishke, stuffed derma [4 kishke (1 cubic inch, cooked)]	72	2.5	334	65%	3	25	1.2
7020	Knish, cheese [1 knish]	60	2.1	208	51%	6	19	0.6
7021	Knish, meat [1 knish]	50	1.8	175	55%	7	13	0.6
7022	Knish, potato [1 knish]	61	2.2	215	52%	5	21	0.9
7023	Kung Pao pork [1 cup]	162	5.7	451	68%	26	11	2.1
7024	Lasagna with meat (Include baked ziti) [1 piece (3½" x 4")]	232	8.2	371	36%	22	38	2.6
7025	Lasagna with meat, canned [1 cup]	250	8.8	218	16%	8	39	1.7
7026	Lasagna with meat and spinach [1 piece (3½" x 4")]	232	8.2	346	35%	21	35	3.0
7027	Lasagna with meat, spinach noodles [1 piece (3½" x 4")]	232	8.2	351	37%	21	34	4.7
7028	Lasagna with meat, whole wheat noodles [1 piece (3½" x 4")]	232	8.2	354	37%	22	36	4.1

Food No.	fat gm	sat fat gm	choles mg	sodium mg	potas mg	% of Daily Value: vit A	vit E	vit C	thia	ribo	niac	vit B-6	fola	vit B-12	calc	phos	mag	iron	zinc
6982	9	3	15	152	428	15	5	22	7	7	8	11	12	5	8	18	11	10	10
6983	12	5	31	256	343	22	5	23	4	9	8	10	3	8	17	21	9	7	12
6984	12	5	25	242	459	22	6	27	7	9	8	12	12	6	16	23	12	10	11
6985	14	7	33	335	300	26	5	22	4	10	4	8	4	4	28	26	9	5	9
6986	7	1	35	197	381	18	5	24	5	8	18	14	3	1	8	20	11	8	9
6987	7	2	17	143	407	15	5	22	6	6	10	11	12	1	7	16	10	8	7
6988	12	5	39	301	382	26	5	27	5	10	12	12	4	3	21	25	10	7	10
6989	11	4	26	234	429	21	6	26	6	8	9	11	11	2	16	22	11	9	8
6990	10	4	25	471	336	20	4	21	10	9	9	10	3	4	17	24	9	6	8
6991	5	1	68	238	396	19	6	26	5	4	10	11	3	7	10	23	13	11	7
6992	18	6	45	316	479	4	8	45	26	18	27	19	6	34	8	24	9	21	23
6993	12	2	39	343	534	6	8	61	28	19	31	19	10	2	10	19	12	18	11
6994	12	2	0	103	275	0	10	2	6	6	3	4	13	0	4	13	13	11	7
6995	28	5	37	68	313	2	21	32	4	8	9	12	3	20	5	18	7	10	23
6996	26	4	35	71	269	3	20	30	3	6	15	11	2	1	5	14	7	5	8
6997	8	2	35	541	166	7	5	0	21	11	19	3	3	4	2	10	6	11	4
6998	9	2	2	653	99	7	6	2	16	2	12	6	1	0	3	7	4	14	5
6999	7	2	1	511	141	4	4	0	9	7	8	3	1	0	8	15	4	5	4
7000	6	1	0	789	304	5	5	2	8	6	18	12	3	0	2	20	17	7	9
7001	3	1	0	672	135	3	3	1	8	3	9	3	2	0	5	10	7	8	6
7002	6	2	3	546	119	8	4	3	17	7	11	6	2	0	5	7	5	13	4
7003	7	2	3	617	135	9	4	3	19	8	12	6	2	0	5	8	6	15	4
7004	24	8	25	217	463	0	3	3	20	8	8	14	64	4	5	21	14	17	13
7005	6	2	162	897	401	7	4	37	30	15	20	20	5	15	5	25	10	12	14
7006	8	3	49	206	51	9	4	0	3	8	2	1	2	4	15	11	2	3	4
7007	13	8	35	141	245	13	1	6	15	10	11	8	3	2	4	8	5	8	3
7008	6	1	0	4	90	26	5	6	2	3	3	4	4	0	5	2	4	4	1
7009	8	2	40	542	446	6	6	23	13	9	23	11	11	40	7	15	10	15	101
7010	8	2	45	607	489	7	7	25	11	10	23	11	13	45	8	16	10	14	112
7011	10	2	38	158	170	3	9	17	9	6	6	6	2	3	2	7	3	5	4
7012	21	7	63	1026	380	0	2	0	1	10	20	8	4	20	2	13	7	21	29
7013	23	8	39	1440	506	10	9	15	48	35	36	13	10	12	14	27	11	28	16
7014	15	6	29	638	358	13	8	13	33	29	23	7	9	3	31	30	10	22	11
7015	22	6	97	341	443	7	3	17	19	12	47	20	3	7	5	23	10	15	15
7016	4	2	74	138	143	13	1	5	6	8	5	6	7	5	6	9	3	3	5
7017	8	3	29	33	228	0	1	2	4	6	13	7	2	11	2	13	12	8	13
7018	14	3	0	614	680	5	14	8	16	6	5	11	48	1	6	22	17	25	11
7019	24	12	26	1	62	0	3	1	14	8	8	2	2	0	1	4	2	8	2
7020	12	3	56	204	62	13	7	0	11	12	6	2	3	3	2	8	2	7	2
7021	11	3	52	107	88	9	6	1	8	9	7	2	2	5	1	6	2	7	7
7022	12	3	59	140	96	13	8	2	11	10	7	3	3	2	2	6	3	7	2
7023	34	7	59	862	541	5	17	13	55	18	35	26	10	9	5	27	15	11	17
7024	15	8	55	370	435	15	5	23	15	19	20	12	5	15	26	28	12	16	21
7025	4	2	13	1404	311	8	2	36	17	10	13	7	4	5	5	10	7	9	7
7026	14	7	51	358	518	27	6	28	15	19	18	11	12	12	26	27	15	18	20
7027	15	8	55	377	440	16	5	23	8	16	16	12	5	13	27	32	20	11	24
7028	15	8	55	372	448	15	5	23	10	16	15	12	4	13	26	32	15	14	23

Mixed Dishes & Fast Foods

Food No.	Food Description & Amount	wt gm	wt oz	cal	% cal fat	prot gm	carbo gm	fiber gm
7029	Lasagna, meatless [1 piece (3½" x 4")]	256	9.0	360	28%	19	46	3.2
7030	Lasagna, meatless, spinach noodles [1 piece (3½" x 4")]	256	9.0	335	29%	18	41	5.8
7031	Lasagna, meatless, whole wheat noodles [1 piece (3½" x 4")]	256	9.0	339	29%	19	44	5.1
7032	Lasagna, meatless, with spinach [1 piece (3½" x 4")]	256	9.0	334	28%	18	43	3.6
7033	Lasagna, with chicken or turkey, and spinach [1 piece (3½"x4")]	232	8.2	327	30%	22	35	3.0
7034	Liver dumpling [1 cup]	250	8.8	783	51%	57	37	1.7
7035	Liver hash (Include liver mush) [1 cup]	225	7.9	286	21%	32	23	1.9
7036	Lo mein with meat [1 cup]	200	7.1	283	43%	20	21	2.7
7037	Lo mein, meatless [1 cup]	200	7.1	135	5%	6	27	3.8
7038	Lo mein with shrimp [1 cup]	200	7.1	218	38%	13	22	4.2
7039	Macaroni, creamed, with cheese [1 cup]	200	7.1	396	39%	15	44	2.6
7040	Macaroni and cheese with egg [1 cup]	243	8.6	475	43%	19	48	1.7
7041	Macaroni or noodles with beans or lentils and tomato sauce [1 cup]	227	8.0	210	5%	9	41	9.0
7042	Macaroni or noodles with cheese (Include macaroni casserole) [1 cup]	243	8.6	478	43%	19	49	1.8
7043	Macaroni or noodles with cheese, canned [1 cup]	239	8.4	210	30%	7	29	1.1
7044	Macaroni or noodles with cheese, made from dry mix [1 cup]	191	6.7	397	43%	11	45	2.0
7045	Macaroni or noodles with cheese, from boxed mix with already prepared cheese sauce [1 cup]	217	7.7	358	28%	14	50	2.2
7046	Macaroni or noodles with cheese and beef (Include Hamburger Helper Cheeseburger Macaroni) [1 cup]	243	8.6	340	40%	28	22	1.1
7047	Macaroni or noodles with cheese and chicken or turkey [1 cup]	243	8.6	466	41%	31	37	1.3
7048	Macaroni or noodles with cheese and frankfurters [1 cup]	243	8.6	551	55%	21	41	1.5
7049	Macaroni or noodles with cheese and pork or ham [1 cup]	243	8.6	445	44%	25	36	1.3
7050	Macaroni or noodles with cheese and tomato [1 cup]	243	8.6	287	10%	12	54	4.0
7051	Macaroni or noodles with cheese and tuna (Include Tuna Helper Cheesy Noodles 'n' Tuna, Tuna Helper Tuna Au gratin) [1 cup]	243	8.6	417	44%	27	30	1.2
7052	Macaroni salad (Include made with celery, cucumber, lettuce, mushroom, olives, onion, peas, green or red pepper, pickles, radish, or relish; Betty Crocker Suddenly Salad) [1 cup]	177	6.2	271	30%	6	43	2.1
7053	Macaroni salad with cheese [1 cup]	177	6.2	348	51%	10	35	3.6
7054	Macaroni salad with chicken (Include made with celery, cucumber, lettuce, mushroom, olives, onion, peas, green or red pepper, pickles, radish, or relish) [1 cup]	177	6.2	304	38%	17	30	1.4
7055	Macaroni salad with crabmeat (Include made with celery, cucumber, lettuce, mushroom, olives, onion, peas, green or red pepper, pickles, radish, or relish) [1 cup]	177	6.2	259	28%	10	37	1.8
7056	Macaroni salad with egg (Include made with celery, cucumber, lettuce, mushroom, olives, onion, peas, green or red pepper, pickles, radish, or relish) [1 cup]	177	6.2	287	39%	8	36	1.6
7057	Macaroni salad with shrimp (Include made with celery, cucumber, lettuce, mushroom, olives, onion, peas, green or red pepper, pickles, radish, or relish) [1 cup]	177	6.2	264	28%	10	38	1.8
7058	Macaroni salad with tuna (Include made with celery, cucumber, lettuce, mushroom, olives, onion, peas, green or red pepper, pickles, radish, or relish) [1 cup]	177	6.2	261	27%	12	36	1.8
7059	Macaroni salad with tuna and egg (Include made with celery, cucumber, lettuce, mushroom, olives, onion, peas, green or red pepper, pickles, radish, or relish) [1 cup]	177	6.2	273	35%	15	30	1.4
7060	Macaroni with tuna, Puerto Rican style (Macarrones con atun) [1 cup]	225	7.9	362	34%	21	38	1.5
7061	Macaroni, creamed (Include fettucine alfredo, macaroni cooked in milk, Noodles Romanoff) [1 cup]	200	7.1	274	35%	8	36	1.4
7062	Macaroni, creamed, with vegetables [1 cup]	200	7.1	232	34%	7	31	2.2
7063	Manapua, filled with bean paste, meatless [1 manapua]	103	3.6	233	15%	6	43	3.7
7064	Manapua, filled with meat [1 manapua]	93	3.3	214	37%	11	22	0.8
7065	Manicotti, cheese-filled, no sauce [1 manicotti]	127	4.5	275	42%	16	23	0.7
7066	Manicotti, cheese-filled, with meat sauce [1 manicotti]	143	5.0	242	42%	15	20	1.1

Food No.	fat gm	sat fat gm	choles mg	sodium mg	potas mg	vit A	vit E	vit C	thia	ribo	niac	vit B-6	fola	vit B-12	calc	phos	mag	iron	zinc
						% of Daily Value													
7029	11	7	38	428	438	18	6	28	18	19	15	10	5	3	31	29	13	15	14
7030	11	7	38	436	445	20	6	28	10	16	11	13	6	3	33	34	22	9	17
7031	11	7	38	431	454	18	6	28	12	16	9	13	5	3	32	33	17	13	17
7032	10	6	34	411	542	33	7	34	17	20	14	12	14	3	31	28	17	18	14
7033	11	6	52	361	509	27	6	28	15	19	21	15	12	4	26	28	15	17	16
7034	44	11	1040	609	527	896	25	78	36	171	77	49	278	1217	11	64	13	58	69
7035	7	2	767	93	463	597	8	70	31	127	35	46	237	393	3	42	11	59	37
7036	14	3	42	142	332	1	9	19	27	16	25	18	13	4	3	19	11	12	12
7037	1	0	0	564	386	13	2	20	16	14	14	10	12	0	5	11	8	11	6
7038	9	2	66	228	400	8	7	14	11	9	14	6	8	7	7	16	13	17	8
7039	17	8	30	416	99	14	5	0	22	15	13	4	3	5	28	25	10	13	10
7040	23	10	74	742	320	24	8	1	20	30	13	6	4	8	38	39	12	16	16
7041	1	0	5	642	538	4	10	11	20	12	15	7	12	0	8	13	12	23	11
7042	23	10	37	756	320	23	8	1	20	29	13	6	4	7	39	38	13	15	16
7043	7	3	14	1058	137	6	2	0	15	13	8	3	2	3	15	14	6	8	6
7044	19	5	9	749	153	16	10	1	21	14	12	4	3	3	15	18	9	11	8
7045	11	6	28	785	109	9	1	0	24	15	14	4	4	3	12	21	9	14	9
7046	15	8	92	736	348	8	1	0	14	18	20	13	4	33	19	34	9	19	31
7047	21	9	78	610	349	18	7	1	16	27	29	12	3	8	30	38	13	15	20
7048	33	14	56	1366	345	18	7	1	23	27	18	8	3	17	32	35	11	16	19
7049	22	9	56	1267	426	20	7	1	30	28	20	13	3	11	32	42	12	12	19
7050	3	2	6	514	526	12	9	30	21	14	18	13	4	2	13	18	14	17	9
7051	21	9	71	874	245	11	7	1	14	20	38	6	4	25	27	40	12	15	15
7052	9	1	6	331	119	3	5	4	15	7	9	4	4	1	2	7	6	10	4
7053	20	5	24	445	135	11	10	8	18	10	9	9	9	3	13	16	8	11	9
7054	13	2	49	870	200	4	6	15	12	10	27	14	4	3	2	14	7	10	9
7055	8	1	29	353	180	2	5	5	15	7	12	5	7	30	4	11	7	10	11
7056	13	2	143	344	134	8	7	3	14	16	8	5	7	7	3	11	5	10	6
7057	8	1	45	327	152	3	5	4	14	7	11	4	4	5	3	12	7	12	6
7058	8	1	13	372	164	3	5	3	14	7	26	8	4	14	2	11	7	11	5
7059	11	2	128	387	182	7	6	2	12	14	26	9	6	21	3	14	7	11	6
7060	14	3	15	309	280	12	8	2	16	18	36	5	3	18	12	28	11	14	9
7061	11	3	7	138	174	12	6	1	18	15	10	4	3	4	11	14	8	9	6
7062	9	3	7	254	275	13	6	70	16	16	11	8	6	3	10	14	8	10	6
7063	4	0	0	174	130	0	3	0	18	12	11	1	7	0	4	9	5	13	3
7064	9	3	28	140	163	0	3	1	25	15	16	4	3	5	2	10	3	10	10
7065	13	7	104	303	121	13	2	0	13	21	8	3	4	8	29	24	5	10	9
7066	11	6	86	447	259	13	4	8	11	18	11	7	4	11	22	21	6	10	11

Mixed Dishes & Fast Foods

Food No.	Food Description & Amount	wt gm	wt oz	cal	% cal fat	prot gm	carbo gm	fiber gm
7067	Manicotti, cheese-filled, with tomato sauce, meatless [1 manicotti]	143	5.0	231	40%	13	22	1.2
7068	Manicotti, vegetable and cheese-filled, with tomato sauce, meatless [1 manicotti]	143	5.0	202	36%	11	22	1.6
7069	Matzo balls [2 matzo balls]	70	2.5	96	32%	4	12	0.4
7070	Meat loaf (Include meatball, with breading, no sauce) [1 slice]	108	3.8	231	54%	18	7	0.4
7071	Meat loaf made with beef, with tomato-based sauce [1 medium slice]	137	4.8	249	53%	19	9	0.9
7072	Meatloaf made with beef and pork (Include meatball or meat patty, made with beef and pork, with breading, no sauce) [1 slice]	108	3.8	214	50%	19	7	0.4
7073	Meatloaf made with beef and pork, with tomato-based sauce (Include meatball or meat patty, made with beef and pork, with breading, tomato-based sauce) [1 slice]	137	4.8	222	46%	20	9	0.9
7074	Meatloaf made with beef, veal and pork (Include meatball or meat patty, made with beef, veal, and pork, with breading, no sauce) [1 slice]	108	3.8	165	33%	20	7	0.4
7075	Meat pie, Puerto Rican style (Pastelon de carne) [1/8 of pie]	139	4.9	680	65%	22	36	1.5
7076	Meat turnovers, Puerto Rican style (Pastelillos de carne; Empanadillas) [2 turnovers]	56	2.0	191	48%	5	19	0.7
7077	Meat with barbecue sauce (Include with Sloppy Joe mix) [1 cup]	263	9.3	427	34%	59	8	0.7
7078	Meat with tomato-based sauce [1 cup]	249	8.8	349	47%	33	12	2.3
7079	Meatballs, Puerto Rican style (Albondigas) [2 meatballs with sauce]	100	3.5	253	65%	14	7	0.8
7080	Meatballs, with breading, with gravy (Incl. sweet and sour meatballs; Danish frikadeller) [2 meatballs with sauce]	86	3.0	131	51%	10	5	0.4
7081	Meatballs, with sauce [2 meatballs with sauce]	86	3.0	175	61%	16	0	0.0
7082	Meatless "chicken" (made with meat substitute) [1 cup]	168	5.9	370	57%	29	12	7.6
7083	Meatless "chicken," breaded, fried (Include Loma Linda brand) [1 cup]	168	5.9	286	64%	18	8	7.4
7084	Meatless luncheon slices, "beef, chicken, salami, or turkey" (Include vegetarian ham, Wham, Loma Linda, Worthington) [4 thin slices]	56	2.0	157	51%	14	5	2.9
7085	Meatless, "fish" stick [2 sticks]	56	2.0	162	56%	13	5	3.4
7086	Meatless, "frankfurter" [2 "frankfurters"]	70	2.5	140	45%	14	6	3.2
7087	Meatless, "meatball" [2 "meatballs"]	72	2.5	144	41%	15	6	3.3
7088	Meatless, "scallops," breaded, fried [1 cup]	168	5.9	507	56%	40	16	10.7
7089	Mexican casserole made with ground beef, beans, tomato sauce, cheese, taco seasonings, and corn chips [1 cup]	144	5.1	316	55%	16	20	3.7
7090	Mexican casserole made with ground beef, tomato sauce, cheese, taco seasonings, and corn chips (Include Frito pie) [1 cup]	144	5.1	358	64%	18	14	1.7
7091	Moo Shi Pork [1 cup]	151	5.3	517	81%	19	5	0.6
7092	Moussaka (eggplant and meat casserole) [1 cup]	203	7.2	300	58%	16	15	2.9
7093	Nachos with beans and cheese [5 nachos]	85	3.0	225	51%	8	20	4.9
7094	Nachos with beans, no cheese [5 nachos]	65	2.3	155	44%	4	18	4.5
7095	Nachos with beef and cheese [5 nachos]	60	2.1	218	61%	14	8	0.8
7096	Nachos with beef, beans, and cheese [5 nachos]	35	1.2	106	55%	5	7	1.4
7097	Nachos with beef, beans, cheese, and sour cream [5 nachos]	80	2.8	248	56%	8	20	3.0
7098	Nachos with beef, beans, cheese, tomatoes and onions [1 cup]	88	3.1	239	59%	6	19	3.1
7099	Nachos with cheese and sour cream [5 nachos]	35	1.2	99	75%	3	4	0.3
7100	Nachos with cheese, meatless, no beans [5 nachos]	35	1.2	156	61%	6	10	1.0
7101	Nachos with chicken and cheese [5 nachos]	60	2.1	173	51%	14	7	0.7
7102	Nachos with chili [1 order]	286	10.1	481	45%	17	55	13.5
7103	Noodle pudding (Include kugel) [1 cup]	144	5.1	298	30%	9	44	2.1
7104	Noodle pudding, with milk [1 cup]	144	5.1	392	36%	8	55	1.1
7105	Paella with seafood [1 cup]	240	8.5	348	28%	21	40	1.8
7106	Pakora (vegetables, dipped in chick-pea flour batter, fried [3 pakoras]	36	1.3	44	35%	2	6	1.6
7107	Panzerotti, with meat, vegetables, and cheese [1 panzerotti]	396	14.0	1071	58%	40	71	4.3
7108	Panzerotti, with vegetables and cheese [1 panzerotti]	402	14.2	992	59%	28	73	5.3
7109	Pasta meat-filled with gravy (Include Chef Boy-ar-dee Mini Chicken Ravioli) [1 cup]	250	8.8	327	21%	12	51	1.9
7110	Pasta salad (macaroni or noodles, vegetables, dressing) [1 cup]	177	6.2	287	49%	5	32	2.2
7111	Pasta salad with meat (macaroni or noodles, vegetables, meat, dressing) [1 cup]	177	6.2	340	51%	12	30	1.9
7112	Pasta with carbonara sauce [1 cup]	201	7.1	356	28%	14	48	2.3

Food No.	fat gm	sat fat gm	choles mg	sodium mg	potas mg	vit A	vit E	vit C	thia	ribo	niac	vit B-6	fola	vit B-12	calc	phos	mag	iron	zinc
						% of Daily Value													
7067	10	6	82	468	245	14	4	8	12	18	8	6	4	6	24	21	6	10	8
7068	8	4	74	416	273	20	5	12	12	17	8	6	7	5	19	17	7	11	7
7069	3	1	73	22	37	3	2	0	4	7	3	2	2	2	1	4	1	4	2
7070	14	5	90	133	295	2	1	1	5	16	20	7	3	28	4	16	6	11	24
7071	15	5	92	320	414	5	3	8	7	18	22	10	4	28	5	17	7	13	25
7072	12	4	87	129	317	2	1	1	12	17	20	9	3	23	4	18	6	10	21
7073	11	4	89	317	441	5	3	8	14	18	23	12	4	23	5	19	7	12	23
7074	6	2	86	125	305	2	1	1	17	17	25	14	4	17	5	18	6	8	17
7075	49	19	97	798	355	1	3	10	24	23	31	9	4	25	16	25	8	22	26
7076	10	2	34	58	83	2	6	2	13	10	8	2	2	2	2	6	2	7	3
7077	16	5	165	620	888	5	4	7	15	33	41	43	4	98	2	50	16	36	97
7078	18	6	100	661	798	5	9	18	40	21	38	28	5	34	5	28	13	17	32
7079	18	6	70	561	330	4	8	7	7	12	16	8	3	17	2	14	5	9	17
7080	7	3	47	244	177	1	0	1	3	9	11	4	2	15	2	9	3	7	15
7081	12	5	88	172	188	2	1	0	2	10	17	8	2	28	1	12	3	9	21
7082	24	4	0	1327	554	0	20	0	123	40	45	59	32	59	6	56	7	12	8
7083	20	3	0	672	504	0	15	0	78	47	39	42	24	59	4	41	5	16	7
7084	9	1	0	482	157	0	8	0	35	18	31	31	14	24	2	25	3	7	6
7085	10	2	0	274	336	0	10	0	41	30	34	42	14	39	5	25	3	6	5
7086	7	1	0	301	105	0	6	0	51	49	56	34	14	28	2	24	3	7	6
7087	6	1	0	396	130	0	6	0	43	25	36	43	14	29	2	25	3	8	9
7088	32	5	0	858	1050	0	31	0	128	93	105	131	45	123	17	79	10	19	16
7089	19	7	47	304	396	6	3	6	6	12	14	10	13	16	11	20	11	14	19
7090	26	9	67	364	345	7	3	6	3	14	18	10	3	23	11	20	9	11	24
7091	47	7	173	385	333	6	39	13	34	22	15	16	5	13	3	21	7	8	12
7092	19	5	45	220	512	9	11	19	11	14	20	11	7	20	10	17	10	12	21
7093	13	6	19	141	275	4	3	3	7	7	2	7	20	2	14	17	10	8	8
7094	8	2	5	51	238	0	3	3	6	3	2	5	18	0	4	9	8	7	4
7095	15	6	49	191	145	5	1	0	2	9	11	7	2	20	14	17	6	7	17
7096	7	3	16	78	102	2	1	1	2	4	3	3	6	5	7	8	4	4	6
7097	15	6	25	211	194	6	3	4	4	8	5	7	8	6	14	16	9	6	9
7098	16	4	13	257	170	2	10	4	3	5	4	7	2	3	11	19	8	6	8
7099	8	5	17	74	50	7	1	0	1	4	0	1	1	2	8	6	2	1	2
7100	11	5	21	203	49	6	1	0	1	6	1	3	1	3	17	13	5	2	6
7101	10	4	44	169	98	5	1	0	2	8	11	7	1	3	12	15	5	4	9
7102	24	8	42	1495	975	9	11	7	10	20	7	22	15	0	18	46	37	50	37
7103	10	2	144	111	193	11	6	4	13	13	8	6	4	5	4	14	7	14	7
7104	16	9	40	173	259	16	3	2	22	19	12	4	3	7	14	17	9	9	6
7105	11	2	47	454	371	13	7	60	20	12	33	13	5	207	4	20	8	35	13
7106	2	0	0	3	93	0	1	2	3	1	1	3	12	0	1	3	3	3	2
7107	69	23	82	2007	647	16	33	13	56	57	48	21	28	32	48	58	15	34	33
7108	66	18	33	2262	496	16	44	45	45	50	34	15	30	9	47	50	14	29	20
7109	8	2	17	1089	197	6	4	0	27	21	25	5	4	2	4	13	6	17	9
7110	16	2	0	951	159	41	16	19	15	7	9	5	5	1	3	7	6	9	4
7111	19	4	24	588	207	30	12	14	17	10	18	9	4	8	2	10	7	10	8
7112	11	4	92	217	154	4	2	1	27	17	17	7	6	6	7	18	9	15	10

Mixed Dishes & Fast Foods

Food No.	Food Description & Amount	wt gm	wt oz	cal	% cal fat	prot gm	carbo gm	fiber gm
7113	Pasta with meat sauce and cheese (Include Cannelloni) [1 cup]	242	8.5	371	44%	19	32	1.9
7114	Pasta with tomato sauce and cheese, meatless [1 cup]	242	8.5	207	14%	8	37	3.0
7115	Pasta with tomato sauce and cheese, canned [1 cup]	249	8.8	187	15%	5	36	1.9
7116	Pasta with tomato sauce and meat or meatballs, canned [1 cup]	249	8.8	256	28%	10	36	1.5
7117	Pasta with tomato sauce and frankfurters or hot dogs, canned [1 cup]	253	8.9	259	40%	8	33	1.3
7118	Pasta with meat sauce (Include American chop suey; made with whole wheat or spinach pasta) [1 cup]	255	9.0	303	30%	21	33	3.5
7119	Pasta with pesto sauce [1 cup]	122	4.3	358	58%	12	27	2.5
7120	Pasta with tomato sauce, meatless [1 cup]	248	8.7	189	4%	7	39	3.2
7121	Pasta, whole wheat, with meat sauce [1 cup]	255	9.0	302	20%	15	49	8.5
7122	Pasta, whole wheat, with tomato sauce, meatless [1 cup]	248	8.7	258	11%	10	53	9.0
7123	Pasta tetrazzini, dry mix prepared with water [1 cup]	202	7.1	187	6%	15	30	3.2
7124	Pastry, cheese-filled [2 pastries]	56	2.0	155	66%	5	8	0.2
7125	Pastry, filled with potatoes and peas, fried [1 samosa]	100	3.5	309	52%	5	33	1.9
7126	Peas cooked with pork [1 cup]	197	6.9	332	36%	16	38	15.0
7127	Pigeon pea asopao (Asopaode grandules) [1 cup]	178	6.3	242	22%	5	41	1.9
7128	Porcupine balls with cream of mushroom soup-based sauce [2 balls with sauce]	70	2.5	124	48%	8	8	0.3
7129	Porcupine balls with tomato-based sauce [2 balls with sauce]	70	2.5	115	41%	8	9	0.3
7130	Pork and beans [1 cup]	253	8.9	248	9%	13	49	12.1
7131	Potato and ham fritters, Puerto Rican style (Frituras de papa y jamon) [1 fritter (2¾" x 2½" x 1")]	70	2.5	139	63%	4	9	0.8
7132	Potato chicken pie, Puerto Rican style (Pastelon de pollo) [¼ of 9" pie]	230	8.1	915	56%	42	58	3.0
7133	Potato salad with egg [1 cup]	193	6.8	280	51%	6	30	2.8
7134	Potato salad, German style [1 cup]	175	6.2	155	17%	4	29	2.6
7135	Puffs, fried, crabmeat and cream cheese filled [1 cup]	77	2.7	273	50%	9	25	0.8
7136	Puerto Rican stew (Sancocho) [1 cup, with bone (yield after bones removed)]	214	7.5	325	41%	17	32	3.8
7137	Puerto Rican style meat loaf (Albondigon) [1 serving (3" x 1" x 2")]	95	3.4	317	61%	19	10	0.6
7138	Puerto Rican style stuffed pot roast (larded meat) (Carne mechada con papas boliche) [1 slice (¾" x 3") with ¼ cup potatoes]	190	6.7	675	62%	46	15	1.5
7139	Puerto-Rican style beef stew (Carne guisada con papas) [1 cup]	212	7.5	457	59%	31	14	1.6
7140	Quesadilla [1 quesadilla]	54	1.9	183	47%	6	18	1.1
7141	Quesadilla with meat and cheese [1 quesadilla]	60	2.1	196	44%	7	20	1.3
7142	Quiche with meat, poultry or fish (Include Quiche Lorraine) [1/8 of 9" dia]	192	6.8	574	70%	16	27	0.8
7143	Quiche, cheese, meatless [1/8 of 9" dia]	192	6.8	569	70%	17	27	0.8
7144	Quiche, spinach, meatless (Include broccoli quiche) [1/8 of 9" dia]	143	5.0	343	69%	11	17	1.2
7145	Rabbit stew with potatoes and vegetables [1 cup]	252	8.9	160	26%	18	12	1.8
7146	Ravioli, cheese and spinach-filled, with cream sauce [1 cup]	250	8.8	370	42%	15	38	1.9
7147	Ravioli, cheese-filled, no sauce [1 cup]	240	8.5	439	34%	21	49	1.7
7148	Ravioli, cheese-filled, with meat sauce [1 cup]	250	8.8	364	42%	17	35	2.1
7149	Ravioli, cheese-filled, with tomato sauce [1 cup]	250	8.8	341	38%	15	38	2.3
7150	Ravioli, cheese-filled, with tomato sauce, canned [1 cup]	246	8.7	234	21%	6	40	1.4
7151	Ravioli, meat-filled, no sauce [1 cup]	240	8.5	489	38%	30	43	1.6
7152	Ravioli, meat-filled, with tomato sauce or meat sauce [1 cup]	250	8.8	393	40%	22	37	2.6
7153	Ravioli, meat-filled, with tomato sauce or meat sauce, canned [1 cup]	251	8.9	220	17%	9	38	1.6
7154	Red beans and rice [1 cup]	224	7.9	251	22%	8	41	7.8
7155	Refried beans [1 cup]	253	8.9	488	43%	17	55	17.7
7156	Refried beans with cheese [1 cup]	253	8.9	502	44%	18	54	17.2
7157	Refried beans with meat (Include Old El Paso Refried Beans with Sausage) [1 cup]	253	8.9	385	46%	18	34	11.5
7158	Rice casserole with cheese (Include risotto) [1 cup]	204	7.2	369	31%	16	47	0.6
7159	Rice dressing (Include combined with bread) [1 cup]	167	5.9	185	27%	3	30	0.9
7160	Rice meal fritters, Puerto Rican style (almojabanas) [2 cruellers (3" x 2" x ½")]	60	2.1	379	78%	6	15	0.4
7161	Rice patty or croquette [1 patty (3¼" dia x 5/8")]	85	3.0	132	38%	3	17	0.8
7162	Rice pilaf [1 cup]	206	7.3	261	24%	4	45	1.3
7163	Rice pudding made with coconut milk, Puerto Rican style [1 cup]	256	9.0	694	60%	7	73	5.6

Food No.	fat gm	sat fat gm	choles mg	sodium mg	potas mg	vit A	vit E	vit C	thia	ribo	niac	vit B-6	fola	vit B-12	calc	phos	mag	iron	zinc
						% of Daily Value													
7113	18	8	162	502	425	20	8	13	18	24	21	12	7	19	15	23	8	18	19
7114	3	2	7	262	345	9	4	27	18	10	13	8	4	1	9	12	9	12	7
7115	3	1	3	997	274	11	3	30	14	9	10	6	4	1	3	8	7	10	4
7116	8	3	28	907	340	6	2	32	14	12	17	8	5	13	2	11	6	12	12
7117	11	4	32	1152	328	7	2	30	11	9	11	11	3	7	6	11	6	8	7
7118	10	4	49	1056	903	16	12	47	23	21	31	20	6	16	4	19	15	21	26
7119	23	5	9	216	188	4	10	3	19	9	10	5	5	3	21	22	15	19	10
7120	1	0	0	231	356	8	4	28	19	9	14	9	4	0	4	9	9	12	6
7121	7	2	20	394	598	11	10	29	16	12	18	18	5	8	4	21	18	17	19
7122	3	0	0	403	560	12	11	31	16	9	13	16	5	0	5	18	18	15	11
7123	1	0	16	740	506	86	2	5	18	19	11	9	9	10	21	26	10	13	9
7124	11	4	48	327	58	10	5	0	6	14	3	4	2	4	11	10	2	4	5
7125	18	4	9	142	174	5	13	5	16	11	11	6	3	1	3	7	4	10	3
7126	13	5	14	228	666	0	4	1	24	6	9	5	29	1	3	19	17	13	13
7127	6	1	2	492	243	2	4	16	19	4	12	8	9	0	2	9	9	11	6
7128	7	2	26	180	114	0	1	1	3	4	10	5	1	14	1	6	2	6	11
7129	5	2	25	319	145	1	2	19	4	4	11	6	1	14	1	6	2	7	11
7130	3	1	18	1113	759	3	6	13	9	7	6	9	14	0	14	30	22	46	99
7131	10	2	36	171	294	1	8	10	9	5	6	9	2	3	1	6	3	3	3
7132	57	15	128	660	651	5	18	15	35	31	74	35	6	6	14	36	15	29	21
7133	16	3	106	214	557	6	11	35	11	9	10	26	7	5	3	11	8	5	5
7134	3	1	5	96	552	1	1	31	12	3	11	20	5	2	1	8	9	4	4
7135	15	8	71	122	125	16	3	0	12	14	10	3	3	8	4	11	5	11	3
7136	15	5	49	249	882	73	8	34	17	15	22	26	6	18	4	23	13	12	19
7137	22	7	155	61	219	4	8	2	14	19	15	8	4	18	2	14	4	11	20
7138	47	16	146	828	1181	0	9	21	16	24	42	36	6	70	2	48	17	26	47
7139	30	9	94	423	933	2	11	27	11	17	30	28	5	49	2	33	13	20	33
7140	10	3	13	230	77	4	5	25	9	8	5	2	1	1	13	11	3	7	4
7141	10	3	15	218	102	3	5	27	10	8	8	3	2	4	10	10	4	8	6
7142	45	21	241	241	261	30	10	1	19	31	11	6	5	11	25	29	7	11	11
7143	44	21	242	199	232	34	10	1	15	32	8	5	5	10	34	32	7	11	12
7144	26	12	158	112	278	42	8	9	12	24	6	7	14	7	25	21	10	12	9
7145	5	1	45	42	447	42	3	11	8	11	25	15	5	57	3	17	6	11	11
7146	17	6	166	236	372	46	9	6	23	33	12	9	17	10	25	26	13	20	11
7147	17	9	251	159	191	21	4	0	28	36	17	6	10	12	24	30	7	21	13
7148	17	7	165	544	423	22	9	14	20	25	18	11	7	14	16	23	8	18	15
7149	15	6	162	574	405	24	9	16	21	25	15	10	8	6	17	22	8	17	10
7150	5	2	8	1112	133	10	4	6	16	12	11	4	2	1	7	9	4	11	4
7151	21	8	251	173	334	9	3	0	26	35	36	14	8	40	8	28	8	28	32
7152	18	6	170	180	528	17	12	12	21	26	30	15	7	28	7	22	10	24	23
7153	4	2	17	1354	337	8	2	36	15	12	14	7	4	8	3	9	6	11	8
7154	6	2	6	477	384	0	1	5	18	7	9	7	16	0	5	15	11	13	7
7155	23	9	21	6	999	0	10	11	24	11	4	19	81	0	11	33	28	29	15
7156	25	10	27	48	979	2	10	11	24	12	4	19	79	1	16	36	28	29	16
7157	20	7	50	1001	672	5	1	22	15	7	12	18	7	3	9	23	19	24	22
7158	13	8	43	254	364	17	1	2	18	24	11	7	3	8	42	36	11	12	14
7159	6	1	0	386	108	5	4	2	13	3	9	4	2	0	4	5	4	10	3
7160	33	7	78	233	50	10	23	0	4	9	3	4	2	4	14	12	3	4	4
7161	6	1	38	32	115	2	4	4	7	4	5	4	3	1	2	5	3	6	3
7162	7	1	0	151	111	6	5	2	18	2	12	6	2	0	3	8	5	13	5
7163	46	41	0	33	665	0	7	8	12	2	13	7	7	0	5	24	21	27	11

Mixed Dishes & Fast Foods

Food No.	Food Description & Amount	wt gm	wt oz	cal	% cal fat	prot gm	carbo gm	fiber gm
7164	Rice with beans and chicken [1 cup]	239	8.4	431	38%	26	39	4.6
7165	Rice with beans and pork [1 cup]	239	8.4	445	40%	25	41	4.9
7166	Rice with beans and tomatoes [1 cup]	239	8.4	308	24%	12	48	6.6
7167	Rice with beans [1 cup]	239	8.4	396	25%	15	60	8.0
7168	Rice with gravy [1 cup]	237	8.4	259	7%	7	52	0.9
7169	Rice with onions, Puerto Rican style (arroz con cebollas) [1 cup]	165	5.8	285	51%	6	31	2.1
7170	Rice with raisins [1 cup]	185	6.5	273	2%	5	62	1.4
7171	Rice with spanish sausage, Puerto Rican style [1 cup]	180	6.3	567	45%	17	59	1.3
7172	Rice with squid, Puerto Rican style (arroz con calamares) [1 cup]	160	5.6	405	37%	14	48	1.5
7173	Rice with stewed beans, Puerto Rican style [1 cup]	188	6.6	251	22%	5	42	1.4
7174	Rice with vienna sausage, Puerto Rican style (arroz con salchichas) [1 cup]	180	6.3	507	41%	12	61	1.3
7175	Rice, brown, with tomato sauce [1 cup]	243	8.6	229	15%	5	44	4.0
7176	Rice, cooked with coconut milk (Arroz con coco) [1 cup]	200	7.1	532	64%	7	46	3.9
7177	Rice, creamed [1 cup]	204	7.2	251	15%	6	45	0.6
7178	Rice, fried, meatless [1 cup]	166	5.9	271	41%	5	34	1.3
7179	Rice, fried, with meat (Include pork or chicken Chinese rice) [1 cup]	198	7.0	329	34%	12	41	1.3
7180	Rice, fried, with shrimp [1 cup]	198	7.0	319	33%	11	42	1.3
7181	Rice-vegetable medley (Include Italian-style rice) [1 cup]	206	7.3	281	33%	5	42	1.9
7182	Ripe plantain meat pie, Puerto Rican style (Pinon) [1 piece (4" x 2" x 2")]	190	6.7	629	61%	24	42	4.8
7183	Roll with meat and/or shrimp, vegetables and rice paper (not fried) [1 roll (4¼" x 1½" dia)]	71	2.5	82	21%	6	10	1.8
7184	Sandwich spread, meat substitute type [2 Tbs]	32	1.1	48	54%	3	3	1.1
7185	Shad creole, with rice [1 cup]	249	8.8	413	50%	25	25	1.1
7186	Shepherd's pie with beef [1 cup]	243	8.6	278	30%	17	32	3.2
7187	Shepherd's pie [1 cup]	243	8.6	298	37%	17	31	3.3
7188	Somen salad [1 cup]	160	5.6	273	27%	20	28	1.6
7189	Soupy rice from Puerto Rican style Asopao de Pollo (chicken parts reported separately) [1 cup]	240	8.5	199	39%	8	22	2.1
7190	Soupy rice mixture with chicken and potatoes, Puerto Rican style [1 cup]	240	8.5	276	34%	18	27	1.5
7191	Soyburger (Include vegetarian burger) [1 patty]	70	2.5	140	41%	15	6	3.2
7192	Soyburger with cheese [1 sandwich]	140	4.9	319	34%	21	31	4.6
7193	Spaghetti sauce with beef, homemade-style (Include canned sauce, extra beef added) [1 cup]	249	8.8	288	52%	16	21	4.2
7194	Spaghetti sauce with combination of meats, homemade-style (Include canned sauce, extra meats added) [1 cup]	249	8.8	287	53%	17	19	3.8
7195	Spaghetti sauce with lamb or mutton, homemade-style [1 cup]	249	8.8	284	53%	15	21	4.2
7196	Spaghetti with corned beef, Puerto Rican style [1 cup]	215	7.6	408	39%	26	36	2.3
7197	Spaghetti with red clam sauce [1 cup]	248	8.7	288	24%	13	41	3.1
7198	Spaghetti with tomato sauce and chicken or turkey [1 cup]	248	8.7	267	20%	18	34	3.3
7199	Spaghetti with tomato sauce and frankfurters [1 cup]	248	8.7	336	44%	11	35	3.3
7200	Spaghetti (spinach noodles) with tomato sauce and meatballs, or with meat sauce, or with meat sauce and meatballs [1 cup]	248	8.7	311	27%	19	36	5.0
7201	Spaghetti with tomato sauce and meatballs or with meat sauce or with meat sauce and meatballs [1 cup]	248	8.7	325	27%	20	38	3.7
7202	Spaghetti (whole wheat noodles) with tomato sauce and meatballs, or with meat sauce, or with meat sauce and meatballs [1 cup]	248	8.7	313	28%	20	37	5.5
7203	Spaghetti with meatless tomato sauce (Include marinara sauce; meatless tomato sauce with cheese, canned) [1 cup]	248	8.7	229	14%	7	41	4.1
7204	Spaghetti (spinach noodles) with meatless tomato sauce [1 cup]	248	8.7	213	14%	7	38	6.0
7205	Spaghetti (whole wheat noodles) with meatless tomato sauce [1 cup]	248	8.7	212	15%	8	40	7.0
7206	Spaghetti with white clam sauce [1 cup]	248	8.7	458	39%	25	43	2.5
7207	Spanakopitta (Include Greek spinach-cheese pie) [1 piece (3" x 3" x 1")]	108	3.8	223	67%	8	11	1.6
7208	Spanish rice (Include Mexican rice) [1 cup]	243	8.6	216	15%	5	42	3.0
7209	Spanish rice with ground beef [1 cup]	230	8.1	306	37%	22	26	2.6
7210	Spanish stew, Puerto Rican style (Cocido Espanol) [1 cup]	242	8.5	204	33%	15	20	4.7

Food No.	fat gm	sat fat gm	choles mg	sodium mg	potas mg	% of Daily Value vit A	vit E	vit C	thia	ribo	niac	vit B-6	fola	vit B-12	calc	phos	mag	iron	zinc
7164	18	4	63	277	567	23	6	1	18	14	26	15	20	11	8	24	16	26	17
7165	20	6	59	251	639	7	6	0	34	13	21	17	16	6	9	23	16	25	24
7166	8	2	0	185	669	11	7	14	18	4	9	11	20	0	11	15	18	26	12
7167	11	2	0	128	717	10	8	0	21	4	9	11	25	0	12	18	22	32	15
7168	2	1	2	359	112	0	1	0	20	3	15	8	2	1	2	9	6	14	10
7169	16	3	0	1111	160	14	11	3	10	3	10	7	5	0	4	7	5	9	7
7170	1	0	0	4	201	0	1	1	20	2	13	10	1	0	3	9	7	13	6
7171	28	9	46	913	338	2	8	8	41	11	28	19	2	15	3	17	8	22	17
7172	17	2	152	88	325	12	14	73	18	17	19	10	3	13	4	21	10	16	11
7173	6	1	2	43	157	0	5	4	17	2	11	8	3	0	2	8	6	12	6
7174	23	7	30	787	217	1	8	7	27	6	21	11	2	7	3	13	7	20	12
7175	4	1	0	463	337	9	12	15	14	5	17	17	3	0	3	16	22	7	8
7176	38	33	4	40	453	1	5	7	21	1	16	6	7	0	4	21	17	25	10
7177	4	1	5	191	145	2	2	1	18	7	12	8	2	3	9	12	7	10	6
7178	12	2	43	261	128	2	11	7	14	6	11	7	5	2	3	9	6	11	6
7179	12	2	102	821	182	5	10	6	20	11	18	12	6	4	4	15	8	15	9
7180	12	2	115	840	169	5	10	6	17	10	16	11	6	6	4	16	8	16	8
7181	10	2	0	906	147	16	8	32	17	4	12	6	3	0	4	7	6	13	4
7182	42	11	248	563	998	24	25	45	13	29	23	28	13	27	6	28	20	19	25
7183	2	1	15	43	183	47	1	14	11	4	6	7	2	2	2	5	3	3	4
7184	3	0	0	202	109	0	3	0	13	13	21	18	8	17	1	7	10	3	3
7185	23	5	97	482	686	13	11	20	24	21	63	31	7	3	9	40	14	15	6
7186	9	3	37	312	764	8	6	27	13	11	19	29	5	21	4	19	12	12	26
7187	12	3	42	649	725	10	8	30	13	12	25	24	7	20	4	18	11	10	20
7188	8	2	218	499	330	10	4	6	19	20	14	14	12	19	5	24	11	10	12
7189	9	4	15	437	254	7	3	36	14	6	8	10	6	3	13	14	6	8	7
7190	10	3	49	188	450	4	2	31	12	7	25	17	4	2	2	14	8	11	11
7191	6	1	0	385	126	0	6	0	42	25	35	42	14	28	2	24	3	8	8
7192	12	4	9	956	251	4	7	1	56	36	43	44	17	30	16	35	7	17	13
7193	17	5	47	872	1103	24	24	63	12	16	30	27	7	24	6	17	16	20	23
7194	17	4	47	889	1038	22	22	55	28	17	29	29	7	16	6	19	15	17	18
7195	17	5	45	866	1108	24	24	63	14	17	31	23	8	19	6	18	16	17	20
7196	18	6	59	1042	266	5	8	31	18	15	19	9	4	17	14	21	10	19	21
7197	8	1	17	170	411	10	6	30	22	15	18	8	5	420	6	17	10	53	10
7198	6	1	37	515	468	5	7	16	15	12	26	15	5	2	4	16	11	15	11
7199	16	5	23	1004	451	4	7	16	19	11	19	11	4	10	4	12	10	14	10
7200	9	3	66	690	636	11	9	25	18	17	21	19	8	16	13	26	19	17	19
7201	10	3	69	711	653	10	10	26	24	19	24	17	7	17	13	24	14	21	18
7202	10	3	69	712	661	10	10	26	19	17	21	19	7	17	14	26	16	19	19
7203	4	1	0	591	455	5	8	19	19	9	16	10	5	0	4	10	11	14	5
7204	3	0	0	565	440	7	8	18	11	6	13	12	6	0	5	15	19	9	8
7205	4	1	0	593	468	5	8	19	13	6	11	12	5	0	5	14	14	12	7
7206	20	3	49	85	514	13	14	27	26	26	24	7	8	1213	8	32	10	126	18
7207	16	8	91	374	322	41	8	16	8	21	5	8	20	5	18	14	11	12	8
7208	4	1	0	295	537	11	6	62	16	5	15	16	5	0	8	9	10	13	6
7209	13	5	63	385	719	11	7	38	12	17	28	17	4	20	5	19	12	19	31
7210	7	3	30	369	627	30	2	40	13	10	16	17	12	16	4	18	11	13	16

Mixed Dishes & Fast Foods

Food No.	Food Description & Amount	wt gm	wt oz	cal	% cal fat	prot gm	carbo gm	fiber gm
7211	Spicy rice pudding, Puerto Rican style (arroz con dulce, arroz con especia) [1 cup]	240	8.5	330	7%	3	74	0.7
7212	Stewed chickpeas with Spanish sausages, Puerto Rican style (Garbanzos guisados con chorizos) [1 cup]	250	8.8	498	65%	15	31	8.7
7213	Stewed chickpeas, Puerto Rican style [1 cup]	260	9.2	233	41%	10	25	7.0
7214	Stewed chickpeas, with potatoes, Puerto Rican style [1 cup]	260	9.2	403	28%	19	57	15.3
7215	Stewed corned beef, Puerto Rican style ("Corned beef" guisado) (Include carne bif guisada) [1 cup]	280	9.9	617	55%	45	22	2.4
7216	Stewed cowpeas, Puerto Rican style (Include frijoles) [1 cup]	260	9.2	281	7%	19	49	8.6
7217	Stewed lima beans, Puerto Rican style [1 cup]	255	9.0	133	55%	6	10	2.2
7218	Stewed dry red beans, Puerto Rican style (Habichuelas coloradas guisadas) [1 cup]	250	8.8	414	34%	21	50	11.2
7219	Stewed green peas with pig's feet and potatoes, Puerto Rican style [1 cup (yield after bones removed)]	230	8.1	321	45%	21	23	6.5
7220	Stewed green peas, Puerto Rican style (Habichuelas del pais) [1 cup]	260	9.2	389	18%	25	57	23.7
7221	Stewed pigeon peas, Puerto Rican style (Gandules guisados, Gandur, Gandules) [1 cup]	260	9.2	254	26%	10	40	6.5
7222	Stewed pink beans with pig's feet, Puerto Rican style [1 cup, with bone (yield after bone removed)]	202	7.1	263	48%	18	16	5.1
7223	Stewed pink beans with viandas, ham, Puerto Rican style (Include pinto beans) [1 cup]	255	9.0	221	33%	11	27	9.2
7224	Stewed red beans with pig's feet and potatoes, Puerto Rican style [1 cup, with bone (yield after bone removed)]	220	7.8	306	45%	20	22	4.2
7225	Stewed red beans with pig's feet, Puerto Rican style [1 cup, with bone (yield after bone removed)]	202	7.1	262	49%	18	16	3.4
7226	Stewed rice, Puerto Rican style (arroz quisado) (Include red rice) [1 cup]	170	6.0	370	31%	7	55	1.2
7227	Stewed seasoned ground beef and pork, Mexican style (Picadillo de carne de rez y puerco) [1 cup]	222	7.8	360	57%	33	3	0.5
7228	Stewed seasoned ground beef and pork, with potatoes, Mexican style (Picadillo de carne de rez y puerco con papas) [1 cup]	222	7.8	334	52%	29	10	1.1
7229	Stewed white beans with pig's feet, Puerto Rican style [1 cup, with bone (yield after bone removed)]	202	7.1	261	49%	18	16	3.4
7230	Stewed white beans, Puerto Rican style [1 cup]	255	9.0	224	26%	8	33	3.6
7231	Stuffed cabbage, Puerto Rican style (Repollo relleno) [1 cup]	234	8.3	531	68%	27	17	4.6
7232	Stuffed cabbage, Syrian dish, Puerto Rican style (Repollo relleno Arabe Mihsy Melful) [1 cabbage roll]	110	3.9	94	37%	4	12	1.8
7233	Stuffed grape leaves with lamb and rice [2 rolls]	42	1.5	111	71%	4	5	1.4
7234	Stuffed pepper, with meat [½ pepper with filling]	149	5.3	286	70%	14	8	1.8
7235	Stuffed pepper, with rice and meat [½ pepper with filling]	149	5.3	220	51%	12	14	1.7
7236	Stuffed pepper, with rice, meatless [½ pepper with filling]	149	5.3	230	57%	6	19	1.8
7237	Stuffed shell, cheese and spinach-filled, no sauce [1 jumbo shell]	60	2.1	115	33%	6	13	0.7
7238	Stuffed shell, cheese-filled, no sauce [1 jumbo shell]	60	2.1	128	39%	7	12	0.4
7239	Stuffed shell, cheese-filled, with meat sauce [1 jumbo shell]	85	3.0	140	39%	8	13	0.9
7240	Stuffed shell, cheese-filled, with tomato sauce, meatless [1 jumbo shell]	85	3.0	130	37%	7	14	0.8
7241	Stuffed shell, with chicken [1 jumbo shell]	83	2.9	117	22%	9	13	0.9
7242	Stuffed shell, with fish and/or shellfish [1 jumbo shell]	83	2.9	103	14%	8	14	0.9
7243	Stuffed tomato, with rice and meat [1 tomato with filling]	149	5.3	151	43%	7	16	1.4
7244	Stuffed tomato, with rice, meatless [1 tomato with filling]	149	5.3	112	22%	2	20	1.5
7245	Sukiyaki [1 cup]	162	5.7	172	40%	19	7	1.3
7246	Sushi (sushi rice w. seaweed, vegetables, raw fish) [2 pieces]	52	1.8	75	3%	2	16	0.4
7247	Sushi rice (rice, vinegar, sugar, rice wine, salt) [1 cup]	145	5.1	256	1%	5	57	0.8
7248	Tabbouleh (Include Tabbuli) [1 cup]	160	5.6	199	68%	3	16	3.7
7249	Tamal in a leaf, Puerto Rican style (Tamales en hoja) [2 tamal (6" x 2" x ½")]	82	2.9	131	50%	8	10	1.3
7250	Tamale casserole with meat [1 cup]	244	8.6	226	42%	14	18	2.4
7251	Tamale casserole, Puerto Rican style (Tamales en cazuela) [1 cup]	237	8.4	392	55%	17	28	3.9
7252	Tamale with meat [1 tamale]	70	2.5	134	48%	6	11	1.5
7253	Tamale, meatless [1 tamale]	72	2.5	199	85%	1	8	1.3

Food No.	fat gm	sat fat gm	choles mg	sodium mg	potas mg	vit A	vit E	vit C	thia	ribo	niac	vit B-6	fola	vit B-12	calc	phos	mag	iron	zinc
						% of Daily Value													
7211	3	1	0	130	194	2	2	0	13	3	9	3	1	0	6	5	6	15	4
7212	36	7	20	440	513	6	18	33	17	10	10	16	23	7	5	19	13	18	15
7213	11	2	9	189	356	2	6	9	11	6	5	10	33	1	5	16	11	14	10
7214	12	2	7	227	776	3	7	20	21	10	9	22	71	1	9	31	22	27	19
7215	38	12	135	1916	882	3	11	36	8	17	28	25	6	39	3	24	13	24	40
7216	2	0	0	18	798	4	4	19	32	10	7	12	81	0	9	32	32	34	17
7217	8	2	9	172	270	5	6	18	6	4	5	6	3	1	3	8	7	8	5
7218	15	3	16	479	1045	3	7	26	26	11	13	19	35	2	7	32	24	26	16
7219	16	5	77	221	543	2	6	21	11	6	9	11	11	2	5	14	9	10	11
7220	8	2	7	158	761	3	5	8	31	10	12	8	38	1	5	33	23	21	18
7221	7	2	8	235	889	9	4	70	28	13	14	12	37	1	6	18	23	12	10
7222	14	4	68	191	448	7	6	14	8	7	5	8	12	2	6	12	9	9	9
7223	8	2	9	203	551	2	4	15	13	6	6	11	23	1	5	17	14	13	8
7224	15	5	74	211	563	2	5	20	9	6	8	12	11	2	5	13	9	11	11
7225	14	4	68	192	464	7	6	14	8	7	6	8	11	2	5	13	8	10	10
7226	13	3	8	363	168	2	8	8	23	3	16	8	2	1	3	10	6	17	7
7227	23	9	115	111	616	2	2	16	33	24	38	22	3	32	3	31	10	15	34
7228	19	7	97	95	731	1	2	24	30	21	34	24	3	27	3	28	11	14	30
7229	14	4	68	193	524	7	7	13	7	6	5	7	11	2	8	11	10	14	11
7230	7	2	8	175	440	1	2	16	14	3	9	9	10	1	5	10	10	15	8
7231	40	11	84	1405	1061	21	22	77	31	21	31	28	14	20	10	28	16	17	26
7232	4	1	8	87	228	2	2	32	5	3	6	5	5	3	4	4	4	6	5
7233	9	2	11	28	82	29	4	5	2	4	6	4	3	4	4	4	4	4	4
7234	22	8	51	276	312	20	10	110	6	10	14	16	6	19	14	17	6	9	17
7235	13	5	68	167	302	6	4	77	7	10	15	12	5	17	3	12	5	10	16
7236	15	5	16	228	203	19	9	102	9	6	6	12	5	1	13	12	5	6	5
7237	4	2	49	111	95	13	1	2	8	11	4	3	6	3	11	10	4	7	4
7238	6	3	52	118	57	6	1	0	7	10	4	2	2	3	11	10	2	5	4
7239	6	3	51	117	172	8	4	4	7	10	7	4	3	6	11	11	4	7	6
7240	5	3	49	259	151	8	3	5	7	10	5	3	3	3	11	11	3	6	4
7241	3	1	53	47	180	5	4	5	8	9	13	6	3	2	2	8	4	8	5
7242	2	0	55	95	201	5	4	5	8	8	13	5	3	7	3	9	5	8	5
7243	7	2	17	379	305	8	4	35	8	5	11	9	4	8	1	8	5	8	8
7244	3	1	0	399	258	8	4	39	9	3	7	8	4	0	2	5	5	6	2
7245	8	3	148	675	463	26	3	8	9	24	16	18	15	25	6	20	12	18	24
7246	0	0	1	42	70	6	0	2	5	2	5	3	2	1	1	3	3	4	2
7247	0	0	0	6	78	0	0	0	20	2	13	5	1	0	2	7	5	15	5
7248	15	2	0	799	246	7	10	48	5	3	6	6	8	0	3	6	9	7	3
7249	7	2	49	110	262	4	4	10	14	9	9	6	4	5	2	10	6	5	8
7250	10	3	40	146	308	8	4	20	10	11	20	10	3	9	3	11	7	12	13
7251	24	8	57	283	506	9	7	68	12	17	24	14	9	22	4	17	11	19	23
7252	7	3	19	84	140	1	2	2	11	8	12	4	1	3	2	7	5	8	6
7253	19	7	17	252	180	5	4	40	2	2	3	4	3	0	1	3	3	4	2

Mixed Dishes & Fast Foods

Food No.	Food Description & Amount	wt gm	wt oz	cal	% cal fat	prot gm	carbo gm	fiber gm
7254	Tamale, plain, meatless, no sauce, Mexican style [1 tamale]	72	2.5	150	47%	3	17	2.2
7255	Taquitoes [1 taquito]	72	2.5	185	49%	10	14	1.9
7256	Tortellini, cheese-filled, meatless, with tomato sauce [1 cup]	250	8.8	338	38%	14	38	2.3
7257	Tortellini, cheese-filled, meatless, with tomato sauce, canned [1 cup]	247	8.7	222	14%	9	39	1.6
7258	Tortellini, cheese-filled, meatless, with vinaigrette dressing [1 cup]	169	6.0	341	50%	12	30	1.1
7259	Tortellini, cheese-filled, meatless, with vegetables and vinaigrette dressing (Include Stouffer's Cheese Tortellini Vinaigrette) [1 cup]	169	6.0	364	63%	12	23	2.4
7260	Tortellini, cheese-filled, with cream sauce [1 cup]	250	8.8	398	43%	16	39	1.3
7261	Tortellini, meat-filled, no sauce [1 cup]	190	6.7	373	36%	25	33	1.1
7262	Tortellini, meat-filled, with tomato sauce [1 cup]	210	7.4	285	32%	15	34	2.0
7263	Tortellini, meat-filled, with tomato sauce, canned [1 cup]	233	8.2	218	17%	9	37	2.5
7264	Tortellini, spinach-filled, no sauce [1 cup]	122	4.3	232	35%	12	25	1.1
7265	Tortellini, spinach-filled, with tomato sauce [1 cup]	200	7.1	241	30%	10	33	2.3
7266	Tostada salad with beef [1 salad]	232	8.2	435	59%	21	24	3.9
7267	Tostada salad, meatless [1 salad]	232	8.2	350	56%	15	25	4.5
7268	Turnover, chicken, with gravy [1 turnover]	112	4.0	316	57%	11	23	0.7
7269	Turnover, chicken or turkey, and cheese-filled, no gravy (Include Hot Pocket) [1 turnover]	128	4.5	453	57%	17	31	1.1
7270	Turnover, chicken- or turkey-, and vegetable-filled [1 turnover]	128	4.5	241	26%	10	34	1.8
7271	Turnover, meat and bean-filled, no gravy [1 turnover]	88	3.1	316	57%	10	23	1.5
7272	Turnover, meat and cheese-filled, no gravy (Include Hot Pockets Ham 'n Cheese, Hot Pockets Beef & Cheddar) [1 turnover]	96	3.4	356	59%	11	25	0.9
7273	Turnover, meat and cheese-filled, tomato-based sauce (Include Hot Pockets Pepperoni Pizza, Hot Pockets Sausage Pizza) [1 turnover]	73	2.6	265	62%	8	17	0.8
7274	Turnover, meat, potato, and vegetable-filled, no gravy [1 turnover]	88	3.1	267	57%	8	20	1.1
7275	Turnover, meat and vegetable- filled (no potatoes, no gravy) [1 turnover]	88	3.1	279	58%	9	20	1.2
7276	Turnover, meat-filled, no gravy [1 turnover]	88	3.1	339	60%	11	23	0.9
7277	Turnover, meat-filled, with gravy [1 turnover]	152	5.4	392	58%	13	27	1.1
7278	Vegetables and cheese in pastry [1 pastry]	103	3.6	327	68%	8	20	2.7
7279	Vegetables in pastry (Include Pepperidge Farm, all varieties) [1 pastry]	103	3.6	320	67%	7	22	3.0
7280	Vegetarian chili (made with meat substitute) [1 cup]	254	9.0	336	13%	45	36	11.8
7281	Vegetarian fillets [1 fillet]	85	3.0	247	56%	20	8	5.2
7282	Vegetarian meat loaf or patties (meat loaf made with meat substitute) [1 slice]	56	2.0	112	41%	12	4	2.6
7283	Vegetarian pot pie (Include beef-like and chicken-like pot pies) [1 pie]	227	8.0	510	57%	14	41	5.2
7284	Vegetarian stew [1 cup]	239	8.4	287	23%	41	17	2.6
7285	Vegetarian stroganoff (made with meat substitute) [1 cup]	125	4.4	231	59%	12	11	2.9
7286	Vienna sausages stewed with potatoes, Puerto Rican style (Salchichas guisadas) [1 cup]	175	6.2	393	68%	9	23	2.3
7287	Welsh rarebit [1 cup]	232	8.2	379	66%	18	14	0.1
7288	White rice with tomato sauce [1 cup]	243	8.6	253	11%	5	50	1.8
7289	Wonton, fried, meat filled [4 wonton]	76	2.7	219	42%	12	19	0.9
	Sandwiches (white bread, unless noted otherwise)							
7400	Bacon and cheese sandwich with mayonnaise [1 sandwich]	121	4.3	401	52%	18	30	1.2
7401	Bacon on biscuit (Include Hardee's) [1 sandwich]	93	3.3	360	47%	8	40	1.1
7402	Bacon and scrambled egg sandwich [1 sandwich]	177	6.2	393	50%	21	27	1.1
7403	Bacon sandwich with mayonnaise [1 sandwich]	91	3.2	351	51%	13	29	1.3
7404	Bacon, chicken, and tomato club sandwich (Includes lettuce, mayonnaise) (Include Arby's Turkey Club, Wendy's Chicken Club) [1 sandwich]	246	8.7	555	42%	31	48	2.8
7405	Bacon, chicken, lettuce, and tomato club sandwich with mayonnaise, on multigrain roll (Include Hardee's Turkey Club) [1 sandwich]	194	6.8	445	47%	32	26	2.5
7406	Bacon, lettuce, and tomato sandwich with mayonnaise [1 sandwich]	164	5.8	350	49%	11	35	2.3
7407	Beef barbecue submarine sandwich, on bun [1 submarine]	192	6.8	421	28%	31	43	2.4
7408	Bologna sandwich with margarine (Include other luncheon meats) [1 sandwich]	83	2.9	256	47%	7	26	1.2
7409	Bologna and cheese sandwich with margarine [1 sandwich]	111	3.9	350	53%	13	28	1.2

						% of Daily Value													
Food No.	fat gm	sat fat gm	choles mg	sodium mg	potas mg	vit A	vit E	vit C	thia	ribo	niac	vit B-6	fola	vit B-12	calc	phos	mag	iron	zinc
7254	8	3	6	115	99	0	1	0	17	10	13	4	1	1	3	6	6	10	3
7255	10	3	27	76	170	3	4	1	3	7	10	8	2	11	6	15	7	7	14
7256	14	6	162	553	406	24	9	16	21	25	15	10	8	6	15	21	8	17	10
7257	4	1	51	737	89	3	1	4	23	12	14	4	3	4	7	13	8	10	7
7258	19	7	148	94	121	12	9	0	16	21	10	4	6	6	14	18	4	12	8
7259	25	6	19	457	210	36	22	66	12	12	8	7	7	4	27	22	8	9	8
7260	19	8	167	378	252	18	7	2	22	31	12	6	7	10	25	27	7	15	11
7261	15	5	240	437	231	13	5	0	31	33	22	11	7	15	18	29	7	17	14
7262	10	3	91	506	277	11	6	9	23	14	17	10	4	7	11	20	10	15	11
7263	4	1	42	745	375	9	2	42	19	10	13	10	5	4	6	15	10	14	7
7264	9	3	158	252	138	18	4	2	16	22	9	5	9	8	14	17	6	13	7
7265	8	2	73	438	297	25	7	12	17	13	11	8	10	5	13	16	12	16	8
7266	29	10	63	455	518	12	10	21	15	20	23	13	15	24	24	26	11	20	24
7267	22	10	40	565	477	19	8	23	18	20	11	10	18	6	38	28	11	15	12
7268	20	4	23	217	146	4	11	1	13	14	15	5	2	3	7	11	4	9	6
7269	29	7	41	197	173	4	14	0	19	18	26	9	3	4	10	18	6	13	9
7270	7	1	31	601	205	15	8	2	19	18	21	8	10	2	11	15	5	14	6
7271	20	5	23	84	133	0	8	0	13	11	11	4	5	12	1	10	4	13	13
7272	24	6	26	125	134	3	11	0	14	15	14	4	2	9	8	12	4	11	11
7273	18	5	24	264	145	2	7	3	16	10	12	5	2	8	4	9	3	8	7
7274	17	4	20	75	133	17	7	2	11	9	10	6	2	10	1	8	3	10	11
7275	18	5	21	78	123	12	8	8	12	10	11	5	3	10	1	8	3	11	12
7276	22	6	26	93	106	0	9	0	14	12	12	4	2	13	1	9	3	13	14
7277	25	7	30	427	160	0	10	0	16	14	15	5	2	15	1	12	3	16	19
7278	25	7	14	180	244	6	23	10	11	18	11	4	5	2	14	18	13	10	7
7279	24	6	6	140	257	4	25	11	12	17	12	4	6	1	8	15	14	10	6
7280	5	1	0	843	868	18	14	22	19	9	14	18	49	0	13	52	21	58	20
7281	15	2	0	417	510	0	13	0	62	45	51	64	22	60	8	38	5	9	8
7282	5	1	0	308	101	0	4	0	34	20	28	34	11	22	2	19	3	7	7
7283	32	9	20	486	378	79	19	17	55	26	26	20	14	17	7	26	8	16	7
7284	7	1	0	956	287	0	5	0	112	84	143	131	62	88	7	53	76	17	18
7285	15	5	11	572	182	5	9	1	33	22	28	31	11	21	6	22	4	8	8
7286	30	8	34	801	765	3	14	44	11	7	15	20	5	9	2	10	8	9	10
7287	28	14	63	480	359	32	8	2	7	30	2	5	4	10	56	42	10	4	14
7288	3	1	0	526	360	11	7	18	21	4	16	14	3	0	3	9	9	14	7
7289	10	3	80	39	204	2	3	1	23	14	13	8	3	4	2	12	4	9	9
7400	23	11	48	1109	244	14	5	0	20	26	13	8	6	12	39	36	8	12	15
7401	19	4	9	1033	235	0	11	0	28	16	18	3	2	5	4	39	4	16	5
7402	22	7	418	781	277	23	8	0	25	42	15	10	13	19	14	28	7	17	12
7403	20	6	27	784	205	0	4	0	31	16	22	7	5	8	7	15	5	12	8
7404	26	6	72	855	463	5	12	16	40	26	60	30	12	9	12	30	12	23	11
7405	23	7	76	843	479	4	5	13	35	20	62	25	8	13	6	31	13	18	15
7406	19	5	20	650	329	6	9	24	26	16	19	10	8	5	8	13	7	14	7
7407	13	4	70	711	506	2	4	3	30	24	33	15	7	49	12	27	11	29	40
7408	13	4	16	598	112	4	3	0	19	12	14	4	5	6	6	7	4	11	6
7409	20	9	35	940	185	10	4	0	20	20	14	6	5	11	22	21	6	12	11

Mixed Dishes & Fast Foods

Food No.	Food Description & Amount	wt gm	wt oz	cal	% cal fat	prot gm	carbo gm	fiber gm
7410	Bologna and cheese submarine sandwich, on bun with lettuce, mayonnaise (Include grinder, poorboy) [1 submarine]	198	7.0	541	62%	21	29	1.6
7411	Cheese sandwich with margarine [1 sandwich]	83	2.9	262	44%	10	27	1.2
7412	Cheese sandwich with margarine, grilled [1 sandwich]	83	2.9	292	49%	10	27	1.2
7413	Cheese sandwich with lettuce, hoagie [1 hoagie]	156	5.5	464	49%	25	33	1.7
7414	Cheese spread sandwich [1 sandwich]	78	2.8	215	32%	9	27	1.2
7415	Chicken barbecue sandwich [1 sandwich]	119	4.2	251	22%	21	27	1.3
7416	Chicken fillet sandwich with lettuce, tomato, mayonnaise [1 sandwich]	174	6.1	466	51%	22	35	2.1
7417	Chicken fillet (fried) sandwich [1 sandwich]	126	4.4	327	34%	29	23	1.2
7418	Chicken fillet (broiled) sandwich, on whole wheat roll with lettuce, tomato, mayonnaise (Include Hardee's Grilled Chicken Sandwich) [1 sandwich]	173	6.1	331	23%	27	39	5.7
7419	Chicken fillet (broiled), sandwich, with lettuce, tomato, and non-mayonnaise type spread (Include Wendy's) [1 sandwich]	175	6.2	343	30%	27	32	1.9
7420	Chicken fillet (broiled), sandwich, on oat bran bun, with lettuce, tomato, spread (Include Burger King) [1 sandwich]	155	5.5	315	32%	30	23	2.4
7421	Chicken fillet (broiled), sandwich with cheese, on whole wheat roll, with lettuce, tomato and non-mayonaise type spread (Include Wendy's) [1 sandwich]	193	6.8	380	27%	34	37	5.3
7422	Chicken fillet (broiled), sandwich with cheese, on bun, with lettuce, tomato and spread (Include Burger King) [1 sandwich]	229	8.1	530	38%	40	41	2.4
7423	Chicken fillet (broiled), sandwich with cheese, on bun, with lettuce, tomato and spread (Include McDonald's) [1 sandwich]	240	8.5	556	38%	41	43	2.5
7424	Chicken patty (battered, fried) sandwich with lettuce, pickles, mayonnaise (Include McDonald's Crispy Chicken Deluxe) [1 sandwich]	208	7.3	595	45%	30	51	2.7
7425	Chicken patty (battered, fried) sandwich or biscuit (Include Jimmy Dean Chicken Biscuit) [1 sandwich]	57	2.0	169	42%	6	18	0.5
7426	Chicken patty (battered, fried) sandwich with cheese, on wheat bun with lettuce, tomato, mayonnaise (Include with onions; Jack-in-the-Box Chicken Supreme) [1 sandwich]	227	8.0	620	47%	35	46	3.9
7427	Chicken patty (battered, fried) sandwich with mayonnaise, miniature (Include Kentucky Fried Chicken Chicken Little) [1 miniature sandwich]	52	1.8	164	47%	6	15	0.7
7428	Chicken salad or chicken spread sandwich [1 sandwich]	113	4.0	268	44%	15	22	1.3
7429	Chicken sandwich with mayonnaise (Include sliced, roast chicken sandwich) [1 sandwich]	112	4.0	267	27%	22	26	1.2
7430	Corned beef sandwich with pickle relish [1 sandwich]	130	4.6	268	33%	19	25	1.7
7431	Crab cake sandwich, on bun [1 sandwich]	140	4.9	312	25%	20	37	1.9
7432	Croissant, filled with creamed chicken and broccoli (Include Sara Lee Le Sanwich with chicken and broccoli) [1 croissant]	128	4.5	347	49%	16	28	1.2
7433	Croissant, filled with creamed ham and cheese (Include Sara Lee Le Sanwich with ham and cheese) [1 croissant]	113	4.0	338	52%	15	25	0.8
7434	Croissant with vegetables and cheese (Include Arby's) [1 croissant]	148	5.2	528	65%	14	33	2.3
7435	Croissant with sausage and egg (Include Arby's) [1 croissant]	142	5.0	497	62%	16	31	1.6
7436	Croissant with bacon and egg (Include Arby's) [1 croissant]	113	4.0	402	56%	14	30	1.6
7437	Croissant with ham, egg, and cheese (Include Burger King) [1 croissant]	144	5.1	402	53%	22	25	1.3
7438	Croissant with sausage, egg, and cheese (Include Burger King) [1 croissant]	159	5.6	538	65%	20	26	1.3
7439	Croissant with bacon, egg, and cheese (Include Burger King) [1 croissant]	118	4.2	386	58%	15	25	1.3
7440	Cuban sandwich, Puerto Rican style (Sandwich cubano) [1 sandwich (6" long)]	255	9.0	704	40%	44	58	3.1
7441	Egg salad sandwich [1 sandwich]	124	4.4	378	66%	11	21	0.9
7442	Scrambled egg sandwich [1 sandwich]	112	4.0	238	35%	11	27	1.2
7443	Egg and bacon on biscuit (Include Hardee's) [1 sandwich]	124	4.4	378	61%	14	24	0.6
7444	Egg and cheese on biscuit [1 sandwich]	140	4.9	425	55%	13	35	0.9
7445	Egg, cheese, bacon on biscuit (Include Swanson Great Starts Egg, Cheese & Bacon on a Biscuit breakfast sandwich) [1 sandwich]	119	4.2	340	50%	13	30	0.8
7446	Egg, cheese, ham on biscuit (Include Hardee's) [1 sandwich]	151	5.3	459	48%	19	43	0.7
7447	Egg, cheese, sausage on biscuit (Include Swanson Great Starts Sausage, Egg and Cheese on a Biscuit breakfast sandwich) [1 sandwich]	176	6.2	573	61%	21	34	0.8
7448	Egg and ham on biscuit (Include Hardee's) [1 sandwich]	138	4.9	317	55%	15	22	0.6

						% of Daily Value													
Food No.	fat gm	sat fat gm	choles mg	sodium mg	potas mg	vit A	vit E	vit C	thia	ribo	niac	vit B-6	fola	vit B-12	calc	phos	mag	iron	zinc
7410	37	15	72	1585	349	8	4	2	27	24	21	12	9	26	25	28	8	18	20
7411	13	6	19	655	135	10	4	0	16	17	10	3	5	5	22	19	5	10	8
7412	16	6	19	696	137	13	6	0	12	16	9	3	3	3	22	19	5	10	8
7413	25	15	68	945	261	21	4	1	20	30	12	6	7	19	73	52	10	13	22
7414	8	4	16	642	127	5	2	0	17	17	10	3	5	2	21	24	5	9	7
7415	6	2	50	422	217	2	2	1	19	16	36	15	5	3	7	16	7	13	10
7416	26	5	67	593	283	5	15	7	24	16	46	22	8	4	10	18	8	16	7
7417	12	3	73	301	260	2	3	0	18	14	59	24	4	5	7	22	8	13	9
7418	9	2	53	699	400	2	6	5	22	14	57	26	13	4	7	32	22	19	14
7419	11	2	63	445	320	2	11	7	22	16	59	23	7	4	9	21	9	15	7
7420	11	2	72	578	290	2	6	2	20	15	68	27	6	5	6	24	10	18	9
7421	11	4	81	591	471	5	8	5	16	15	68	33	8	7	17	41	22	15	17
7422	22	7	100	889	461	9	9	6	30	27	76	34	9	11	29	42	13	21	15
7423	23	8	104	931	484	10	10	6	31	29	79	35	9	11	30	44	14	22	16
7424	29	7	93	1042	327	4	13	1	34	26	51	21	9	5	14	23	10	23	15
7425	8	2	15	579	64	0	5	0	9	7	11	3	1	1	6	7	2	6	3
7426	33	10	108	1151	413	10	12	5	30	28	50	22	12	9	29	41	16	23	21
7427	9	2	18	284	97	1	5	0	9	6	13	6	2	2	4	7	2	6	3
7428	13	2	42	333	181	2	7	2	15	13	21	11	6	2	6	11	5	10	8
7429	8	2	51	346	201	1	4	0	19	14	45	20	5	4	6	17	7	12	7
7430	10	4	46	1177	187	0	1	5	16	15	16	5	5	15	7	11	5	15	15
7431	9	2	97	637	341	6	7	7	27	17	25	8	13	69	18	22	10	18	22
7432	19	10	72	627	219	17	3	6	16	17	24	10	6	4	12	20	6	11	10
7433	20	11	65	877	234	17	2	0	27	19	17	6	4	6	16	26	5	10	11
7434	38	16	73	945	293	17	15	2	19	25	14	6	7	11	25	28	6	12	13
7435	34	15	242	878	207	19	5	2	28	24	14	7	10	13	5	20	5	15	12
7436	25	12	223	732	185	19	4	2	23	23	11	7	10	13	5	20	5	14	10
7437	24	12	265	1080	271	23	5	3	30	30	14	14	11	17	13	31	7	15	16
7438	39	17	281	1034	259	23	6	3	27	29	14	8	11	17	14	29	6	16	17
7439	25	12	252	751	199	23	5	3	18	26	8	8	10	15	13	26	5	14	12
7440	31	10	93	1466	591	17	12	1	99	44	52	31	10	19	37	48	14	26	28
7441	28	5	263	433	130	12	17	0	15	26	8	12	10	12	8	15	4	11	6
7442	9	3	213	447	145	12	4	0	18	26	10	5	9	8	10	15	5	13	6
7443	26	7	291	826	207	4	8	4	7	11	10	6	6	14	16	20	5	17	9
7444	26	7	174	1153	270	19	15	0	21	29	12	6	5	11	18	47	6	16	9
7445	19	6	135	1204	255	11	10	0	22	24	13	6	4	9	15	42	5	14	8
7446	25	14	145	1593	263	12	12	0	33	29	17	9	4	7	25	64	7	17	15
7447	39	12	201	1649	413	18	15	2	42	34	21	12	5	23	19	53	7	19	16
7448	19	4	215	994	229	17	7	0	32	25	7	10	6	14	16	23	6	18	11

Mixed Dishes & Fast Foods

Food No.	Food Description & Amount	wt gm	wt oz	cal	% cal fat	prot gm	carbo gm	fiber gm
7449	Egg and sausage on biscuit (Include Hardee's) [1 biscuit]	150	5.3	485	60%	16	34	0.8
7450	Egg and sausage on biscuit [1 sandwich]	162	5.7	523	60%	17	37	0.8
7451	Egg and sausage on biscuit (Include McDonald's) [1 biscuit]	175	6.2	565	60%	19	40	0.9
7452	Egg and steak on biscuit (Include Hardee's) [1 sandwich]	179	6.3	547	48%	20	50	1.3
7453	Egg, cheese, and bacon on English muffin [1 sandwich]	135	4.8	377	48%	19	29	1.5
7454	Egg, cheese, beef on English muffin (Include Swanson Great Starts Beefsteak, Egg & Cheese on a Muffin breakfast sandwich) [1 sandwich]	147	5.2	416	49%	22	30	1.6
7455	Egg, cheese, ham on English muffin (Include Egg McMuffin; Swanson Great Starts Egg, Canadian Style Bacon & Cheese on a Muffin breakfast sandwich) [1 sandwich]	125	4.4	288	40%	19	24	1.3
7456	Egg, cheese, sausage on English muffin (Include Sausage and Egg McMuffin) [1 egg muffin]	165	5.8	476	58%	20	29	1.5
7457	Fajeta-style beef sandwich with cheese, lettuce on pita bread (Include with onions; Jack-in-the-Box Original Pita Pocket Sandwich) [1 pita sandwich]	207	7.3	292	35%	19	28	2.5
7458	Fajeta-style chicken sandwich with cheese, lettuce on pita bread (Include with onions; Jack-in-the-Box Chicken Pita Pocket Sandwich) [1 pita sandwich]	207	7.3	311	35%	22	28	2.5
7459	Finger sandwich (tuna-egg-mayonnaise filling) [2 finger sandwiches]	46	1.6	104	24%	6	13	0.6
7460	Fish (coated, fried) sandwich, on bun, with tartar sauce [1 sandwich]	140	4.9	376	36%	18	41	1.9
7461	Fish sandwich, on bun, with cheese and spread (Include Hardee's) [1 sandwich]	207	7.3	537	35%	30	56	2.8
7462	Fried egg sandwich [1 sandwich]	96	3.4	226	34%	10	26	1.2
7463	Gyro sandwich (pita bread, beef, lamb, tomato, and condiments) [1 gyro]	105	3.7	170	21%	12	21	1.0
7464	Ham on biscuit (Include Hardee's) [1 sandwich]	106	3.7	363	43%	13	41	0.7
7465	Ham and cheese on English muffin [1 ham and cheese muffin]	96	3.4	251	42%	17	18	1.0
7466	Ham and cheese sandwich with lettuce, margarine [1 sandwich]	155	5.5	380	46%	20	30	1.4
7467	Ham and cheese sandwich, grilled [1 sandwich]	141	5.0	381	46%	21	30	1.2
7468	Ham and cheese sandwich, on bun with lettuce, mayonnaise (Include ham and cheese hero sandwich) [1 sandwich]	154	5.4	352	48%	19	25	1.5
7469	Ham and cheese submarine sandwich, on multigrain roll with lettuce and tomato (Include Hardee's Ham 'N' Cheese Supreme) [1 submarine]	219	7.7	476	60%	24	25	2.3
7470	Hot ham and cheese sandwich, on bun, with tomato, lettuce, mayonnaise (Include Arby's or Burger King Hot Ham and Cheese Sandwich) [1 sandwich]	230	8.1	519	50%	30	34	2.2
7471	Ham and fried egg sandwich [1 sandwich]	124	4.4	277	38%	15	27	1.2
7472	Ham and tomato club sandwich with lettuce, french dressing [1 sandwich]	254	9.0	594	48%	30	47	2.2
7473	Ham salad sandwich [1 sandwich]	107	3.8	246	44%	13	20	1.2
7474	Ham sandwich, with spread [1 sandwich]	112	4.0	282	41%	14	27	1.2
7475	Ham sandwich with lettuce, margarine [1 sandwich]	127	4.5	285	38%	15	29	1.4
7476	Meat spread or potted meat sandwich [1 sandwich]	107	3.8	268	39%	8	32	1.3
7477	Meatball and spaghetti sauce sandwich [1 sandwich]	189	6.7	438	42%	29	32	2.3
7478	Midnight sandwich, Puerto Rican style (Media noche) [1 sandwich]	201	7.1	483	35%	34	42	2.2
7479	Pastrami sandwich [1 sandwich]	134	4.7	331	49%	14	27	1.7
7480	Pork barbecue or Sloppy Joe, on bun [1 sandwich]	186	6.6	322	27%	23	34	2.2
7481	Pork sandwich [1 sandwich]	136	4.8	324	26%	26	32	1.5
7482	Pork sandwich, with gravy [1 sandwich]	218	7.7	326	25%	25	34	1.7
7483	Pork, barbeque sauce, onions, dill pickles on white roll (Include McRib sandwich) [1 sandwich]	189	6.7	421	32%	28	40	2.5
7484	Puerto Rican sandwich (Sandwich criollo) (Includes cheese, mortadella, margarine) [1 sandwich]	160	5.6	550	50%	17	50	2.6
7485	Reuben sandwich (corned beef sandwich with sauerkraut and cheese) [1 sandwich]	181	6.4	464	56%	21	30	3.4
7486	Roast beef sandwich (Incl. Arby's or Hardee's or RAX or Roy Rogers Roast Beef Sandwich) [1 sandwich]	136	4.8	343	36%	27	26	1.2
7487	Roast beef sandwich dipped in egg, fried in butter, with gravy [1 sandwich]	258	9.1	521	51%	33	30	1.5
7488	Roast beef sandwich with bacon and cheese sauce (Include RAX Beef, Bacon and Cheddar) [1 sandwich]	189	6.7	588	47%	38	37	1.9
7489	Roast beef sandwich with cheese (Include Arby's Beef 'N Swiss) [1 sandwich]	175	6.2	460	41%	36	29	1.3
7490	Roast beef sandwich, with gravy [1 sandwich]	222	7.8	388	36%	30	30	1.5

Food No.	fat gm	sat fat gm	choles mg	sodium mg	potas mg	vit A	vit E	vit C	thia	ribo	niac	vit B-6	fola	vit B-12	calc	phos	mag	iron	zinc
						% of Daily Value													
7449	32	12	252	951	267	14	11	0	28	22	15	8	8	19	13	41	5	18	12
7450	35	13	272	1027	288	15	11	0	30	24	16	9	9	21	14	44	6	20	13
7451	38	15	294	1110	312	16	12	0	33	26	18	10	10	22	15	48	6	21	14
7452	29	6	161	1544	410	13	20	0	33	33	24	12	5	22	8	58	8	27	19
7453	20	8	242	908	258	17	5	0	22	31	15	8	9	15	25	32	7	14	14
7454	22	8	183	900	289	18	8	0	17	28	20	9	8	22	25	30	7	16	22
7455	13	5	204	898	237	14	4	0	24	27	15	11	7	12	21	28	6	12	13
7456	31	12	207	1060	279	19	7	0	24	30	16	7	8	14	29	33	7	14	16
7457	11	4	39	778	464	9	7	56	22	18	21	21	9	28	18	25	10	14	18
7458	12	5	51	784	372	10	7	56	20	17	26	15	9	6	19	22	9	12	13
7459	3	1	21	213	66	1	2	0	8	7	14	3	3	8	3	5	2	6	2
7460	15	3	45	577	320	2	13	1	27	17	23	8	6	14	12	18	9	15	5
7461	21	5	75	1032	446	4	12	0	36	27	36	16	10	18	32	43	15	25	12
7462	9	2	207	433	120	11	4	0	18	24	10	5	9	7	8	14	4	12	6
7463	4	2	34	272	209	1	1	6	16	13	16	7	4	15	5	12	5	10	15
7464	17	11	23	1344	184	3	10	0	32	17	16	6	2	1	15	52	5	14	10
7465	12	7	46	739	170	9	1	0	25	17	15	9	5	8	28	26	6	8	13
7466	19	8	53	1449	350	11	5	1	51	27	26	14	7	13	23	34	8	14	16
7467	20	8	54	1465	337	11	5	0	48	26	25	13	4	14	23	34	8	13	16
7468	19	8	51	1357	357	11	5	2	47	24	23	13	7	13	23	32	7	12	16
7469	31	12	73	1587	496	16	11	13	46	30	24	20	9	17	35	46	13	16	21
7470	29	9	77	2016	592	10	11	9	63	35	39	22	9	15	25	44	11	20	22
7471	12	3	224	800	213	11	4	0	34	28	18	10	9	11	8	20	6	14	10
7472	32	12	76	2099	480	15	15	10	72	33	37	21	9	16	30	43	11	20	21
7473	12	2	29	817	226	1	7	2	31	14	18	14	5	5	5	13	5	9	9
7474	13	3	36	1033	245	1	5	0	47	18	24	13	5	8	6	18	6	12	10
7475	12	3	34	1103	276	4	4	1	51	20	26	12	6	8	7	20	6	13	11
7476	12	4	22	841	122	1	5	0	23	15	15	5	5	11	6	8	4	11	6
7477	20	7	86	591	497	2	5	6	22	22	41	17	7	47	10	23	10	25	36
7478	19	7	76	1379	458	8	5	1	74	32	39	26	7	13	22	36	10	19	22
7479	18	6	51	1335	243	0	1	6	19	16	24	7	5	16	7	14	6	15	18
7480	10	3	51	948	426	7	6	9	50	22	28	17	5	8	9	20	10	16	15
7481	9	3	62	392	343	0	2	0	60	27	31	17	7	9	9	23	9	15	17
7482	9	3	58	805	337	0	2	1	57	27	30	17	6	9	9	23	9	15	16
7483	15	5	81	891	460	3	4	5	57	30	30	14	6	12	13	20	9	22	29
7484	31	10	31	1285	251	21	12	0	33	27	21	5	7	10	32	26	8	19	13
7485	29	10	82	1348	261	9	4	7	16	21	17	11	9	22	30	29	10	16	27
7486	14	5	68	338	377	0	1	0	21	21	28	13	6	41	6	23	8	22	41
7487	29	9	173	973	478	15	10	0	23	30	30	15	9	47	8	30	9	27	48
7488	31	12	93	1047	549	4	3	0	39	31	39	16	7	47	20	39	11	28	47
7489	21	9	96	696	471	5	2	0	23	27	31	15	7	51	25	43	11	25	52
7490	16	6	70	821	446	0	1	0	22	23	31	13	6	42	7	25	9	25	47

Mixed Dishes & Fast Foods

Food No.	Food Description & Amount	wt gm	wt oz	cal	% cal fat	prot gm	carbo gm	fiber gm
7491	Roast beef submarine sandwich, on multigrain roll with lettuce, tomato, mayonnaise (Include Hardee's Roast Beef Supreme) [1 sandwich]	202	7.1	440	46%	24	35	2.5
7492	Roast beef submarine sandwich, on roll, au jus (Include French Dip sandwich) [1 sandwich]	193	6.8	363	32%	25	34	1.8
7493	Salami sandwich with margarine [1 sandwich]	82	2.9	234	43%	8	25	1.1
7494	Sardine sandwich (filling of sardine in tomato sauce, celery, egg, mayonnaise, pickle, onion) with lettuce [1 sandwich]	214	7.5	492	52%	27	31	1.9
7495	Sausage and spaghetti sauce sandwich [1 sandwich]	189	6.7	469	49%	23	35	2.3
7496	Sausage on biscuit [1 sandwich]	124	4.4	485	59%	12	40	1.4
7497	Sausage on biscuit, diet (Include Weight Watchers) [1 sandwich]	85	3.0	220	46%	10	19	0.6
7498	Sausage and cheese on English muffin (Include McDonald's McMuffin) [1 sandwich]	135	4.8	462	56%	18	34	1.8
7499	Sausage sandwich [1 sandwich]	107	3.8	343	51%	15	26	1.2
7500	Steak and cheese submarine sandwich, on roll [1 submarine]	170	6.0	448	41%	34	30	1.5
7501	Steak and cheese submarine sandwich, on roll [1 submarine]	197	6.9	538	48%	41	27	1.2
7502	Steak and cheese submarine sandwich, with fried peppers. onions, on roll (Include Philadelphia-style cheese steak submarine sandwich; Arby's Philly Beef N' Swiss) [1 submarine]	204	7.2	491	39%	37	35	2.3
7503	Steak and cheese submarine sandwich, with tomato, lettuce on roll [1 submarine]	214	7.5	474	41%	35	33	2.0
7504	Steak on biscuit (Include Jimmy Dean Steak Biscuit) [1 sandwich]	57	2.0	170	37%	8	18	0.6
7505	Steak sandwich, plain, on roll [1 sandwich]	142	5.0	349	36%	30	24	1.3
7506	Steak submarine sandwich, with tomato and tomato, on roll [1 sandwich]	186	6.6	378	33%	30	31	2.1
7507	Tomato sandwich with lettuce, mayonnaise [1 sandwich]	134	4.7	237	39%	5	31	2.1
7508	Tuna salad sandwich [1 sandwich]	152	5.4	278	23%	19	35	1.6
7509	Tuna salad sandwich [1 sandwich]	172	6.1	297	23%	20	37	1.9
7510	Tuna salad submarine sandwich, on roll with lettuce [1 sandwich]	190	6.7	373	22%	20	51	2.9
7511	Turkey salad or turkey spread sandwich [1 sandwich]	92	3.2	216	42%	13	18	1.0
7512	Turkey sandwich, with mayonnaise [1 sandwich]	143	5.0	331	31%	29	26	1.2
7513	Turkey sandwich, with gravy [1 sandwich]	284	10.0	392	23%	41	32	1.7
7514	Turkey submarine sandwich, on roll, with cheese, lettuce, tomato and spread (Include Arby's) [1 submarine]	277	9.8	583	38%	37	51	3.1
	Frozen Meals							
7600	Beans and franks [1 frozen meal]	340	12.0	531	33%	18	74	8.2
7601	Beef and noodles with meat sauce and cheese (diet meal) (Include Weight Watcher's Ziti Macaroni) [1 frozen meal]	319	11.3	404	33%	28	40	3.4
7602	Beef and pork cannelloni (diet meal) (Include Lean Cuisine Beef and Pork Cannelloni) [1 frozen meal]	273	9.6	242	29%	18	25	2.2
7603	Beef chop suey with rice (Include Stouffer's) [1 frozen meal]	340	12.0	327	24%	17	44	1.2
7604	Beef enchilada, chili gravy, rice, refried beans (Include Mexican meal) [1 frozen meal]	425	15.0	634	43%	22	68	8.1
7605	Beef enchilada, chili gravy, rice, refried beans [1 frozen meal]	227	8.0	516	55%	18	40	2.6
7606	Beef pot pie (Include Greek meat pie, sirloin burger pie) [1 frozen pie]	298	10.5	389	41%	28	30	4.6
7607	Beef sirloin tips with gravy, potatoes, vegetable in cheese sauce (Include LeMenu Beef Sirloin Tips) [1 frozen meal]	326	11.5	378	36%	32	29	4.8
7608	Beef steak with rice, vegetable (diet meal) (Include Classic Lite Beef Pepper Steak) [1 frozen meal]	284	10.0	306	27%	25	29	2.4
7609	Beef steak, with noodles and vegetables in soy-based sauce (Include Lean Cuisine Szechwan Beef) [1 frozen meal]	262	9.2	338	32%	22	35	3.0
7610	Beef with noodles, vegetable (Include Armour Dinner Classics Beef Burgundy) [1 frozen meal]	298	10.5	407	31%	14	59	2.7
7611	Beef with potatoes (Include Swanson entrees: Gravy and Sliced Beef) [1 frozen meal]	227	8.0	523	47%	24	45	4.2
7612	Beef with potatoes (large meat portion) (Include Salisbury steak) [1 frozen meal]	340	12.0	634	48%	39	44	5.8
7613	Beef with spaetzle or rice, vegetable (Include Budget Gourmet Peppersteak with Rice) [1 frozen meal]	284	10.0	279	28%	22	28	2.5
7614	Beef with vegetable (diet meal) [1 frozen meal]	284	10.0	371	54%	28	14	2.4

Food No.	fat gm	sat fat gm	choles mg	sodium mg	potas mg	% of Daily Value													
						vit A	vit E	vit C	thia	ribo	niac	vit B-6	fola	vit B-12	calc	phos	mag	iron	zinc
7491	22	6	59	482	455	4	9	13	26	21	27	16	11	32	10	21	9	23	33
7492	13	5	54	616	380	0	2	0	26	22	30	11	6	34	10	21	8	23	34
7493	11	3	19	612	117	4	3	0	20	16	15	5	4	18	6	8	4	13	6
7494	29	5	228	895	480	12	14	4	23	30	31	16	13	117	37	47	12	24	11
7495	26	8	65	1295	472	2	5	9	56	24	32	18	6	18	11	21	9	19	16
7496	32	14	35	1071	198	1	14	0	26	17	16	6	2	8	13	45	5	14	10
7497	11	4	30	534	179	1	0	1	26	13	14	6	1	10	4	11	3	8	7
7498	28	12	69	1216	252	10	3	2	55	17	24	9	5	13	20	22	7	15	13
7499	19	6	47	998	262	0	1	2	44	19	23	11	5	16	7	15	5	12	11
7500	20	9	89	718	462	6	3	0	24	30	26	19	6	45	25	38	10	24	45
7501	29	14	116	1054	552	14	4	0	21	37	25	22	6	53	42	55	12	25	54
7502	21	8	93	616	421	7	6	20	26	29	30	19	8	39	28	40	11	28	37
7503	21	10	93	752	553	9	3	8	26	32	28	21	9	47	26	41	12	26	48
7504	7	2	17	376	140	0	4	0	11	10	10	5	1	9	5	18	3	9	9
7505	14	5	77	326	409	0	2	0	21	23	26	19	5	44	7	26	8	23	43
7506	14	5	74	391	481	2	3	8	26	25	28	20	9	42	9	26	10	25	42
7507	10	2	6	368	217	5	7	20	20	13	13	7	8	1	7	7	5	12	3
7508	7	1	21	687	233	2	5	2	18	13	47	12	6	28	7	15	7	14	5
7509	8	1	22	731	264	3	5	3	19	14	51	14	8	30	7	16	8	16	6
7510	9	2	18	851	296	3	6	3	29	19	50	12	9	26	13	17	9	20	7
7511	10	2	32	271	188	1	6	2	13	11	16	12	5	3	5	11	5	10	9
7512	11	3	69	376	316	1	6	0	20	19	33	23	6	6	8	23	9	17	20
7513	10	3	89	1045	529	0	3	0	23	28	49	28	7	9	9	32	11	25	32
7514	25	7	70	2408	552	8	12	8	35	29	62	27	11	40	32	51	13	22	18
7600	20	6	62	1619	731	5	6	15	23	16	12	13	21	10	11	27	23	22	13
7601	15	7	61	1224	660	19	13	18	20	24	31	17	6	21	25	34	16	22	31
7602	8	3	39	608	454	51	2	6	20	22	18	14	11	18	15	23	13	17	22
7603	9	3	33	1185	292	1	4	13	18	8	20	16	5	20	3	19	9	18	18
7604	30	9	38	1689	568	8	18	11	31	18	22	16	32	11	18	33	18	31	22
7605	31	7	36	562	409	45	16	14	24	19	24	13	6	22	2	19	8	20	17
7606	18	8	78	579	841	13	5	29	13	15	23	25	10	43	6	26	16	25	44
7607	15	5	79	1124	784	21	8	73	15	23	27	35	12	40	12	34	16	23	42
7608	9	3	67	1062	514	8	6	58	11	17	21	27	7	34	5	24	13	18	35
7609	12	4	81	1008	370	30	4	47	17	17	22	17	8	22	4	24	12	23	24
7610	14	5	31	2756	466	31	6	28	16	15	17	10	10	15	12	21	11	11	15
7611	27	8	72	815	749	0	3	20	15	14	38	30	7	39	4	25	12	22	32
7612	34	12	105	1503	1146	1	3	18	23	26	26	33	19	41	11	44	25	34	61
7613	9	3	51	865	571	7	5	118	15	14	23	24	8	34	4	23	12	20	24
7614	22	9	96	828	715	92	6	53	8	22	36	27	6	54	7	26	12	19	40

Mixed Dishes & Fast Foods

Food No.	Food Description & Amount	wt gm	wt oz	cal	% cal fat	prot gm	carbo gm	fiber gm
7615	Beef, oriental style, with vegetable, rice (diet meal) (Include Lean Cuisine Oriental Beef, Benihana Oriental Lites Beef and Mushrooms in sauce with Vegetables and Rice) [1 frozen meal]	245	8.6	290	20%	21	35	1.4
7616	Beef, sliced, with gravy, barley and wild rice, vegetables (diet meal) [1 frozen meal]	311	11.0	367	11%	20	64	9.1
7617	Beef, oriental style, with vegetable, rice, and fruit dessert (diet meal) (Include Healthy Choice) [1 frozen meal]	311	11.0	306	22%	23	37	3.3
7618	Vegetable and beef in soy-based sauce, reduced fat and sodium (diet meal) [1 frozen meal]	255	9.0	127	21%	10	16	4.9
7619	Beef, sliced, with gravy, hash brown potatoes, vegetable, soup, dessert [1 frozen meal]	425	15.0	596	39%	33	61	4.5
7620	Beef, sliced, with gravy, potatoes, vegetable (Include LeMenu Yankee Pot Roast) [1 frozen meal]	312	11.0	424	51%	25	24	2.9
7621	Beef, sliced, with gravy, potatoes, vegetable, dessert [1 frozen meal]	326	11.5	372	28%	29	37	4.2
7622	Beef, sliced, with vegetable in sauce, au gratin potatoes (Include Banquet Gourmet Sliced Beef and Fresh Vegetables in Sauce with Au Gratin Potatoes) [1 frozen meal]	284	10.0	388	47%	28	24	3.1
7623	Broiled steak with potatoes, vegetable [1 frozen meal]	312	11.0	336	38%	29	23	3.6
7624	Burrito with beef and beans, refried beans, salsa [1 frozen meal]	305	10.8	540	37%	24	62	8.2
7625	Cannelloni, cheese-filled, with tomato sauce (diet meal) (Include Lean Cuisine Cheese Cannelloni with Tomato Sauce) [1 frozen meal]	259	9.1	298	38%	22	24	1.5
7626	Cheese enchilada (Include Old El Paso Cheese Enchiladas with Sauce) [1 frozen meal]	284	10.0	587	40%	24	67	13.8
7627	Cheese enchilada with beans and rice [1 frozen meal]	340	12.0	515	31%	19	71	13.8
7628	Chicken enchilada with salsa, rice, vegetable, and dessert (diet meal) [1 frozen meal]	311	11.0	296	12%	8	61	4.6
7629	Chicken a la king with rice (Include LeMenu and Stouffer's Chicken a la King) [1 frozen meal]	269	9.5	454	46%	20	40	1.3
7630	Chicken and noodles with vegetable, dessert [1 frozen meal]	291	10.3	393	32%	17	50	3.5
7631	Chicken with noodles and cheese sauce (diet meal) (Include Weight Watchers) [1 frozen meal]	234	8.3	257	14%	26	27	1.6
7632	Chicken with noodles and cheese sauce (diet meal) (Include Healthy Choice) [1 frozen meal]	241	8.5	265	14%	27	27	1.6
7633	Chicken and vegetable entree with noodles (diet meal) (Include Lean Cuisine Chicken and Vegetables with Vermicelli) [1 frozen meal]	361	12.7	301	21%	27	33	5.8
7634	Chicken and vegetable entree with noodles (Include Banquet Gourmet Chicken Cacciatore and Vermicelli) [1 frozen meal]	284	10.0	274	19%	19	36	2.9
7635	Chicken and vegetable entree with noodles and cream sauce (Include Budget Gourmet Chicken and Egg Noodles with Broccoli) [1 frozen meal]	284	10.0	349	37%	25	30	2.7
7636	Chicken and vegetable entree with rice, Oriental (diet meal) (Include Benihana Oriental Lites Chicken in Spicy Garlic Sauce with Vegetables and Rice) [1 frozen meal]	255	9.0	483	27%	32	59	5.3
7637	Chicken and vegetable entree with rice, Oriental (Include Green Giant Stir Fry Cashew Chicken, Chun King Crunchy Walnut Chicken, Green Giant Chicken and Pea Pods) [1 frozen meal]	284	10.0	311	24%	19	40	3.6
7638	Chicken and vegetable entree, oriental (diet meal) (Include Weight Watcher's Sweet and Sour Chicken) [1 frozen meal]	255	9.0	206	18%	17	26	3.5
7639	Chicken and vegetables au gratin with rice-vegetable mixture (diet meal) (Include Budget Gourmet Chicken au Gratin) [1 frozen meal]	258	9.1	317	37%	30	19	2.2
7640	Chicken and vegetables in cream or white sauce (diet meal) (Include Weight Watcher's Chicken Ala King) [1 frozen meal]	255	9.0	244	30%	27	15	2.0
7641	Chicken burritos (diet meal) (Include Weight Watchers Chicken Burritos) [1 frozen meal]	284	10.0	516	21%	27	74	5.8
7642	Chicken cacciatore with noodles (diet meal) (Include Lean Cuisine Chicken Cacciatore with Vermicelli) [1 frozen meal]	308	10.9	311	29%	22	33	3.4
7643	Chicken chow mein with rice (diet meal) (Include Lean Cuisine Chicken Chow Mein with Rice) [1 frozen meal]	319	11.3	290	20%	19	38	2.0

Food No.	fat gm	sat fat gm	choles mg	sodium mg	potas mg	vit A	vit E	vit C	thia	ribo	niac	vit B-6	fola	vit B-12	calc	phos	mag	iron	zinc
						% of Daily Value													
7615	6	2	55	1218	303	36	2	11	12	13	18	16	6	31	4	20	9	21	35
7616	5	2	45	334	471	6	2	33	12	14	20	17	7	23	6	24	18	21	34
7617	8	3	57	617	596	15	7	103	15	18	21	26	10	28	8	24	12	19	30
7618	3	1	11	379	523	9	6	138	13	12	8	17	14	6	8	13	13	19	10
7619	26	10	88	1249	823	6	3	32	27	28	36	28	12	36	6	37	16	28	34
7620	24	7	67	816	671	106	9	9	10	14	24	28	5	43	3	26	11	18	27
7621	12	3	75	1294	694	8	5	18	21	19	30	29	12	44	3	31	14	20	31
7622	20	8	86	955	714	35	5	66	12	19	25	30	8	32	10	31	12	19	31
7623	14	4	74	932	774	12	8	86	14	21	27	31	12	38	8	30	14	23	38
7624	22	9	49	881	685	8	7	33	33	26	29	15	34	18	14	35	18	31	24
7625	12	7	42	1221	226	19	6	7	11	17	8	6	5	7	27	26	7	9	11
7626	26	14	61	1752	787	24	19	30	18	22	14	22	39	8	57	59	24	19	20
7627	18	8	32	1967	645	13	8	10	21	16	11	16	28	3	29	41	25	24	18
7628	4	1	9	543	549	17	3	65	28	12	20	13	12	1	4	16	14	18	6
7629	23	8	131	740	307	23	10	6	20	16	32	18	5	7	11	25	9	15	14
7630	14	4	51	1081	439	2	5	1	23	16	25	8	10	4	4	21	14	18	8
7631	4	1	60	250	209	1	2	0	15	10	55	22	2	4	3	21	9	11	8
7632	4	1	62	257	215	1	2	0	15	10	57	22	2	4	3	22	10	12	8
7633	7	2	62	813	673	45	5	63	21	21	38	22	14	3	7	25	15	18	16
7634	6	1	43	710	442	7	5	45	17	14	28	16	5	2	3	16	11	14	12
7635	14	6	100	156	336	18	5	38	7	17	21	14	8	6	16	27	13	9	15
7636	14	3	71	631	694	48	10	19	12	16	68	51	8	5	11	31	20	26	13
7637	8	3	43	727	483	3	4	54	23	15	47	24	7	3	4	22	12	20	11
7638	4	1	45	893	483	57	5	67	8	13	31	22	8	3	6	16	11	11	11
7639	13	7	88	1113	509	40	3	21	11	19	52	29	18	8	28	35	18	16	14
7640	8	2	65	649	437	13	5	53	10	19	30	16	8	6	12	25	9	11	15
7641	12	2	45	4400	739	66	10	45	39	28	39	21	11	2	16	27	15	28	14
7642	10	2	59	934	596	9	5	43	19	23	40	21	8	3	3	22	12	18	18
7643	6	2	47	1069	336	5	2	33	14	11	28	17	7	2	4	16	9	14	12

Mixed Dishes & Fast Foods

Food No.	Food Description & Amount	wt gm	wt oz	cal	% cal fat	prot gm	carbo gm	fiber gm
7644	Chicken cordon bleu with vegetables (diet meal) [1 frozen meal]	227	8.0	224	39%	21	14	3.2
7645	Chicken chow mein with rice, reduced fat and sodium (diet meal) (Include Healthy Choice) [1 frozen meal]	241	8.5	231	20%	15	30	2.7
7646	Chicken cordon bleu with vegetable, rice (Include LeMenu Chicken Cordon Bleu) [1 frozen meal]	312	11.0	495	26%	32	59	4.1
7647	Chicken divan (Include Stouffer's Chicken Divan) [1 frozen meal]	241	8.5	353	57%	22	14	1.1
7648	Chicken enchilada (diet meal) (Include Weight Watchers Chicken Enchilada) [1 frozen meal]	241	8.5	355	39%	27	29	2.5
7649	Chicken fajitas (diet meal) [1 frozen meal]	191	6.7	234	19%	17	30	2.8
7650	Chicken in butter sauce with potatoes and vegetable (diet meal) (Include Le Menu Lite Style Herb Roasted Chicken) [1 frozen meal]	262	9.2	312	19%	49	12	2.3
7651	Chicken in cheese sauce with Spanish rice (Include Top Shelf Breast of Chicken Acapulco) [1 frozen meal]	284	10.0	386	24%	34	36	0.8
7652	Chicken in cream sauce with noodles and vegetable (Include Budget Gourmet Chicken Fricassee Dinner) [1 frozen meal]	340	12.0	437	29%	31	44	3.2
7653	Chicken in cream sauce, with brown and wild rice, vegetable, and fruit dessert (diet meal) (Include Healthy Choice) [1 frozen meal]	312	11.0	310	25%	22	37	5.0
7654	Chicken in mushroom sauce, white and wild rice, vegetable (Include Armour Dinner Classics Chicken with Wine and Mushroom Sauce) [1 frozen meal]	305	10.8	369	41%	24	29	3.3
7655	Chicken in orange sauce with almond rice (diet meal) (Include Lean Cuisine Chicken a l'Orange) [1 frozen meal]	227	8.0	302	15%	26	37	1.1
7656	Chicken kiev with rice-vegetable mixture (Include Le Menu Chicken Kiev with Rice, Vegetable, and Fruit Medley) [1 frozen meal]	227	8.0	504	54%	26	31	2.1
7657	Chicken patty parmigiana, breaded, with vegetable (diet meal) (Include Weight Watcher's Breaded Chicken Patty Parmigiana with Vegetable Medley) [1 frozen meal]	226	8.0	301	50%	23	15	2.7
7658	Chicken patty with vegetable (diet meal) (Include Weight Watchers Southern Fried Chicken Patty with Vegetable Medley) [1 frozen meal]	184	6.5	255	51%	21	10	2.0
7659	Chicken patty, breaded, with tomato sauce and cheese, fettuccine alfredo, vegetable (Include Le Menu Breast of Chicken Parmigiana) [1 frozen meal]	326	11.5	396	41%	31	28	3.9
7660	Chicken patty or nuggets, boneless, breaded, potatoes, vegetable (Include Banquet Favorite Boneless Chicken Pattie Platter) [1 frozen meal]	213	7.5	443	36%	26	46	3.8
7661	Chicken patty or nuggets, boneless, breaded, with pasta and tomato sauce, fruit, dessert [1 frozen meal]	193	6.8	327	33%	10	45	2.5
7662	Chicken teriyaki with rice, vegetable (Include Budget Gourmet Sweet and Sour Chicken with Rice) [1 frozen meal]	284	10.0	365	35%	24	34	3.3
7663	Chicken in soy-based sauce, rice and vegetables [1 frozen meal]	255	9.0	277	7%	17	46	2.6
7664	Chicken with barbeque sauce, beans, vegetable, dessert (Include Swanson Chicken in Barbecue Sauce) [1 frozen meal]	333	11.7	509	31%	28	61	6.8
7665	Chicken in barbecue sauce, with rice, vegetable and dessert, reduced fat and sodium (diet meal) (Include Healthy Choice) [1 frozen meal]	298	10.5	329	13%	21	52	3.3
7666	Chicken with rice-vegetable mixture (diet meal) (Include Lean Cuisine Glazed Chicken with Vegetable Rice) [1 frozen meal]	241	8.5	272	26%	25	25	2.0
7667	Chicken with rice and vegetable, reduced fat and sodium (diet meal) (Include Weight Watchers meal, Healthy Choice) [1 frozen meal]	241	8.5	242	18%	20	29	2.7
7668	Chicken, boneless, with gravy, dressing, rice, vegetable, dessert (large meat portion) (Include Swanson Hungry Man Boneless Chicken Dinner) [1 frozen meal]	503	17.7	878	30%	47	105	7.4
7669	Chicken, boneless, with gravy, potatoes, vegetable, dessert (large meat portion) [1 frozen meal]	539	19.0	709	43%	44	56	6.2
7670	Chicken, fried in honey sauce, with Oriental style rice and vegetables, in soy-based sauce (Include Tyson Chicken Peking) [1 frozen meal]	276	9.7	397	30%	30	38	2.2
7671	Chicken, fried, with potatoes (Include Swanson Fried Chicken Entree) [1 frozen meal]	227	8.0	470	52%	25	31	2.7
7672	Chicken, fried, with potatoes (frozen meal, large meat portion) (Include Swanson Hungry Man Fried Chicken) [1 frozen meal]	361	12.7	720	49%	37	54	4.3

Food No.	fat gm	sat fat gm	choles mg	sodium mg	potas mg	% of Daily Value													
						vit A	vit E	vit C	thia	ribo	niac	vit B-6	fola	vit B-12	calc	phos	mag	iron	zinc
7644	10	5	54	804	357	71	6	23	7	14	25	16	8	7	30	36	10	8	12
7645	5	1	37	622	397	6	3	36	11	9	26	19	7	2	5	15	8	11	10
7646	14	5	69	1280	452	110	6	20	32	27	48	26	8	7	31	36	17	24	21
7647	22	9	86	678	404	22	5	38	9	25	23	13	9	12	27	30	10	9	14
7648	15	9	75	1018	413	17	3	153	7	17	23	20	6	6	37	41	14	9	15
7649	5	1	36	585	320	25	5	118	18	14	29	21	7	2	4	17	7	15	9
7650	6	2	132	245	574	4	2	18	15	14	109	51	6	9	5	38	16	12	12
7651	10	5	93	1245	319	10	3	34	17	12	51	25	3	6	11	31	11	14	13
7652	14	6	114	1395	360	27	4	6	12	14	37	18	7	6	13	30	14	13	15
7653	9	4	62	397	367	16	4	10	15	12	45	24	8	4	8	26	16	10	12
7654	17	10	99	977	464	119	7	97	17	12	52	31	10	4	7	25	13	12	10
7655	5	1	61	676	289	23	2	13	5	8	34	19	4	3	4	18	10	7	10
7656	30	12	104	697	299	40	6	13	16	15	41	17	4	5	6	21	11	12	8
7657	17	6	57	937	355	24	8	78	9	17	18	12	9	6	27	27	9	10	15
7658	14	3	54	979	230	39	8	26	7	12	31	19	6	4	5	14	5	11	10
7659	18	7	110	894	494	22	8	25	16	18	60	29	10	6	14	31	18	16	12
7660	18	5	58	818	735	5	5	9	16	10	60	34	11	5	3	29	14	11	9
7661	12	3	35	716	317	3	8	7	12	10	22	10	3	2	3	14	8	13	6
7662	14	4	69	1976	417	180	4	5	14	13	42	29	5	4	5	22	13	16	15
7663	2	1	40	902	315	4	1	13	10	11	42	20	5	2	4	17	9	12	8
7664	18	5	75	904	592	7	11	19	16	16	28	16	19	3	5	25	16	18	20
7665	5	1	48	459	447	13	3	9	17	9	47	23	7	3	4	22	13	12	8
7666	8	2	62	812	345	2	3	6	6	11	52	27	5	4	4	22	9	9	10
7667	5	1	47	392	276	3	2	3	10	11	35	18	6	3	4	20	14	11	16
7668	29	8	113	1663	723	9	8	19	52	37	85	43	28	6	12	45	25	37	29
7669	34	10	122	2032	795	23	16	27	36	31	78	32	14	9	10	41	19	25	24
7670	13	2	70	645	406	32	12	51	18	10	67	34	7	4	4	27	13	15	11
7671	27	8	76	1247	388	11	16	11	20	17	39	16	4	5	7	23	11	13	13
7672	39	12	135	2261	595	15	18	18	32	28	58	23	7	9	12	35	17	20	20

Mixed Dishes & Fast Foods

Food No.	Food Description & Amount	wt gm	wt oz	cal	% cal fat	prot gm	carbo gm	fiber gm
7673	Chicken, fried, with potatoes, vegetable (Include Banquet Fried Chicken Dinner) [1 frozen meal]	312	11.0	543	48%	33	38	5.9
7674	Chicken, fried, with potatoes, vegetable, cornbread, dessert [1 frozen meal]	425	15.0	665	37%	27	81	9.1
7675	Chicken, fried, with potatoes, vegetable, dessert (Include Morton Chicken Patty Dinner, Morton and Swanson Fried Chicken Dinner) [1 frozen meal]	326	11.5	585	45%	33	48	5.8
7676	Chicken, fried, with potatoes, vegetable, dessert (large meat portion) (Include Swanson Hungry Man Fried Chicken Dinner) [1 frozen meal]	432	15.2	948	45%	49	84	7.1
7677	Chicken, fried, with potatoes, vegetable, vegetable soup, dessert [1 frozen meal]	425	15.0	704	40%	38	69	5.4
7678	Cod in cheese sauce with vegetable (diet meal) (Include Weight Watcher's Fillet of Fish Au Gratin) [1 frozen meal]	262	9.2	283	29%	31	19	2.8
7679	Cod with vegetable (diet meal) (Include Weight Watcher's Oven Fried Fish) [1 frozen meal]	191	6.7	230	49%	20	9	2.9
7680	Corned beef hash with apple slices, vegetable [1 frozen meal]	284	10.0	406	39%	20	44	5.1
7681	Fish and chips (Include Swanson Fish and Chips) [1 frozen meal]	156	5.5	310	41%	13	33	3.3
7682	Fish and chips (large portion) [1 frozen meal]	447	15.8	908	41%	38	97	9.5
7683	Fish and chips with vegetable, potatoes, tomatoes [1 frozen meal]	291	10.3	463	41%	30	40	3.8
7684	Fish, breaded, or fish sticks, with pasta, vegetable and dessert [1 frozen meal]	208	7.3	371	35%	10	51	2.1
7685	Fish in lemon-butter sauce with rice, vegetable [1 frozen meal]	284	10.0	298	33%	17	32	3.8
7686	Fish parmesan [1 frozen meal]	284	10.0	528	41%	44	31	2.4
7687	Fish, batter-dipped or fish cake, with vegetable, potatoes (Include Taste-O-Sea Haddock Dinner) [1 frozen meal]	255	9.0	450	44%	28	35	5.2
7688	Fish, batter-dipped, or fish cake, with vegetable, potatoes, dessert (Include Swanson Fish and Chips) [1 frozen meal]	298	10.5	580	44%	25	57	6.9
7689	Flounder in cream sauce with potatoes, carrots (diet meal) (Include Le Menu Light Style Flounder Vin Blanc) [1 frozen meal]	298	10.5	286	19%	25	30	3.1
7690	Flounder with chopped broccoli (diet meal) (Include Lean Cuisine Filet of Fish Divan) [1 frozen meal]	351	12.4	239	19%	32	17	2.6
7691	Grilled cheese sandwich with potato, vegetable, and dessert [1 frozen meal]	184	6.5	290	40%	8	38	3.2
7692	Haddock with chopped spinach (diet meal) (Include Lean Cuisine Filet of Fish Florentine) [1 frozen meal]	255	9.0	211	29%	26	11	0.9
7693	Shrimp and noodles in tomato-based sauce, with vegetable and fruit dessert (diet meal) (Include Healthy Choice) [1 frozen meal]	298	10.5	232	8%	11	43	3.1
7694	Ham, glazed, with sweetpotatoes, vegetable (Include LeMenu Ham Steak Dinner) [1 frozen meal]	284	10.0	319	26%	16	44	3.5
7695	Lasagna with cheese and meat sauce (diet meal) (Include Weight Watcher's Lasagna with meat, tomato sauce, and cheese, Budget Gourmet Lasagna with Meat Sauce) [1 frozen meal]	340	12.0	389	33%	24	41	3.5
7696	Lasagna with cheese and meat sauce, reduced fat and sodium (diet meal) (Include Healthy Choice) [1 frozen meal]	255	9.0	247	16%	16	37	2.5
7697	Lasagna with cheese and sauce (diet meal) (Include Weight Watcher's Italian Cheese Lasagna) [1 frozen meal]	340	12.0	447	33%	19	58	4.5
7698	Lasagna with cheese, tomato sauce, vegetable, dessert [1 frozen meal]	369	13.0	460	30%	20	63	5.2
7699	Linguini with clam sauce (diet meal) (Include Lean Cuisine Linguini with Clam Sauce) [1 frozen meal]	273	9.6	476	29%	22	62	4.8
7700	Linguini with vegetables and seafood in white wine sauce (diet meal) (Include Budget Gourmet Linguini with Scallops and Clams) [1 frozen meal]	269	9.5	298	32%	22	29	2.9
7701	Livers, chicken, with vegetable (diet meal) [1 frozen meal]	298	10.5	203	26%	29	11	6.0
7702	Macaroni or noodles, spinach, with chicken and cheese sauce (diet meal) (Include Ultra Slim Fast Chicken Fettucini) [1 frozen meal]	340	12.0	398	26%	33	38	3.3
7703	Macaroni and beef in tomato-based sauce, vegetable, and dessert (Include Swanson's Macaroni and Beef Dinner) [1 frozen meal]	340	12.0	378	29%	15	53	4.1
7704	Macaroni and cheese (diet meal) [1 frozen meal]	255	9.0	313	28%	15	40	1.6
7705	Macaroni and cheese with apples, vegetable (Include Swanson Macaroni and Cheese Dinner) [1 frozen meal]	347	12.2	421	35%	14	55	5.5
7706	Macaroni with veal, cheese, and sauce (diet meal) [1 frozen meal]	369	13.0	364	24%	27	42	3.5

Food No.	fat gm	sat fat gm	choles mg	sodium mg	potas mg	% of Daily Value													
						vit A	vit E	vit C	thia	ribo	niac	vit B-6	fola	vit B-12	calc	phos	mag	iron	zinc
7673	29	10	128	1571	621	32	12	23	22	22	52	23	8	8	10	30	16	14	18
7674	28	10	103	1133	743	77	14	36	40	27	42	20	12	7	18	42	17	19	15
7675	29	10	124	1523	605	32	12	21	22	23	51	23	8	7	12	30	15	15	18
7676	47	11	183	1480	959	11	18	19	34	31	81	45	15	11	8	48	23	25	27
7677	31	10	137	1183	677	55	12	21	32	27	63	27	9	8	10	34	17	20	19
7678	9	3	68	669	590	19	11	97	15	19	20	21	14	19	21	30	19	12	11
7679	13	2	44	498	570	61	19	39	9	8	13	17	10	14	6	25	12	6	5
7680	18	7	61	2360	413	4	2	22	13	11	14	15	12	18	5	16	10	13	19
7681	14	2	23	620	529	1	12	11	12	6	15	17	3	8	2	20	10	9	5
7682	42	6	66	2180	1446	4	26	29	34	18	41	47	10	22	7	57	30	25	14
7683	21	5	109	214	888	5	14	26	17	22	34	30	9	59	11	40	28	13	8
7684	14	3	42	445	235	4	9	9	12	13	13	4	6	11	4	13	8	11	5
7685	11	4	39	1221	484	8	13	17	21	9	18	18	11	9	4	24	14	12	9
7686	24	8	222	922	972	18	18	13	21	42	42	28	8	76	41	61	34	21	16
7687	22	6	91	1965	819	6	14	21	27	17	26	21	14	40	8	46	22	15	11
7688	29	5	42	956	821	6	31	21	22	10	23	25	13	13	4	34	18	14	10
7689	6	2	59	133	710	85	14	24	14	13	23	21	6	26	8	28	14	8	7
7690	5	2	68	585	918	23	18	109	15	24	22	20	15	34	27	43	19	9	10
7691	13	4	12	521	314	11	6	10	12	13	12	8	5	2	14	16	7	9	7
7692	7	3	73	507	636	29	4	5	8	16	22	21	13	24	26	36	21	14	9
7693	2	1	75	222	416	22	4	117	10	7	11	13	5	10	4	12	10	15	7
7694	9	2	36	1587	521	116	11	78	41	15	18	25	7	7	5	19	10	11	16
7695	14	7	55	840	759	24	16	21	19	23	25	16	7	15	26	31	16	21	25
7696	4	2	13	466	484	9	3	47	15	15	12	13	8	7	14	22	10	11	9
7697	16	6	28	788	675	23	20	27	21	19	21	15	7	3	35	34	17	20	14
7698	15	8	63	1099	566	21	7	28	15	24	11	11	10	8	44	38	17	15	16
7699	15	6	51	3406	765	34	9	41	29	26	22	22	12	810	17	31	15	119	18
7700	11	6	66	734	569	24	7	45	18	20	15	9	9	540	15	33	13	63	18
7701	6	2	582	101	730	482	22	280	17	109	26	41	203	298	11	41	17	53	32
7702	12	5	127	790	298	7	3	0	26	19	64	31	8	9	11	31	16	13	13
7703	12	4	28	743	518	5	6	15	19	17	25	13	8	13	8	19	14	17	17
7704	10	6	29	640	176	12	1	0	15	18	10	3	3	3	29	27	9	11	12
7705	16	8	33	1308	279	90	6	9	19	17	12	11	9	3	27	27	11	12	13
7706	10	5	66	608	700	19	12	36	23	26	34	21	7	15	28	37	17	17	25

Mixed Dishes & Fast Foods

Food No.	Food Description & Amount	wt gm	wt oz	cal	% cal fat	prot gm	carbo gm	fiber gm
7707	Manicotti, cheese-filled, with tomato sauce (diet meal) (Include Weight Watcher's Cheese Manicotti) [1 frozen meal]	262	9.2	317	40%	20	29	1.8
7708	Meat loaf in tomato sauce with potatoes, vegetable [1 frozen meal]	312	11.0	372	42%	20	34	3.8
7709	Meat loaf with tomato sauce, vegetable, applesauce [1 frozen meal]	312	11.0	374	40%	18	39	3.6
7710	Meat loaf with tomato sauce, vegetable, potatoes, dessert (Include Swanson and Morton Meat Loaf Dinner) [1 frozen meal]	312	11.0	480	39%	19	57	5.7
7711	Meatballs, Swedish, in sauce, with noodles (Include Budget Gourmet Swedish Meatballs with noodles) [1 frozen meal]	284	10.0	502	50%	25	36	1.5
7712	Meatballs, Swedish, in gravy, with noodles (diet meal) [1 frozen meal]	258	9.1	303	29%	25	28	2.3
7713	Meatballs, Swedish, in sauce, with noodles and vegetable medley [1 frozen meal]	241	8.5	285	24%	18	33	1.7
7714	Mexican dinner with fried beans [1 frozen meal]	510	18.0	775	44%	28	81	9.7
7715	Mosticolli with meatballs, sauce, bread [1 frozen meal]	312	11.0	433	37%	23	44	2.7
7716	Noodles and chicken with gravy, vegetable, dessert (Include Swanson's Noodles and Chicken Dinner) [1 frozen meal]	298	10.5	316	30%	15	40	4.5
7717	Noodles with vegetables in tomato-based sauce (diet meal) [1 frozen meal]	284	10.0	186	21%	10	29	4.3
7718	Pasta, spinach, with vegetables, cheese sauce (diet meal) (Include Ultra Slim Fast Pasta Primavera) [1 frozen meal]	340	12.0	348	23%	13	55	7.2
7719	Pasta with vegetable, cheese sauce (diet meal) (Include Weight Watchers) [1 frozen meal]	227	8.0	306	21%	15	45	2.3
7720	Pork with rice, vegetable, in soy-based sauce (diet meal) (Include Benihana Oriental Lites Roast Pork and Mushrooms) [1 frozen meal]	255	9.0	261	24%	15	34	2.3
7721	Pork, sliced, with gravy, mashed potatoes, vegetable, dessert (Include Swanson Loin of Pork Dinner) [1 frozen meal]	319	11.3	458	40%	27	42	4.0
7722	Pork, sliced, with sweetpotatoes, vegetable, dessert [1 frozen meal]	319	11.3	407	24%	22	55	5.1
7723	Ravioli, cheese-filled, with tomato sauce (diet meal) (Include Weight Watcher's Baked Cheese Ravioli) [1 frozen meal]	229	8.1	251	33%	15	27	2.2
7724	Ravioli, cheese-filled, with vegetable, fruit [1 frozen meal]	248	8.7	264	27%	7	44	3.6
7725	Rice, with broccoli, cheese sauce (frozen side dish) (Include Green Giant) [1 frozen meal]	128	4.5	190	40%	7	22	1.4
7726	Rice, with green beans, water chestnuts, in sherry mushroom sauce (frozen side dish) (Include Green Giant Microwave Garden Gourmet) [1 cup]	179	6.3	172	30%	5	26	2.3
7727	Rigatoni with meat sauce and cheese (diet meal) [1 frozen meal]	276	9.7	256	36%	18	25	3.1
7728	Salisbury steak with gravy, macaroni and cheese (Include Swanson Salisbury Steak in Gravy with Macaroni and Cheese) [1 frozen meal]	284	10.0	567	37%	31	56	2.4
7729	Salisbury steak with gravy, macaroni and cheese, vegetable (Include Budget Gourmet Sirloin Salisbury Steak Dinner) [1 frozen meal]	326	11.5	490	50%	31	31	3.1
7730	Salisbury steak with gravy, potatoes, vegetable (Include Armour Dinner Classics Salisbury Steak) [1 frozen meal]	312	11.0	469	52%	21	36	4.3
7731	Salisbury steak with gravy, potatoes, vegetable, dessert (large meat portion) (Include Swanson Hungry Man Salisbury Steak Dinner) [1 frozen meal]	468	16.5	880	43%	56	68	7.5
7732	Salisbury steak with gravy, potatoes, vegetable, soup or macaroni and cheese, dessert [1 frozen meal]	439	15.5	518	40%	31	48	6.2
7733	Salisbury steak with gravy, whipped potatoes, vegetable, dessert (Include Swanson Salisbury Steak Dinner, Morton Salisbury Steak Dinner) [1 frozen meal]	312	11.0	470	45%	23	43	3.4
7734	Salisbury steak with vegetables in tomato-based sauce, noodles (diet meal) (Include Weight Watcher's Beef Salisbury Steak Romana) [1 frozen meal]	248	8.7	323	30%	26	30	2.6
7735	Salisbury steak, baked, with tomato sauce, vegetable (diet meal) (Include Lean Cuisine Salisbury Steak) [1 frozen meal]	269	9.5	293	48%	24	14	2.5
7736	Salisbury steak, potatoes, vegetable, dessert (diet meal) (Include Healthy Choice Salisbury Steak Dinner) [1 frozen meal]	326	11.5	313	27%	17	42	4.3
7737	Sausage and french toast (Include Swanson French Toast and Sausage) [1 frozen meal]	184	6.5	432	47%	22	34	1.2
7738	Sausage and pancakes (Include Swanson Pancakes and Sausage) [1 frozen meal]	170	6.0	477	47%	15	47	1.1
7739	Sausage rice links and whole wheat pancakes [1 frozen meal]	156	5.5	367	53%	16	28	3.4
7740	Scallops with potatoes, vegetable [1 frozen meal]	227	8.0	402	38%	25	37	5.2

Food No.	fat gm	sat fat gm	choles mg	sodium mg	potas mg	vit A	vit E	vit C	thia	ribo	niac	vit B-6	fola	vit B-12	calc	phos	mag	iron	zinc
						% of Daily Value													
7707	14	7	47	809	394	20	6	36	13	20	9	8	7	8	42	35	10	10	15
7708	17	7	60	1112	729	12	10	30	20	20	30	15	9	31	15	24	14	21	25
7709	16	6	50	941	604	40	8	20	15	14	30	19	9	28	5	20	11	16	24
7710	21	6	79	1532	920	18	10	37	19	22	30	21	12	20	8	24	16	24	22
7711	28	12	113	838	433	8	2	2	22	27	32	18	5	35	12	27	12	22	32
7712	10	3	42	672	382	1	2	4	15	22	28	11	8	20	6	25	9	21	24
7713	8	3	35	683	618	89	2	3	14	32	17	15	6	21	31	33	12	9	18
7714	38	11	49	2030	695	9	22	13	28	21	22	19	39	15	22	41	21	32	28
7715	18	7	63	2168	576	8	8	23	21	21	37	16	6	32	7	21	12	24	29
7716	10	2	40	941	253	4	7	8	23	13	25	9	9	3	3	16	9	16	10
7717	4	2	8	409	713	13	8	30	9	17	21	13	8	2	18	22	13	14	9
7718	9	4	69	500	450	92	5	26	32	26	22	21	17	7	15	23	16	16	13
7719	7	3	67	557	133	7	2	16	21	14	13	5	5	5	25	26	11	16	11
7720	7	2	33	1056	432	3	4	43	28	16	23	21	5	13	3	19	9	11	29
7721	20	7	76	971	658	101	10	16	65	23	32	26	5	12	9	28	12	10	16
7722	11	4	65	1253	568	166	4	31	42	24	24	26	13	8	5	26	12	12	17
7723	9	5	29	934	424	18	10	18	12	16	11	8	5	3	31	27	10	11	11
7724	8	3	74	552	397	13	3	28	12	15	9	9	6	4	7	13	8	10	5
7725	8	4	15	545	154	11	6	57	9	6	6	7	6	1	12	12	5	7	6
7726	6	2	4	386	292	5	4	8	11	11	10	7	5	2	8	11	6	10	5
7727	10	4	40	835	608	17	8	42	14	14	22	15	7	16	14	23	12	15	20
7728	23	9	70	1010	393	17	6	2	31	29	31	13	6	23	36	39	14	33	29
7729	27	11	94	887	623	21	9	43	17	32	30	14	13	29	22	36	14	23	39
7730	27	13	131	871	617	17	3	31	17	15	29	24	14	33	4	23	13	15	28
7731	42	15	146	1623	1445	49	5	19	47	51	55	52	27	82	12	57	37	53	65
7732	23	10	101	1702	838	6	7	28	27	23	43	18	13	43	12	34	19	25	35
7733	24	9	80	1853	596	3	5	14	24	22	34	11	10	31	8	24	15	20	26
7734	11	4	74	1088	505	11	9	15	7	16	18	17	6	22	14	31	13	17	27
7735	16	6	77	727	704	11	5	35	11	23	28	19	9	27	13	26	13	17	32
7736	9	4	51	446	557	4	2	17	9	15	22	19	7	22	4	16	11	13	25
7737	23	7	251	1068	373	8	4	2	41	36	21	13	9	26	15	26	8	16	15
7738	25	7	90	1197	294	13	9	2	39	25	20	9	4	17	9	19	6	14	11
7739	22	6	100	713	354	5	9	2	36	19	18	13	5	19	19	27	14	12	15
7740	17	4	62	624	719	7	14	23	21	13	20	20	15	25	8	37	24	15	13

Mixed Dishes & Fast Foods

Food No.	Food Description & Amount	wt gm	wt oz	cal	% cal fat	prot gm	carbo gm	fiber gm
7741	Scrambled eggs, sausage, hash brown potatoes (Include Swanson Scrambled Eggs and Sausage with Hash Brown Potatoes) [1 frozen meal]	177	6.2	419	68%	16	19	1.1
7742	Scrambled eggs, bacon, home fried potatoes [1 frozen meal]	149	5.3	352	64%	16	16	1.0
7743	Scrambled eggs, sausage, pancakes [1 frozen meal]	147	5.2	311	50%	14	24	0.9
7744	Seafood newburg with rice, vegetable (Include Dinner Classics Seafood Newburg) [1 frozen meal]	298	10.5	288	30%	14	35	2.9
7745	Seafood platter with fish cake, fish fillet, scallops, shrimp, potatoes (Include Taste-O-Sea Seafood Platter) [1 frozen meal]	255	9.0	523	44%	27	49	3.8
7746	Shrimp and clams in tomato-based sauce, with noodles (Include Budget Gourmet Linguini with Shrimp and Clams Marinara) [1 frozen meal]	284	10.0	292	22%	23	34	3.6
7747	Shrimp and vegetables in sauce with noodles (diet meal) (Include Mrs. Paul's Shrimp Primavera with Fettucini Pasta) [1 frozen meal]	312	11.0	282	17%	17	40	4.5
7748	Shrimp chow mein with egg rolls, pepper oriental [1 frozen meal]	369	13.0	443	24%	15	68	3.2
7749	Shrimp creole with rice, peppers (diet meal) (Include Light and Elegant Shrimp Creole with Rice and Peppers) [1 frozen meal]	284	10.0	250	9%	10	47	2.2
7750	Shrimp with potatoes, vegetable (Include Taste-O-Sea Shrimp Dinner) [1 frozen meal]	198	7.0	367	40%	23	32	3.5
7751	Shrimp with rice, vegetable (Include Benihana Oriental Shrimp and Vegetables in Sauce with Rice) [1 frozen meal]	312	11.0	288	12%	13	50	4.1
7752	Sirloin beef with gravy, potatoes, vegetable (Include Armour Dinner Classics Sirloin Roast) [1 frozen meal]	312	11.0	279	32%	27	21	3.7
7753	Sirloin enchilada with tomatoes, zucchini and chilies (diet entree) (Include Budget Gourmet Slim Select Sirloin Enchilada Ranchero) [1 frozen entree]	248	8.7	275	33%	17	30	3.0
7754	Sirloin tips with gravy, potatoes, vegetable (Include Budget Gourmet Sirloin Tips with Country Style Vegetables) [1 frozen meal]	284	10.0	334	47%	23	22	3.4
7755	Sirloin tips and mushrooms in wine sauce with rotini (diet entree) [1 frozen entree]	213	7.5	247	31%	20	22	2.0
7756	Sirloin tips, potato, vegetable, fruit (diet meal) (Include Healthy Choice Sirloin Tips Dinner) [1 frozen meal]	333	11.7	289	18%	25	34	3.2
7757	Sirloin, chopped, or swiss steak with gravy, vegetable, potatoes, dessert or muffin (Include Swanson Chopped Sirloin Beef Dinner) [1 frozen meal]	326	11.5	432	38%	23	44	5.6
7758	Sirloin, chopped, with gravy, mashed potatoes, vegetable (Include LeMenu Chopped Sirloin Beef) [1 frozen meal]	347	12.2	551	47%	27	47	5.8
7759	Sole with vegetable (diet meal) [1 frozen meal]	241	8.5	218	12%	34	14	3.7
7760	Spaghetti and meatballs dinner [1 frozen meal]	354	12.5	364	24%	16	53	4.8
7761	Spaghetti and meatballs with tomato sauce, sliced apples, bread (Include Morton Spaghetti and Meatballs Dinner) [1 frozen meal]	326	11.5	446	29%	25	55	4.9
7762	Spaghetti and meatballs with vegetable, dessert [1 frozen meal]	354	12.5	366	23%	15	56	5.4
7763	Spaghetti with meat and mushroom sauce (diet meal) (Include Lean Cuisine Spaghetti with Beef and Mushroom Sauce) [1 frozen meal]	326	11.5	364	23%	19	52	4.8
7764	Spaghetti with meat sauce (diet meal) (Include Weight Watcher's Spaghetti with meat sauce) [1 frozen meal]	298	10.5	335	24%	17	47	4.5
7765	Stuffed cabbage, with meat and tomato sauce (diet meal) (Include Lean Cuisine Stuffed Cabbage) [1 frozen meal]	305	10.8	247	39%	16	22	3.1
7766	Stuffed green pepper (diet meal) (Include Weight Watcher's Stuffed Pepper with Veal and Tomato Sauce) [1 frozen meal]	333	11.7	292	26%	23	31	3.3
7767	Stuffed green pepper (Include Green Giant Stuffed Green Pepper) [1 frozen meal]	397	14.0	410	47%	18	39	5.0
7768	Tuna lasagna (diet meal) (Include Lean Cuisine Tuna Lasagna with Spinach Noodles and Vegetables) [1 frozen meal]	276	9.7	275	25%	19	32	3.7
7769	Turbot with vegetable (diet meal) [1 frozen meal]	241	8.5	330	53%	21	19	3.3
7770	Turkey and vegetables, in sauce (diet meal) (Include Lean Cuisine Turkey Dijon) [1 frozen meal]	269	9.5	263	36%	22	18	2.7
7771	Turkey breast with gravy, long-grain and wild rice, vegetable (Include LeMenu Sliced Turkey Breast Dinner) [1 frozen meal]	319	11.3	449	47%	27	31	3.2
7772	Turkey tetrazzini (Include Stouffer's Turkey Tetrazzini) [1 frozen meal]	340	12.0	526	50%	25	38	2.8
7773	Turkey with dressing, gravy, potato (Include Swanson Turkey Entree) [1 frozen meal]	248	8.7	272	44%	15	22	1.9

Food No.	fat gm	sat fat gm	choles mg	sodium mg	potas mg	% of Daily Value													
						vit A	vit E	vit C	thia	ribo	niac	vit B-6	fola	vit B-12	calc	phos	mag	iron	zinc
7741	32	9	257	843	463	10	11	7	24	23	15	13	6	18	6	22	6	11	11
7742	25	9	292	662	425	15	6	5	15	24	14	10	7	15	7	23	6	11	10
7743	17	5	303	607	178	17	7	1	18	36	13	6	7	12	9	34	5	16	10
7744	10	5	80	964	330	12	4	7	6	11	14	11	6	19	8	19	14	11	9
7745	25	7	96	880	809	4	10	14	20	15	27	28	6	18	7	32	19	15	10
7746	7	3	87	635	789	22	7	78	22	23	26	15	12	661	9	31	15	81	15
7747	5	2	80	1105	329	85	6	40	16	11	20	10	8	9	6	20	12	18	9
7748	12	3	49	591	456	36	11	72	25	14	24	18	9	11	5	18	11	21	14
7749	3	0	39	826	391	8	7	84	18	6	18	17	5	4	4	14	10	16	8
7750	16	4	182	513	479	45	12	17	19	11	22	15	7	16	8	28	14	23	11
7751	4	1	52	1219	489	14	6	122	20	12	24	15	10	7	6	19	11	20	10
7752	10	4	75	977	774	109	5	65	13	19	24	32	10	35	5	26	13	21	39
7753	10	4	40	599	512	12	7	44	16	16	19	17	7	18	14	24	13	17	20
7754	17	7	68	754	780	23	3	38	16	17	23	29	9	37	3	24	13	20	28
7755	8	2	45	897	317	0	4	2	14	12	19	16	5	23	2	20	9	17	27
7756	6	2	67	475	590	68	2	9	11	16	23	26	5	37	3	23	10	17	34
7757	18	6	67	800	682	85	5	30	24	21	25	26	13	30	5	26	14	23	34
7758	29	14	141	1982	812	16	4	38	29	23	29	33	18	40	5	33	18	23	33
7759	3	1	76	1779	776	2	14	60	18	14	29	22	15	38	8	34	17	10	7
7760	10	3	25	1050	604	18	5	58	29	19	26	15	11	14	7	21	15	20	17
7761	14	5	55	2202	492	0	1	2	22	17	30	16	11	30	5	23	14	23	27
7762	9	3	22	1012	589	20	5	53	27	19	23	15	12	11	9	22	15	18	16
7763	9	3	36	1348	718	10	7	46	26	25	34	18	9	15	5	22	15	23	23
7764	9	3	31	1041	681	14	14	23	23	19	31	16	7	12	5	19	14	23	20
7765	11	4	49	691	553	33	5	44	16	14	20	18	8	21	5	16	10	12	21
7766	9	4	78	1605	847	26	14	184	16	24	51	32	10	18	4	26	14	17	22
7767	21	6	49	1217	811	25	10	113	14	14	27	29	11	27	15	20	16	41	25
7768	8	3	19	935	439	76	7	30	16	19	28	14	17	17	31	27	18	14	12
7769	19	4	53	1201	488	77	7	13	25	12	18	27	7	16	5	25	13	13	7
7770	10	3	55	877	476	71	5	8	11	18	22	19	7	6	15	24	12	12	17
7771	23	5	53	1218	496	74	17	58	17	12	37	32	10	6	5	25	12	15	15
7772	29	9	86	1013	490	9	7	6	22	24	29	17	7	6	16	28	13	19	18
7773	13	5	40	1449	401	7	7	11	10	10	26	9	3	16	5	21	7	8	11

Mixed Dishes & Fast Foods

Food No.	Food Description & Amount	wt gm	wt oz	cal	% cal fat	prot gm	carbo gm	fiber gm
7774	Turkey with dressing, gravy, potato (large meat portion) (Include Swanson Turkey Entree) [1 frozen meal]	376	13.3	415	39%	31	31	3.2
7775	Turkey with dressing, gravy, vegetable and fruit (diet meal) (Include Healthy Choice Breast of Turkey Dinner) [1 frozen meal]	298	10.5	291	17%	21	40	5.9
7776	Turkey with gravy, dressing, potatoes, vegetable (Include Banquet Turkey Dinner) [1 frozen meal]	312	11.0	498	40%	30	44	4.5
7777	Turkey with gravy, dressing, potatoes, vegetable, cream of tomato soup, dessert [1 frozen meal]	454	16.0	788	38%	45	76	4.4
7778	Turkey with gravy, dressing, potatoes, vegetable, dessert (Include Swanson and Morton Turkey Dinner) [1 frozen meal]	326	11.5	331	35%	26	27	4.8
7779	Turkey with gravy, dressing, potatoes, vegetable, dessert (large meat portion) (Include Swanson Hungry Man Turkey Dinner) [1 frozen meal]	524	18.5	565	29%	34	68	8.4
7780	Turkey with vegetable, stuffing (diet meal) (Include Weight Watcher's Sliced Breast of Turkey) [1 frozen meal]	454	16.0	424	14%	43	48	6.7
7781	Veal lasagna (diet meal) (Include Lean Cuisine Veal Lasagna) [1 frozen meal]	291	10.3	271	24%	22	30	3.8
7782	Veal parmigiana with potatoes, vegetable [1 frozen meal]	312	11.0	440	31%	35	40	5.3
7783	Veal parmigiana with vegetable (diet meal) (Include Weight Watcher's Veal Patty Parmigiana with Zucchini) [1 frozen meal]	255	9.0	190	41%	20	9	2.1
7784	Veal parmigiana with vegetable, fettuccine alfredo, dessert (Include Swanson's Veal Parmigiana Dinner) [1 frozen meal]	361	12.7	502	44%	23	49	4.1
7785	Veal parmigiana with vegetable, muffin, dessert [1 frozen meal]	347	12.2	486	37%	28	50	5.7
7786	Veal parmigiana with vegetable, spaghetti in butter sauce (Include Armour Dinner Classics Veal Parmigiana) [1 frozen meal]	305	10.8	382	45%	17	38	6.5
7787	Veal parmigiana with vegetable, tortellini in butter sauce (Include Budget Gourmet Veal Parmigiana Dinner) [1 frozen meal]	340	12.0	771	54%	37	52	3.8
7788	Veal with peppers in sauce, rice (diet meal) [1 frozen meal]	369	13.0	298	22%	26	33	3.7
7789	Veal with vegetable, potato wedges (diet meal) (Include Classic Lite Veal Pepper Steak) [1 frozen meal]	312	11.0	276	24%	27	26	5.1
7790	Veal, breaded, with spaghetti, in tomato sauce (Include Swanson Spaghetti with Breaded Veal) [1 frozen meal]	234	8.3	298	44%	15	27	2.5
7791	Vegetable lasagna (Include Le Menu Vegetable Lasagna) [1 frozen meal]	312	11.0	372	53%	14	33	5.0
7792	Zucchini lasagna (diet meal) (Include Lean Cuisine Zucchini Lasagna, Light and Elegant Lasagna Florentine) [1 frozen meal]	312	11.0	301	26%	17	40	4.5
	Hamburgers and Hot Dogs							
7900	Bacon cheeseburger, ¼ lb meat, with tomato and/or catsup, lettuce, pickles, onions, and/or mustard; Roy Rogers Bacon Cheeseburger; Wendy's Bacon Cheeseburger) [1 burger]	208	7.3	557	52%	32	34	2.1
7901	Cheeseburger, ¼ lb meat (beef modified in fat content), with tomato and/or catsup, on bun [1 burger]	219	7.7	409	35%	31	34	2.5
7902	Cheeseburger (hamburger with cheese sauce), ¼ lb meat, with grilled onions, on rye bun, with lettuce, pickles, onions, and/or mustard; McDonald's Cheddar Melt) [1 burger]	183	6.5	411	47%	23	30	3.8
7903	Bacon cheeseburger with tomato, lettuce, pickle, onion, mayonnaise) [1 burger]	288	10.2	751	51%	37	52	3.4
7904	Cheeseburger with tomato and/or catsup, on bun (Incl. with lettuce, pickles, onions, and/or mustard; McDonald's Cheeseburger; Roy Rogers Kid's Meal Cheeseburger) [1 burger]	127	4.5	299	40%	16	29	1.8
7905	Cheeseburger, ¼ lb meat, plain, on bun (Include Hardee's ¼ Pound Cheeseburger; Roy Rogers Cheeseburger) [1 burger]	184	6.5	543	48%	33	36	1.8
7906	Cheeseburger, ¼ lb meat, with ham, on bun (Include Roy Rogers Double R Bar Burger) [1 burger]	219	7.7	600	48%	41	35	1.8
7907	Cheeseburger, ¼ lb meat, with mayonnaise or salad dressing and tomatoes, on bun (Include with lettuce, pickles, onions, and/or mustard; Jack-in-the-Box Jumbo-Jack with Cheese; McDonald's McDLT; Wendy's Cheeseburger) [1 burger]	274	9.7	698	54%	37	43	2.8
7908	Cheeseburger, ¼ lb meat, with mayonnaise or salad dressing, on bun (Include with lettuce, pickles, onions, and/or mustard; Hardee's Big Deluxe) [1 burger]	228	8.0	636	54%	33	38	2.3

Food No.	fat gm	sat fat gm	choles mg	sodium mg	potas mg	% of Daily Value													
						vit A	vit E	vit C	thia	ribo	niac	vit B-6	fola	vit B-12	calc	phos	mag	iron	zinc
7774	18	7	112	2914	679	12	9	21	16	20	36	21	5	10	11	31	13	15	20
7775	5	2	41	433	480	7	3	26	21	16	26	20	12	4	7	21	11	18	16
7776	22	7	82	1219	612	75	12	20	17	16	38	28	10	8	8	29	14	14	17
7777	33	9	234	714	733	24	17	17	24	40	44	30	17	35	12	41	16	33	35
7778	13	4	63	1775	569	8	6	24	18	14	35	24	12	6	7	27	13	13	16
7779	18	6	105	1894	792	14	11	35	26	23	41	30	17	8	10	36	19	21	26
7780	7	2	105	858	936	114	7	21	13	22	60	47	11	9	11	39	20	27	20
7781	7	3	68	947	507	34	3	25	9	20	26	15	9	13	24	27	12	17	18
7782	15	6	122	1324	797	10	8	35	23	31	39	25	16	29	17	40	19	16	47
7783	9	5	70	459	657	12	7	24	7	19	28	18	7	14	23	32	13	8	20
7784	25	9	101	1345	607	26	16	32	17	25	31	18	9	10	29	35	16	18	18
7785	20	7	96	984	608	15	7	42	23	27	39	19	15	13	19	34	15	17	23
7786	19	5	43	1247	583	82	13	23	14	18	27	18	11	10	17	27	16	16	16
7787	46	18	306	1494	670	35	21	17	32	48	46	21	14	20	42	52	17	29	25
7788	7	3	94	904	856	27	10	120	18	23	48	40	11	21	6	29	16	17	30
7789	7	2	88	730	751	77	6	65	10	22	41	31	11	20	7	28	14	14	29
7790	15	4	74	1738	466	30	14	21	16	18	27	14	7	10	6	17	10	13	12
7791	22	9	39	1091	595	70	18	114	15	23	17	14	16	3	29	28	14	16	11
7792	9	5	24	900	611	57	5	41	16	19	12	15	10	4	36	36	17	12	15
7900	32	13	93	1323	533	7	5	5	29	28	38	16	8	43	23	36	11	23	36
7901	16	7	77	1021	525	8	4	9	25	27	26	18	10	35	23	35	12	25	40
7902	21	7	68	727	387	5	5	2	19	22	31	13	11	36	9	23	11	19	30
7903	43	15	101	1436	638	9	9	14	45	36	48	21	13	44	29	41	13	31	38
7904	13	5	40	676	272	4	3	3	18	17	21	8	6	20	15	18	6	15	17
7905	29	13	98	811	426	7	3	0	24	30	39	15	7	48	27	35	10	25	39
7906	32	13	119	1388	578	7	4	0	43	36	50	21	7	51	27	46	12	27	44
7907	42	15	116	1169	578	11	11	10	28	34	44	22	11	53	31	41	13	30	43
7908	38	14	106	1072	478	9	9	2	25	31	39	19	9	49	29	37	11	27	40

Mixed Dishes & Fast Foods

Food No.	Food Description & Amount	wt gm	wt oz	cal	% cal fat	prot gm	carbo gm	fiber gm
7909	Cheeseburger, ¼ lb meat, with mushrooms in sauce, on bun (Include with lettuce, pickles, onions, and/or mustard; Hardee's Mushroom 'N' Swiss Burger) [1 burger]	205	7.2	464	50%	27	30	2.6
7910	Cheeseburger, ¼ lb meat, with tomato and/or catsup, on bun (Include with lettuce, pickles, onions, and/or mustard; McDonald's ¼-Pounder with Cheese) [1 burger]	220	7.8	526	46%	31	39	2.5
7911	Cheeseburger, plain, on bun (Include Wendy's Kid's Meal Cheeseburger) [1 burger]	107	3.8	314	41%	17	28	1.5
7912	Cheeseburger, with mayonnaise or salad dressing and tomatoes, on bun (Include with lettuce, pickles, onions, and/or mustard; Burger King Whopper Jr. with Cheese; Jack-in-the-Box Cheeseburger Deluxe) [1 burger]	167	5.9	379	45%	18	34	2.2
7913	Cheeseburger, with mayonnaise or salad dressing, on bun (Include with lettuce, pickles, onions, and/or mustard; Jack-in-the-Box Cheeseburger) [1 burger]	129	4.6	345	46%	17	29	1.7
7914	Triple cheeseburger (3 patties, ¼ lb meat each), with mayonnaise or salad dressing and tomatoes, on bun (Include with lettuce, pickles, onions, and/or mustard; Wendy's Triple Cheeseburger) [1 burger]	400	14.1	1055	60%	66	38	2.5
7915	Chiliburger, on bun (Include hamburger with chili) [1 burger]	159	5.6	401	45%	24	30	2.8
7916	Double bacon cheeseburger (2 patties, ¼ lb meat each), on bun (Include with lettuce, pickles, onions, and/or mustard; Burger King Double Bacon Cheeseburger) [1 burger]	290	10.2	838	56%	53	36	2.1
7917	Double bacon cheeseburger (2 patties, ¼ lb meat each), with mayonnaise or salad dressing and tomatoes, on bun (Incl. with lettuce, pickles, onions, and/or mustard; Burger King Deluxe Bacon Cheeseburger) [1 burger]	335	11.8	973	60%	56	39	2.4
7918	Double cheeseburger (2 patties), plain, on bun [1 burger]	158	5.6	466	46%	27	34	1.7
7919	Double cheeseburger (2 patties), plain, on double-decker bun [1 burger]	186	6.6	548	46%	32	40	2.0
7920	Double cheeseburger (2 patties), with mayonnaise or salad dressing and tomatoes, on bun (Include with lettuce, pickles, onions, and/or mustard) [1 burger]	225	7.9	575	52%	30	39	2.4
7921	Double cheeseburger (2 patties), with mayonnaise or salad dressing, on bun (Include with lettuce, pickles, onions, and/or mustard; Jack-in-the-Box Bonus-Jack Hamburger) [1 burger]	187	6.6	523	52%	27	34	2.0
7922	Double cheeseburger (2 patties), with mayonnaise or salad dressing, on double-decker bun (Include with lettuce, pickles, onions, and/or mustard; Burger Chef Big Chef; McDonald's Big Mac) [1 burger]	224	7.9	615	52%	32	41	2.4
7923	Double cheeseburger (2 patties), with tomato and/or catsup, on bun with lettuce, pickles, onions, and/or mustard; (Include Burger Chef, McDonald's Double Cheeseburger) [1 burger]	192	6.8	463	46%	27	34	2.1
7924	Double cheeseburger (2 patties, ¼ lb meat each), with mayonnaise or salad dressing, on bun (Include with lettuce, pickles, onions, and/or mustard; Jack-in-the-Box Ultimate Cheeseburger) [1 burger]	272	9.6	790	58%	46	35	2.0
7925	Double hamburger (2 patties), plain, on bun [1 burger]	130	4.6	374	45%	23	27	1.4
7926	Double hamburger (2 patties), with mayonnaise or salad dressing and tomatoes, on bun (Include with lettuce, pickles, onions, and/or mustard) [1 burger]	197	6.9	478	52%	25	31	2.1
7927	Double hamburger (2 patties), with mayonnaise or salad dressing and tomatoes, on double-decker bun (Include with lettuce, pickles, onions, and/or mustard; Wendy's Double Hamburger) [1 burger]	241	8.5	593	49%	30	45	2.9
7928	Double hamburger (2 patties), with mayonnaise or salad dressing, on bun (Include with lettuce, pickles, onions, and/or mustard) [1 burger]	159	5.6	430	53%	22	27	1.7
7929	Double hamburger (2 patties), with tomato and/or catsup, on bun (Include with lettuce, pickles, onions, and/or mustard) [1 burger]	164	5.8	378	42%	22	31	1.9
7930	Double hamburger (2 patties, ¼ lb meat each), with tomato and/or catsup, on bun (Include with lettuce, pickles, onions, and/or mustard) [1 burger]	314	11.1	780	48%	51	48	2.9
7931	Hamburger, ¼ lb meat (beef modified in fat content), with tomato and/or catsup, on bun [1 burger]	206	7.3	347	27%	28	34	2.7
7932	Hamburger, 1 oz meat, with tomato and/or catsup, on miniature bun (Include with lettuce, pickles, onions, and/or mustard; Burger King Burger Bundles) [1 baby burger]	47	1.7	97	36%	6	10	0.7
7933	Hamburger, ¼ lb meat, plain, on bun (Include Roy Rogers Hamburger) [1 burger]	156	5.5	449	45%	28	32	1.7

Food No.	fat gm	sat fat gm	choles mg	sodium mg	potas mg	% of Daily Value													
						vit A	vit E	vit C	thia	ribo	niac	vit B-6	fola	vit B-12	calc	phos	mag	iron	zinc
7909	26	10	80	993	398	9	5	1	21	22	33	12	8	38	26	36	10	21	33
7910	27	12	90	1204	516	9	5	6	24	28	37	16	9	44	27	34	11	25	37
7911	14	6	44	505	226	3	2	0	19	18	22	7	5	22	16	18	6	15	18
7912	19	7	49	737	355	6	6	10	21	20	24	11	8	23	17	20	7	18	20
7913	18	6	46	601	251	4	5	1	19	18	22	9	6	21	16	18	6	16	18
7914	70	29	227	1577	952	19	13	13	26	51	70	38	13	107	49	73	19	42	84
7915	20	7	72	523	409	1	3	1	19	20	32	13	7	37	10	22	10	25	32
7916	52	22	170	1458	733	11	5	2	33	42	59	26	10	80	38	59	15	34	63
7917	65	25	185	1598	811	14	13	8	35	44	62	32	11	84	40	62	16	36	66
7918	24	10	79	708	357	5	3	0	23	26	33	12	6	39	23	29	8	22	32
7919	28	12	93	833	420	6	3	0	27	30	39	15	7	45	28	35	10	26	37
7920	33	12	90	1168	466	9	9	8	26	28	36	17	9	42	26	33	10	25	34
7921	30	11	83	888	386	7	8	1	23	26	33	15	8	38	24	30	9	22	31
7922	36	13	97	1044	460	8	9	2	27	30	38	18	10	45	28	35	11	26	37
7923	24	10	80	1034	453	8	4	5	21	25	33	14	8	39	23	30	10	22	32
7924	51	20	155	1192	621	12	11	1	23	37	50	26	10	72	36	51	13	31	57
7925	19	7	69	364	299	0	2	0	19	18	33	12	5	37	8	18	7	20	29
7926	28	8	79	614	406	3	8	8	21	21	35	17	8	40	9	20	8	23	31
7927	32	10	88	800	484	3	9	9	30	27	44	19	11	45	13	24	10	29	35
7928	25	8	71	555	325	1	7	1	19	18	31	14	7	36	9	18	7	20	28
7929	18	7	66	677	391	2	3	5	19	19	32	13	7	36	9	18	8	20	28
7930	41	16	161	1014	775	3	5	7	32	37	69	29	12	88	14	39	15	40	66
7931	10	3	64	771	488	3	4	9	26	23	28	17	10	33	10	24	10	25	37
7932	4	1	14	160	101	1	1	1	7	5	8	3	3	6	3	4	2	5	7
7933	22	8	82	437	358	0	2	0	23	22	39	14	6	45	10	21	8	24	34

Mixed Dishes & Fast Foods

Food No.	Food Description & Amount	wt gm	wt oz	cal	% cal fat	prot gm	carbo gm	fiber gm
7934	Hamburger, ¼ lb meat, with mayonnaise or salad dressing and tomatoes, on bun (Include with lettuce, pickles, onions, and/or mustard; Burger King Whopper; Jack-in-the-Box Jumbo Jack ; Wendy's Single; Wendy's Big Classic) [1 burger]	244	8.6	595	51%	30	41	2.8
7935	Hamburger, ¼ lb meat, with mayonnaise or salad dressing, on bun (Include with lettuce, pickles, onions, and/or mustard) [1 burger]	200	7.1	542	51%	28	36	2.3
7936	Hamburger, ¼ lb meat, with tomato and/or catsup, on bun (Include with lettuce, pickles, onions, and/or mustard; McDonald's ¼-Pounder) [1 burger]	192	6.8	446	41%	26	38	2.3
7937	Hamburger, 2½ oz meat, with mayonnaise or salad dressing and tomatoes, on bun (Include with lettuce, pickles, onions, and/or mustard) [1 burger]	178	6.3	395	46%	20	32	2.3
7938	Hamburger, plain, on bun (Include Wendy's Kid's Meal Hamburger) [1 burger]	93	3.3	267	36%	14	27	1.5
7939	Hamburger, plain, on miniature bun (Include Jimmy Dean Mini Burger; White Castle Miniature) [1 baby burger]	49	1.7	137	37%	8	13	0.7
7940	Hamburger, with mayonnaise or salad dressing and tomatoes, on bun (Include with lettuce, pickles, onions, and/or mustard; Burger King Whopper Jr.; Jack-in-the-Box Hamburger Deluxe) [1 burger]	153	5.4	342	43%	16	32	2.2
7941	Hamburger, with mayonnaise or salad dressing, on bun (Include with lettuce, pickles, onions, and/or mustard) [1 burger]	115	4.1	298	43%	14	28	1.7
7942	Hamburger, with catsup, pickles, mustard (Include Burger Chef Hamburger, Hardee's Hamburger, McDonald's Hamburger, Roy Rogers Kid's Meal Hamburger) [1burger]	113	4.0	261	35%	13	28	1.7
7943	Pizzaburger (hamburger, cheese, sauce) on ½ bun [1 burger]	137	4.8	327	47%	22	20	1.3
7944	Pizzaburger (hamburger, cheese, sauce) on whole bun [1 burger]	165	5.8	409	40%	24	36	2.2
7945	Steak patty (breaded, fried) sandwich, with mayonnaise or salad dressing, lettuce, and tomato, on bun (Include Jack-in-the-Box Country Fried Steak Sandwich) [1 sandwich]	153	5.4	440	51%	15	39	2.3
7946	Taco burger, on bun (Include chiliburger with cheese; Wendy's Chili, Cheese, and Beef) [1 burger]	127	4.5	286	33%	13	34	2.9
7947	Pochito (frankfurter and beef chili wrapped in tortilla) [1 pochito]	122	4.3	280	62%	10	18	3.1
7948	Chili dogs (frankfurters with chili con carne, no bun) [1 frankfurter with sauce]	125	4.4	248	70%	10	10	3.2
7949	Chili dog (frankfurter, with chili, on bun) [1 hot dog]	152	5.4	349	53%	13	28	3.7
7950	Chili cheese dog (frankfurter with chili and cheese on bun) [1 hot dog]	147	5.2	400	57%	16	26	2.4
7951	Corn dog (frankfurter with cornbread coating) (Include beef, pork, chicken, turkey) [1 corn dog]	88	3.1	274	58%	9	20	1.1
7952	Corny dog, with chili, on bun [1 corny dog]	162	5.7	431	44%	13	47	4.1
7953	Hot dog (frankfurter, plain, on bun) [1 hot dog]	85	3.0	260	55%	9	20	1.0
7954	Hot dog (frankfurter with catsup and/or mustard on bun) [1 hot dog]	105	3.7	295	54%	10	24	1.3
7955	Hot dog with cheese (frankfurter, with cheese, plain, on bun) [1 hot dog]	118	4.2	368	59%	14	23	1.1
7956	Hot dog (chicken frankfurter, plain, on bun) [1 hot dog]	85	3.0	229	44%	9	22	1.0
7957	Frankfurter, beef [1 frankfurter, thick (8 per lb)]	57	2.0	186	81%	7	1	0.0
7958	Frankfurter, beef, lowfat [1 frankfurter]	57	2.0	136	74%	7	1	0.0
7959	Frankfurter, beef and pork (Include Smokie Links) [1 frankfurter (8 per lb)]	57	2.0	189	81%	7	2	0.0
7960	Frankfurter, beef and pork, lowfat [1 frankfurter]	57	2.0	92	58%	7	3	0.0
7961	Frankfurter, chicken [1 frankfurter (10 per lb)]	45	1.6	119	67%	6	3	0.0
7962	Frankfurter, low salt [1 frankfurter (10 per lb)]	45	1.6	146	81%	6	1	0.0
7963	Frankfurter, meat and poultry [1 frankfurter (8 per 12 oz package)]	43	1.5	132	77%	6	2	0.0
7964	Frankfurter, meat and poultry, lowfat (Include Healthy Choice Frankfurter) [1 frankfurter (8 per lb)]	57	2.0	72	20%	9	5	0.1
7965	Frankfurter, meat and poultry, fat free [1 frankfurter]	50	1.8	40	0%	7	3	0.0
7966	Frankfurter, turkey [1 frankfurter (10 per lb)]	45	1.6	104	69%	7	1	0.0
7967	Frankfurters and sauerkraut [1 frankfurter with sauerkraut]	120	4.2	140	74%	5	4	2.0
7968	Frankfurter, bacon and cheese-filled [1 frankfurter (10 per lb)]	45	1.6	147	80%	6	1	0.0
7969	Frankfurters with tomato-based sauce (Include frankfurters with barbecue sauce or chili sauce) [1 frankfurter in sauce]	68	2.4	130	77%	5	3	0.4
7970	Frankfurter, breaded, baked [1 frankfurter]	51	1.8	176	75%	6	4	0.1

Food No.	fat gm	sat fat gm	choles mg	sodium mg	potas mg	% of Daily Value: vit A	vit E	vit C	thia	ribo	niac	vit B-6	fola	vit B-12	calc	phos	mag	iron	zinc
7934	34	10	94	779	498	4	10	10	28	26	44	20	11	48	12	25	10	28	37
7935	31	9	87	713	404	2	9	2	25	23	40	17	9	44	11	22	9	25	34
7936	21	8	74	802	452	3	4	6	24	22	38	15	9	41	11	21	9	24	32
7937	20	6	58	596	355	3	5	9	22	19	30	13	8	30	10	17	7	20	24
7938	11	4	35	336	190	0	2	0	18	14	22	7	5	19	8	11	5	15	16
7939	6	2	20	161	107	0	1	0	9	8	11	4	2	9	4	6	3	7	9
7940	16	5	42	494	294	2	5	9	22	17	25	10	8	21	9	14	6	18	18
7941	14	4	37	435	215	1	4	1	18	14	21	8	6	19	8	12	5	15	16
7942	10	4	33	478	240	1	2	3	18	14	21	7	6	18	8	11	5	15	15
7943	17	7	69	629	387	7	4	7	14	18	27	13	5	34	16	23	7	17	27
7944	18	8	66	790	420	7	4	6	24	24	32	13	7	33	20	25	9	22	28
7945	25	6	38	910	262	3	12	7	25	17	24	11	8	17	11	13	6	18	15
7946	11	4	30	638	266	5	5	9	21	16	20	7	8	13	14	14	6	15	13
7947	19	7	35	851	278	2	2	1	9	7	9	8	4	10	7	19	10	13	14
7948	19	7	38	964	353	2	3	2	9	8	8	8	5	11	4	16	10	17	16
7949	21	8	36	1125	361	2	3	2	22	15	16	8	7	12	9	17	10	22	16
7950	25	11	49	1277	318	7	3	1	21	19	15	8	5	16	23	25	8	17	17
7951	18	7	47	609	140	2	3	0	10	11	11	5	2	13	10	11	3	10	9
7952	21	8	49	1284	320	4	8	9	25	19	21	9	9	15	15	16	6	18	11
7953	16	6	24	747	132	0	1	0	18	10	14	4	3	11	6	7	3	10	7
7954	18	6	27	963	185	1	2	2	21	11	15	5	4	12	7	9	4	11	9
7955	24	10	44	1127	212	6	2	0	20	18	15	6	4	16	21	21	5	11	13
7956	11	3	49	868	92	2	1	0	14	10	15	8	3	2	10	8	3	12	5
7957	17	7	36	591	96	0	0	0	2	3	7	3	1	13	1	5	0	5	9
7958	11	5	24	600	74	0	0	1	2	3	6	2	1	12	0	11	2	4	8
7959	17	6	30	645	96	0	1	0	7	4	7	3	1	11	1	5	1	4	7
7960	6	2	26	716	86	0	0	0	6	4	6	2	1	11	1	8	1	4	8
7961	9	3	48	623	38	2	0	0	2	3	7	6	0	2	5	5	1	5	3
7962	13	6	29	141	75	0	0	0	1	3	5	2	0	10	1	4	0	4	7
7963	11	4	32	509	60	0	0	0	3	3	6	3	0	7	2	4	1	4	5
7964	2	1	25	532	141	0	1	0	10	5	8	6	0	4	1	8	2	3	7
7965	0	0	15	525	110	0	0	0	5	5	9	5	1	9	3	7	2	5	10
7966	8	3	51	649	81	0	1	0	1	5	9	4	1	2	5	6	2	5	10
7967	12	4	20	973	203	0	1	20	6	4	6	8	5	8	3	5	4	9	6
7968	13	5	31	487	93	2	1	0	7	4	7	3	0	13	3	8	1	3	7
7969	11	4	19	605	175	3	2	6	6	4	7	4	1	8	1	4	2	4	5
7970	15	5	36	583	94	1	1	0	8	5	8	3	1	10	2	5	2	5	6

Mixed Dishes & Fast Foods

Food No.	Food Description & Amount	wt gm	wt oz	cal	% cal fat	prot gm	carbo gm	fiber gm
7971	Frankfurter, cheese-filled (Include pork, beef, chicken, turkey) [1 frankfurter (8 per 12 oz package)]	43	1.5	147	79%	6	1	0.0
7972	Frankfurter, chili-filled [1 frankfurter (8 per lb)]	57	2.0	155	77%	6	3	0.8
7973	Pig in a blanket (frankfurter wrapped in dough) [1 pig in blanket]	85	3.0	283	69%	7	15	0.4
	Pizza and Other Fast Foods							
8100	Burrito with beans and cheese, meatless [1 burrito]	99	3.5	285	45%	12	27	4.5
8101	Burrito with beans, meatless [1 burrito]	72	2.5	173	31%	5	24	4.1
8102	Burrito with beans and rice, meatless [1 burrito]	99	3.5	202	16%	6	36	3.5
8103	Burrito with rice, beans, cheese, sour cream, lettuce, tomato and guacamole (Include Taco Bell 7 Layer Burrito) [1 burrito]	234	8.3	457	42%	18	49	7.6
8104	Burrito with beef and beans [1 burrito]	110	3.9	289	39%	14	30	5.0
8105	Burrito with beef and cheese, no beans [1 burrito]	132	4.7	468	55%	29	23	1.3
8106	Burrito with beef and potato, no beans [1 burrito]	110	3.9	262	37%	12	28	1.9
8107	Burrito with beef, beans, and cheese [1 burrito]	132	4.7	384	48%	20	30	4.9
8108	Burrito with beef, beans, cheese, and sour cream (Include Taco Bell Burrito Supreme) [1 burrito]	234	8.3	578	48%	31	43	6.5
8109	Burrito with beef, no beans [1 burrito]	110	3.9	351	41%	22	28	1.7
8110	Burrito with chicken and beans [1 burrito]	106	3.7	247	32%	14	28	4.6
8111	Burrito with chicken and cheese [1 burrito]	130	4.6	355	48%	26	19	1.2
8112	Burrito with chicken [1 burrito]	148	5.2	287	26%	25	26	1.9
8113	Burrito with chicken, beans, and cheese [1 burrito]	134	4.7	329	43%	19	27	4.6
8114	Burrito with chicken, no beans [1 burrito]	148	5.2	355	27%	32	30	1.8
8115	Burrito with eggs, no beans (Include Breakfast Burrito; Huevos Rancheros) [1 burrito]	188	6.6	386	53%	20	24	1.6
8116	Burrito with eggs, sausage, cheese and vegetables (Include McDonald's Breakfast Burrito) [1 burrito]	105	3.7	262	52%	10	21	1.3
8117	Burrito with pork and beans [1 burrito]	110	3.9	275	37%	14	29	4.8
8118	Pizza rolls (Include Pizza Bites) [4 miniature rolls]	56	2.0	168	41%	7	17	0.9
8119	Pizza with beans and vegetables, thick crust (Include Pizza Hut taco pizza) [1/8 of 12" dia]	87	3.1	237	30%	8	33	2.3
8120	Pizza with beans and vegetables, thin crust (Include Pizza Hut taco pizza) [1/8 of 12" dia]	79	2.8	192	34%	8	24	2.3
8121	Pizza with meat and fruit, thick crust (Include ham and pineapple, Canadian bacon and pineapple) [1/8 of 12" dia]	79	2.8	194	30%	8	26	1.3
8122	Pizza with meat and fruit, thin crust (Include ham and pineapple, Canadian bacon and pineapple) [1/8 of 12" dia]	71	2.5	152	34%	8	18	1.1
8123	Pizza with meat and vegetables, thick crust [1/8 of 12" dia]	87	3.1	235	37%	9	28	1.6
8124	Pizza with meat and vegetables, thin crust [1/8 of 12" dia]	79	2.8	194	44%	9	19	1.4
8125	Pizza with meat and vegetables, lowfat, thin crust [1 piece]	130	4.6	264	38%	12	28	1.4
8126	Pizza with meat, thick crust (Include sausage, ground beef, pepperoni, ham, bacon, salami) [1/8 of 12" dia]	79	2.8	245	37%	9	29	1.3
8127	Pizza with meat, thin crust (Include sausage, ground beef, pepperoni, ham, bacon, salami) [1/8 of 12" dia]	71	2.5	210	44%	10	19	1.1
8128	Pizza with seafood, thin crust [1 piece]	83	2.9	271	33%	14	30	1.0
8129	Pizza with seafood, thick crust [1 piece]	92	3.2	308	29%	13	41	1.4
8130	Pizza, cheese, thick crust (Include English muffin; pizza) [1/8 of 12" dia]	71	2.5	204	30%	8	28	1.3
8131	Pizza, cheese, thin crust (Include Weight Watcher's) [1/8 of 12" dia]	63	2.2	163	34%	7	19	1.1
8132	Pizza, cheese, with fruit, thick crust [1/8 of 12" dia]	78	2.8	207	29%	7	29	1.4
8133	Pizza, cheese, with vegetables, thick crust [1/8 of 12" dia]	78	2.8	193	30%	7	27	1.5
8134	Pizza, cheese, with vegetables, thin crust [1/8 of 12" dia]	70	2.5	149	35%	7	18	1.3
8135	Pizza, deep dish, with ground beef and tomato sauce on a crust (Include Pizzabake) [1/6 of 13" x 9" x 2"]	146	5.1	462	37%	27	44	1.9
8136	Pizza, no cheese, thick crust (Include tomato pie) [1/8 of 12" dia]	71	2.5	189	23%	4	32	1.5
8137	Pizza, no cheese, thin crust (Include tomato pie) [1/8 of 12" dia]	63	2.2	140	25%	3	23	1.3
8138	White pizza, thin crust [1 piece]	63	2.2	234	31%	10	30	1.1

						% of Daily Value													
Food No.	fat gm	sat fat gm	choles mg	sodium mg	potas mg	vit A	vit E	vit C	thia	ribo	niac	vit B-6	fola	vit B-12	calc	phos	mag	iron	zinc
7971	13	5	31	470	88	1	1	0	6	4	6	2	0	11	3	8	1	3	7
7972	13	5	24	542	132	1	1	0	5	4	5	3	1	8	1	6	3	6	8
7973	22	7	22	672	128	1	6	0	12	9	10	3	1	10	13	11	3	8	7
8100	14	7	28	281	264	7	4	2	15	12	6	5	17	3	22	22	9	12	9
8101	6	2	4	124	217	0	3	2	13	6	5	4	15	0	5	9	7	10	4
8102	4	1	3	403	164	0	3	4	17	8	10	5	2	0	7	9	7	13	6
8103	21	10	45	734	508	15	5	16	23	20	14	12	10	5	34	32	16	21	17
8104	13	4	31	176	352	0	4	2	17	11	15	9	19	14	7	16	10	16	15
8105	28	14	101	536	261	15	4	0	15	24	23	10	4	32	40	39	9	17	31
8106	11	3	30	203	303	0	5	9	16	10	19	11	3	16	5	12	6	12	14
8107	21	10	57	328	370	8	5	2	17	16	15	9	20	17	25	29	11	17	20
8108	31	15	101	813	513	16	5	9	21	25	24	15	7	28	42	45	16	26	34
8109	16	5	64	303	275	0	4	0	19	17	30	10	3	33	7	18	7	19	27
8110	9	3	28	160	297	0	4	2	15	10	15	8	17	1	6	15	9	13	8
8111	19	10	83	521	223	14	4	3	13	20	22	9	4	7	34	32	8	11	17
8112	8	2	63	392	310	10	5	8	18	16	33	13	3	3	7	18	8	14	13
8113	16	7	50	364	350	8	5	5	16	15	15	9	18	4	22	26	11	14	13
8114	11	3	83	341	299	1	4	0	23	19	53	23	3	5	8	25	9	16	16
8115	23	10	333	644	294	33	8	10	17	36	8	9	9	14	33	35	8	15	14
8116	15	5	130	565	165	10	8	10	15	18	8	5	4	7	13	17	5	10	7
8117	11	4	28	161	366	0	4	3	27	12	13	10	18	2	7	16	9	14	9
8118	8	3	13	424	125	4	3	4	11	10	9	3	4	3	10	11	3	7	5
8119	8	3	7	82	188	5	6	6	19	13	12	4	8	1	10	12	5	12	6
8120	7	3	9	102	209	6	5	8	13	11	9	4	8	1	12	13	5	10	6
8121	6	2	10	198	146	4	4	7	18	12	11	4	3	2	10	12	4	9	5
8122	6	2	12	232	152	4	4	9	14	9	9	5	2	2	12	12	4	7	5
8123	10	4	13	238	172	5	5	13	17	13	12	4	4	3	12	13	4	11	6
8124	10	4	16	282	183	5	5	15	12	11	10	5	3	4	14	13	4	8	7
8125	11	4	18	488	215	6	4	21	20	16	14	6	4	6	13	19	5	11	8
8126	10	4	14	230	151	4	5	4	17	13	13	3	4	4	12	13	4	11	7
8127	10	4	18	287	164	5	4	6	13	11	10	4	3	4	15	14	4	8	7
8128	10	4	35	246	95	6	4	0	17	16	11	3	4	7	21	22	6	12	9
8129	10	4	25	174	97	4	5	0	23	18	15	2	5	5	15	19	6	15	8
8130	7	3	7	120	125	4	5	4	16	12	11	3	3	1	12	12	4	10	5
8131	6	3	9	153	135	5	4	6	11	10	8	3	3	1	15	13	4	7	5
8132	7	2	7	118	136	4	5	6	16	12	11	3	3	1	12	12	4	10	5
8133	6	2	7	133	144	4	5	12	15	12	10	4	4	1	11	11	4	10	5
8134	6	2	8	160	153	5	4	15	10	9	7	4	3	1	13	12	4	7	5
8135	19	7	81	82	402	1	4	5	27	25	41	16	15	44	2	22	8	25	37
8136	5	1	0	24	129	2	5	5	18	11	12	3	4	0	1	5	3	11	3
8137	4	1	0	32	147	3	5	7	13	8	9	3	3	0	1	4	3	9	2
8138	8	4	18	153	65	5	2	0	17	15	10	2	4	2	18	16	4	11	6

Mixed Dishes & Fast Foods

Food No.	Food Description & Amount	wt gm	wt oz	cal	% cal fat	prot gm	carbo gm	fiber gm
8139	White pizza, thick crust [1 piece]	71	2.5	261	29%	10	35	1.3
8140	Taco filling: beef, cheese, tomato, taco sauce [1 cup]	204	7.2	382	58%	26	15	3.7
8141	Taco or tostada with beans, meatless [1 taco or tostada]	80	2.8	146	38%	4	20	4.6
8142	Taco or tostada with beans and cheese, meatless [1 taco or tostada]	88	3.1	174	43%	6	20	4.7
8143	Taco or tostada with beans, cheese, and meat (Include beef or chicken taco, beef or chicken tostada, Taco Bell Prizzaz pizza) [1 taco or tostada]	83	2.9	167	44%	8	16	3.2
8144	Taco or tostada with beef [1 taco or tostada]	76	2.7	138	48%	8	11	1.7
8145	Taco or tostada with beef and cheese (Include Taco Bell Grande) [1 taco or tostada]	83	2.9	180	48%	9	14	2.4
8146	Taco or tostada with beef, cheese and lettuce (Include Taco Bell taco) [1 taco]	78	2.8	225	52%	11	16	2.1
8147	Taco or tostada with chicken or turkey [1 taco or tostada]	72	2.5	125	34%	8	13	2.1
8148	Taco or tostada with chicken and cheese [1 taco or tostada]	79	2.8	153	41%	10	13	2.1
8149	Taco or tostada with fish, lettuce, tomato, salsa [1 taco or tostada]	76	2.7	100	32%	8	10	1.5
8150	Taco with crab meat, Puerto Rican style (Tacos de jueyes) [1 taco (4½" dia)]	121	4.3	270	49%	16	19	2.3
8151	Taco salad [1 cup]	122	4.3	198	57%	11	11	1.7
8152	Soft taco with beef, cheese, and lettuce (IncludeTaco Bell Soft Taco) [1 taco]	92	3.2	256	38%	13	25	1.6
8153	Soft taco with beef, cheese, lettuce, tomato and sour cream (Include Taco Bell Soft Taco Supreme) [1 taco]	124	4.4	304	46%	15	26	1.7
8154	Soft taco with chicken, cheese, and lettuce (IncludeTaco BellTaco) [1 taco]	128	4.5	252	31%	22	20	1.5
	Your Additions							
	Phillip Cheesesteak c mushrooms			737				
	" turkey sandwich			376				
	" Italian			996				
	Latte fudge			240	60			
	Berry smoothy			290	0			
	Berry sundae			410	0			

Food No.	fat gm	sat fat gm	choles mg	sodium mg	potas mg	vit A	vit E	vit C	thia	ribo	niac	vit B-6	fola	vit B-12	calc	phos	mag	iron	zinc
						% of Daily Value													
8139	9	4	18	150	72	5	2	0	20	17	12	2	4	2	18	17	4	12	7
8140	25	12	93	948	522	16	10	26	7	18	24	16	13	36	25	31	8	14	30
8141	6	2	3	233	259	2	5	9	7	3	3	7	16	0	4	9	8	7	4
8142	8	3	10	277	271	4	6	9	7	4	3	7	16	1	8	12	9	8	5
8143	8	3	21	317	219	5	5	9	6	5	7	8	9	4	8	12	7	6	7
8144	7	2	20	117	173	3	3	10	4	5	8	8	3	9	4	8	6	6	11
8145	10	4	28	363	212	5	5	9	5	7	9	8	5	9	8	13	7	7	12
8146	13	4	35	462	174	3	4	1	5	6	11	10	4	17	8	15	9	9	15
8147	5	1	21	286	164	3	5	8	4	4	10	8	4	1	3	8	6	5	5
8148	7	2	28	329	171	5	5	8	5	5	10	8	4	2	8	12	6	5	6
8149	4	1	39	164	174	3	4	10	4	2	5	6	4	4	5	11	7	6	7
8150	15	5	79	416	317	9	8	21	11	11	13	10	9	51	16	23	9	9	18
8151	13	4	35	166	310	21	2	17	3	8	11	9	6	16	8	13	7	7	14
8152	11	4	33	593	170	3	3	1	18	14	15	5	4	11	13	15	5	13	14
8153	16	7	44	605	223	9	4	5	18	17	15	6	5	12	17	18	6	13	15
8154	9	3	59	556	203	3	3	1	15	14	26	10	5	3	9	17	7	11	12

Mixed Dishes & Fast Foods

	Food No.	Food Description & Amount	wt gm	wt oz	cal	% cal fat	prot gm	carbo gm	fiber gm
		Your Additions							
1	90	egg							
15	90	toast							
1	39	½ & ½ (2TBS)							
½	20	" (1TBS)							
0	102	butter (1TBS)							
0	28	ham							
0	109	fontina							
0	46	bacon							
0	70	tuna(¼c)							
12	90	milk							
13	70	Activia							
4	80	non-fat cottage cheese(½c)							
3-4	15-20	tomato							
5	21	carrot							
4	19	cucumber							
21	81	apple							
18	75	blackberries							
8	60	chicken-noodle soup(½c)							
6	164	low fat cottage cheese							

Food No.	fat gm	sat fat gm	choles mg	sodium mg	potas mg	% of Daily Value													
						vit A	vit E	vit C	thia	ribo	niac	vit B-6	fola	vit B-12	calc	phos	mag	iron	zinc

Index

C

D

E

F

H

I

J

K

L

M

N

O

P

T

U

V

W

Y

Z

Order Form

for this 1997 edition of

Are You Eating Right?

$29.95 per book (sales tax for Calif. addresses and domestic postage included).

Mail this entire form
and a check made out to *Orange Grove Publishing* to: Orange Grove Publishing
1239 Bellair Way
Menlo Park, CA 94025-6612

Order for ____ copies X $29.95/copy = $________ (check enclosed)

Your name: ____

Street Address: ____

City: ____________________ State: ______ Zip: __________-________

Phone and/or e-mail address: ________________________________

Please fill out your mailing label:

Orange Grove Publishing
1239 Bellair Way
Menlo Park, CA 94025-6612

____

____

____

____

Thank you!

Order Form

for this 1997 edition of

Are You Eating Right?

$29.95 per book (sales tax for Calif. addresses and domestic postage included).

Mail this entire form
and a check made out to *Orange Grove Publishing* to:

Orange Grove Publishing
1239 Bellair Way
Menlo Park, CA 94025-6612

Order for ____ copies X $29.95/copy = $________ (check enclosed)

Your name: ______________________________

Street Address: ______________________________

City: ____________________ State: ______ Zip: __________-________

Phone and/or e-mail address: ______________________________

Please fill out your mailing label:

Orange Grove Publishing
1239 Bellair Way
Menlo Park, CA 94025-6612

____

____

____

____

Thank you!